Theoretical Neuroscience: Computational and Mathematical Modeling of Neural Systems

Theoretical Neuroscience: Computational and Mathematical Modeling of Neural Systems

Editor: Lucio Johnston

AMERICAN
MEDICAL PUBLISHERS
www.americanmedicalpublishers.com

AMERICAN
MEDICAL PUBLISHERS
www.americanmedicalpublishers.com

Cataloging-in-Publication Data

Theoretical neuroscience : computational and mathematical modeling of neural systems / edited by Lucio Johnston.
p. cm.
Includes bibliographical references and index.
ISBN 979-8-88740-504-9
1. Neurosciences. 2. Nervous system. 3. Computational neuroscience. 4. Neurosciences--Data processing.
5. Neurosciences--Mathematical models. I. Johnston, Lucio.
RC341 .T44 2023
612.8--dc23

American Medical Publishers,
41 Flatbush Avenue,
1st Floor, New York,
NY 11217, USA

ISBN 979-8-88740-504-9 (Hardback)

Contents

Preface

Over the recent decade, advancements and applications have progressed exponentially. This has led to the increased interest in this field and projects are being conducted to enhance knowledge. The main objective of this book is to present some of the critical challenges and provide insights into possible solutions. This book will answer the varied questions that arise in the field and also provide an increased scope for furthering studies.

Theoretical neuroscience refers to a subfield of neuroscience which makes use of brain abstractions, mathematical models and theoretical analysis. It provides a quantitative foundation to explain what nervous systems do, determines how they work and discovers the underlying general principles of their operation. Computational modelling and theoretical analysis are useful tools for describing what nervous systems do, figuring out how they work and understanding why they do so in a specific manner. Neuroscience includes a wide range of methods from molecular and cellular research as well as human, psychophysics and psychology. Theoretical neuroscience promotes cross-disciplinary collaboration through creating compact representations of what has been learned, bridging the gap among different levels of description and recognizing unifying concepts and principles. The basic function of computational modeling neuroscience is to understand the principles governing the development, structure, physiology and cognitive abilities of the nervous system. The goal of models in theoretical neuroscience is to capture the key characteristics of the biological system at multiple spatial-temporal scales. This book is a valuable compilation of topics, ranging from the basic to the most complex advancements in the field of theoretical neuroscience. It aims to shed light on the computational and mathematical modeling of neural systems. The book is appropriate for those seeking detailed information in this area.

I hope that this book, with its visionary approach, will be a valuable addition and will promote interest among readers. Each of the authors has provided their extraordinary competence in their specific fields by providing different perspectives as they come from diverse nations and regions. I thank them for their contributions.

Editor

1

Reproducibility vs. Replicability: A Brief History of a Confused Terminology

Hans E. Plesser[1,2*]

[1] *Faculty of Science and Technology, Norwegian University of Life Sciences, Ås, Norway,* [2] *Institute for Neuroscience and Medicine (INM-6), Jülich Research Centre, Jülich, Germany*

***Correspondence:**
Hans E. Plesser
hans.ekkehard.plesser@nmbu.no

A cornerstone of science is the possibility to critically assess the correctness of scientific claims made and conclusions drawn by other scientists. This requires a systematic approach to and precise description of experimental procedure and subsequent data analysis, as well as careful attention to potential sources of error, both systematic and statistic. Ideally, an experiment or analysis should be described in sufficient detail that other scientists with sufficient skills and means can follow the steps described in published work and obtain the same results within the margins of experimental error. Furthermore, where fundamental insights into nature are obtained, such as a measurement of the speed of light or the propagation of action potentials along axons, independent confirmation of the measurement or phenomenon is expected using different experimental means. In some cases, doubts about the interpretation of certain results have given rise to new branches of science, such as Schrödinger's development of the theory of first-passage times to address contradictory experimental data concerning the existence of fractional elementary charge (Schrödinger, 1915). Experimental scientists have long been aware of these issues and have developed a systematic approach over decades, well-established in the literature and as international standards.

When scientists began to use digital computers to perform simulation experiments and data analysis, such attention to experimental error took back stage. Since digital computers are exact machines, practitioners apparently assumed that results obtained by computer could be trusted, provided that the principal algorithms and methods employed were suitable to the problem at hand. Little attention was paid to the correctness of implementation, potential for error, or variation introduced by system soft- and hardware, and to how difficult it could be to actually reconstruct after some years—or even weeks—how precisely one had performed a computational experiment. Stanford geophysicist Jon Claerbout was one of the first computational scientists to address this problem (Claerbout and Karrenbach, 1992). His work was followed up by David Donoho and Victoria Stodden (Donoho et al., 2009) and introduced to a wider audience by Peng (2011).

Claerbout defined "reproducing" to mean "running the same software on the same input data and obtaining the same results" (Rougier et al., 2017), going so far as to state that "[j]udgement of the reproducibility of computationally oriented research no longer requires an expert—a clerk can do it" (Claerbout and Karrenbach, 1992). As a complement, replicating a published result is then defined to mean "writing and then running new software based on the description of a computational model or method provided in the original publication, and obtaining results that are similar enough ..." (Rougier et al., 2017). I will refer to these definitions of "reproducibility" and "replicability" as *Claerbout terminology*; they have also been recommended in social, behavioral and economic sciences (Bollen et al., 2015).

Unfortunately, this use of "reproducing" and "replicating" is at odds with the terminology long established in experimental sciences. A standard textbook in analytical chemistry states (Miller and Miller, 2000, p. 6, emphasis in the original)

Keywords: computational science, repeatability, replicability, reproducibility, artifacts

> ... modern convention makes a careful distinction between **reproducibility** and **repeatability**. ... student A ... would do the five replicate titrations in rapid succession ... . The same set of solutions and the same glassware would be used throughout, the same temperature, humidity and other laboratory conditions would remain much the same. In such circumstances, the precision measured would be the within-run precision: this is called the **repeatability**. Suppose, however, that for some reason the titrations were performed by different staff on five different occasions in different laboratories, using different pieces of glassware and different batches of indicator ... . This set of data would reflect the between-run precision of the method, i.e. its **reproducibility**.

and further on p. 95

> A crucial requirement of a [collaborative test] is that it should distinguish between the repeatability standard deviation, s_r, and the reproducibility standard deviation, s_R. At each analyte level these are related by the equation
>
> $$s_R^2 = s_r^2 + s_L^2$$

where s_L^2 is the variance due to inter-laboratory differences,.... Note that in this context reproducibility refers to errors arising in different laboratories and equipment, but using the same method: this is a more restricted definition of reproducibility than that used in other instances.

Further, the International Vocabulary of Metrology (Joint Committee for Guides in Metrology, 2006) and the corresponding standard ISO 5725-2 define as *repeatability condition of a measurement* (§2.21)

> a set of conditions that includes the same measurement procedure, same operators, same measuring system, same operating conditions and same location, and replicate measurements on the same or similar objects over a short period of time

and as *reproducibility condition of a measurement* (§2.23)

> a set of conditions that includes the same measurement procedure, same location, and replicate measurements on the same or similar objects over an extended period of time, but may include other conditions involving changes.

Based on these definitions, the *Association for Computing Machinery* has adopted the following definitions (Association for Computing Machinery, 2016)

> **Repeatability** (Same team, same experimental setup): The measurement can be obtained with stated precision by the same team using the same measurement procedure, the same measuring system, under the same operating conditions, in the same location on multiple trials. For computational experiments, this means that a researcher can reliably repeat her own computation.
>
> **Replicability** (Different team, same experimental setup): The measurement can be obtained with stated precision by a different team using the same measurement procedure, the same measuring system, under the same operating conditions, in the same or a different location on multiple trials. For computational experiments, this means that an independent group can obtain the same result using the author's own artifacts.
>
> **Reproducibility** (Different team, different experimental setup): The measurement can be obtained with stated precision by a different team, a different measuring system, in a different location on multiple trials. For computational experiments, this means that an independent group can obtain the same result using artifacts which they develop completely independently.

I will refer to this definition as the *ACM terminology*. Together with some colleagues, I proposed similar definitions some years ago (Crook et al., 2013). The different terminologies are summarized in **Table 1**.

The debate about which terminology is the proper one is heated at times, as witnessed by a discussion on "R-words" on Github (Rougier et al., 2016). One reason for the intensity of that debate may be a paper by Drummond (2009). He attempted to bring terminology in computational science in line with the experimental sciences, but at the same time argued that one should not focus on collecting computer-experimental artifacts to ensure that simulations and analyses can be re-run. While I agree with Drummond on the choice of terminology, I consider it to be essential to preserve artifacts such as software, scripts, and input data underlying computational science publications. Where re-running is successful, the published artifacts allow others to build on earlier work. Where re-running fails, which may happen due to subtle differences in system software (Glatard et al., 2015) as well as through genuine errors in problem-specific code written by researchers, well-preserved and accessible artifacts provide a basis to identify the cause of errors; Baggerly and Coombes (2009) give a high-profile example of such forensic bioinformatics.

In recent years, a number of authors have attempted to resolve this disagreement on terminology. Patil et al. (2016; see especially the Supplementary Material) give a precise definition of reproducibility, of different types of replicability, and of related terms in the form of a σ-algebra. They follow Claerbout terminology, but encounter conflicts with their own choice of terms when discussing one specific example (Patil et al., 2016; Supplementary Material, p. 6):

> In this case, data and code for the original study were made available but were incomplete and/or incorrect. An independent group ... examined what was provided and engineered **a new set of code which reproduced** the original results. ... This differs from our definition of reproducibility because the second set of analysts ... were unable to use the original code, and had to apply [modified code] instead.

Nichols et al. (2017) suggest best practices for neuroimaging based on a detailed discussion of different levels of reproducibility and replicability. They provide an informative table of which aspects of a study are fixed and which may vary at the different levels, using a terminology closer to Claerbout than to the ACM. But also these authors appear to confuse terminology slightly, since they state

TABLE 1 | Comparison of terminologies. See text for details.

Goodman	Claerbout	ACM
		Repeatability
Methods reproducibility	Reproducibility	Replicability
Results reproducibility	Replicability	Reproducibility
Inferential reproducibility		

that "Peng reproducibility" allows for variation in code, experimenter and data analyst, while Peng's definition of reproducibility only allows for a different data analyst (Peng, 2011)—a case which Nichols et al label "Collegial analysis replicability".

To solve the terminology confusion, Goodman et al. (2016) propose a new *lexicon for research reproducibility* with the following definitions:

- *Methods reproducibility*: provide sufficient detail about procedures and data so that the same procedures could be exactly repeated.
- *Results reproducibility*: obtain the same results from an independent study with procedures as closely matched to the original study as possible.
- *Inferential reproducibility*: draw the same conclusions from either an independent replication of a study or a reanalysis of the original study.

These definitions make explicit which aspects of trustworthiness of a study we focus on and avoid the ambiguity caused by the fact that "reproducible", "replicable," and "repeatable" have very similar meaning in everyday language (Goodman et al., 2016).

Applying the terminology of Goodman and colleagues to computational neuroscience, we need to consider two types of studies in particular: simulation experiments and advanced analyses of experimental data. In the latter case, we assume that the experimental data is fixed. In both types of study, methods reproducibility amounts to obtaining the same results when running the same code again; access to simulation specifications, experimental data and code is essential. Results reproducibility, on the other hand will require access to the experimental data for analysis studies, but may use different code, e.g., different analysis packages or neural simulators.

The lexicon proposed by Goodman et al. (2016) is an important step out of the terminology quagmire in which the active and fruitful debate about the trustworthiness of research has been stuck for the past decade, because it sidesteps confounding common language associations of terms by explicit labeling (explicit is better than implicit; Peters, 2004). One can only wish that it will be adopted widely so that the debate can once more focus on scientific rather than language issues.

AUTHOR CONTRIBUTIONS

The author confirms being the sole contributor of this work and approved it for publication.

ACKNOWLEDGMENTS

I am grateful to the reviewers for constructive criticism and to Sharon Crook, Andrew Davison, and Robert McDougal for discussions and comments on a draft of this manuscript. My work was partly supported by the European Union's Horizon 2020 research and innovation programme under grant agreement no. 720270 (HBP SGA1).

REFERENCES

Association for Computing Machinery (2016). *Artifact Review and Badging.* Available online at: https://www.acm.org/publications/policies/artifact-review-badging (Accessed November 24, 2017).

Baggerly, K. A., and Coombes, K. R. (2009). Deriving chemosensitivity from cell lines: forensic bioinformatics and reproducible research in high-throughput biology *Ann. Appl. Stat.* 3, 1309–1334. doi: 10.1214/09-AOAS291

Bollen, K., Cacioppo, J. T., Kaplan, R., Krosnick, J., and Olds, J. L. (2015). *Social, Behavioral, and Economic Sciences Perspectives on Robust and Reliable Science.* Arlington, VA: National Science Foundation. Available online at: https://www.nsf.gov/sbe/SBE_Spring_2015_AC_Meeting_Presentations/Bollen_Report_on_Replicability_SubcommitteeMay_2015.pdf (Accessed December 8, 2017).

Claerbout, J. F., and Karrenbach, M. (1992). Electronic documents give reproducible research a new meaning. *SEG Expanded Abstracts* 11, 601–604. doi: 10.1190/1.1822162

Crook, S., Davison, A. P., and Plesser, H. E. (2013). "Learning from the past: approaches for reproducibility in computational neuroscience," in *20 Years in Computational Neuroscience*, ed J. M. Bower (New York, NY: Springer Science+Business Media), 73–102. doi: 10.1007/978-1-4614-1424-7_4

Donoho, D. L., Maleki, A., Rahman, I. U., Shahram, M., and Stodden, V. (2009). 15 Years of reproducible research in computational harmonic analysis. *Comput. Sci. Eng.* 11, 8–18. doi: 10.1109/MCSE.2009.15

Drummond, C. (2009). "Replicability is not reproducibility: nor is it good science," in *Proceedings of the Evaluation Methods for Machine Learning Workshop at the 26th ICML* (Montreal, QC). Available online at: http://www.site.uottawa.ca/~cdrummon/pubs/ICMLws09.pdf (Accessed September 24, 2017).

Glatard, T., Lewis, L. B., Ferreira da Silva, R., Adalat, R., Beck, N., Lepage, C., et al. (2015). Reproducibility of neuroimaging analyses across operating systems. *Front. Neuroinform.* 9:12. doi: 10.3389/fninf.2015.00012

Goodman, S. N., Fanelli, D., and Ioannidis, J. P. A. (2016). What does research reproducibility mean? *Sci. Transl. Med.* 8:341ps12. doi: 10.1126/scitranslmed.aaf5027

Joint Committee for Guides in Metrology (2006). *International Vocabulary of Metrology – Basic and General Concepts and Associated Terms, 3rd Edn.* Joint Committee for Guides in Metrology/Working Group 2. Available online at: https://www.nist.gov/sites/default/files/documents/pml/div688/grp40/International-Vocabulary-of-Metrology.pdf (Accessed September 24, 2017).

Miller, J. N., and Miller, J. C. (2000). *Statistics and Chemometrics for Analytical Chemistry. 4th Edn.* Harlow: Pearson.

Nichols, T. E., Das, S., Eickhoff, S. B., Evans, A. C., Glatard, T., Hanke, M., et al. (2017). Best practices in data analysis and sharing in neuroimaging using MRI. *Nat. Neurosci.* 20, 299–303. doi: 10.1038/nn.4500

Patil, P., Peng, R. D., and Leek, J. T. (2016). A statistical definition for reproducibility and replicability. *bioRxiv.* doi: 10.1101/066803. [Epub ahead of print].

Peng, R. D. (2011). Reproducible research in computational science. *Science* 334, 1226–1227. doi: 10.1126/science.1213847

Peters, T. (2004). *PEP20—The Zen of Python*. Available online at: https://www.python.org/dev/peps/pep-0020/ (Accessed December 8, 2017).

Rougier, N. P., et al. (2016). *R-words*. Available online at: https://github.com/ReScience/ReScience-article/issues/5 (Accessed September 24, 2017).

Rougier, N. P., Hinsen, K., Alexandre, F., Arildsen, T., Barba, L. A., Benureau, F. C. Y., et al. (2017). *Sustainable Computational Science: The ReScience Initiative*. Available online at: https://arxiv.org/abs/1707.04393

Schrödinger, E. (1915). Zur Theorie der Fall- und Steigversuche an Teilchen mit Brownscher Bewegung. *Physik. Z.* 16, 289–295.

2

Challenges in Reproducibility, Replicability and Comparability of Computational Models and Tools for Neuronal and Glial Networks, Cells and Subcellular Structures

Tiina Manninen[1,2*], *Jugoslava Aćimović*[1,2*], *Riikka Havela*[1,2], *Heidi Teppola*[1,2] *and Marja-Leena Linne*[1,2*]

[1] *Computational Neuroscience Group, BioMediTech Institute and Faculty of Biomedical Sciences and Engineering, Tampere University of Technology, Tampere, Finland,* [2] *Laboratory of Signal Processing, Tampere University of Technology, Tampere, Finland*

Correspondence:
Tiina Manninen
tiina.manninen@tut.fi
Jugoslava Aćimović
jugoslava.acimovic@tut.fi
Marja-Leena Linne
marja-leena.linne@tut.fi

The possibility to replicate and reproduce published research results is one of the biggest challenges in all areas of science. In computational neuroscience, there are thousands of models available. However, it is rarely possible to reimplement the models based on the information in the original publication, let alone rerun the models just because the model implementations have not been made publicly available. We evaluate and discuss the comparability of a versatile choice of simulation tools: tools for biochemical reactions and spiking neuronal networks, and relatively new tools for growth in cell cultures. The replicability and reproducibility issues are considered for computational models that are equally diverse, including the models for intracellular signal transduction of neurons and glial cells, in addition to single glial cells, neuron-glia interactions, and selected examples of spiking neuronal networks. We also address the comparability of the simulation results with one another to comprehend if the studied models can be used to answer similar research questions. In addition to presenting the challenges in reproducibility and replicability of published results in computational neuroscience, we highlight the need for developing recommendations and good practices for publishing simulation tools and computational models. Model validation and flexible model description must be an integral part of the tool used to simulate and develop computational models. Constant improvement on experimental techniques and recording protocols leads to increasing knowledge about the biophysical mechanisms in neural systems. This poses new challenges for computational neuroscience: extended or completely new computational methods and models may be required. Careful evaluation and categorization of the existing models and tools provide a foundation for these future needs, for constructing multiscale models or extending the models to incorporate additional or more detailed biophysical mechanisms. Improving the quality of publications in computational neuroscience, enabling progressive building of advanced computational models and tools, can be achieved only through adopting publishing standards which underline replicability and reproducibility of research results.

Keywords: astrocyte, computational model, glial cell, neuron, neuronal network, replicability, reproducibility, subcellular structure

1. INTRODUCTION

All areas of science are facing problems with reproducibility and replicability (Baker, 2016; Eglen et al., 2017; Munafò et al., 2017; Rougier et al., 2017), and computational neuroscience is no exception. We aim to contribute to the ongoing discussion on reproducibility and replicability by presenting several efforts to systematize and compare, rerun and replicate, as well as reimplement, simulate, and reproduce models and knowledge within our fields of expertise. By comparability, we mean comparing either the simulation results of different simulation tools when the same model has been implemented in them or the simulation results of different models. By replicability, we mean rerunning the publicly available code developed by the authors of the study and replicating the original results from the study. By reproducibility, we mean reimplementing the model using the knowledge from the original study, often in a different simulation tool or programming language from the one reported in the study, and simulating it to verify the results from the study. These definitions are consistent with the terminology on replicability and reproducibility used in the literature (see also Crook et al., 2013; McDougal et al., 2016). However, there is an ongoing discussion on optimal use of terminology and several alternatives have been proposed (see e.g., Goodman et al., 2016; Rougier et al., 2017; Benureau and Rougier, 2018). The lack of universally accepted terminology, solutions proposed in other scientific disciplines, and possible solutions for computational neuroscience are also discussed by Plesser (2018). In order to focus on our findings and conclusions rather than terminology, we will adopt the definitions described above without further discussion about the alternatives.

There is an evident need to evaluate, compare, and systematize tools and models. With the increasing number of published models, it is becoming difficult to evaluate the unique contribution in each of them or assess the scientific rigor. The published articles might provide incomplete information, due to accidental mistakes or limited space and publication format. The original model implementations are not always available. The overhead of model reimplementation and reproduction of the results could be significant. More systematic model description (Nordlie et al., 2009), publishing the code in addition to the article (Eglen et al., 2017; Rougier et al., 2017), and efforts on independent reproduction and replication of the published models (Manninen et al., 2017; Rougier et al., 2017) improve quality and reliability of results in computational neuroscience. Better systematization and classification of the models provide more straightforward recommendations for the scientists initiating new projects or for the training of young researchers entering the field (see also Akil et al., 2016; Amunts et al., 2016; Nishi et al., 2016). All these can better support the reuse and extension of the published models which is often necessary when building models of complex phenomena. The development of new experimental techniques and the new experimental findings also pose new questions for the computational neuroscience. The models that address these questions are often built on top of the existing ones, and heavily depend on the reusability and reliability of the published work. These issues become even more important with the increasing interest and current intensive development of multiscale models. Multiscale models include fine details of all levels of physical organization (molecular reaction networks, individual cells, local neuronal networks, glial networks, large-scale networks, and even complete functional brain systems), and naturally such complex and demanding models must rely even more on the existing knowledge and models. Furthermore, as the complexity of the models increases it becomes more difficult to duplicate the original work even if only one parameter value is mistyped, or completely omitted.

The listed challenges have been extensively discussed within the computational neuroscience and neuroinformatics community. Several publications have proposed improvements in model development and description recommending a clear and compact tabular format for model description (see e.g., Nordlie et al., 2009; Topalidou et al., 2015; Manninen et al., 2017). The issue of reproducibility in computational neuroscience has been emphasized through development of model description and simulation tools: the standardization of tools significantly accelerates development of new models and reproduction of the published models. An overview of the existing simulation tools, their features and strengths, as well as a discussion on future developments are presented in recent publications (Brette et al., 2007; Crook et al., 2013; McDougal et al., 2016). In addition, journals rarely explicitly state that they accept replicability and reproducibility studies (Yeung, 2017). However, the ReScience initiative was started to encourage researchers to reimplement published models and reproduce the research results (Rougier et al., 2017). During the review process in the ReScience Journal, both the manuscript and the reimplementation of the model are tested and checked by the reviewers, and both are made publicly available for the scientific community. In our previous study (Manninen et al., 2017), we addressed the reproducibility of a small set of computational glial models. Based on this study, we emphasize the necessity for giving out all information about the models, such as the inputs, equations, parameters, and initial conditions, in a tabular format, in addition to making the model code publicly available. Similar holds for complex network-level models composed of many interacting neurons where every small error might lead to a large deviation in the simulation outcome.

Equally important concept that should be discussed in the context of reproducibility and replicability is the development of validation strategies for comparability of various computational models. Better mathematical and computational tools are needed to provide easy and user-friendly evaluation and comparison. As can be seen from the reviews of previous modeling work in the field (Manninen et al., 2010, 2018a,b), many new models are built on top of pre-existing models, with some further parameter estimation based on experimental data. Often the validation against existing similar models is too tedious to do and, consequently, is skipped. To facilitate the usability of models, future computational neuroscience research should pay more attention to the questions of reproducibility, replicability, and validation of simulation results. As indicated, this issue becomes even more important with the current trends toward developing multiscale models.

In this study, we evaluate a number of computational models describing a very diverse set of neural systems and phenomena, as well as simulation tools dedicated to these models. We evaluate and discuss a versatile choice of simulation tools, from simulation tools of biochemical reactions, to relatively new simulation tools of growth in cell cultures, to relatively mature and widely adopted tools for modeling spiking neuronal networks. The computational models are equally diverse, including the models of intracellular signal transduction for neurons and glial cells, in addition to single glial cells, neuron-glia interactions, and neuronal networks. Although we take into account a range of models, some classes of models are not considered in this study. We omit single neuron models which are already well developed, compared, and systematized in the literature (Izhikevich, 2004; Sterratt et al., 2011). Furthermore, we do not intend to provide any extensive evaluation of neuronal network models, which are numerous in the literature, but instead discuss an illustrative data-driven modeling example and specific reproducibility, replicability, and comparability issues that emerge in this type of studies. The models for glial networks and the larger models of neuron-glia networks are also excluded from this work and might be subject of future studies. Through the evaluation of examples under consideration, we present the state-of-the-art in reproducibility and replicability of computational models of neuronal and glial systems, summarize our recent findings about reproducibility in computational neuroscience, and propose some good practices based on our present and previous work.

2. MATERIAL AND METHODS

2.1. Simulation Tools

In this section, we describe a range of simulation tools utilized to simulate the spiking neuronal networks, biochemical reactions, and neuronal growth. Simulation tools that allow constructing, simulating, and analyzing whole-cell and neuronal circuit models attracted the most attention in the past and are among the most developed tools used in computational neuroscience. Typical models range from multicompartmental neurons integrating some level of morphological and physiological details of the certain neuron type to the highly abstract models containing large number of low-dimensional model neurons and statistical description of connectivity rules. In computational systems biology, the simulation tools developed for different kinds of biological systems, such as gene regulatory networks, metabolic networks, and signal transduction, have been the focus of development. These tools are relatively mature, standardized, and well-known in the research community. On the other hand, the simulation tools for neurodevelopment are not so well-known, and thus we give more details about these tools in the upcoming sections. All the simulation tools tested and compared in this work are listed in **Table 1**.

2.1.1. Simulation Tools for Biochemical Reactions

Mathematical modeling of biochemistry is important for understanding complex biochemical processes that underlie many neuronal, glial, and synaptic phenomena. Recent interest in modeling biochemical networks in systems biology and in neuroscience have provided several tools that can be used to simulate time-series behavior of the networks (see e.g., Lemerle et al., 2005; Pettinen et al., 2005; Alves et al., 2006; Gilbert et al., 2006; Strömbäck et al., 2006; Wierling et al., 2007; Bergmann and Sauro, 2008; Blackwell, 2013; Schöneberg et al., 2014; Bartocci and Lió, 2016; Olivier et al., 2016). In this study, we used the following simulation tools: GENESIS/Kinetikit (Wilson et al., 1989; Bower and Beeman, 1998; Bhalla and Iyengar, 1999; Bhalla, 2001, 2002), Gepasi (Mendes, 1993, 1997; Mendes and Kell, 1998), Jarnac/JDesigner (Sauro, 2000, 2001), XPPAUT (Ermentrout, 2002), SimTool (Aho, 2003), Dizzy (Ramsey et al., 2005), Copasi (Hoops et al., 2006), NEURON (Carnevale and Hines, 2006), Systems Biology Toolbox (Schmidt and Jirstrand, 2006), and Narrator (Mandel et al., 2007) (see **Table 1**). Here, we do not provide any detailed overview of the simulation tools, because the topic has been already extensively discussed previously. However, we want to point out the differences in these tools by providing information about the methods used for modeling and simulation.

In the listed simulation tools, the model is often implemented using chemical reactions presented by the law of mass action and Michaelis-Menten kinetics. These reactions form coupled ordinary differential equations (ODEs) presenting the biochemical network, and these equations are then solved numerically when simulating the model. However, for example, in XPPAUT, the model is directly implemented using the ODEs and not the chemical reactions. Several of the tools also provide stochastic approaches to model and simulate the reactions (see e.g., Manninen et al., 2006a; Gillespie, 2007), such as the discrete-state Gillespie stochastic simulation algorithm (Gillespie, 1976, 1977) and τ-leap method (Gillespie, 2001), as well as continuous-state chemical Langevin equation (Gillespie, 2000) and several other stochastic differential equations (SDEs, Manninen et al., 2006a,b). Few simulation tools providing hybrid approaches also exist. They combine either deterministic and stochastic methods or different stochastic methods (see e.g., Salis et al.,

TABLE 1 | List of simulation tools and model repositories.

Tool/Repository	Website	References
SIMULATION TOOL		
Brian	http://brian2.readthedocs.io/en/stable/index.html	Goodman and Brette, 2008
Copasi	http://copasi.org/	Hoops et al., 2006
Cortex3D	https://www.ini.uzh.ch/~amw/seco/cx3d/	Zubler and Douglas, 2009
Dizzy	http://magnet.systemsbiology.net/software/Dizzy/	Ramsey et al., 2005
GENESIS/ Kinetikit	http://genesis-sim.org/, https://www.ncbs.res.in/faculty/bhalla-kinetikit	Wilson et al., 1989; Bower and Beeman, 1998; Bhalla and Iyengar, 1999; Bhalla, 2001, 2002
Gepasi	http://www.gepasi.org/	Mendes, 1993, 1997; Mendes and Kell, 1998
Jarnac/JDesigner	http://jdesigner.sourceforge.net/	Sauro, 2000, 2001
Narrator	https://omictools.com/narrator-tool	Mandel et al., 2007
NEST	http://www.nest-simulator.org/	Eppler et al., 2015
NETMORPH	http://www.netmorph.org/Home, http://www.scholarpedia.org/article/NETMORPH	Koene et al., 2009
NEURON	https://www.neuron.yale.edu/neuron/	Carnevale and Hines, 2006
PyNN	http://neuralensemble.org/PyNN/	Davison et al., 2009
SimTool	Request from the author	Aho, 2003
Systems Biology Toolbox	http://www.sbtoolbox.org/	Schmidt and Jirstrand, 2006
XPPAUT	http://www.math.pitt.edu/~bard/xpp/xpp.html	Ermentrout, 2002
MODEL REPOSITORY		
DOQCS	http://doqcs.ncbs.res.in/	Sivakumaran et al., 2003
DRYAD	http://datadryad.org/	
ModelDB	http://senselab.med.yale.edu/modeldb/	Migliore et al., 2003; Hines et al., 2004

This table lists the names of the simulation tools and model repositories as well as their websites and references.

2006; Lecca et al., 2017). The increased computing power has recently made it possible also to take into account diffusion processes. The reaction-diffusion simulation tools often use combined Gillespie algorithm or τ-leap method for both reaction and diffusion processes, such as STEPS (Wils and De Schutter, 2009; Hepburn et al., 2012) and NeuroRD (Oliveira et al., 2010), or track each molecule individually in a certain volume with Brownian dynamics combined with a Monte Carlo procedure for reaction events, such as MCell (Stiles and Bartol, 2001; Kerr et al., 2008) and Smoldyn (Andrews et al., 2010). Few studies to compare different reaction-diffusion tools exist (Dobrzyński et al., 2007; Oliveira et al., 2010; Schöneberg et al., 2014). In this study, however, we were only interested in comparing simulation tools with simple reaction models, and thus reaction-diffusion tools and models were not tested. The more detailed testing of reaction-diffusion tools remains for future work and will most probably be accelerated once more models for reaction-diffusion systems become available. The simulation tools for biochemical reactions addressed in this work have been studied in detail in our previous work (Pettinen et al., 2005; Manninen et al., 2006c; Mäkiraatikka et al., 2007) and the here presented results are a summary of our previous work. We recommend to consult the earlier studies for more details.

2.1.2. Simulation Tools for Neurodevelopment

We examined relatively new and promising tools for modeling neurodevelopment. They facilitate exploring through computational means individual biophysical mechanisms involved in development and growth of neuronal circuits and analyzing the properties that arise from those mechanisms. We examined two simulation tools, NETMORPH (Koene et al., 2009) and Cortex3D (Zubler and Douglas, 2009), the full references and links to these tools are given in **Table 1**. Because these tools are newer, less known and used than the other simulation tools presented in this study, we describe them with additional details.

NETMORPH implements a phenomenological model of neurite growth (in 2D or 3D) based on extensive statistical characterization of dendritic morphology in developing circuits conducted by the authors of the simulation tool (van Pelt and Uylings, 2003; Koene et al., 2009). It can simulate formation of synaptic contacts based on morphology and the proximity between axonal and dendritic segments. The simulation tool was developed in C++ under Unix/Linux and can be installed straightforwardly under the same environment. In Windows, it can be installed using Cygwin. The inputs are text files containing a list of model components and the belonging parameters. The components include description of neuronal population, morphology for each neuron type, parameters determining synapse formation, and a set of flags describing the format of simulation outputs. Model equations are evaluated at fixed time steps, and the output can be generated either at specified time points or at the end of a simulation. Three types of outputs are possible: visualization of neuronal morphologies and networks, raw data containing the list of all generated model components, and the statistics computed from the raw data.

Cortex3D is a simulation platform that supports modeling biophysical and mechanistic details of neural development. As such it does not specify any particular model but rather a set of underlying mechanisms that can be used to implement and simulate user-defined models. The mechanisms embedded into the simulation tool include discretization of space occupied by a model, production, diffusion, degradation, and reactions between chemical species, the effect of mechanical and chemical forces between components of the model, and movement of objects inside the model. The model is solved at a fixed time grid. Parts of the model represented by dynamical equations are solved using Euler method, but numerical integration is replaced by analytical solution whenever possible to avoid overshoot for large time steps. The simulation tool is organized into layers of abstraction, with the discretization of space mapped into the lowest layer, the physical properties of the objects being specified one layer above, and the biological properties mapped into the top two layers. Most of the user-defined model properties can be specified in the top "cell" layer (Zubler and Douglas, 2009). The simulation tool was implemented in Java and is easy to install on any platform. A parallelized version of the simulation tool is also available (Zubler et al., 2011, 2013). Recently, a new simulation tool capable of modeling neuronal tissue development, inspired by Cortex3D and based on the same computational principles, was proposed (https://biodynamo.web.cern.ch/). To specify a model in Cortex3D, a user should write Java module containing the description of model components, interactions between the components, and model parameters. The output of the simulation tool is an Extensible Markup Language (XML) schema compatible with NeuroML containing the details of the obtained model. The simulation tool also integrates Java packages that allow visualization of the simulation evolution. We tested and compared NETMORPH and Cortex3D by implementing and running the same model compatible with both tools and evaluating the simulated data. In addition to tool evaluation, we were interested in promoting the usefulness of these new and underutilized simulation tools.

2.1.3. Simulation Tools for Neuronal Networks

Computational studies of individual neurons and neuronal circuits were the first attempts at computational modeling in neuroscience, have the longest history, and are still the most represented level of abstraction when addressing the function and organization of neuronal systems. They originate from the experimentally verified models of neurons, the ground truth of neuron electrophysiology based on Hodgkin-Huxley (HH, Hodgkin and Huxley, 1952) formalism and the mathematical description of ion channel dynamics. Individual neurons can be described either as single compartmental models representing the somatic membrane potential or as multicompartmental models including parts of dendritic and axonal arbors. In addition, the simulation tools provide a number of simpler and computationally less demanding neuron models based on an integrate-and-fire (IF) modeling formalism. They also provide mechanisms to construct networks of model neurons, from generic random networks to specific brain circuits. Some of these simulation tools also have a capacity to implement subcellular models (NEURON, XPPAUT, and GENESIS). Consequently, these simulation tools are widely accepted and well known within the scientific community and can be considered mature. All of these simulation tools implement deterministic methods to solve the systems of ODEs, and some of them also have possibility to implement SDE models (see e.g., Stimberg et al., 2014). Deterministic integration methods for solving ODEs use either a fixed or adaptable integration step size. For some neurons of IF type, it is possible to solve the ODE exactly between the spike times and update the model at each spike time, thus significantly increasing the accuracy of numerical integration. The extensive discussion about numerical methods can be found in the literature (Rotter and Diesmann, 1999; Lytton and Hines, 2005; Carnevale and Hines, 2006; Brette et al., 2007; Stimberg et al., 2014). Here, we do not aim at giving an overview of simulation tools or comparing their properties, these topics have been extensively discussed elsewhere (see e.g., Brette et al., 2007; McDougal et al., 2016). Instead, we will present our unpublished user experiences from describing and simulating spiking neuronal networks using NEST (Eppler et al., 2015), Brian (Goodman and Brette, 2008; Stimberg et al., 2014), and PyNN (Davison et al., 2009).

2.2. Models

In this section, we give an overview of computational models used in our reproducibility, replicability, and comparability studies. These include the models of intracellular signal transduction for neurons and glial cells, in addition to single glial cells, neuron-glia interactions, and neuronal networks. We tabulated the following properties for the models whenever suitable:

- **Neuron model:** Multicompartmental or point neuron models adopted from the literature.
- **Synapse model:** Types of synaptic models and receptors.
- **Neuron-astrocyte synapse model:** Types of synaptic models and receptors.
- **Connectivity:** Statistical description of connectivity schemes.
- **Intracellular signaling;** Intracellular calcium signaling (e.g., leaks, pumps, and receptors that are not named under other categories) in addition to different intracellular chemical species taken into account either in neurons or astrocytes.
- **Data analysis:** Description of the methods used to analyze *in silico* data from spiking neuronal network models.

Some of the models we used in this study were found available in model repositories. These repositories are listed in **Table 1**.

2.2.1. Neuronal Signal Transduction Models

More than a hundred intracellular biochemical species are important in synaptic plasticity. Hundreds of neuronal signal transduction models have been developed to test the criticality of different chemical species. Several reviews of the models exist, some focus on just a few different models whereas others give an overview of more than hundred models (Brown et al., 1990; Neher, 1998; Hudmon and Schulman, 2002a,b; Bi and Rubin, 2005; Holmes, 2005; Wörgötter and Porr, 2005; Ajay and Bhalla, 2006; Klipp and Liebermeister, 2006; Zou and Destexhe, 2007; Morrison et al., 2008; Ogasawara et al., 2008; Bhalla, 2009; Ogasawara and Kawato, 2009; Tanaka and Augustine,

2009; Urakubo et al., 2009; Castellani and Zironi, 2010; Gerkin et al., 2010; Graupner and Brunel, 2010; Hellgren Kotaleski and Blackwell, 2010; Manninen et al., 2010; Shouval et al., 2010). The models range from a simple models with just a single reversible reaction to very detailed models with several hundred reactions. In **Table 2**, we list the neuronal signal transduction models for plasticity that we evaluated in this study. The models by d'Alcantara et al. (2003) and Delord et al. (2007) were the simplest with just a few reactions, whereas the model by Zachariou et al. (2013) had both pre- and postsynaptic single-compartmental neurons and rest of the models had very detailed intracellular signaling pathways taken into account. The models by d'Alcantara et al. (2003), Delord et al. (2007), and Zachariou et al. (2013) we used in the reproducibility studies. In the comparability studies (Manninen and Linne, 2008; Manninen et al., 2011), we tested the models by d'Alcantara et al. (2003), Hayer and Bhalla (2005), Lindskog et al. (2006), Delord et al. (2007), Nakano et al. (2010), and Kim et al. (2010).

2.2.2. Astrocyte Models

Similarly to neuronal signal transduction models, hundreds of single astrocyte, astrocytic network, and neuron-astrocyte interaction models have been developed to study different phenomena. Several reviews of computational astrocyte and neuron-astrocyte models have appeared during the last few years, some focusing only to a few models and some giving a general overview of the field (see e.g., Jolivet et al., 2010; Mangia et al., 2011; De Pittà et al., 2012, 2016; Fellin et al., 2012; Min et al., 2012; Volman et al., 2012; Wade et al., 2013; Linne and Jalonen, 2014; Tewari and Parpura, 2014; Manninen et al., 2018a,b). In **Table 3**, we list the models that we evaluated in this study. We chose five single astrocyte and signal transduction models (Di Garbo et al., 2007; Lavrentovich and Hemkin, 2008; De Pittà et al., 2009; Dupont et al., 2011; Riera et al., 2011a,b) and four neuron-astrocyte interaction models (Nadkarni and Jung, 2003; Silchenko and Tass, 2008; Wade et al., 2011, 2012). Silchenko and Tass (2008) used a two-compartmental neuron model, whereas the other three (Nadkarni and Jung, 2003; Wade et al., 2011, 2012) used single-compartmental models. The models by Nadkarni and Jung (2003), Di Garbo et al. (2007), Silchenko and Tass (2008), Lavrentovich and Hemkin (2008), De Pittà et al. (2009), Riera et al. (2011a,b), Dupont et al. (2011), and Wade et al. (2011, 2012) were tested in the reproducibility studies (see also Manninen et al., 2017, 2018b). In addition, the models by Lavrentovich and Hemkin (2008), De Pittà et al. (2009), Riera et al. (2011a,b), and our modified version of the model by Dupont et al. (2011) were used in the comparability study (see also Manninen et al., 2017).

2.2.3. Spiking Neuronal Network Models

Spiking neuronal network models are numerous in the literature and used to model various phenomena and brain structures. In order to constrain this evaluation to a reasonable set of models, we selected only those models which are developed for the spontaneously synchronized population activity from dissociated neuronal cultures *in vitro* (for more details, see Robinson et al., 1993; Teppola et al., 2011). The focus on data-driven models gives us an opportunity to emphasize the need for reproduction of both model and data analysis tools. We compared several publications (Latham et al., 2000; Giugliano et al., 2004; French and Gruenstein, 2006; Gritsun et al., 2010, 2011; Baltz et al., 2011; Maheswaranathan et al., 2012; Mäki-Marttunen et al., 2013; Masquelier and Deco, 2013; Yamamoto et al., 2016; Lonardoni et al., 2017), that use similar models, address similar questions, and should converge toward similar conclusions. Some differences emerge from the experimental preparation, from the recording technology, or variations in model composition. The publications by Gritsun et al. (2010, 2011) present two parts of the same study. They are considered as one study, but are presented separately in **Table 4** due to the small differences in model construction and data analysis. The publication by Mäki-Marttunen et al. (2013) is not, strictly speaking, modeling the experimental data but rather uses the theoretical concepts to explore models and synthetic data typical for this same type of experiments. All of the studies under consideration implement networks of point-neurons (a few hundred to few thousand neurons) with none or short-term plasticity in synapses and statistical description of connectivity. Similar models have been extensively analyzed in theoretical studies exploring feasible dynamical regimes, and some of them are available in public repositories dedicated to reproducible model development (see OpenSourceBrain; http://www.opensourcebrain.org/). In this study, we do not consider recent attempts to model the effects of non-neuronal cells, and we also leave out the mean field approaches to modeling the same type of experiments and data. The 10 selected studies are summarized in **Table 4**.

3. RESULTS

We here evaluate first the simulation tools we used for biochemical reactions, growth in cell cultures, and spiking neuronal networks, and last the computational models for signal transduction in neurons, astrocytes, and spiking neuronal networks.

3.1. Evaluation of Simulation Tools

3.1.1. Simulation Tools for Biochemical Reactions

In our previous studies, we have extensively used and evaluated both deterministic and stochastic simulation tools for biochemical reactions (see **Table 1**), categorized their basic properties, benefits, and drawbacks, as well as tested the tools by implementing test cases and running simulations (Pettinen et al., 2005; Manninen et al., 2006c; Mäkiraatikka et al., 2007). At first, we tested four deterministic simulation tools, GENESIS/Kinetikit (versions 2.2 and 2.2.1 of the GENESIS and versions 8 and 9 of the Kinetikit), Jarnac/JDesigner (version 2.0 of Jarnac and version 1.8k of JDesigner), Gepasi (version 3.30), and SimTool, by implementing the same test case for every simulation tool and running simulations (Pettinen et al., 2005). Next, we tested three stochastic simulation tools, Dizzy (version 1.11.2), Copasi (release candidate 1, build 17), and Systems Biology Toolbox (version 1.5), the same way (Manninen et al., 2006c; Mäkiraatikka et al., 2007). Last, we tested the possibility to

TABLE 2 | Summary of the neuronal signal transduction models.

Model	Neuron model	Synapse model	Intracellular signaling
d'Alcantara et al., 2003	No	AMPAR	CaM, CaMKII, CaN, DARPP32 or I1, PP1
Hayer and Bhalla, 2005	No	AMPAR, NMDAR	AC1, AC2, AMP, Ca^{2+}, CaM, CaMKII, cAMP, CaN, I1, Ng, PDE1, PKA, PKC, PP1, PP2A
Lindskog et al., 2006	No	D_1R	AC5, AMP, ATP, CaM, CaMKII, cAMP, CaN, Cd5k, DARPP32, G protein, PDE1, PDE4, PKA, PP1, PP2A
Delord et al., 2007	No	No	Kinase, phosphatase, substrate
Nakano et al., 2010	No	AMPAR, D_1R	AC5, AMP, ATP, Ca^{2+}, CaM, CaMKII, cAMP, CaN, Cd5k, CK1, DARPP32, G protein, I1, PDE1, PDE2, PKA, PP1, PP2A, PP2C
Kim et al., 2010	No	D_1R	AC1, AC8, AMP, ATP, Ca^{2+}, CaM, CaMKII, cAMP, CaN, G protein, I1, PDE1B, PDE4, PKA, PP1
Zachariou et al., 2013	Presyn.: HH (Kdr, Na, N-type VGCC), postsyn.: HH (Kdr, L-type VGCC, Na)	Presyn.: CB_1, postsyn.: AMPAR, $GABA_AR$	Postsyn.: 2-AG, Ca^{2+} (Ca^{2+} leak from ER into cyt, Ca^{2+} leak from ext into cyt, PMCA, SERCA), Ca^{2+}_{ER}, DAG

Neuron model: *pre- and postsynaptic point neuron models.* ***Synapse model:*** *pre- and postsynaptic receptors.* ***Intracellular signaling:*** *intracellular calcium signaling (e.g., leaks and pumps that are not named under other categories) in addition to different intracellular chemical species in pre- and postsynaptic neurons. 2-AG, 2-arachidonoylglycerol; AC1, adenylyl cyclase type 1; AC2, AC type 2; AC5, AC type 5; AC8, AC type 8; AMP, adenosine monophosphate; AMPAR, α-amino-3-hydroxy-5-methyl-4-isoxazolepropionic acid receptor; ATP, adenosine triphosphate;* Ca^{2+}*, calcium ion; CaM, calmodulin; CaMKII,* Ca^{2+}*/CaM-dependent protein kinase II; cAMP, cyclic AMP; CaN, calcineurin;* CB_1*, cannabinoid type 1 receptor; Cdk5, cyclin-dependent kinase 5; CK1, casein kinase 1; cyt, cytosol;* D_1R*, dopamine receptor; DAG, diacylglycerol; DARPP32, dopamine- and cAMP-regulated neuronal phosphoprotein of 32 kDa; ER, endoplasmic reticulum; ext, extracellular space;* $GABA_AR$*, gamma-aminobutyric acid type A receptor; HH, Hodgkin-Huxley; I1, inhibitor 1; Kdr, delayed rectifier potassium current; Na, sodium current; Ng, neurogranin; NMDAR, N-methyl-D-aspartate receptor; PDE1, phosphodiesterase type 1; PDE1B, PDE type 1B; PDE2, PDE type 2; PDE4, PDE type 4; PKA, cAMP-dependent protein kinase; PKC, protein kinase C; PMCA, plasma membrane* Ca^{2+} *ATPase; PP1, protein phosphatase 1; PP2A, PP type 2A; PP2C, PP type 2C; SERCA, sarco/endoplasmic reticulum* Ca^{2+}*-ATPase; VGCC, voltage-gated* Ca^{2+} *channel.*

easily exchange models between stochastic simulation tools using Systems Biology Markup Language (SBML) (Mäkiraatikka et al., 2007). As a surprise, only a few of the tools that were supposed to support SBML import were capable of simulating the selected test case when imported as SBML file (Mäkiraatikka et al., 2007). Of the tools that we tested for that study, only Dizzy, Narrator, and XPPAUT succeeded in simulating the imported SBML file. We found out in all of our studies (Pettinen et al., 2005; Manninen et al., 2006c; Mäkiraatikka et al., 2007) that the simulation results between the tools were convergent. Using the same test case as by Pettinen et al. (2005), we also found out in a separate set of tests that NEURON produced similar results as the other tools mentioned above. Based on our studies, we concluded that the comparability of the simulation results needed several requirements to be fulfilled. First, the usability of the simulation tools and existence of proper manuals were crucial. For example, even beginners were able to use Dizzy, Gepasi, Copasi, and Jarnac/JDesigner, but former experience in MATLAB® was required for Systems Biology Toolbox and SimTool. Second, the lack of standards and interfaces between tools also made the comparability problematic. For example related to SBML import, graphical user interfaces designed to help the SBML import were not intuitive, the error messages were not informative enough, and not all the SBML levels were supported. Furthermore, for stochastic simulations with the Gillespie stochastic simulation algorithm, all the chemical reactions in the model had to be implemented as irreversible. Although the test case was implemented and exported with only irreversible reactions, we found simulation tools that mistook some of the irreversible reactions for reversible reactions during the SBML import and thus, we were not able to run stochastic simulations with these tools (Mäkiraatikka et al., 2007). In addition, problems arose when having various biochemical and physiological units because during manual conversion the chance of making errors was significant. Third, the utilization of realistic external stimuli was not possible in all simulation tools. Out of the tested simulation tools, GENESIS/Kinetikit was one of the good examples where external stimuli were enabled. Fourth, only a few of the tools had built-in automated parameter estimation methods to tune the models and their unknown parameter values. However, several methodology improvements have been made in the field in order to perform sophisticated parameter estimation. The use may, however, require some more detailed knowledge in computer science. Thus, all these difficulties and deficiencies present in simulation tools can make the comparison of simulation results difficult.

3.1.2. Simulation Tools for Neurodevelopment

We tested two simulation tools dedicated to modeling neurodevelopmental mechanisms, NETMORPH and Cortex3D (Aćimović et al., 2011). While other simulation tools (e.g., NEURON) can be used to implement models at particular developmental age, NETMORPH and Cortex3D implement the mechanisms behind developmental changes. NETMORPH and Cortex3D can be used to address the same questions, but they are fundamentally different in methodology, approach, and philosophy of modeling being therefore complementary rather than competing. NETMORPH and Cortex3D were implemented using different programming languages. Running simulations beyond making simple changes to the provided examples required a deeper understanding of the tools.

In short, we implemented a phenomenological model, compatible with both simulation tools, of neurite growth and

TABLE 3 | Summary of the astrocyte and neuron-astrocyte models.

Model	Neuron model	Neuron-astrocyte synapse model	Intracellular signaling in neuron	Intracellular signaling in astrocyte
Nadkarni and Jung, 2003	Postsyn.: HH (Kdr, Na)	Postsyn. voltage ↦ astro IP_3, astro Ca^{2+} ↦ postsyn. current	No	Ca^{2+} (CICR via IP_3R, Ca^{2+} leak from ER into cyt, SERCA), IP_3, active fraction of IP_3R
Di Garbo et al., 2007	No	Astro: P2XR, P2YR	No	Ca^{2+} (CCE, CICR via IP_3R, Ca^{2+} efflux, Ca^{2+} leak from ER into cyt, Ca^{2+} leak from ext into cyt, SERCA), Ca^{2+}_{ER}, IP_3, active fraction of IP_3R
Silchenko and Tass, 2008	Postsyn.: Pinsky-Rinzel, HH (AHP, Kdr, L-type VGCC, Na)	Postsyn.: AMPAR, NMDAR, astro: mGluR	Ca^{2+}	Ca^{2+} (CICR via IP_3R, Ca^{2+} efflux, glutamate-dependent Ca^{2+} influx, Ca^{2+} influx, Ca^{2+} leak from ER into cyt, SERCA), Ca^{2+}_{ER}, IP_3, vesicle cycle, glutamate release
Lavrentovich and Hemkin, 2008	No	No	No	Ca^{2+} (CICR via IP_3R, Ca^{2+} efflux, Ca^{2+} influx, Ca^{2+} leak from ER into cyt, SERCA), Ca^{2+}_{ER}, IP_3
De Pittà et al., 2009	No	No	No	Ca^{2+} (CICR via IP_3R, Ca^{2+} leak from ER into cyt, SERCA), IP_3, active fraction of IP_3R
Riera et al., 2011a,b	No	No	No	Ca^{2+} (CCE, CICR via IP_3R, Ca^{2+} efflux, Ca^{2+} influx via channels, Ca^{2+} leak from ER into cyt, SERCA), Ca^{2+}_{free}, IP_3, active fraction of IP_3R
Dupont et al., 2011	No	Astro: mGluR	No	Ca^{2+} (CICR via IP_3R, Ca^{2+} efflux, Ca^{2+} influx, Ca^{2+} leak from ER into cyt, SERCA), DAG, IP_3, fraction of Ca^{2+}-inhibited IP_3R, active fraction of PKC
Wade et al., 2011	Postsyn.: LIF	Tsodyks ↦ astro IP_3 and syn. current, astro Ca^{2+} ↦ postsyn. NMDAR, astro glutamate ↦ Tsodyks	No	Ca^{2+} (CICR via IP_3R, Ca^{2+} leak from ER into cyt, SERCA), IP_3, active fraction of IP_3R, glutamate release
Wade et al., 2012	Postsyn.: LIF	Postsyn. 2-AG ↦ astro IP_3, astro glutamate ↦ syn. current	Postsyn.: 2-AG, depression, potentiation	Ca^{2+} (CICR via IP_3R, Ca^{2+} leak from ER into cyt, SERCA), IP_3, active fraction of IP_3R, glutamate release

Neuron model: *postsynaptic multicompartmental and point neuron models.* ***Neuron-astrocyte synapse model:*** *Tsodyks-Pawelzik-Markram model; postsynaptic and astrocytic receptors.* ***Intracellular signaling in neuron:*** *intracellular chemical species in postsynaptic neuron.* ***Intracellular signaling in astrocyte:*** *intracellular calcium signaling (e.g., leaks, pumps, and receptors that are not named under other categories) in addition to different intracellular chemical species in astrocyte. We only implemented the astrocyte component of the model by Di Garbo et al. (2007), and not the neuron component at all. 2-AG, 2-arachidonoylglycerol; AHP, after-hyperpolarization current; AMPAR, α-amino-3-hydroxy-5-methyl-4-isoxazolepropionic acid receptor; ATP, adenosine triphosphate;* Ca^{2+}*, calcium ion; CCE, capacitive* Ca^{2+} *entry; CICR,* Ca^{2+}*-induced* Ca^{2+} *release; cyt, cytosol; DAG, diacylglycerol; ER, endoplasmic reticulum; ext, extracellular space; HH, Hodgkin-Huxley;* IP_3*, inositol trisphosphate;* IP_3R*,* IP_3 *receptor; Kdr, delayed rectifier potassium current; LIF, leaky integrate-and-fire; mGluR, metabotropic glutamate receptor; Na, sodium current; NMDAR, N-methyl-D-aspartate receptor; P2XR, ionotropic purinergic ATP receptor; P2YR, purinergic G-protein-coupled metabotropic receptor; PKC, protein kinase C; SERCA, sarco/ER* Ca^{2+}*-ATPase; VGCC, voltage-gated* Ca^{2+} *channel.*

formation of synaptic contacts based on morphology criteria (for more details see Aćimović et al., 2011). The choice is determined by model components and mechanisms available in NETMORPH. To analyze the simulation results, we wrote own MATLAB® code which converted both simulated data sets to the same format and computed the statistics from the data. We examined the simulated morphologies, analyzed the number of generated synapses at different simulation times, and compared the synapse counts to the experimental data extracted from the literature (see **Figure 1**). As a conclusion, the two simulation tools produced qualitatively similar growth dynamics. The simulated results were consistent with the experimental data in the early phase of growth but deviated in the latter phase. Cortex3D gave somewhat shorter neurites with less synaptic contacts and less precise control of the orientation of neurite segments than NETMORPH. While NETMORPH implements a set of equations derived to produce precise statistics for all relevant parameters of neurite morphology, Cortex3D focuses on the underlying mechanisms of growth, for example the tensions resulting from elongation and the production of resources needed for growth. These mechanisms affect neurite morphology in a complex and not fully predictable way. The computational model used for testing and comparing the simulation tools was a natural choice for NETMORPH and therefore easier to implement, faster to simulate, and less memory consuming. However, Cortex3D offers more flexibility to implement user-defined models for various phases of neurodevelopment, and can be used to study many other mechanisms in addition to neurite growth.

3.1.3. Simulation Tools for Spiking Neuronal Networks

We present our user experience with three common tools for simulation of large spiking networks of point neuron models. In addition to testing and comparing the simulation tools, we discuss the flexibility of simulation tools to implement user-defined model components. We tested the common tools, NEST (version 2.8.0) with PyNN (version 0.8.0) used as an interface and Brian (version 2.0). All of the tested packages are well documented and additional support is offered through user groups. The general tendency to develop Python based simulation tools or Python interface to simulation tools saves time when analyzing the obtained simulation results, since the

TABLE 4 | Summary of the spiking neuronal network models.

Model	Neuron model	Synapse model	Connectivity	Data analysis
Latham et al., 2000	QIF/Theta, AHP, Ref, excitatory and inhibitory	exp-cond.	Nonstructured, distance-based	Burst detection: none; Measures: rasterplot, GFR
Giugliano et al., 2004	LIFa, excitatory	exp-curr.	Nonstructured	Burst detection: not given; Measures: burst structure, burst count/freq.
French and Gruenstein, 2006	LIF, AHP, Ref, T-type VGCC	alpha-curr., depression	SW	Burst detection: none; Measures: burst size (number of active neurons), speed of burst propagation
Gritsun et al., 2010	Izhikevich, excitatory and inhibitory	exp-curr., Tsodyks	Nonstructured	Burst detection: GFR; Measures: burst structure
Gritsun et al., 2011	Izhikevich, excitatory and inhibitory	exp-curr., Tsodyks	Nonstructured, intense neurons	Burst detection: ISI-cell.; Measures: burst count/freq.
Baltz et al., 2011	LIF, AHP, Ref, T-type VGCC, excitatory	AMPAR, NMDAR, Tsodyks	Nonstructured	Burst detection: ISI-cell.; Measures: rasterplots, GFR, burst structure, burst count/freq.
Maheswaranathan et al., 2012	Izhikevich, excitatory and inhibitory	exp	SW	Burst detection: GFR; Measures: rasterplots, GFR, burst structure, spectral analysis, PCA
Mäki-Marttunen et al., 2013	LIF, HH (Kdr, K-slow, Na, NaP), excitatory and inhibitory	(with LIF) exp-curr., Tsodyks; (with HH) AMPAR, NMDAR, $GABA_AR$	Nonstructured, distance-based, SW, complex, simulated	Burst detection: ISI-pop.; Measures: rasterplots, burst structure, connectivity, graph measures
Masquelier and Deco, 2013	LIF, AHP, excitatory	AMPAR, NMDAR, Tsodyks	Nonstructured	Burst detection: GFR; Measures: burst count/freq.
Yamamoto et al., 2016	LIF, AHP, Ref, T-type VGCC, excitatory	biexp-cond.	Nonstructured	Burst detection: not clear; Measures: rasterplots, burst count/freq., connectivity
Lonardoni et al., 2017	AdExp, excitatory and inhibitory	biexp-cond., AMPAR, $GABA_AR$, NMDAR, Tsodyks	Distance-based (alternatives considered)	Burst detection: GFR; Measures: burst structure, burst count/freq., GFR, connectivity, burst propagation, graph measures

Neuron model: *point neuron model, one (excitatory) or two (excitatory and inhibitory) neuronal populations.* ***Synapse model:*** *exponential (exp.), bi-exponential (biexp.), or alpha postsynaptic current (curr.) or conductance (cond.); Tsodyks-Markram model; synaptic receptors.* ***Connectivity:*** *network connectivity, nonstructured (equal probability of connection for every pair of neurons), distance-based (probability of connection decreases with the distance between somata), small-world and other complex connectivity schemes, intense neurons (nonstructured, but a subset of neurons has particularly strong synapses), simulated (morphology-based connectivity simulated using NETMORPH).* ***Data analysis:*** *burst detection (identifying periods of global synchronization from the data), categories: from inter-spike-intervals of individual neurons (ISI-cell.), from inter-spike-intervals of the population (ISI-pop.), from global firing rates (GFR). Data measures: burst structure (length, number of spikes per burst etc.), burst count or frequency or statistics of inter-burst-intervals, frequency analysis, burst propagation through network, analysis of connectivity (physical or functional/from spike trains), graph measures of connectivity. AdExp, adaptive exponential; AHP, after-hyperpolarization current; AMPAR, α-amino-3-hydroxy-5-methyl-4-isoxazolepropionic acid receptor; $GABA_AR$, gamma-aminobutyric acid type A receptor; HH, Hodgkin-Huxley; Kdr, delayed rectifier potassium current; K-slow, slow potassium current; LIF and LIFa, leaky integrate and fire without and with adaptation; Na, sodium current; NaP, persistent sodium current; NMDAR, N-methyl-D-aspartate receptor; PCA, principal component analysis; QIF, quadratic integrate-and-fire; Ref, refractory current; SW, small-world connectivity; Theta, theta model; T-type VGCC, T-type voltage-gated Ca^{2+} channel (in bursting neurons).*

same Python modules for analysis and visualization of data can be combined with each simulation tool. Parallelization is supported by NEST and PyNN, however it is still under development in Brian. An earlier version of Brian offers a model fitting method for tuning the statistics of the interspike intervals in spiking neuron models. In Brian version 2.0, this option is under development. NEST and PyNN do not provide direct tools for model fitting. However, both Brian and NEST can easily be combined with external Python modules for model fitting. For fast exploration of models, for example in the early phase of model development, or for incorporating nonstandard biophysical mechanisms in the model, Brian offered more flexibility. In NEST and PyNN, the components of the model have to be either selected from the list of existing models or implemented by extending the simulation tool to include new models. Brian provides more flexible framework for implementation of user-defined models. Model components are specified directly as strings of ODEs. Various models can easily be implemented, however they still rely on the existing functionalities of the simulation tool.

3.2. Evaluation and Comparison of Computational Models

3.2.1. Neuronal Signal Transduction Models

Based on our large review of postsynaptic signal transduction models for long-term potentiation and depression (Manninen et al., 2010), we found out that it would have been often time consuming or even impossible to try to reproduce the simulations results. First, not all the details of the models, such as equations, variables, inputs, outputs, compartments, parameters, and initial conditions, were given in the original publications. For example, even just missing to give the inputs in the publications makes the reimplementation and reproduction of the simulation results difficult or impossible with signal transduction models. Second, most of the models were not available in model databases or were not open access, and sometimes even the simulation tool or programming language used was not named in the publications. Third, comparison to previous models was non-existent. Even qualitative comparison was difficult because only a few publications provided graphical illustrations of the model components or the graphical illustrations were

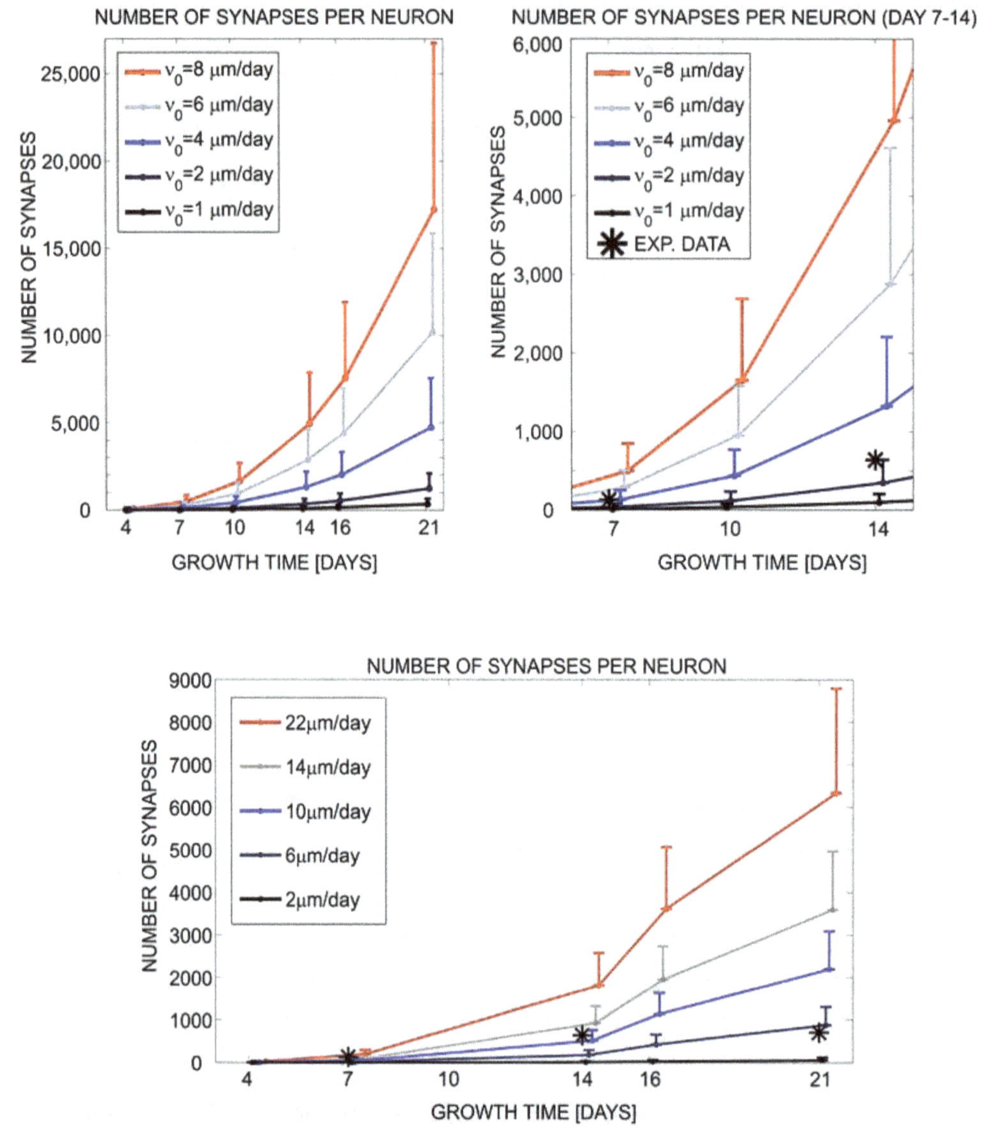

FIGURE 1 | Evaluation and comparison of the neuronal growth simulation tools (NETMORPH and Cortex3D). Panels illustrate the increase in synapse counts during simulation time equivalent to 4–21 days *in vitro*. The number and position of somata were fixed. For each neuron, the neurites grew according to the implemented model and formed synaptic contacts based on proximity between axonal and dendritic branches. In this figure, we varied one of the parameters that controlled neurite growth, the elongation rate ν_0 (see legend), and different colors correspond to different parameter values. The results show mean (line) and standard deviation (bar) for the number of synapses per neuron, averaged over all neurons in the culture. Stars indicate experimental values extracted from the literature (Ichikawa et al., 1993). **(Top left)** Synapse counts obtained from NETMORPH, elongation rates equal to 1, 2, 4, 6, and 8 μm/day. **(Top right)** Zoomed interval 7–14 days from the panel (Top left). **(Bottom)** Synapse counts obtained from Cortex3D, elongation rates equal to 2, 6, 10, 14, and 22 μm/day. x axis—growth time in days, y axis—number of synapses per neuron. For days 4–14 and $\nu_0 = 2\,\mu$m/day (NETMORPH) or $\nu_0 = 10\,\mu$m/day (Cortex3D), the simulated values corresponded to the experimental ones. After 14 days the simulated values increased while the experimental values saturated as no synaptic pruning was implemented in this test. The neurite growth was slower for Cortex3D which was visible from the values for ν_0.

misleading by having also components that were not actually modeled. We concluded that the value of computational models for understanding molecular mechanisms of synaptic plasticity would be increasing only with detailed descriptions of the published models and sharing the codes online.

We listed the models we tried to reimplement, resimulate, and compare based on the information in the original publications in **Tables 2, 5.** In **Table 5**, we can see that four out of seven models were available in the model repositories but this is because four of the models were chosen to this study because of the availability of the code. Thus, the ratio of models available online is generally not this high. In addition, most of the publications gave all the details of the models as text, tabular format, supplementary material, or at least in the model code. We were able to reproduce Figure 1C of the publication by Delord et al. (2007). From the publication by d'Alcantara et al. (2003), we decided to reproduce

TABLE 5 | Evaluation of the neuronal signal transduction models.

Model	Online	Language	Equations	Parameters	Init. cond.	Repro., Repli.	Compa.
d'Alcantara et al., 2003	No	MATLAB®	All appendix	Most text	Most appendix, text	++	Tested
Hayer and Bhalla, 2005	DOQCS	GENESIS/Kinetikit, MATLAB®, SBML	All code, suppl, tab	All code, suppl, tab	All code, suppl, tab	Not tried	Tested
Lindskog et al., 2006	ModelDB	XPPAUT	All code, tab, text	All code, tab	All code	Not tried	Tested
Delord et al., 2007	No	Not given	All text	All text	All text	+++	Tested
Nakano et al., 2010	ModelDB	GENESIS/Kinetikit	All code, suppl, tab, text	All code, suppl, tab	All code, suppl, tab	Not tried	Tested
Kim et al., 2010	ModelDB	XPPAUT	All code, tab, text	All code, tab, text	All code	Not tried	Tested
Zachariou et al., 2013	No	XPPAUT	Most text	Most tab, text	Some text	–	Not tried

Online: *availability of the model implementation in a model repository by the original authors.* ***Language/Simulation tool:*** *programming language or simulation tool used by the original authors to implement the model.* ***Equations:*** *availability and format of equations—embedded in the text, appendix, or supplementary material, presented in a table, or described in the publicly available model implementation (code).* ***Parameters:*** *availability and format of model parameters (same categories as for Equations).* ***Init. cond.:*** *availability and format of initial conditions (same categories as for Equations).* ***Repro., Repli.:*** *reproducibility or replicability of the original results with the information given in the original publication.* ***Compa.:*** *comparability of the models to each other. We described model implementation in the original publication using the following categories: none, some (at least about one third of the details necessary for model reimplementation is given), most (at least about two thirds are given), or all. Models for which we were not able to reproduce any results are marked by – sign. Models for which we reproduced at least some of the results are marked by one to three + signs depending how well we reproduced the results. We implemented the chosen models with MATLAB®. See more details in section 3 and in our previous publications (Manninen and Linne, 2008; Manninen et al., 2011).*

only Figures 3D–F. After fixing one mistake in the equations by d'Alcantara et al. (2003), we were able to reproduce most of the simulation results. We were able to reproduce all the other curves, except our maximum value for α-amino-3-hydroxy-5-methylisoxazole-4-propionic acid receptor (AMPAR) activity was about 220 % whereas the original maximum value in Figure 3D was about 280 %. The reason behind the different value might be that not all parameter and initial values were given in the original publication. We were not able to completely implement the model by Zachariou et al. (2013) because not all the information of the model was given in the original publication. More information about the reproducibility issues of the models can be found in our previous publications (Manninen and Linne, 2008; Manninen et al., 2011).

We were the first ones to provide a computational comparison of postsynaptic signal transduction models for synaptic plasticity (Manninen et al., 2011). We evaluated altogether five models, of which two were developed for hippocampal CA1 neurons (d'Alcantara et al., 2003; Kim et al., 2010), two were developed for striatal medium spiny neurons (Lindskog et al., 2006; Nakano et al., 2010), and one was a generic model (Hayer and Bhalla, 2005) (see **Tables 2, 5**). The model by d'Alcantara et al. (2003), we implemented ourselves in MATLAB®, but the others we took from model databases. The models by Kim et al. (2010) and Lindskog et al. (2006) we took from ModelDB (Migliore et al., 2003; Hines et al., 2004) in XPPAUT format. The codes were properly commented and clearly written, which made it easy to find the values we wanted to modify. The model by Nakano et al. (2010) we took from ModelDB in GENESIS/Kinetikit format. The model codes were neither intuitive nor commented. However, the database and simulation tool provided helpful explanation files to ease the use of the model files (see more details in Manninen et al., 2011). The model by Hayer and Bhalla (2005) we took from the Database of Quantitative Cellular Signaling (DOQCS, Sivakumaran et al., 2003) in MATLAB® format. However, the MATLAB® implementation of the model was hard to modify due to issues with parameter handling. Precisely, it was challenging to identify model parameters as the authors opted to hard code numerical values to the MATLAB® script instead of using parameter names (see more details in Manninen et al., 2011). We compared the simulation results of the models by using the same input for the models. We ran a set of six simulations with different total concentrations of calcium/calmodulin-dependent protein kinase II and protein phosphatase 1 to see how the behavior of the models changed. Our study showed that when using the same input for all the models, models describing the plasticity phenomenon in the very same neuron type produced partly different responses. On the other hand, the models by d'Alcantara et al. (2003) and Nakano et al. (2010) produced partly similar responses even though they had been built for neurons in different brain areas, and Nakano et al. (2010) did not report using the details of the model by d'Alcantara et al. (2003) when building their model. The models by Lindskog et al. (2006) and Kim et al. (2010) produced also partly similar responses even though they had been built for neurons in different brain areas, but Kim et al. (2010) stated that they used the details of the model by Lindskog et al. (2006) when building their model. Based on these results, we concluded that there is a demand for a general setup to objectively compare the models (see more details in Manninen et al., 2011). In our other study (Manninen and Linne, 2008), we compared the models by d'Alcantara et al. (2003) and Delord et al. (2007) with the same input and the total concentration of AMPARs. We verified that the model by d'Alcantara et al. (2003) was only able to explain the induction of plastic modifications, whereas the model by Delord et al. (2007) was able to explain both induction and maintenance (see also d'Alcantara et al., 2003; Delord et al., 2007).

3.2.2. Astrocyte Models

After categorization of astrocyte and neuron-astrocyte models in our previous studies (Manninen et al., 2018a,b), we realized that these models have the same shortcomings as listed in the previous section for neuronal signal transduction models, such as several publications lacked important model details, model codes were rarely available online, graphical illustrations of these models were misleadingly plotting also model components that were not part of the actual model, mathematical equations were sometimes incorrect, and selected model components were not often justified.

In our previous studies (Manninen et al., 2017, 2018b), we tried to reimplement altogether seven astrocyte models. In the present study, we tried to reimplement two more models. None of the models were available in model repositories by the original authors. However, the model by Lavrentovich and Hemkin (2008) is in ModelDB submitted by someone else (Accession number: 112547). We have provided our implementation for four out of nine models in ModelDB [the models by Lavrentovich and Hemkin (2008), De Pittà et al. (2009), and Riera et al. (2011a,b), and modified version of the model by Dupont et al. (2011), Accession number: 223648]. Most of the publications provided all the details of the models, except the initial conditions, either in text, tabular format, appendix, supplementary material, or in corrigendum. We were able to reproduce all of the chosen original results by Di Garbo et al. (2007) and Lavrentovich and Hemkin (2008) (see **Table 6**). We reproduced Figures 2, 5, and 8 by Di Garbo et al. (2007) and Figures 3, 4, 5, 7, and 9 by Lavrentovich and Hemkin (2008). We were not able to reproduce any of the important features of the original results by Riera et al. (2011a,b) with the original equations, but after we fixed the found error in one of the equations we were able to reproduce some of the original results in Figure 4B by Riera et al. (2011a) when X_{IP3} was 0.43 μM/s between 100 and 900 s and 0 otherwise and all of the original results when X_{IP3} was 0.43 μM/s between 100 and 900 s and 0.2 μM/s otherwise. We were able to reproduce most of the original results in Figure 12 by De Pittà et al. (2009). We were able to reproduce well the amplitude modulation but not the frequency modulation part of the figure. Thus the problem might be that the original authors did not provide all the model details correctly for the frequency modulation. We were not able to reproduce any of the important features of the original results in Figures 2 and 3 by Dupont et al. (2011) with the original equations. After we tested our implementation, we realized that there had to be a mistake in the original calcium equation. We tested several different calcium equations based on the equations published by the same authors and were able to reproduce most of the original results with one of the tested equations. At first, we were not able to reproduce Figure 2 by Nadkarni and Jung (2003). After we fixed mistakes in one of the original equations and parameter values, we were able to reproduce most of the original results in Figure 2 by Nadkarni and Jung (2003). Due to several deficiencies in the original model descriptions, we were not able to reproduce the simulation results of the models by Wade et al. (2011, 2012) (see **Table 6**). In addition, we were not able to completely implement the model by Silchenko and Tass (2008) because not all the information of the model was given in the original publication. More details about the reproducibility issues of the astrocyte models can be found in our previous publications (Manninen et al., 2017, 2018b).

In addition to testing reproducibility, we also addressed the comparability of the astrocyte models in our previous study (Manninen et al., 2017). We compared the model by Riera et al. (2011a,b) to the model by Lavrentovich and Hemkin (2008), and the model by De Pittà et al. (2009) to our modified version of the model by Dupont et al. (2011). We chose these models because they described similar biological processes. The models by Riera et al. (2011a,b) and Lavrentovich and Hemkin (2008) were spontaneously oscillating models, whereas the other two models used glutamate as stimulus. The overall dynamical behaviors of the models were relatively different. The model by Lavrentovich and Hemkin (2008) oscillated less frequently than the model by Riera et al. (2011a,b). We found out that both models were sensitive to parameter values. Especially, when using the parameter values from the model by Riera et al. (2011a,b) in the model by Lavrentovich and Hemkin (2008), the model by Lavrentovich and Hemkin (2008) behaved differently compared to the behavior with its own parameter values. With a constant glutamate stimulus, the models by De Pittà et al. (2009) and our modified version of the model by Dupont et al. (2011) showed partly similar kind of behavior but there were a few exceptions. First, a higher constant glutamate stimulus value produced higher calcium concentrations with the model by De Pittà et al. (2009) and lower calcium concentrations with our modified version of the model by Dupont et al. (2011). Second, the higher the constant glutamate stimulus value, the faster the model by De Pittà et al. (2009) ceased to oscillate. With pulse wave stimuli, the model by De Pittà et al. (2009) and our modified version of the model by Dupont et al. (2011) produced differing results. In our modified version of the model by Dupont et al. (2011), the calcium concentration oscillated even with the minimum concentration value of the glutamate stimulus pulse. This did not happen with the model by De Pittà et al. (2009). More details about the comparability issues of the astrocyte models can be found in our previous publication (Manninen et al., 2017).

3.2.3. Spiking Neuronal Network Models

We evaluated 10 models listed in **Table 4**. The majority of the examined publications presented a complete set of equations describing the neuron and synapse models, either in the methods section, appendices, or supplementary material. We found an incomplete set of equations in two of the publications. All model parameters were presented, however not in an easily tractable format. Only one publication presented all the parameters in a tabular format, 6/10 (7/10 if the supplementary material was included) publications partially summarized parameters in a tabular format. None of the publications used the recommendable model description format introduced by Nordlie et al. (2009). Non-systematic model description increases the chance of errors both in the publication and when reimplementing the model. We found several minor errors: wrong naming of parameters, same name used for different parameters in the same article, missing to define some relevant parameters before using them, ambiguities in defining probability distributions used to randomize some of the parameters (e.g., using the wrong name for probability distribution, ambiguity about implementation of probability distribution in the utilized simulation tool), and ambiguities in

TABLE 6 | Evaluation of the astrocyte and neuron-astrocyte models.

Model	Online	Language	Equations	Parameters	Init. cond.	Repro.	Compa.
Nadkarni and Jung, 2003	No	Not given	All text	All text	No	−/++	Not tried
Di Garbo et al., 2007	No	Not given	All text	All tab	No	+++	Not tried
Silchenko and Tass, 2008	No	Not given	Most appendix, text	Most appendix, tab, text	No	−	Not tried
Lavrentovich and Hemkin, 2008	No (ModelDB by us and others)	Fortran (Python by us, XPP by others)	All text	All corrigendum, text	All text	+++	Tested
De Pittà et al., 2009	No (ModelDB by us)	Not given (Python by us)	All appendix, text	All tab	No	++	Tested
Riera et al., 2011a,b	No (ModelDB by us)	MATLAB® (Python by us)	All suppl, tab, text	All suppl, tab, text	No	−/+/+++	Tested
Dupont et al., 2011	No (ModelDB by us)	MATLAB® (Mod. model with Python by us)	All text	All tab, text	No	−/++	Tested
Wade et al., 2011	No	MATLAB®	All text	Most tab, text	Some text	−	Not tried
Wade et al., 2012	No	MATLAB®	All text	All appendix, tab, text	Most appendix, tab, text	−	Not tried

Online: *availability of the model implementation in a model repository by the original authors, by us, or by someone else.* ***Language/Simulation tool:*** *programming language or simulation tool used by the original authors, by us, or by someone else to implement the model.* ***Equations:*** *availability and format of equations—embedded in the text, appendix, supplementary material, or corrigendum, or presented in a table.* ***Parameters:*** *availability and format of model parameters (same categories as for Equations).* ***Init. cond.:*** *availability and format of initial conditions (same categories as for Equations).* ***Repro.:*** *reproducibility of the original results with the information given in the original publication.* ***Compa.:*** *comparability of the models to each other. We described model implementation in the original publication using the following categories: none, some (at least about one third of the details necessary for model reimplementation is given), most (at least about two thirds are given), or all. Models for which we were not able to reproduce any results are marked by − sign. Models for which we reproduced at least some of the results are marked by one to three + signs depending how well we reproduced the results. We implemented all the models with Python and/or MATLAB®, and made some of the models available in ModelDB (Accession number: 223648). We marked the language we used only if we made the model available in ModelDB. See more details in section 3 and in our previous publications (Manninen et al., 2017, 2018b).*

describing the connectivity scheme. In addition, most of the publications did not give the initial conditions.

Description of network connectivity scheme is equally important part in presentation of network models. The unstructured connectivity is used in 6/10 studies, thus each pair of neurons was connected with equal probability. The other studies included additional connectivity schemes, often distance-dependent connectivity, where the probability of connection decreased with the distance between the pair of neurons, or the small-world connectivity that allows the majority of local and a few long-distance connections. A careful description of the connectivity generating algorithm is advisable for all but the simplest (unstructured) connectivity in order to avoid implementation errors. For example, in one of the publications the authors described network connectivity as "scale-free random" but then assigned a number of outputs to each neuron using a uniform random instead of a power-law distribution. The two studies by Mäki-Marttunen et al. (2013) and Lonardoni et al. (2017) paid additional attention to the generation of connectivity matrix. Both included supplementary material to describe implementations and implications of different connectivity schemes.

The comparison between simulated and experimental data requires extensive data analysis. The lack of standardization of methodology and the ambiguity in presentation of the applied algorithms pose additional obstacles to reproducibility and replicability. All of the models under consideration generated the same type of data, the spontaneous activity exhibiting network-wide bursts, thus the intervals of intensive spiking activity reflecting global synchronization. The analysis of this data often consists of two steps: bursts detection, segmenting the population spike-data into intervals containing bursts, and computing the statistics of different quantitative measures based on the burst detection or on original non-segmented data. Burst detection itself might not be very reliable. A recent review article conducted evaluation of a broad range of burst detection methods and tested them against a carefully crafted benchmark data (Cotterill et al., 2016). The authors concluded that none of the algorithms performed ideally, and suggested a combination of several methods for improving the precision. The issue was not so dramatic in studies that we examined. All of them focused on relatively large bursting events that were easier to identify, compared to the study by Cotterill et al. (2016). Typically, burst detection algorithms depend on free parameters that are manually tuned to the data. However, the fact that methods used in various studies differ and that authors rarely provide the implementation of the algorithms creates an additional obstacle in reproducing the published results. Even bigger variability is presented in selection of methodology to quantify bursting dynamics. The last column in **Table 4** illustrates this variability and lists the data measures used in different publications. In the table, burst detection methods are classified into three categories: methods based on spike-data of individual electrodes/neurons, based on population spike-data, and based on global/population firing rate. The measures used to quantify data include analysis of the spike-data statistics, analysis of burst profiles or frequency

TABLE 7 | Evaluation of the spiking network models.

Model	Online	Language	Equations	Parameters	Init. cond.	Repli.
Latham et al., 2000	No	Not given	All text	All tab, text	No	Not tried
Giugliano et al., 2004	No	Not given	All text	All tab, text	No	Not tried
French and Gruenstein, 2006	No	MATLAB®	All text	All text	No	Not tried
Gritsun et al., 2010	No	C++, MATLAB®	Most appendix, text	All tab, text	No	Not tried
Gritsun et al., 2011	No	C++, MATLAB®	Some text	Some tab, text	No	Not tried
Baltz et al., 2011	No	Brian v2, Python	All text	All text	No	Not tried
Maheswaranathan et al., 2012	No	C++, MATLAB®	Most text	Most tab, text	No	Not tried
Mäki-Marttunen et al. (2013)	ModelDB	MATLAB®, NEST	All code, text	All code, tab, text	All code	+++
Masquelier and Deco, 2013	ModelDB	Brian v1, Python	All code, text	All code, tab, text	All code	++
Yamamoto et al., 2016	No	Not given	All text	All text	No	Not tried
Lonardoni et al., 2017	DRYAD	NEURON, Python	All code, suppl, text	All code, suppl, tab, text	All code	++

***Online:** availability of the model implementation in a model repository by the original authors. **Language/Simulation tool:** programming language or simulation tool used by the original authors to implement the model. **Equations:** availability and format of equations—embedded in the text, appendix, or supplementary material, presented in a table, or described in the publicly available model implementation (code). **Parameters:** availability and format of model parameters (same categories as for Equations). **Init. cond.:** availability and format of initial conditions (same categories as for Equations). **Repli.:** replicability of the original results with the information given in the original publication. We described model implementation in the original publication using the following categories: none, some (at least about one third of the details necessary for model reimplementation is given), most (at least about two thirds are given), or all. Models for which we replicated at least some of the results are marked by one to three + signs depending how well we replicated the results.*

of their occurrences, frequency analysis, principal component analysis applied to global firing rates, spatial burst propagation, extraction of connectivity from the spike-data of individual neurons, as well as graph theoretic analysis of the extracted connectivity. This lack of standardization in data representation somewhat hinders the comparison between different studies. Reproducibility of the model requires reimplementation of the model equations, burst detection method, and measures used to quantify the data.

The simulation tools range from the custom-made software in MATLAB® or C++ to the public simulation tools of spiking neuronal networks (e.g., Brian, NEST, and NEURON). Three out of 10 listed studies provide the full model implementation, namely Masquelier and Deco (2013), Mäki-Marttunen et al. (2013), and Lonardoni et al. (2017). From these studies, we attempted to replicate the results that demonstrate time evolution of model variables and the global dynamical regime of the model, for example adaptation variables, cell membrane potential, and spike raster plots. The replicability of the three studies is summarized in **Table 7**. The model by Masquelier and Deco (2013) is available in Brian version 1.4.0 and Python version 2.6, and we ran it in Brian version 1.4.1 and Python version 2.7. The code contains model implementation, the list of parameters, and the plotting function sufficient to replicate Figures 4, 5 from the article. The replication of Figure 4, the illustration of neuron and network dynamics, was straightforward. In Figure 5, the neuronal adaptation mechanism was examined and the basic model was tested for two different values of the adaptation time constant τ_a. We replicated the result obtained for $\tau_a = 1.6$ s but failed to replicate the results for $\tau_a = 1.2$ s. This might be caused by different versions of Python and Brian used in the original study and in our replicability test. The model by Lonardoni et al. (2017) is available in NEURON/Python format (versions of the software not indicated). It required installation of an additional nonstandard Python package. The model is well documented and supported by many implementation details. The code downloaded from DRYAD repository included model implementation, the code for generating connectivity matrices, as well as three test examples and three examples of connectivity matrices. The first attempt to run the model using Neuron 7.1. produced errors. After contacting the authors, we obtained the correct version for the simulation tool (Neuron 7.3) and Python packages, as well as valuable instructions how to use the code. Under Neuron 7.3, all three test examples worked. We were able to use two out of three connectivity matrices, but not the biggest one (N = 4,096 neurons) used in the article. Attempt to run the biggest matrix failed most likely due to memory issues. However, we managed to replicate the rasterplots in Figure 2A by Lonardoni et al. (2017) using a smaller matrix (N = 1,024 neurons) and after modifying one parameter. In a smaller network, the burst propagation in Figure 2B by Lonardoni et al. (2017) was somewhat less evident. Thus, we were able to replicate most of the original results by Lonardoni et al. (2017). The study by Mäki-Marttunen et al. (2013) contains two models, a network of HH neurons and a network of leaky-IF (LIF) neurons. We replicated Figure 3 from the article. The first, HH model, is available in MATLAB® format (version R2010a/R2011b) using own code and it was possible to replicate it. The second, LIF model, is available in PyNEST format (Python version 2.4.3 and NEST version 2.0.0). The software versions are indicated in the code. We managed to replicate the result using Python version 2.7 and NEST version 2.2.1. Running the same code in a newer version of the simulation tool, NEST version 2.8.0, failed to produce any bursting dynamics. All of the studies provided well-documented models and full set of parameters. However, the replicability of the results was hindered by common problems related to versions of the utilized software. These

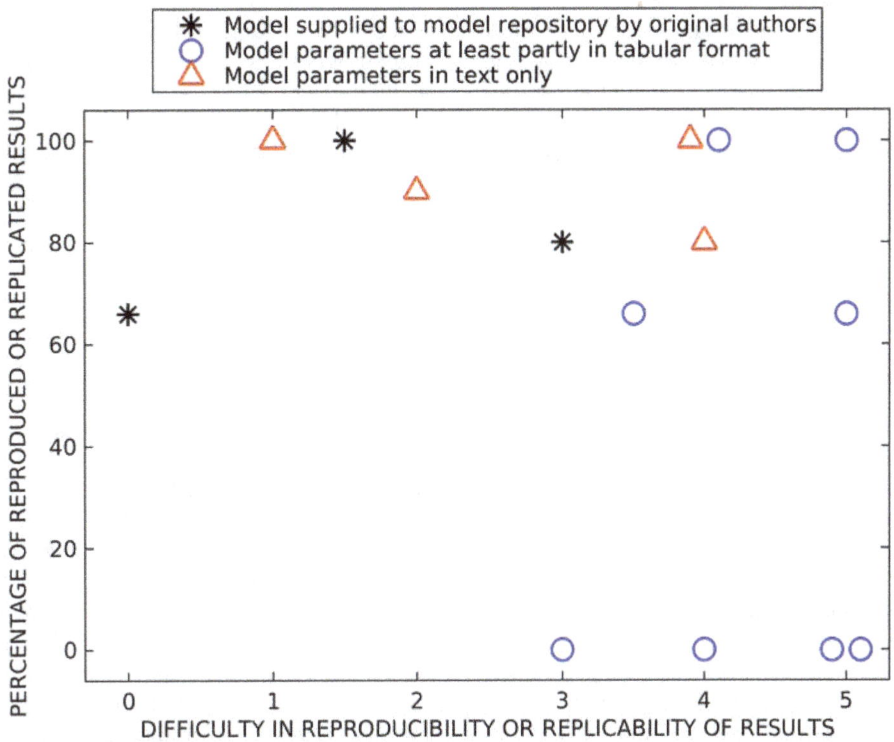

FIGURE 2 | Summary of reproducibility and replicability studies. Both x- and y-values are based on subjective estimation. On the x-axis, we present the difficulty to reimplement, simulate, and reproduce or rerun and replicate previous results (numbers mean the following: 0—immediately, 1—after a few hours of working on the model, 2—after 1 day, 3—after a few days, 4–after 1 week, and 5—after 2 weeks or more). On the y-axis, we present the percentage of reproduced or replicated results. The models are separated into three categories based on were they supplied in model repositories by original authors, were at least part of the parameter values given in a tabular format, and were parameter values given only in text format.

examples illustrate the need to provide detailed information about simulation environment, in addition to model description and implementation.

3.2.4. Summary of Reproducibility and Replicability Studies

Figure 2 shows our subjective evaluation of the difficulty in timewise to reproduce and replicate the original simulation results and the percentage of reproduced and replicated original results. The list of issues affecting the evaluation of models included: (1) complexity of the reproduced/replicated model, (2) model description in the original publication (in a tabular format, as text, or as a supplementary material, and the amount of details given), (3) possible errors in the model description, (4) report of versions of the simulation tools and packages, (5) person who reimplemented the model, thus the experience of the researcher, and (6) user support from the authors of the model.

We separated all tested reproducibility and replicability models (see **Tables 5–7**) into three classes according to presentation in related publications: models described fully in the text (all parameters embedded in the text), models with parameters at least partially (and in some cases entirely) given in a tabular format, and the studies which supplied model implementation to the public repositories. We carried out reproducibility studies for the first two categories and replicability studies for the last category. As expected, the replicability studies were less difficult than most of the reproducibility studies, the replication times ranged from working immediately to 2 days. The percentage of replicated results was high in all studies (more than 60 %), and the main obstacle was incompatibility of simulation tool versions. Reproduction time for models described entirely in text ranged from a few hours to a week. Surprisingly, we were able to reproduce on average better the results from these models than the rest of the models, including the three models that we tried to replicate by rerunning the available model implementations (see **Figure 2**). The reason might be a difference in complexity of models, as these models tended to be simpler than others. The majority of the reproduced models presented most or all the parameter values in a tabular format. The time needed for reproducing these models ranged from a few days to more than 2 weeks. Even though parameter values were given, at least partly, in a tabular format for eight models, we were able to reproduce the original results completely only with two of these models and none of the original results with four of these models. Thus, this category of models had a huge variation in percentage of reproduced results, indicating that some other issues, in addition to model presentation in the article, determined the success of reproduction. The difficulty to reproduce the results increased even when only one parameter value was missing or one mistake in equations. Our results showed that the four models for which we were able to reproduce all the original results gave all the equations and parameter values in the original publication, including corrigenda and supplementary material. However, one of the completely reproduced models had a mistake in one of the equations that we had to fix, for all the other completely reproduced models all the details were given correctly in the publications. Moreover, if all the details of the models were given in the original publication, it did not mean that we were able to reproduce all the results. The reason was that often the models had mistakes in parameter values or equations. We should emphasize that small number of model examples in some categories affected the conclusions (only three replication tests and four tests with models fully described in text are shown).

Figure 2 shows some level of correlation between difficulty and accuracy of reproduction/replication studies: all studies that were done relative fast (up to a few days) achieved relatively high reproduction/replication of the original results. The studies that required more time ranged from no reproduction to perfect reproduction. This also reflects the way how these studies were carried out, some models immediately gave good results while others required long time and numerous tests without guarantee of success. The distribution of values reflecting the success was somewhat bimodal, the reproduction results either failed or succeeded with over 60 % reproduced results. The percentage of replicated results were over 60 % for all models. Finally, the large distribution of precisions for some classes of models indicated that additional issues affect the success of reproduction, particularly the complexity and the accuracy of the model description. This should be emphasized in the light of increasing interest for very complex and biophysically accurate multiscale models. While simpler models provide solid reproducibility in relatively short time, complex models require detailed description of the model, preferably with model implementation made publicly available.

4. DISCUSSION

We have continually evaluated computational neuroscience and systems biology software and computational models since 2004 while developing new methods and models for computational neuroscience. In this study, we partly summarized results from our previous studies and partly presented new results. We examined selected simulation tools that are intended for simulation of biochemical reactions and subcellular networks in neuronal and glial cells (see also Pettinen et al., 2005; Manninen et al., 2006c; Mäkiraatikka et al., 2007) and for studying the growth and development of neocortical cultures (see also Mäki-Marttunen et al., 2010; Aćimović et al., 2011) and the dynamics of spiking neuronal networks. We have previously provided an extensive overview of more than hundred computational models for postsynaptic signal transduction pathways in synaptic plasticity (Manninen et al., 2010) and more than hundred computational models for astrocytes and neuron-astrocyte interactions (Manninen et al., 2018a,b), where our purpose was to categorize the models in order to make their similarities and differences more readily apparent. In this study, we provided reproducibility and comparability results for some of these models (see also Manninen et al., 2011, 2017, 2018b) with an aim to present the state-of-the-art in the field and to provide solutions for better reproducibility. Additionally, we provided replicability results for spiking neuronal network models.

Our results show that the different simulation tools we tested were able to provide same simulation results when the same models were implemented in them. On the other hand, it was somewhat difficult to reproduce the original simulated results after reimplementing and simulating the models based on the information in the original publications. We were able to reproduce all the original simulation results of four models out of 12 models we tested. The more complete and correct description the model had in the original publication, the more likely we were able to reimplement the model and reproduce the original results. When the parameter values were in a tabular format, it was much easier to reimplement the model because there was no need to go through the whole article looking for the possible values. Mistyped or missing equations and parameter values in the original publications made the reproducibility of the simulation results most difficult. In our replicability studies, we were able to replicate one study and most of the results from the other two studies. The issues encountered while rerunning the models can be attributed to mismatch in versions of the software used for replication and for original model development. Our experiences emphasize the need to supply not only the model description and implementation but also the details of simulation environment, the versions of the software, and the list of necessary packages. The need for better tracking and documentation of the simulation environment and possible solutions are discussed by Crook et al. (2013).

When developing new simulation tools, a multitude of questions should be asked. Naturally, every simulation tool is limited with the adopted modeling framework but should aim at providing the maximal flexibility within that framework. In that context, the following challenges and questions are relevant:

- How big programming load is needed to implement new biological mechanisms?
- How easy is it to incorporate the model components into the existing models from the literature and public databases?
- Does the simulation tool allow flexible level of details when describing different model components?
- Do the version of the simulation tool and packages needed to run the simulations pose a problem for replicability?

Most of the existing simulation tools of spiking neuronal networks impose strict constraint on selection of model components. Those components are implemented as part of the model source code, and the new ones can be added only through extension of the source code which prevents fast modification of model components. Simulation tools that provide basic mechanisms for model implementation and allow flexible description of details, for example directly implementing the model as either ODEs or SDEs (Brian, XPPAUT), by providing interface for adding new components (NEURON), or by providing unit checks (Brian), offer easier manipulation and modification of the model. For the same reason, the simulation tools of this type allow easier extension and reuse of the published models. Several existing tools support development of multiscale models [MOOSE (Ray et al., 2008), GENESIS, NEURON] or implementation of models using more than one standard simulation tool (MUSIC, Djurfeldt et al., 2010). These tools support models where different mechanisms are represented at different level of details. The different versions of the simulation tools and the packages needed can make replicability problematic. It is very important for the tool developers to take this into account.

Our findings on a specific set of published models for different biological systems stress the importance of a variety of aspects of model development. The following challenges and questions are relevant:

- Has the model been checked carefully in the review process and can it produce the results in the publication?
- Is the quality of the code sufficient?
- Is the model properly validated against experimental wet-lab data and correctly representing the biological findings?
- What new biological, modeling, and computational aspects the model provides on top of the previously published models?
- Are all the details of the model equations and biological components given in the publication in a clear way, preferably in a tabular format?
- Which programming language or simulation tool was used to implement the model, which data analysis methods were used, and are the implementation of the model and data analysis methods available online?

It is important to emphasize that a good-quality model implementation supplied with the original publication improves not only replicability of the study but also understanding of the model itself. This is already important during the review process. Reviewers should have the possibility to rerun the model code, check the simulated results, and compare the simulated and experimental data during the review process (see also Eglen et al., 2017; Rougier et al., 2017). Equally important is to clearly explain what new components the model has in comparison to previously published models and what old and new results the model can show. Verbal description is a suboptimal way to present complex mathematical formalisms and algorithms. It often turns out to be incomplete and a number of ambiguities emerge when attempting to reimplement a model, usually not evident at first. More systematic and compact description of all model details, such as equations, parameter values, initial conditions, and stimuli, using, for example, a tabular format proposed by Nordlie et al. (2009) and Manninen et al. (2017) and a supplementary material presenting a metadata and meta-code are needed for successful reproduction of the published scientific results. Tools to manage, share, and, most importantly, analyze and understand large amounts of both experimental and simulated data are still needed (Bouchard et al., 2016). However, suggestions how to design workflows for electrophysiological data analysis (Denker and Grün, 2016) and how to structure, collect, and distribute metadata of neurophysiological data (Zehl et al., 2016) has already been proposed. Our example of replicability of spiking network models points at a bottleneck in reproducibility and replicability created by the lack of commonly adopted methodology and publicly available code for analysis of simulated data. Following the good practices in development of data-analysis methods, careful description of the methods in the article, and supplying the code with method implementation in addition to the model implementation are necessary steps to ensure model reproducibility and replicability.

Best practices for description of neuronal network models (Nordlie et al., 2009) and minimum information requirements for reproduction (Le Novère et al., 2005; Waltemath et al., 2011a) have been suggested. Moreover, many XML-based model and simulation representation formats, such as SBML (Hucka et al., 2003), CellML (Lloyd et al., 2004), NeuroML (Gleeson et al., 2010), SED-ML (Waltemath et al., 2011b), and LEMS (Cannon et al., 2014), have been developed. On the other hand, Jupyter Notebook (earlier known as IPython Notebook) could be a potential solution to enhance reproducibility and accessibility. In addition to giving all the details needed for model implementation, it is equally important to categorize the biological details of the models, such as neuron models, ion channels, pumps, receptors, signaling pathways, synapse models, in tabular format in publications (see e.g., Manninen et al., 2010, 2018a,b). If not possible to publish via journal due to page limitations, providing the implementation of the model and data-analysis method in a public and widely adopted simulation tool or programming language (e.g., Python) in some of the available model repositories, for example in ModelDB and BioModels database (Le Novère et al., 2006), is a must. Regardless of all the available formats and tools, many authors do not publish their models in a format that is easily exchangeable between different simulation platforms or provide their models at all in model repositories. All these issues should be carefully considered in the training of both experimental and computational neuroscientists (see also Akil et al., 2016).

Throughout this study, we evaluated, reimplemented and reproduced, and replicated a range of models incorporating different levels of biological details and modeling scales. The models and biological mechanisms included some relatively conventional examples but also some that only recently attracted larger attention within the computational community. As the experimental methodology and protocols advance and various neurobiological mechanisms become better understood, the new challenges for computational modeling emerge. Few examples are molecular diffusion in synaptic clefts, dendritic spines, and in other neural compartments (Chay et al., 2016; Hepburn et al., 2017), models of neurodevelopmental phenomena (Tetzlaff et al., 2010; van Ooyen, 2011), or wider range of plasticity mechanisms explored using conventional spiking networks (Miner and Triesch, 2016). Finally, one can aim beyond network modeling formalism and include extracellular space, for example similarly to the approach adopted in the Cortex3D simulation tool (Zubler and Douglas, 2009).

All the above suggestions would greatly improve the replicability and reproducibility of the published results, reduce the time needed to compare the model details and results, and support model reuse in complementary studies or in the studies extending the range of biophysical mechanisms and experimental data.

AUTHOR CONTRIBUTIONS

TM: Designed the study, acquired and reimplemented the neuronal signal transduction and astrocyte models, simulated the models, evaluated and tabulated the results, and coordinated the production of the final version; JA: Designed the study, evaluated the simulation tools for growth and spiking neuronal networks, acquired and reran the spiking neuronal network models, and evaluated and tabulated the results; RH: Contributed to the design of the study, reimplemented, simulated, and evaluated an astrocyte model, contributed to the testing of the simulation tools for growth, and interpreted biological terminology and knowledge; HT: Contributed to the design of the study, contributed to the interpretation of network growth and activity studies, and interpreted biological terminology; M-LL: Conceived, funded, and designed the study, took part in the selection and evaluation of all models and tools, and interpreted the results in terms of replicability and reproducibility. All contributed to the drafting of the manuscript and approved the final version of the manuscript. All other work reported in the present publication, as motivation for the topic, is cited and is based on the work done previously in Computational Neuroscience Research Group in Tampere, Finland.

FUNDING

This project received funding from the European Union's Seventh Framework Programme (FP7) under grant agreement No. 604102 (HBP RUP), the European Union's Horizon 2020 research and innovation programme under grant agreement No. 720270 (HBP SGA1), and the Academy of Finland (decision No. 297893).

ACKNOWLEDGMENTS

The authors wish to thank Tampere University of Technology Graduate School, Emil Aaltonen Foundation, The Finnish Concordia Fund, and Ulla Tuominen Foundation for support for RH and Tampere University of Technology Graduate School, Finnish Foundation for Technology Promotion, Finnish Cultural Foundation, Pirkanmaa Regional Fund of Finnish Cultural Foundation, and Finnish Brain Foundation sr. for HT.

REFERENCES

Aćimović, J., Mäki-Marttunen, T., Havela, R., Teppola, H., and Linne, M.-L. (2011). Modeling of neuronal growth *in vitro*: comparison of simulation tools NETMORPH and CX3D. *EURASIP J. Bioinf. Syst. Biol.* 2011:616382. doi: 10.1155/2011/616382

Aho, T. (2003). *Simulation Tool for Genetic Regulatory Networks.* Master's thesis, Department of Information Technology, Tampere University of Technology, Tampere.

Ajay, S. M., and Bhalla, U. S. (2006). Synaptic plasticity *in vitro* and *in silico*: insights into an intracellular signaling maze. *Physiology* 21, 289–296. doi: 10.1152/physiol.00009.2006

Akil, H., Balice-Gordon, R., Cardozo, D. L., Koroshetz, W., Norris, S. M. P., Sherer, T., et al. (2016). Neuroscience training for the 21st century. *Neuron* 90, 917–926. doi: 10.1016/j.neuron.2016.05.030

Alves, R., Antunes, F., and Salvador, A. (2006). Tools for kinetic modeling of biochemical networks. *Nat. Biotechnol.* 24, 667–672. doi: 10.1038/nbt0606-667

Amunts, K., Ebell, C., Muller, J., Telefont, M., Knoll, A., and Lippert, T. (2016). The Human Brain Project: creating a European research infrastructure to decode the human brain. *Neuron* 92, 574–581. doi: 10.1016/j.neuron.2016.10.046

Andrews, S. S., Addy, N. J., Brent, R., and Arkin, A. P. (2010). Detailed simulations of cell biology with Smoldyn 2.1. *PLoS Comput. Biol.* 6:e1000705. doi: 10.1371/journal.pcbi.1000705

Baker, M. (2016). 1,500 scientists lift the lid on reproducibility. *Nature* 533, 452–454. doi: 10.1038/533452a

Baltz, T., Herzog, A., and Voigt, T. (2011). Slow oscillating population activity in developing cortical networks: models and experimental results. *J. Neurophysiol.* 106, 1500–1514. doi: 10.1152/jn.00889.2010

Bartocci, E., and Lió, P. (2016). Computational modeling, formal analysis, and tools for systems biology. *PLoS Comput. Biol.* 12:e1004591. doi: 10.1371/journal.pcbi.1004591

Benureau, F., and Rougier, N. (2018). Re-run, repeat, reproduce, reuse, replicate: transforming code into scientific contributions. *Front. Neuroinform.* 11:69. doi: 10.3389/fninf.2017.00069

Bergmann, F. T., and Sauro, H. M. (2008). Comparing simulation results of SBML capable simulators. *Bioinformatics* 24, 1963–1965. doi: 10.1093/bioinformatics/btn319

Bhalla, U. S. (2001). "Modeling networks of signaling pathways," in *Computational Neuroscience: Realistic Modeling for Experimentalists*, ed E. De Shutter (New York, NY: CRC Press LLC), 25–48.

Bhalla, U. S. (2002). "Use of Kinetikit and GENESIS for modeling signaling pathways," in *Methods in Enzymology, Vol. 345*, eds J. D. Hildebrandt and R. Iyengar (San Diego, CA: Academic Press), 3–23.

Bhalla, U. S. (2009). "Molecules, networks, and memory," in *Systems Biology: The Challenge of Complexity*, eds S. Nakanishi, R. Kageyama, and D. Watanabe (Tokyo: Springer), 151–158.

Bhalla, U. S., and Iyengar, R. (1999). Emergent properties of networks of biological signaling pathways. *Science* 283, 381–387. doi: 10.1126/science.283.5400.381

Bi, G.-Q., and Rubin, J. (2005). Timing in synaptic plasticity: from detection to integration. *Trends Neurosci.* 28, 222–228. doi: 10.1016/j.tins.2005.02.002

Blackwell, K. T. (2013). Approaches and tools for modeling signaling pathways and calcium dynamics in neurons. *J. Neurosci. Methods* 220, 131–140. doi: 10.1016/j.jneumeth.2013.05.008

Bouchard, K. E., Aimone, J. B., Chun, M., Dean, T., Denker, M., Diesmann, M., et al. (2016). High-performance computing in neuroscience for data-driven discovery, integration, and dissemination. *Neuron* 92, 628–631. doi: 10.1016/j.neuron.2016.10.035

Bower, J. M., and Beeman, D. (1998). *The Book of GENESIS: Exploring Realistic Neural Models with the GEneral NEural SImulation System, 2nd Edn.* New York, NY: Telos; Springer-Verlag.

Brette, R., Rudolph, M., Carnevale, T., Hines, M., Beeman, D., Bower, J. M., et al. (2007). Simulation of networks of spiking neurons: a review of tools and strategies. *J. Comput. Neurosci.* 23, 349–398. doi: 10.1007/s10827-007-0038-6

Brown, T. H., Kairiss, E. W., and Keenan, C. L. (1990). Hebbian synapses: biophysical mechanisms and algorithms. *Annu. Rev. Neurosci.* 13, 475–511. doi: 10.1146/annurev.ne.13.030190.002355

Cannon, R. C., Gleeson, P., Crook, S., Ganapathy, G., Marin, B., Piasini, E., et al. (2014). LEMS: a language for expressing complex biological models in concise and hierarchical form and its use in underpinning NeuroML 2. *Front. Neuroinform.* 8:79. doi: 10.3389/fninf.2014.00079

Carnevale, T., and Hines, M. (2006). *The NEURON Book, 1st Edn*. Cambridge, UK: Cambridge University Press.

Castellani, G. C., and Zironi, I. (2010). "Biophysics-based models of LTP/LTD," in *Hippocampal Microcircuits: A Computational Modelers Resource Book*, eds V. Cutsuridis, B. Graham, S. Cobb, and I. Vida (New York, NY: Springer), 555–570.

Chay, A., Zamparo, I., Koschinski, A., Zaccolo, M., and Blackwell, K. T. (2016). Control of βAR- and N-methyl-D-aspartate (NMDA) receptor-dependent cAMP dynamics in hippocampal neurons. *PLoS Comput. Biol.* 12:e1004735. doi: 10.1371/journal.pcbi.1004735

Cotterill, E., Charlesworth, P., Thomas, C. W., Paulsen, O., and Eglen, S. J. (2016). A comparison of computational methods for detecting bursts in neuronal spike trains and their application to human stem cell-derived neuronal networks. *J. Neurophysiol.* 116, 306–321. doi: 10.1152/jn.00093.2016

Crook, S. M., Davison, A. P., and Plesser, H. E. (2013). "Learning from the past: approaches for reproducibility in computational neuroscience," in *20 Years of Computational Neuroscience*, ed J. M. Bower (New York, NY: Springer), 73–102.

d'Alcantara, P., Schiffmann, S. N., and Swillens, S. (2003). Bidirectional synaptic plasticity as a consequence of interdependent Ca^{2+}-controlled phosphorylation and dephosphorylation pathways. *Eur. J. Neurosci.* 17, 2521–2528. doi: 10.1046/j.1460-9568.2003.02693.x

Davison, A., Brüderle, D., Eppler, J., Kremkow, J., Muller, E., Pecevski, D., et al. (2009). PyNN: a common interface for neuronal network simulators. *Front. Neuroinform.* 2:11. doi: 10.3389/neuro.11.011.2008

De Pittà, M., Brunel, N., and Volterra, A. (2016). Astrocytes: orchestrating synaptic plasticity? *Neuroscience* 323, 43–61. doi: 10.1016/j.neuroscience.2015.04.001

De Pittà, M., Goldberg, M., Volman, V., Berry, H., and Ben-Jacob, E. (2009). Glutamate regulation of calcium and IP_3 oscillating and pulsating dynamics in astrocytes. *J. Biol. Phys.* 35, 383–411. doi: 10.1007/s10867-009-9155-y

De Pittà, M., Volman, V., Berry, H., Parpura, V., Volterra, A., and Ben-Jacob, E. (2012). Computational quest for understanding the role of astrocyte signaling in synaptic transmission and plasticity. *Front. Comput. Neurosci.* 6:98. doi: 10.3389/fncom.2012.00098

Delord, B., Berry, H., Guigon, E., and Genet, S. (2007). A new principle for information storage in an enzymatic pathway model. *PLoS Comput. Biol.* 3:e124. doi: 10.1371/journal.pcbi.0030124

Denker, M., and Grün, S. (2016). "Designing workflows for the reproducible analysis of electrophysiological data," in *Brain-Inspired Computing. BrainComp 2015. Lecture Notes in Computer Science, Vol. 10087*, eds K. Amunts, L. Grandinetti, T. Lippert, and N. Petkov (Cham: Springer), 58–72.

Di Garbo, A., Barbi, M., Chillemi, S., Alloisio, S., and Nobile, M. (2007). Calcium signalling in astrocytes and modulation of neural activity. *Biosystems* 89, 74–83. doi: 10.1016/j.biosystems.2006.05.013

Djurfeldt, M., Hjorth, J., Eppler, J. M., Dudani, N., Helias, M., Potjans, T. C., et al. (2010). Run-time interoperability between neuronal network simulators based on the MUSIC framework. *Neuroinformatics* 8, 43–60. doi: 10.1007/s12021-010-9064-z

Dobrzyński, M., Rodríguez, J. V., Kaandorp, J. A., and Blom, J. G. (2007). Computational methods for diffusion-influenced biochemical reactions. *Bioinformatics* 23, 1969–1977. doi: 10.1093/bioinformatics/btm278

Dupont, G., Lokenye, E. F. L., and Challiss, R. A. J. (2011). A model for Ca^{2+} oscillations stimulated by the type 5 metabotropic glutamate receptor: an unusual mechanism based on repetitive, reversible phosphorylation of the receptor. *Biochimie* 93, 2132–2138. doi: 10.1016/j.biochi.2011.09.010

Eglen, S. J., Marwick, B., Halchenko, Y. O., Hanke, M., Sufi, S., Gleeson, P., et al. (2017). Toward standard practices for sharing computer code and programs in neuroscience. *Nat. Neurosci.* 20, 770–773. doi: 10.1038/nn.4550

Eppler, J. M., Pauli, R., Peyser, A., Ippen, T., Morrison, A., Senk, J., et al. (2015). *NEST 2.8.0*. Zenodo. doi: 10.5281/zenodo.32969

Ermentrout, B. (2002). *Simulating, Analyzing, and Animating Dynamical Systems: A Guide to XPPAUT for Researchers and Students, 1st Edn*. Philadelphia, PA: Society for Industrial & Applied Mathematics (SIAM).

Fellin, T., Ellenbogen, J. M., De Pittà, M., Ben-Jacob, E., and Halassa, M. M. (2012). Astrocyte regulation of sleep circuits: experimental and modeling perspectives. *Front. Comput. Neurosci.* 6:65. doi: 10.3389/fncom.2012.00065

French, D. A., and Gruenstein, E. I. (2006). An integrate-and-fire model for synchronized bursting in a network of cultured cortical neurons. *J. Comput. Neurosci.* 21, 227–241. doi: 10.1007/s10827-006-7815-5

Gerkin, R. C., Bi, G.-Q., and Rubin, J. E. (2010). "A phenomenological calcium-based model of STDP," in *Hippocampal Microcircuits: A Computational Modelers Resource Book*, eds V. Cutsuridis, B. Graham, S. Cobb, and I. Vida (New York, NY: Springer), 571–591.

Gilbert, D., Fuß, H., Gu, X., Orton, R., Robinson, S., Vyshemirsky, V., et al. (2006). Computational methodologies for modelling, analysis and simulation of signalling networks. *Brief. Bioinform.* 7, 339–353. doi: 10.1093/bib/bbl043

Gillespie, D. T. (1976). A general method for numerically simulating the stochastic time evolution of coupled chemical reactions. *J. Comput. Phys.* 22, 403–434. doi: 10.1016/0021-9991(76)90041-3

Gillespie, D. T. (1977). Exact stochastic simulation of coupled chemical reactions. *J. Phys. Chem.* 81, 2340–2361. doi: 10.1021/j100540a008

Gillespie, D. T. (2000). The chemical Langevin equation. *J. Chem. Phys.* 113, 297–306. doi: 10.1063/1.481811

Gillespie, D. T. (2001). Approximate accelerated stochastic simulation of chemically reacting systems. *J. Chem. Phys.* 115, 1716–1733. doi: 10.1063/1.1378322

Gillespie, D. T. (2007). Stochastic simulation of chemical kinetics. *Annu. Rev. Phys. Chem.* 58, 35–55. doi: 10.1146/annurev.physchem.58.032806.104637

Giugliano, M., Darbon, P., Arsiero, M., Lüscher, H.-R., and Streit, J. (2004). Single-neuron discharge properties and network activity in dissociated cultures of neocortex. *J. Neurophysiol.* 92, 977–996. doi: 10.1152/jn.00067.2004

Gleeson, P., Crook, S., Cannon, R. C., Hines, M. L., Billings, G. O., Farinella, M., et al. (2010). NeuroML: a language for describing data driven models of neurons and networks with a high degree of biological detail. *PLoS Comput. Biol.* 6:e1000815. doi: 10.1371/journal.pcbi.1000815

Goodman, D., and Brette, R. (2008). Brian: a simulator for spiking neural networks in Python. *Front. Neuroinform.* 2:5. doi: 10.3389/neuro.11.005.2008

Goodman, S. N., Fanelli, D., and Ioannidis, J. P. A. (2016). What does research reproducibility mean? *Sci. Transl. Med.* 8:341ps12. doi: 10.1126/scitranslmed.aaf5027

Graupner, M., and Brunel, N. (2010). Mechanisms of induction and maintenance of spike-timing dependent plasticity in biophysical synapse models. *Front. Comput. Neurosci.* 4:136. doi: 10.3389/fncom.2010.00136

Gritsun, T., le Feber, J., Stegenga, J., and Rutten, W. L. C. (2011). Experimental analysis and computational modeling of interburst intervals in spontaneous activity of cortical neuronal culture. *Biol. Cybern.* 105, 197–210. doi: 10.1007/s00422-011-0457-3

Gritsun, T. A., Le Feber, J., Stegenga, J., and Rutten, W. L. C. (2010). Network bursts in cortical cultures are best simulated using pacemaker neurons and adaptive synapses. *Biol. Cybern.* 102, 293–310. doi: 10.1007/s00422-010-0366-x

Hayer, A., and Bhalla, U. S. (2005). Molecular switches at the synapse emerge from receptor and kinase traffic. *PLoS Comput. Biol.* 1:e20. doi: 10.1371/journal.pcbi.0010020

Hellgren Kotaleski, J., and Blackwell, K. T. (2010). Modelling the molecular mechanisms of synaptic plasticity using systems biology approaches. *Nat. Rev. Neurosci.* 11, 239–251. doi: 10.1038/nrn2807

Hepburn, I., Chen, W., Wils, S., and De Schutter, E. (2012). STEPS: efficient simulation of stochastic reaction-diffusion models in realistic morphologies. *BMC Syst. Biol.* 6:36. doi: 10.1186/1752-0509-6-36

Hepburn, I., Jain, A., Gangal, H., Yamamoto, Y., Tanaka-Yamamoto, K., and De Schutter, E. (2017). A model of induction of cerebellar long-term depression including RKIP inactivation of Raf and MEK. *Front. Mol. Neurosci.* 10:19. doi: 10.3389/fnmol.2017.00019

Hines, M. L., Morse, T., Migliore, M., Carnevale, N. T., and Shepherd, G. M. (2004). ModelDB: a database to support computational neuroscience. *J. Comput. Neurosci* 17, 7–11. doi: 10.1023/B:JCNS.0000023869.22017.2e

Hodgkin, A. L., and Huxley, A. F. (1952). A quantitative description of membrane current and its application to conduction and excitation in nerve. *J. Physiol.* 117, 500–544. doi: 10.1113/jphysiol.1952.sp004764

Holmes, W. R. (2005). "Calcium signaling in dendritic spines," in *Modeling in the Neurosciences: From Biological Systems to Neuromimetic Robotics, 2nd Edn*, eds G. N. Reeke, R. R. Poznanski, K. A. Lindsay, J. R. Rosenberg, and O. Sporns (Boca Raton, FL: CRC Press), 25–60.

Hoops, S., Sahle, S., Gauges, R., Lee, C., Pahle, J., Simus, N., et al. (2006). COPASI – a complex pathway simulator. *Bioinformatics* 22, 3067–3074. doi: 10.1093/bioinformatics/btl485

Hucka, M., Finney, A., Sauro, H. M., Bolouri, H., Doyle, J. C., Kitano, H., et al. (2003). The systems biology markup language (SBML): a medium for representation and exchange of biochemical network models. *Bioinformatics* 19, 524–531. doi: 10.1093/bioinformatics/btg015

Hudmon, A., and Schulman, H. (2002a). Neuronal Ca^{2+}/calmodulin-dependent protein kinase II: the role of structure and autoregulation in cellular function. *Annu. Rev. Biochem.* 71, 473–510. doi: 10.1146/annurev.biochem.71.110601.135410

Hudmon, A., and Schulman, H. (2002b). Structure-function of the multifunctional Ca^{2+}/calmodulin-dependent protein kinase II. *Biochem. J.* 364, 593–611. doi: 10.1042/BJ20020228

Ichikawa, M., Muramoto, K., Kobayashi, K., Kawahara, M., and Kuroda, Y. (1993). Formation and maturation of synapses in primary cultures of rat cerebral cortical cells: an electron microscopic study. *Neurosci. Res.* 16, 95–103. doi: 10.1016/0168-0102(93)90076-3

Izhikevich, E. M. (2004). Which model to use for cortical spiking neurons? *IEEE Trans. Neural Netw.* 15, 1063–1070. doi: 10.1109/TNN.2004.832719

Jolivet, R., Allaman, I., Pellerin, L., Magistretti, P. J., and Weber, B. (2010). Comment on recent modeling studies of astrocyte–neuron metabolic interactions. *J. Cereb. Blood Flow Metab.* 30, 1982–1986. doi: 10.1038/jcbfm.2010.132

Kerr, R. A., Bartol, T. M., Kaminsky, B., Dittrich, M., Chang, J.-C. J., Baden, S. B., et al. (2008). Fast Monte Carlo simulation methods for biological reaction-diffusion systems in solution and on surfaces. *SIAM J. Sci. Comput.* 30, 3126–3149. doi: 10.1137/070692017

Kim, M. S., Huang, T., Abel, T., and Blackwell, K. T. (2010). Temporal sensitivity of protein kinase A activation in late-phase long term potentiation. *PLoS Comput. Biol.* 6:e1000691. doi: 10.1371/journal.pcbi.1000691

Klipp, E., and Liebermeister, W. (2006). Mathematical modeling of intracellular signaling pathways. *BMC Neurosci.* 7(Suppl 1):S10. doi: 10.1186/1471-2202-7-S1-S10

Koene, R. A., Tijms, B., van Hees, P., Postma, F., de Ridder, A., Ramakers, G. J. A., et al. (2009). NETMORPH: a framework for the stochastic generation of large scale neuronal networks with realistic neuron morphologies. *Neuroinformatics* 7, 195–210. doi: 10.1007/s12021-009-9052-3

Latham, P. E., Richmond, B. J., Nelson, P. G., and Nirenberg, S. (2000). Intrinsic dynamics in neuronal networks. I. Theory. *J. Neurophysiol.* 83, 808–827. doi: 10.1152/jn.2000.83.2.808

Lavrentovich, M., and Hemkin, S. (2008). A mathematical model of spontaneous calcium (II) oscillations in astrocytes. *J. Theor. Biol.* 251, 553–560. doi: 10.1016/j.jtbi.2007.12.011

Le Novère, N., Bornstein, B., Broicher, A., Courtot, M., Donizelli, M., Dharuri, H., et al. (2006). BioModels Database: a free, centralized database of curated, published, quantitative kinetic models of biochemical and cellular systems. *Nucleic Acids Res.* 34, D689–D691. doi: 10.1093/nar/gkj092

Le Novère, N., Finney, A., Hucka, M., Bhalla, U. S., Campagne, F., Collado-Vides, J., et al. (2005). Minimum information requested in the annotation of biochemical models (MIRIAM). *Nat. Biotechnol.* 23, 1509–1515. doi: 10.1038/nbt1156

Lecca, P., Bagagiolo, F., and Scarpa, M. (2017). Hybrid deterministic/stochastic simulation of complex biochemical systems. *Mol. BioSyst.* 13, 2672–2686. doi: 10.1039/C7MB00426E

Lemerle, C., Di Ventura, B., and Serrano, L. (2005). Space as the final frontier in stochastic simulations of biological systems. *FEBS Lett.* 579, 1789–1794. doi: 10.1016/j.febslet.2005.02.009

Lindskog, M., Kim, M., Wikström, M. A., Blackwell, K. T., and Hellgren Kotaleski, J. (2006). Transient calcium and dopamine increase PKA activity and DARPP-32 phosphorylation. *PLoS Comput. Biol.* 2:e119. doi: 10.1371/journal.pcbi.0020119

Linne, M.-L., and Jalonen, T. O. (2014). Astrocyte–neuron interactions: from experimental research-based models to translational medicine. *Prog. Mol. Biol. Transl. Sci.* 123, 191–217. doi: 10.1016/B978-0-12-397897-4.00005-X

Lloyd, C. M., Halstead, M. D. B., and Nielsen, P. F. (2004). CellML: its future, present and past. *Prog. Biophys. Mol. Biol.* 85, 433–450. doi: 10.1016/j.pbiomolbio.2004.01.004

Lonardoni, D., Amin, H., Di Marco, S., Maccione, A., Berdondini, L., and Nieus, T. (2017). Recurrently connected and localized neuronal communities initiate coordinated spontaneous activity in neuronal networks. *PLoS Comput. Biol.* 13:e1005672. doi: 10.1371/journal.pcbi.1005672

Lytton, W. W., and Hines, M. L. (2005). Independent variable time-step integration of individual neurons for network simulations. *Neural Comput.* 17, 903–921. doi: 10.1162/0899766053429453

Maheswaranathan, N., Ferrari, S., VanDongen, A., and Henriquez, C. (2012). Emergent bursting and synchrony in computer simulations of neuronal cultures. *Front. Comput. Neurosci.* 6:15. doi: 10.3389/fncom.2012.00015

Mäki-Marttunen, T., Aćimović, J., Ruohonen, K., and Linne, M.-L. (2013). Structure-dynamics relationships in bursting neuronal networks revealed using a prediction framework. *PLoS ONE* 8:e69373. doi: 10.1371/journal.pone.0069373

Mäki-Marttunen, T., Havela, R., Aćimović, J., Teppola, H., Ruohonen, K., and Linne, M.-L. (2010). "Modeling growth in neuronal cell cultures: network properties in different phases of growth studied using two growth simulators," in *Proceeding of the 7th International Workshop on Computational System Biology (WCSB 2010)*, eds M. Nykter, P. Ruusuvuori, C. Carlberg, and O. Yli-Harja (Luxemburg), 75–78.

Mäkiraatikka, E., Manninen, T., Saarinen, A., Ylipää, A., Teppola, H., Hituri, K., et al. (2007). "Stochastic simulation tools for cellular signaling: survey, evaluation, and quantitative analysis," in *Proceedings of the 2nd Conference on Foundations of Systems Biology in Engineering (FOSBE 2007)*, eds F. Allgöwer and M. Reuss (Stuttgart), 171–176.

Mandel, J. J., Fuß, H., Palfreyman, N. M., and Dubitzky, W. (2007). Modeling biochemical transformation processes and information processing with Narrator. *BMC Bioinformatics* 8:103. doi: 10.1186/1471-2105-8-103

Mangia, S., DiNuzzo, M., Giove, F., Carruthers, A., Simpson, I. A., and Vannucci, S. J. (2011). Response to 'comment on recent modeling studies of astrocyte–neuron metabolic interactions': much ado about nothing. *J. Cereb. Blood Flow Metab.* 31, 1346–1353. doi: 10.1038/jcbfm.2011.29

Manninen, T., Havela, R., and Linne., M.-L. (2017). Reproducibility and comparability of computational models for astrocyte calcium excitability. *Front. Neuroinform.* 11:11. doi: 10.3389/fninf.2017.00011

Manninen, T., Havela, R., and Linne., M.-L. (2018a). Computational models for calcium-mediated astrocyte functions. *Front. Comput. Neurosci.* 12:14. doi: 10.3389/fncom.2018.00014

Manninen, T., Havela, R., and Linne, M.-L. (2018b). "Computational models of astrocytes and astrocyte-neuron interactions: characterization, reproducibility, and future perspectives," in *Mathematical Methods in Modeling of Neuron-Glia Interactions*, eds M. De Pittà and H. Berry (Springer), 2018.

Manninen, T., Hituri, K., Hellgren Kotaleski, J., Blackwell, K. T., and Linne, M.-L. (2010). Postsynaptic signal transduction models for long-term potentiation and depression. *Front. Comput. Neurosci.* 4:152. doi: 10.3389/fncom.2010.00152

Manninen, T., Hituri, K., Toivari, E., and Linne, M.-L. (2011). Modeling signal transduction leading to synaptic plasticity: evaluation and comparison of five models. *EURASIP J. Bioinf. Syst. Biol.* 2011:797250. doi: 10.1155/2011/797250

Manninen, T., and Linne, M.-L. (2008). "Stochastic kinetic simulations of activity-dependent plastic modifications in neurons," in *Proceedings of the 5th International Workshop on Computational Systems Biology (WCSB 2008)*, eds M. Ahdesmäki, K. Strimmer, N. Radde, J. Rahnenfuhrer, K. Klemm, H. Lähdesmäki, and O. Yli-Harja (Leipzig), 101–104.

Manninen, T., Linne, M.-L., and Ruohonen, K. (2006a). Developing Itô stochastic differential equation models for neuronal signal transduction pathways. *Comput. Biol. Chem.* 30, 280–291. doi: 10.1016/j.compbiolchem.2006.04.002

Manninen, T., Linne, M.-L., and Ruohonen, K. (2006b). A novel approach to model neuronal signal transduction using stochastic differential equations. *Neurocomputing* 69, 1066–1069. doi: 10.1016/j.neucom.2005.12.047

Manninen, T., Mäkiraatikka, E., Ylipää, A., Pettinen, A., Leinonen, K., and Linne, M.-L. (2006c). "Discrete stochastic simulation of cell signaling: comparison of computational tools," in *Proceedings of the 28th Annual International Conference of the IEEE Engineering in Medicine and Biology Society (EMBC 2006)* (New York, NY), 2013–2016.

Masquelier, T., and Deco, G. (2013). Network bursting dynamics in excitatory cortical neuron cultures results from the combination of different adaptive mechanisms. *PLoS ONE* 8:e75824. doi: 10.1371/journal.pone.0075824

McDougal, R. A., Bulanova, A. S., and Lytton, W. W. (2016). Reproducibility in computational neuroscience models and simulations. *IEEE Trans. Biomed. Eng.* 63, 2021–2035. doi: 10.1109/TBME.2016.2539602

Mendes, P. (1993). GEPASI: a software package for modelling the dynamics, steady states and control of biochemical and other systems. *Comput. Appl. Biosci.* 9, 563–571. doi: 10.1093/bioinformatics/9.5.563

Mendes, P. (1997). Biochemistry by numbers: simulation of biochemical pathways with Gepasi 3. *Trends Biochem. Sci.* 22, 361–363. doi: 10.1016/S0968-0004(97)01103-1

Mendes, P., and Kell, D. B. (1998). Non-linear optimization of biochemical pathways: applications to metabolic engineering and parameter estimation. *Bioinformatics* 14, 869–883. doi: 10.1093/bioinformatics/14.10.869

Migliore, M., Morse, T. M., Davison, A. P., Marenco, L., Shepherd, G. M., and Hines, M. L. (2003). ModelDB: making models publicly accessible to support computational neuroscience. *Neuroinformatics* 1, 135–139. doi: 10.1385/NI:1:1:135

Min, R., Santello, M., and Nevian, T. (2012). The computational power of astrocyte mediated synaptic plasticity. *Front. Comput. Neurosci.* 6:93. doi: 10.3389/fncom.2012.00093

Miner, D., and Triesch, J. (2016). Plasticity-driven self-organization under topological constraints accounts for non-random features of cortical synaptic wiring. *PLoS Comput. Biol.* 12:e1004759. doi: 10.1371/journal.pcbi.1004759

Morrison, A., Diesmann, M., and Gerstner, W. (2008). Phenomenological models of synaptic plasticity based on spike timing. *Biol. Cybern.* 98, 459–478. doi: 10.1007/s00422-008-0233-1

Munafò, M. R., Nosek, B. A., Bishop, D. V. M., Button, K. S., Chambers, C. D., du Sert, N. P., et al. (2017). A manifesto for reproducible science. *Nat. Hum. Behav.* 1:0021. doi: 10.1038/s41562-016-0021

Nadkarni, S., and Jung, P. (2003). Spontaneous oscillations of dressed neurons: a new mechanism for epilepsy? *Phys. Rev. Lett.* 91:268101. doi: 10.1103/PhysRevLett.91.268101

Nakano, T., Doi, T., Yoshimoto, J., and Doya, K. (2010). A kinetic model of dopamine- and calcium-dependent striatal synaptic plasticity. *PLoS Comput. Biol.* 6:e1000670. doi: 10.1371/journal.pcbi.1000670

Neher, E. (1998). Usefulness and limitations of linear approximations to the understanding of Ca^{2+} signals. *Cell Calcium* 24, 345–357. doi: 10.1016/S0143-4160(98)90058-6

Nishi, R., Castañeda, E., Davis, G. W., Fenton, A. A., Hofmann, H. A., King, J., et al. (2016). The global challenge in neuroscience education and training: the MBL perspective. *Neuron* 92, 632–636. doi: 10.1016/j.neuron.2016.10.026

Nordlie, E., Gewaltig, M.-O., and Plesser, H. E. (2009). Towards reproducible descriptions of neuronal network models. *PLoS Comput. Biol.* 5:e1000456. doi: 10.1371/journal.pcbi.1000456

Ogasawara, H., Doi, T., and Kawato, M. (2008). Systems biology perspectives on cerebellar long-term depression. *Neurosignals* 16, 300–317. doi: 10.1159/000123040

Ogasawara, H., and Kawato, M. (2009). "Computational models of cerebellar long-term memory," in *Systems Biology: The Challenge of Complexity, 1st Edn*, eds S. Nakanishi, R. Kageyama, and D. Watanabe (Tokyo: Springer), 169–182.

Oliveira, R. F., Terrin, A., Di Benedetto, G., Cannon, R. C., Koh, W., Kim, M., et al. (2010). The role of type 4 phosphodiesterases in generating microdomains of cAMP: large scale stochastic simulations. *PLoS ONE* 5:e11725. doi: 10.1371/journal.pone.0011725

Olivier, B. G., Swat, M. J., and Moné, M. J. (2016). "Modeling and simulation tools: from systems biology to systems medicine," in *Systems Medicine. Methods in Molecular Biology, Vol. 1386*, eds U. Schmitz and O. Wolkenhauer (New York, NY: Humana Press), 441–463.

Pettinen, A., Aho, T., Smolander, O.-P., Manninen, T., Saarinen, A., Taattola, K.-L., et al. (2005). Simulation tools for biochemical networks: evaluation of performance and usability. *Bioinformatics* 21, 357–363. doi: 10.1093/bioinformatics/bti018

Plesser, H. E. (2018). Reproducibility vs. replicability: a brief history of a confused terminology. *Front. Neuroinform.* 11:76. doi: 10.3389/fninf.2017.00076

Ramsey, S., Orrell, D., and Bolouri, H. (2005). Dizzy: stochastic simulation of large-scale genetic regulatory networks. *J. Bioinform. Comput. Biol.* 3, 415–436. doi: 10.1142/S0219720005001132

Ray, S., Deshpande, R., Dudani, N., and Bhalla, U. S. (2008). A general biological simulator: the multiscale object oriented simulation environment, MOOSE. *BMC Neurosci.* 9:P93. doi: 10.1186/1471-2202-9-S1-P93

Riera, J., Hatanaka, R., Ozaki, T., and Kawashima, R. (2011a). Modeling the spontaneous Ca^{2+} oscillations in astrocytes: inconsistencies and usefulness. *J. Integr. Neurosci.* 10, 439–473. doi: 10.1142/S0219635211002877

Riera, J., Hatanaka, R., Uchida, T., Ozaki, T., and Kawashima, R. (2011b). Quantifying the uncertainty of spontaneous Ca^{2+} oscillations in astrocytes: particulars of Alzheimer's disease. *Biophys. J.* 101, 554–564. doi: 10.1016/j.bpj.2011.06.041

Robinson, H. P., Kawahara, M., Jimbo, Y., Torimitsu, K., Kuroda, Y., and Kawana, A. (1993). Periodic synchronized bursting and intracellular calcium transients elicited by low magnesium in cultured cortical neurons. *J. Neurophysiol.* 70, 1606–1616. doi: 10.1152/jn.1993.70.4.1606

Rotter, S., and Diesmann, M. (1999). Exact digital simulation of time-invariant linear systems with applications to neuronal modeling. *Biol. Cybern.* 81, 381–402. doi: 10.1007/s004220050570

Rougier, N. P., Hinsen, K., Alexandre, F., Arildsen, T., Barba, L. A., Benureau, F. C. Y., et al. (2017). Sustainable computational science: the ReScience initiative. *PeerJ Comput. Sci.* 3:e142. doi: 10.7717/peerj-cs.142

Salis, H., Sotiropoulos, V., and Kaznessis, Y. N. (2006). Multiscale Hy3S: hybrid stochastic simulation for supercomputers. *BMC Bioinformatics* 7:93. doi: 10.1186/1471-2105-7-93

Sauro, H. M. (2000). "JARNAC: a system for interactive metabolic analysis," in *Animating the Cellular Map: Proceegings of the 9th International Meeting on BioThermoKinetics* (Stellenbosch: Stellenbosch University Press), 221–228.

Sauro, H. M. (2001). *JDesigner: A Simple Biochemical Network Designer*. Technical report.

Schmidt, H., and Jirstrand, M. (2006). Systems Biology Toolbox for MATLAB: a computational platform for research in systems biology. *Bioinformatics* 22, 514–515. doi: 10.1093/bioinformatics/bti799

Schöneberg, J., Ullrich, A., and Noé, F. (2014). Simulation tools for particle-based reaction-diffusion dynamics in continuous space. *BMC Biophys.* 7:11. doi: 10.1186/s13628-014-0011-5

Shouval, H. Z., Wang, S. S. H., and Wittenberg, G. M. (2010). Spike timing dependent plasticity: a consequence of more fundamental learning rules. *Front. Comput. Neurosci.* 4:19. doi: 10.3389/fncom.2010.00019

Silchenko, A. N., and Tass, P. A. (2008). Computational modeling of paroxysmal depolarization shifts in neurons induced by the glutamate release from astrocytes. *Biol. Cybern.* 98, 61–74. doi: 10.1007/s00422-007-0196-7

Sivakumaran, S., Hariharaputran, S., Mishra, J., and Bhalla, U. S. (2003). The Database of Quantitative Cellular Signaling: management and analysis of chemical kinetic models of signaling networks. *Bioinformatics* 19, 408–415. doi: 10.1093/bioinformatics/btf860

Sterratt, D., Graham, B., Gillies, A., and Willshaw, D. (2011). *Principles in Computational Modeling in Neuroscience*. New York, NY: Cambridge University Press.

Stiles, J. R., and Bartol, T. M. (2001). "Monte Carlo methods for simulating realistic synaptic microphysiology using MCell," in *Computational Neuroscience: Realistic Modeling for Experimentalists*, ed E. De Schutter (Boca Raton, FL: CRC Press), 87–127.

Stimberg, M., Goodman, D. F. M., Benichoux, V., and Brette, R. (2014). Equation-oriented specification of neural models for simulations. *Front. Neuroinform.* 8:6. doi: 10.3389/fninf.2014.00006

Strömbäck, L., Jakoniene, V., Tan, H., and Lambrix, P. (2006). Representing, storing and accessing molecular interaction data: a review of models and tools. *Brief. Bioinform.* 7, 331–338. doi: 10.1093/bib/bbl039

Tanaka, K., and Augustine, G. J. (2009). "Systems biology meets single-cell physiology: role of a positive-feedback signal transduction network in cerebellar long-term synaptic depression," in *Systems Biology: The Challenge of Complexity, 1st Edn*, eds S. Nakanishi, R. Kageyama, and D. Watanabe (Tokyo: Springer), 159–168.

Teppola, H., Okujeni, S., Linne, M.-L., and Egert, U. (2011). "AMPA, NMDA and $GABA_A$ receptor mediated network burst dynamics in cortical cultures *in vitro*," in *Proceedings of the 8th International Workshop on Computational Systems Biology (WCSB 2011)*, eds H. Koeppl, J. Aćimović, J. Kesseli, T. Mäki-Marttunen, A. Larjo, and O. Yli-Harja (Zurich), 181–184.

Tetzlaff, C., Okujeni, S., Egert, U., Wörgötter, F., and Butz, M. (2010). Self-organized criticality in developing neuronal networks. *PLoS Comput. Biol.* 6:e1001013. doi: 10.1371/journal.pcbi.1001013

Tewari, S., and Parpura, V. (2014). Data and model tango to aid the understanding of astrocyte-neuron signaling. *Front. Comput. Neurosci.* 8:3. doi: 10.3389/fncom.2014.00003

Topalidou, M., Leblois, A., Boraud, T., and Rougier, N. P. (2015). A long journey into reproducible computational neuroscience. *Front. Comput. Neurosci.* 9:30. doi: 10.3389/fncom.2015.00030

Urakubo, H., Honda, M., Tanaka, K., and Kuroda, S. (2009). Experimental and computational aspects of signaling mechanisms of spike-timing-dependent plasticity. *HFSP J.* 3, 240–254. doi: 10.2976/1.3137602

van Ooyen, A. (2011). Using theoretical models to analyse neural development. *Nat. Rev. Neurosci.* 12, 311–326. doi: 10.1038/nrn3031

van Pelt, J., and Uylings, H. B. M. (2003). Growth functions in dendritic outgrowth. *Brain Mind* 4, 51–65. doi: 10.1023/A:1024160131897

Volman, V., Bazhenov, M., and Sejnowski, T. J. (2012). Computational models of neuron-astrocyte interaction in epilepsy. *Front. Comput. Neurosci.* 6:58. doi: 10.3389/fncom.2012.00058

Wade, J., McDaid, L., Harkin, J., Crunelli, V., and Kelso, S. (2012). Self-repair in a bidirectionally coupled astrocyte-neuron (AN) system based on retrograde signaling. *Front. Comput. Neurosci.* 6:76. doi: 10.3389/fncom.2012.00076

Wade, J., McDaid, L., Harkin, J., Crunelli, V., and Kelso, S. (2013). Biophysically based computational models of astrocyte ~ neuron coupling and their functional significance. *Front. Comput. Neurosci.* 7:44. doi: 10.3389/fncom.2013.00044

Wade, J. J., McDaid, L. J., Harkin, J., Crunelli, V., and Kelso, J. A. S. (2011). Bidirectional coupling between astrocytes and neurons mediates learning and dynamic coordination in the brain: a multiple modeling approach. *PLoS ONE* 6:e29445. doi: 10.1371/journal.pone.0029445

Waltemath, D., Adams, R., Beard, D. A., Bergmann, F. T., Bhalla, U. S., Britten, R., et al. (2011a). Minimum information about a simulation experiment (MIASE). *PLoS Comput. Biol.* 7:e1001122. doi: 10.1371/journal.pcbi.100 1122

Waltemath, D., Adams, R., Bergmann, F. T., Hucka, M., Kolpakov, F., Miller, A. K., et al. (2011b). Reproducible computational biology experiments with SED-ML - the simulation experiment description markup language. *BMC Syst. Biol.* 5:198. doi: 10.1186/1752-0509-5-198

Wierling, C., Herwig, R., and Lehrach, H. (2007). Resources, standards and tools for systems biology. *Brief. Funct. Genomic. Proteomic.* 6, 240–251. doi: 10.1093/bfgp/elm027

Wils, S., and De Schutter, E. (2009). STEPS: modeling and simulating complex reaction-diffusion systems with Python. *Front. Neuroinform.* 3:15. doi: 10.3389/neuro.11.015.2009

Wilson, M. A., Bhalla, U. S., Uhley, J. D., and Bower, J. M. (1989). "GENESIS: a system for simulating neural networks," in *Advances in Neural Information Processing Systems*, ed D. S. Touretzky (San Francisco, CA: Morgan Kaufmann Publishers Inc.), 485–492.

Wörgötter, F., and Porr, B. (2005). Temporal sequence learning, prediction, and control: a review of different models and their relation to biological mechanisms. *Neural Comput.* 17, 245–319. doi: 10.1162/0899766053011555

Yamamoto, H., Kubota, S., Chida, Y., Morita, M., Moriya, S., Akima, H., et al. (2016). Size-dependent regulation of synchronized activity in living neuronal networks. *Phys. Rev. E* 94:012407. doi: 10.1103/PhysRevE.94.012407

Yeung, A. W. K. (2017). Do neuroscience journals accept replications? A survey of literature. *Front. Hum. Neurosci.* 11:468. doi: 10.3389/fnhum.2017.00468

Zachariou, M., Alexander, S. P. H., Coombes, S., and Christodoulou, C. (2013). A biophysical model of endocannabinoid-mediated short term depression in hippocampal inhibition. *PLoS ONE* 8:e58926. doi: 10.1371/journal.pone.0058926

Zehl, L., Jaillet, F., Stoewer, A., Grewe, J., Sobolev, A., Wachtler, T., et al. (2016). Handling metadata in a neurophysiology laboratory. *Front. Neuroinform.* 10:26. doi: 10.3389/fninf.2016.00026

Zou, Q., and Destexhe, A. (2007). Kinetic models of spike-timing dependent plasticity and their functional consequences in detecting correlations. *Biol. Cybern.* 97, 81–97. doi: 10.1007/s00422-007-0155-3

Zubler, F., and Douglas, R. (2009). A framework for modeling the growth and development of neurons and networks. *Front. Comput. Neurosci.* 3:25. doi: 10.3389/neuro.10.025.2009

Zubler, F., Hauri, A., Pfister, S., Bauer, R., Anderson, J. C., Whatley, A. M., et al. (2013). Simulating cortical development as a self constructing process: a novel multi-scale approach combining molecular and physical aspects. *PLoS Comput. Biol.* 9:e1003173. doi: 10.1371/journal.pcbi.1003173

Zubler, F., Hauri, A., Pfister, S., Whatley, A., Cook, M., and Douglas, R. (2011). An instruction language for self-construction in the context of neural networks. *Front. Comput. Neurosci.* 5:57. doi: 10.3389/fncom.2011.00057

3

FindSim: A Framework for Integrating Neuronal Data and Signaling Models

Nisha A. Viswan[1,2†], *Gubbi Vani HarshaRani*[1†], *Melanie I. Stefan*[3,4] *and Upinder S. Bhalla*[1*]

[1]*National Centre for Biological Sciences, Tata Institute of Fundamental Research, Bangalore, India,* [2]*The University of Trans-Disciplinary Health Sciences and Technology, Bangalore, India,* [3]*Centre for Discovery Brain Sciences, University of Edinburgh, Edinburgh, United Kingdom,* [4]*ZJU-UoE Institute, Zhejiang University, Hangzhou, China*

Correspondence:
Upinder S. Bhalla
bhalla@ncbs.res.in

[†]*Joint first authors.*

Current experiments touch only small but overlapping parts of very complex subcellular signaling networks in neurons. Even with modern optical reporters and pharmacological manipulations, a given experiment can only monitor and control a very small subset of the diverse, multiscale processes of neuronal signaling. We have developed FindSim (Framework for Integrating Neuronal Data and SIgnaling Models) to anchor models to structured experimental datasets. FindSim is a framework for integrating many individual electrophysiological and biochemical experiments with large, multiscale models so as to systematically refine and validate the model. We use a structured format for encoding the conditions of many standard physiological and pharmacological experiments, specifying which parts of the model are involved, and comparing experiment outcomes with model output. A database of such experiments is run against successive generations of composite cellular models to iteratively improve the model against each experiment, while retaining global model validity. We suggest that this toolchain provides a principled and scalable way to tackle model complexity and diversity of data sources.

Keywords: simulation, signaling pathway, systems biology, biochemistry, pharmacology, LTP, synaptic signaling

INTRODUCTION

Neuronal signaling is a complex, multiscale phenomenon which includes genetic, biochemical, transport, structural, protein synthesis, electrical and network components. There is an abundance of models of specific parts of this landscape, with a special focus on electrophysiological properties of neurons (Hodgkin and Huxley, 1952; Bhalla and Bower, 1993; De Schutter and Bower, 1994; Narayanan and Johnston, 2010) and biochemical signaling in plasticity (Lisman, 1985; Bhalla and Iyengar, 1999; Shouval et al., 2002; Hayer and Bhalla, 2005; Smolen et al., 2006; Kim et al., 2010; Manninen et al., 2010; Li et al., 2012; Stefan et al., 2012). Each of these models has its own parameterization idiosyncrasies, and even when the data sources are described in some detail (e.g., Bhalla and Iyengar, 1999) the derivation of specific rate terms and parameters is something of an individualistic art form. Further, each of these models typically incorporates far more knowledge about the biological system than is apparent from a plain listing of data sources. While this has resulted in high quality, hand-crafted models for specific processes, there are several major drawbacks of this almost universal modeling process. First, it is idiosyncratic. Second, most models are highly specific for individual questions posed by the developers. Third, by necessity, all such models are tiny subsets of known signaling (Heil et al., 2018). Fourth, models rarely venture across scales, that is cross electrical and biochemical, or structural and genetic.

There are some counter-currents to this highly personalized modeling process. The first has been the emergence of a range of standards for model specification (Hucka et al., 2003; Gleeson et al., 2010), experiments (Waltemath et al., 2011; Garcia et al., 2014; Teeters et al., 2015), and model output (Ray et al., 2016). The continued development of community-based standards is overseen by the COMBINE initiative (Hucka et al., 2015). These standards mean that even though individual model development may remain personalized, models can be much more readily shared. Numerous databases now host such models (Migliorc et al., 2003; Sivakumaran et al., 2003; HarshaRani et al., 2005; Le Novère et al., 2006; Gleeson et al., 2015). With this set of resources, the models, simulation experiments performed on them, and their output, can each be specified in a platform-neutral and unambiguous manner.

A second recent development has been the emergence of simulators designed for multiscale signaling (Ray and Bhalla, 2008; Wils and De Schutter, 2009) as well as the incorporation of multiscale features in existing simulators (Bhalla, 2002b; Brown et al., 2011; McDougal et al., 2013). With these developments the most common scale crossover, between spatially detailed electrical and chemical models, is greatly facilitated.

A third major counter-current to this highly personalized modeling process is the development of model specification pipelines. The CellML project has developed data pipelines for model composition, annotation, model reduction and linkage to databases (Beard et al., 2009). The Allen Brain Project (Gouwens et al., 2018) and the Human Brain Project (Markram et al., 2015) have each developed systematic approach to parameterizing neuronal models, and the availability of such open resources has enabled development of independent efforts for experiment-driven modeling workflows (Stockton and Santamaria, 2017). These models build on previously developed ion-channel specifications and the parameter tuning is typically by way of assigning experimentally-driven passive properties and scaling channel densities, both in reduced and in detailed cellular morphologies. There are several related approaches to specify experimental data and metadata. For example, Silva and colleagues (Silva and Müller, 2015; Matiasz et al., 2017) have come up with frameworks for defining neurobiological experiments. Much more structured experiments such as microarrays (Brazma et al., 2001), next-generation sequencing, e.g., (Kent et al., 2010) or proteomics (Taylor et al., 2006, 2007) have their own metadata formats. In neuroscience, several such initiatives exist, for various types of neurobiological data (Garcia et al., 2014; Rübel et al., 2016; Stead and Halford, 2016). These specification formats are very powerful ways to ensure experimental consistency and reproducibility. However, our objectives were distinct, and more restricted, in two important ways. First, we needed not to reproduce experiments, but to be able to map them to simulations. Second, we needed to do this for a wide range of "legacy" style experiments, where structured metadata was neither available, nor easily specified. We therefore selected a small core subset of metadata and experimental data of direct relevance to simulation development.

The current study examines how to systematically use experimental data to parameterize multiscale neuronal signaling models reproducibly, scalably, openly, and in a generally applicable manner. It is clearly desirable to have a standard for facile mapping between experiments and models, especially in the rapidly expanding domain of neural physiology and signaling. We envision the role of FindSim as a first key step towards a standard, by demonstrating a functional implementation of experiment-driven simulation specification in a production environment. We examine the requirements for such an eventual standard by exploring a diverse and challenging set of use cases. We report two core developments: how to unambiguously and scalably match experimental observations to models, and how to manage development of very large models having thousands of components needing thousands of experimental constraints. Both are combined in FindSim, the Framework for Integration of Neuronal Data and SIgnaling Models. We explain FindSim and illustrate a model development pipeline capable of handling such models and their associated experiments.

METHODS AND RESULTS

General Approach

We illustrate our approach using a large core model of biochemical signaling which is designed to be embedded in a single-compartment electrical model (**Figure 1**). The biochemical model has over 300 molecular species and a similar number of reactions and is drawn from several neuronal signaling models (Bhalla and Iyengar, 1999; Hayer and Bhalla, 2005; Jain and Bhalla, 2009). While large by current standards, this model is, of course, far from the current known complexity of synaptic signaling (Bayés et al., 2011; Heil et al., 2018). Even though reduced, the current models explore many of the technical challenges for model specification that will arise in more complete future models and serve as a good test-bed for the current analysis.

Based on experience with development of neuronal signaling models, both within our groups and from the published literature, we chose three categories of experiments for our initial set. These were time-series, dose-response and multi-stimulus response. It was our observation that a large fraction (typically well over half) of data panels from the articles that were used for prior model development studies in this domain (Bhalla and Iyengar, 1999; Shouval et al., 2002; Lindskog et al., 2006; Stefan et al., 2008; Kim et al., 2010) fell into these three categories. As such, these were easy targets with substantial value for model development. Further, we were able to generalize effectively within each category. For example, there are many variations of dose-response experiments. These may use different initial conditions, different ways of controlling the stimulus (dose), absolute or relative scaling for measuring the response, and so on. These variations were readily accommodated within our framework. As we discuss below, this approach also generalizes to the electrophysiological domain, and commonly used current and voltage-clamp experiments also fall into this framework.

Model Development and Parameterization Pipeline

The first of the core advances in this study is the definition of a model development and parameterization pipeline that takes the model and subjects it to a battery of experimental tests, defined in an open, extendable and structured form. In brief, any of a set

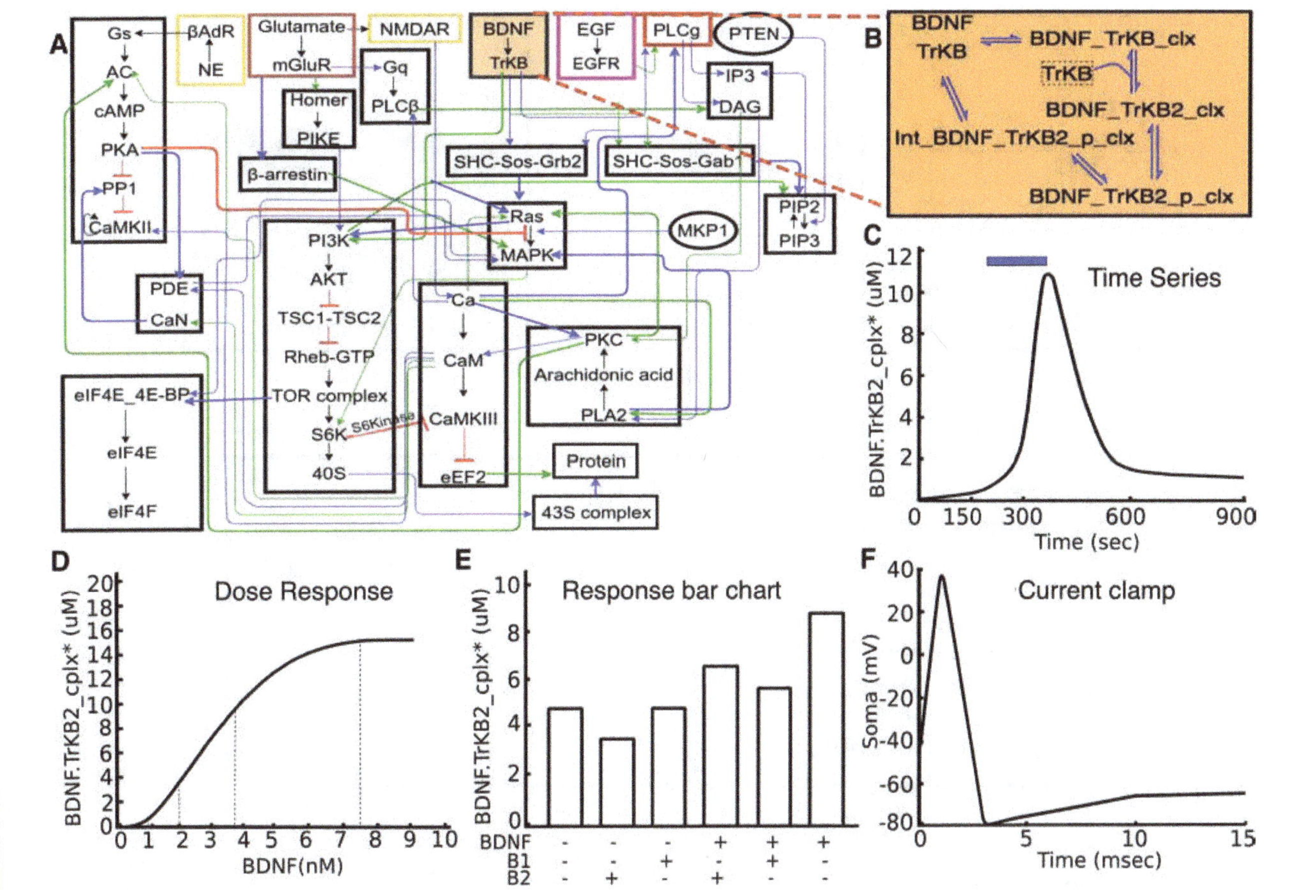

FIGURE 1 | Signaling model and experiments on it. **(A)** Block diagram of model. **(B)** Expanded reaction scheme for one of the reaction blocks. The experiments typically act on similar small subsets of the full model. **(C–F)**: Typical kinds of experiments on the model. **(C)** Time-series experiment with stimulus pulse (brain-derived neurotrophic factor (BDNF), blue) leading to signaling response (TrkB receptor activation, black). **(D)** Dose-response experiment, where defined BDNF stimuli lead to receptor activation. **(E)** Schematic of drug interaction experiment, where different combinations of stimuli are examined for their response, as shown by the bar chart. **(F)** Schematic voltage trace following a step current clamp stimulus.

of models is simulated according to instructions derived from the experimental dataset, and the outcome for each such simulation is scored according to how well the model fits the data. The models may be variants of the reference model, updated with progressively improved parameters or reaction schemes. They may also be specifically altered "mutant" or "disease" versions of the reference, for example, representing known mutants through the loss of a given molecular species. Our reference model is a composite of several modeling studies linked together based on known interactions.

Each structured experiment entry in the dataset is drawn from one of the three categories illustrated above: time-series, dose-response, or multi-stimulus response (**Figure 1**). The ~40 experiments in our initial database are all variants of these three categories, though further categories can readily be implemented. The experiment definitions specify which part of the model to use, which stimuli to deliver, and what results to expect (**Figures 2, 3**). The structured form of these definitions makes them independent of the exact model implementation.

To run through the models, we have implemented a Python-based script that reads the model and experiment definitions and launches the MOOSE simulator to execute the experiment. This wrapper script then examines the outputs from MOOSE and compares these with those expected from experiment (**Figure 2**). This comparison is scored according to a user-defined scoring function specified as part of the experiment definition. In order to improve cross-platform testability, the pipeline can also generate an SBML file for execution of the model on alternate platforms. This SBML file contains the model definition for that subpart or version of the reference model upon which the experiment is carried out, and where feasible, the definition of the stimulus that is applied to the model.

Stepping back, this entire pipeline can be run successively with different models, different experiments, and different scoring schemes. This is an embarrassingly parallel problem, so it is relatively easy to decompose the entire experiment set onto different processors on a cluster. Further, the structure of the scoring pipeline lends itself to an optimization step (dashed line in **Figure 2**) in which the model parameters are tweaked to improve the match to experiment as reflected in the model score.

In summary, we have implemented a model, a database and structure for experiment specification, and a pipeline to

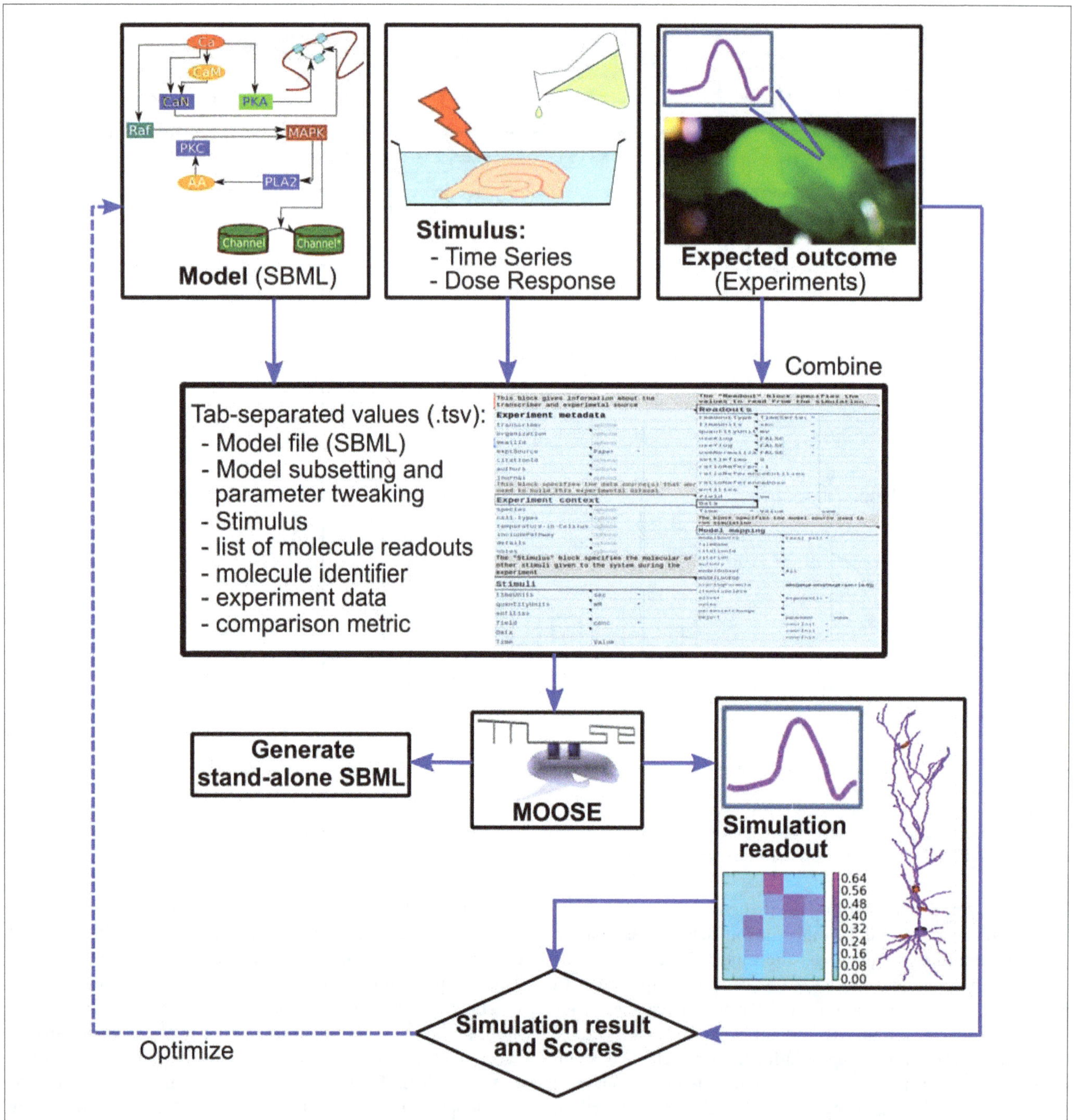

FIGURE 2 | Block diagram of the FindSim pipeline. Top: the inputs to the pipeline. Left: Model specification, typically in SBML. Middle: experimental stimuli. Right: experimental outcomes. Middle from top: the two experimental inputs and the metadata for how to apply these to the model are specified in a structured experiment definition in a tab-separated text file (.tsv file). This may be manipulated by an enhanced spreadsheet, or through a GUI. Below: the experiment definition and model are read in and executed by a Python/MOOSE script. This may either run the simulation and compare with experiment (right, lowermost) or emit SBML output so that the experiment can be run on other simulators. There are options to utilize the score from the simulation comparison as part of a model optimization cycle.

systematically test the model against each experiment. Each of these is in an open format and is accessible for other models and simulation tools[1].

[1]https://github.com/BhallaLab/FindSim

Experiment Specification and Mapping

The second core development in this study is a methodology for mapping experiments to large models. The conceptual challenge is how to merge many pathway-specific readouts into a consistent, cell-wide model. One could do so either by assembly

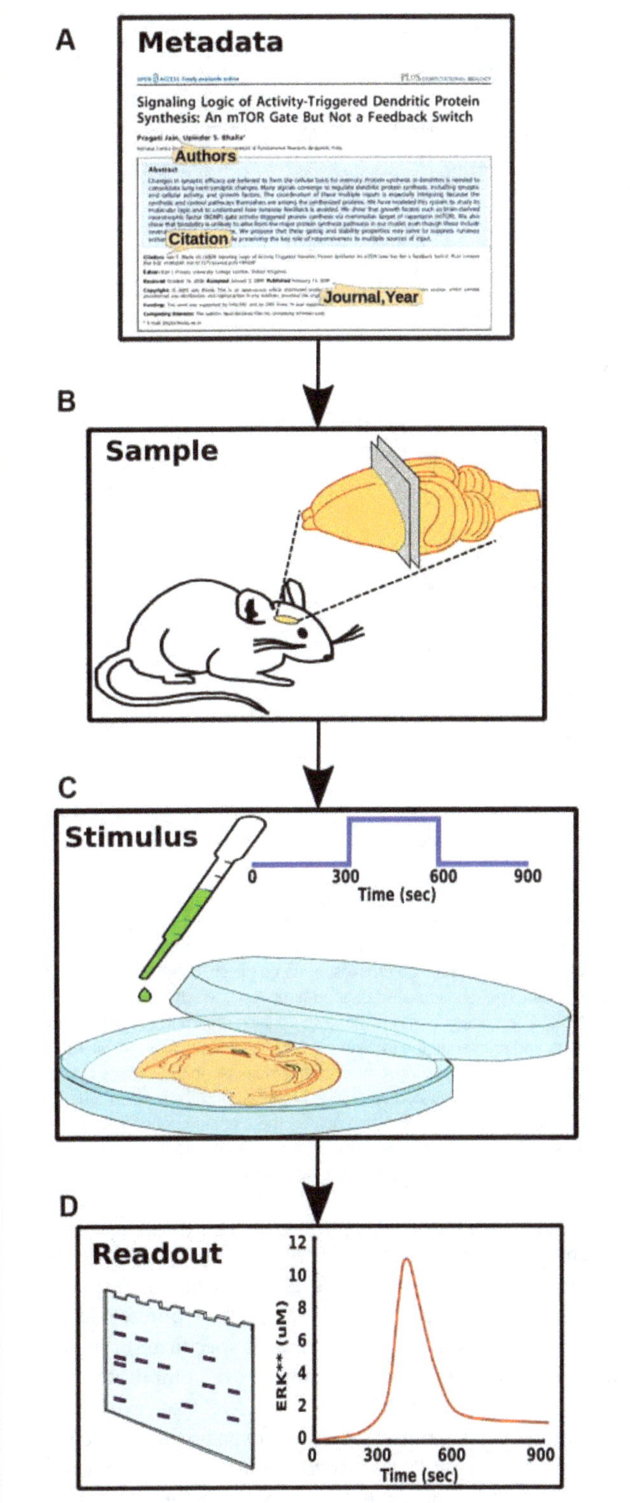

FIGURE 3 | Components of experiment specification. **(A)** Experiment metadata, including citation information and authorship. **(B)** Experimental context, including species, preparation and conditions. **(C)** Stimulus information such as molecular identity and concentration of a pharmacological agent. **(D)** Readouts from the experiment, such as a gel or time-course, each representing a set of measurables that should have a direct mapping to the model.

of small models into a large composite one, or by extraction of small sub-models from the reference composite model. The first approach maps closely to the individual experiments and modular perspectives of pathway function (Bhalla and Iyengar, 2001). We have described composition of large models from small modules for the first approach in previous work (Bhalla, 2002a), but with a topological rather than parameterization emphasis. The second approach incorporates interactions and takes a systems-level view.

The problems with the first approach are: (a) it is just as important and difficult to parameterize interactions *between* pathways as it is to parameterize the pathways themselves; (b) modifications to one pathway are likely to have knock-on effects on many others. The second approach (which we adopt here) handles pathway modularity by running the experiment on just that sub-portion of the model that is addressed in the experiment. It addresses point (a) by building in the pathway interactions into the composite model. This facilitates model comparison with experiments that span interacting pathways, and hence provides a process to parameterize the interactions. It does pose a specific technical issue of cleanly extracting small sub-models from the large one, which is addressed below. Point (b) remains relevant even in the second approach using a composite model. However, the larger model is amenable to "clean-up" of knock-on effects by running through all the subsequent experiments to fine-tune sub-models that may be impacted by the original change.

We now describe the structured experiment definition that implements the mapping of experiments to a large composite model (**Figure 3**). The goal of this definition is to provide a standardized, model-independent specification of experimental context, inputs, observed experimental results, and support for mapping each of these to model definitions. Some portions of such a definition have been formalized in the Simulation Experiment Definition Markup Language (Waltemath et al., 2011). Other aspects have been implemented in individual projects (Wolstencroft et al., 2017). SBML itself has support for delivery of specific inputs within the model definition markup file (Hucka et al., 2003). To our knowledge there is no unified specification standard that supports all of the elements essential to developing a model pipeline of the kind we envisage.

The key parts of the structured experiment definition are: (1) Experiment metadata. This specifies who did the experiment, citations, and other context. (2) Experiment context. This specifies species, cell-types, sample extraction methods, and the pathways expected to be relevant to the experiment. It also includes temperature, pH and other conditions pertinent to reproducibility. (3) Stimuli. These are the specific manipulations performed in the course of the experiment. This section can be quite diverse, and currently represents three main classes of experiments (**Figure 1**). For example, in the case of a time-series experiments, the inputs section would specify which molecule(s) were added to the preparation, at what times, and at what concentration. (4) Readouts. These are the readouts from the experimental preparation. This too is specific for each class of experiment. For example, in a time-series experiment the output would specify which molecule(s) were monitored, the observed concentration, and where available, the standard error for each observation.

The above four sections are all purely in the experimental domain and could in principle be filled in without any reference to the modeling. Part 5 (Model mapping) is special in that it explicitly sets up the mapping of experimental entities to model entities. Several of these are straightforward, such as identifying the mapping between input/output molecules in the experiment and in the model. The crucial and novel part of the experiment definition is the extraction of the relevant pathways from the composite model. While the experimentalist will provide some indication of the relevant pathways when describing the experiment (**Figure 3B**), it requires some understanding of model structure to formally define which pathways should be used. In brief, we impose a hierarchical organization onto our reference composite models, thus facilitating grouping of molecules and reactions into pathways, and even further groupings of related pathways into larger pathway circuits. In most experiments, the extraction of sub-models is a simple matter of specifying which pathways need to be used. Further fine-tuning of the sub-model may involve addition or removal of specific molecules or reactions from the final subset for extraction (**Figure 4**). In the current implementation, the extracted subset is defined as a string in the familiar directory/file format, which is also similar to the XPATH format used in XML.

While this key step is conceptually simple, the implementation of pathway extraction has a number of subtleties (**Figure 4B**). First, there is the problem of "dangling" reactions, which occur when model extraction has removed one or more of the substrates of a reaction. This admits of a technical solution by way of explicit tests and warnings for such situations. Second, extracted pathways may lose key regulatory inputs, leading to uncontrolled build-up of signals at run-time. This requires human inspection of the outcome of each experiment, and subsequent reconsideration of the extraction procedure. Third, experimental conditions frequently modify the base model not just by removal of pathways, but also by addition of buffers and inhibitors to the medium. This is addressed by expansion of Part 5 of the experiment specification to include such manipulations. Fourth, the mapping of experiment to model entities is not always clean. For example, there may be multiple protein isoforms in the experiment, the model, or both. In essence, this is a problem of model detail, and the modeler and experimentalist have to get together to decide the appropriate mapping, given the detail in any given composite model.

One of the key design decisions for the current pipeline implementation was *not* to try to automate too much of the mapping of entities that comprises part 5 of the experiment definition. For example, one could envisage using extensive Gene Ontology (GO) markup of each pathway or molecule to automatically obtain the appropriate mapping between experiment and model (Ashburner et al., 2000). This is the approach taken in existing tools for model merging (Neal et al., 2015), model feature extraction (Alm et al., 2015; Neal et al., 2015), or combination of models with experimental datasets (Cooper et al., 2011) based on semantic annotation. All those tools rely on high-quality expert annotation. For our purposes,

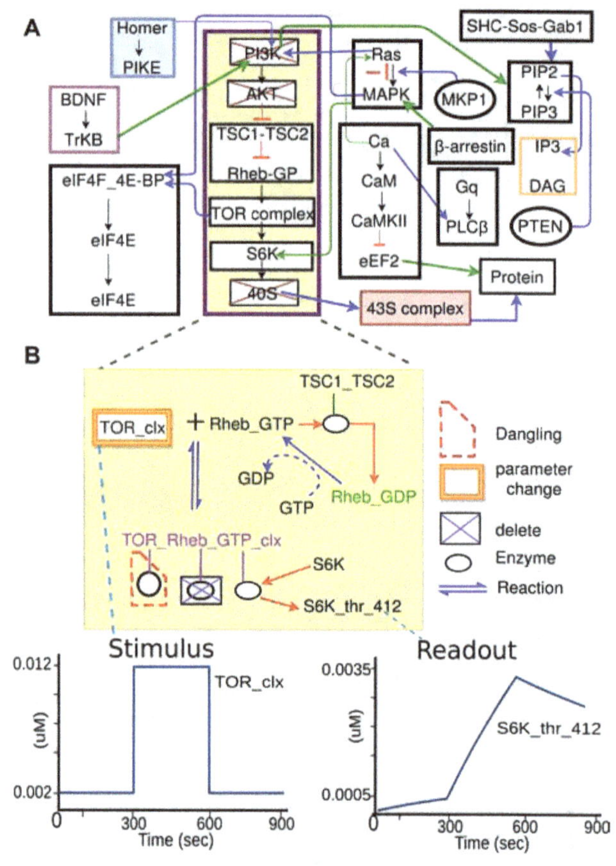

FIGURE 4 | Specification of model sub-parts. **(A)** Original full model, from which a few pathways are selected. **(B)** Further selections of reactions from the subset of pathways. Deleted molecules, reactions, and enzymes are indicated by boxes with blue crosses. In some cases, deleting molecules leads to dangling reactions (red dashed boundary), which lack one or more reactants. The system identifies these. In addition to removal of extraneous reactions and reactants, the experiment specification may involve alteration of parameters, such as the concentration of a molecule that is buffered in the experiment. This is illustrated as orange boxes around the molecule TOR_clx. Finally, the model specification also defines the mapping between the experimental names for stimulus or readout molecules, to the corresponding names for these molecules as used in the model.

our analysis was that the GO, or any other markup, would typically fall short of specifying all the details of experiments or model implementation. Thus, in practice one would almost always have to layer on further explicit specification of entities, and thus have to fall back on some more complicated version of our current "part 5". We also felt that extensive GO annotation from the outset would impose a further burden on the experimentalist as well as on anyone adapting existing models.

This effectively means that part 5 of the experiment definition requires curation by human experts. This is an opportunity for experimentalists and modelers to collaborate and provides a framework for clarifying assumptions on both sides and reaching agreement on the model. It is also worth noting that once this work has been done once for a specific combination of sub-model and experiment, it can be used for testing and validating future versions of the model.

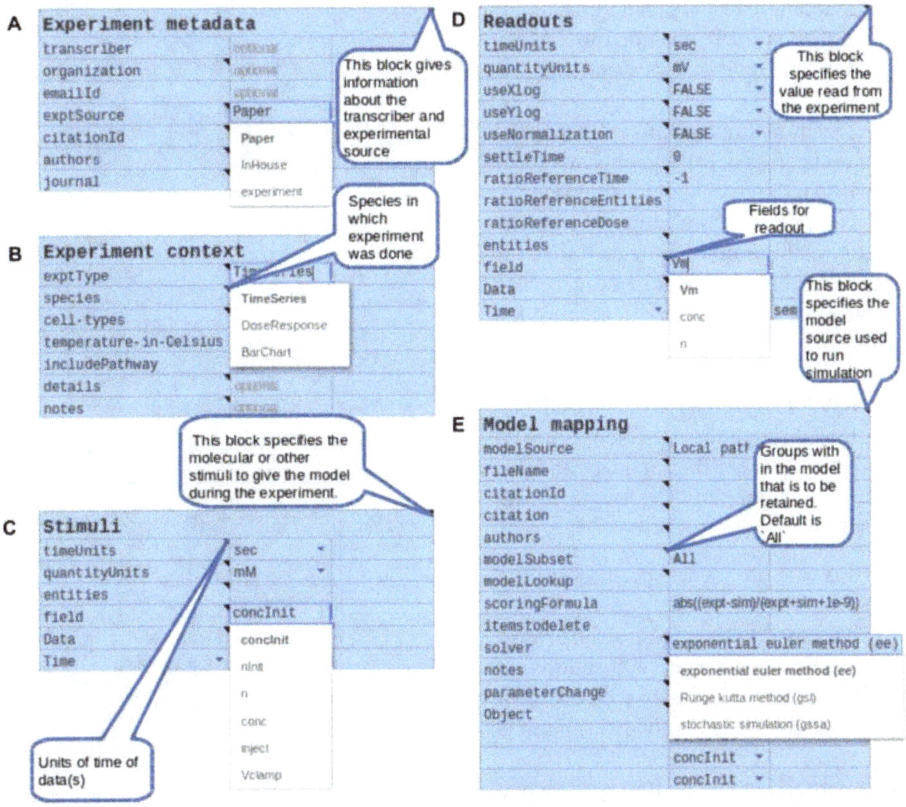

FIGURE 5 | Components of the structured specification of experiment and its mapping to the simulation, implemented as a spreadsheet. In all sections the top line specifies a block of data, and the left column specifies fields to fill in that block. All fields and block titles support tool-tips, that is, pop-up help windows with an explanation of the block and field. These are illustrated here as speech balloons. Fields having a restricted set of options, such as quantity units, are specified with pull-down menus. In several cases there are tabulated sections, which contain value-range limited entries and which can be extended for additional data points. **(A)** Experiment metadata section. This specifies data about the experiment source and who transcribed it. A menu item is illustrated for the "exptSource" field. **(B)** Experiment context section. This specifies biological context for the experiment. **(C)** Stimuli. This section specifies inputs that were given during the experiment: which entity or molecule to change, which parameter was altered, and finally a series of time-value pairs that specifies the stimulus. **(D)** Readouts. This specifies which entities (such as molecules) were monitored during the experiment, and what values were obtained at each readout time. It may include error bars for each value. **(E)** Model mapping. This section is the only model-specific part. It indicates a reference model for which the experiment was first tested. For that model it specifies how to obtain the appropriate subset of pathways, molecules and other model entities to use in the simulated "experiment". The model map next specifies which numerical methods to use. There follows a dictionary of entity names, which maps the experimenter's naming scheme to unique entity names in the simulation. Finally, there is a table of parameters that have to be changed so that the model matches the experimental conditions. For example, some of the molecules in the experiment may now be buffered to specified values.

Having determined the components of the structured experiment specification, we next explain its implementation. Drawing upon lessons from existing projects that implement some parts of these requirements (Wolstencroft et al., 2011, 2017), we chose an enhanced spreadsheet interface as our initial interface (**Figure 5**). Our interface is implemented and exported in Google Docs[2] and additional versions are provided for Microsoft Excel and Open Office. The contents of these spreadsheets are exported to tab-separated value (tsv) files for use by FindSim. We provide a schema for these tsv files[3].

There were several reasons for a first implementation as a spreadsheet. First, spreadsheets are easy to set up and familiar to users. Our spreadsheet interface supports key features such as bounds checking on entered data, for example to ensure that only positive values are used. It also supports pull-down menu options for restricted choices, such as concentration units. Explanatory tool-tips are readily incorporated to provide immediate online help. Spreadsheets are inherently extendable with additional data rows or columns and can easily export data into the standard tab-separated value (tsv) format we use for driving the simulations. Finally, spreadsheets are highly portable, including in the cloud.

Based on a pilot set of ∼40 experiments, we have found that a large range of biochemical experiments can be specified with just three kinds of very similar spreadsheets: time-series, dose-response, and multi-stimulus response. In all cases there are identical panels for experiment metadata and context. There

[2]https://www.ncbs.res.in/faculty/bhalla-findsim/worksheet
[3]https://github.com/BhallaLab/FindSim

are slightly specialized blocks for experimental stimulus and readouts. The final, model mapping panel (**Figure 5E**) is again almost identical. This framework is easily extended to further kinds of experiments, including electrophysiological and imaging data.

In summary, we have designed and implemented a framework for specifying the design and outcomes of experiments in a form which maps directly to corresponding simulation experiments. This supports validation, scoring and optimization of models. The key innovations are formalization of a wide range of experiments and a procedure for defining how to extract parts of a large model that are necessary and sufficient to account for any given experiment.

Example of Data Flow Through the Pipeline

We now illustrate the data flow through the pipeline (**Figure 2**) using a specific example of a pre-existing model, and an experiment to be applied to it (**Figure 6**). The stages in the pipeline are:

1. Model specification. In this case the model specification is a pre-existing SBML file.
2. Experimental details. The experiment is a straightforward stimulus-response experiment in which the 40S subunit of the translation complex is applied to a solution with a known amount of eIF4E-mRNA, and the formation of 43S subunit is monitored.
3. Mapping between experiment and model. As the experimental pathways are a small subset of the larger model, we select a few relevant pathways, and further we remove from the pathway models those reactions that are not present in the experiment.
4. Simulation control. Here we take those molecules that are buffered in the experiment and change the model accordingly. We then run the simulation, applying the stimulus to one of the molecules at the specified times.
5. We now compare experiment and simulation readouts, using a scoring equation defined in the model mapping section from **Figure 5**.
6. At this stage we could use the score to do a local optimization of parameters using manual or automated optimization. This would give us a version of the main model where the local parameters for this pathway have been matched to experiment.
7. We now repeat steps 2 to 6 for different experiments, to obtain a global score for the model. Additionally, local optimizations will need validation from experiments that involve larger subsets of the overall model.

At the end of this process, we will have a model that is a better fit to specific experiments, and we also have a score that can be given to the model as a whole. Note that it is entirely up to the modeler-experimentalist team to decide how much weight should be given to different experiments.

Cross-Experiment Model Reproducibility

A key goal of the FindSim pipeline is to expose models to a range of experiments so that the model is a good fit to all of them, not just a single case. This is a particularly tough constraint when

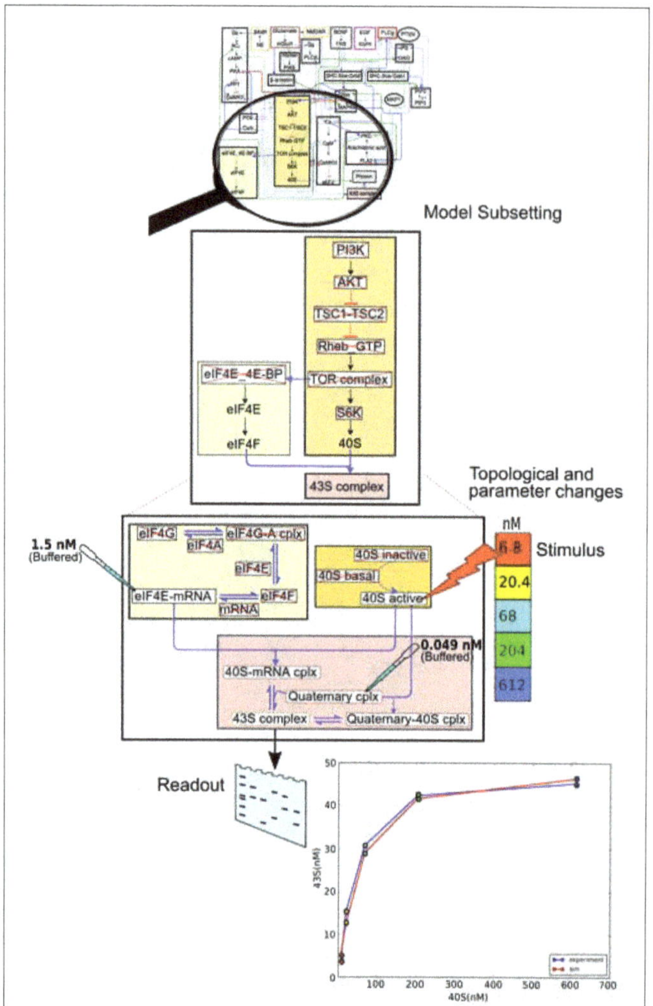

FIGURE 6 | Data flow using the model specification, experiment specification, model subset extraction, simulation and comparison with output.

we have multiple experiments that probe responses of the same and overlapping signaling pathways. In this section we describe how the model database can include just this kind of overlapping experiment, to show how the modeler and experimentalist can together examine reproducibility and generalizability of the core model.

Here we focused our attention on the MAPK signaling pathway. We first considered reproducibility of the core part of this pathway, in which MAPK is stimulated by an epidermal growth factor (EGF) signal in PC12 cells (**Figure 7A**, green boundary; Teng et al., 1995). The simulation approximates the experiment quite closely (**Figure 7B**). We next illustrate a fundamental limitation on being able to reproducibly fit data: the observation that different experiments with very similar contexts may give mutually inconsistent results (**Figures 7B,C**). We then considered experiments involving overlap of the core (MAPK) pathway but distinct input signaling via brain-derived neurotrophic factor (BDNF) in E18 primary embryonic hippocampal neurons (Ji et al., 2010). In the case of BDNF, the core model behavior of a transient strong response followed by

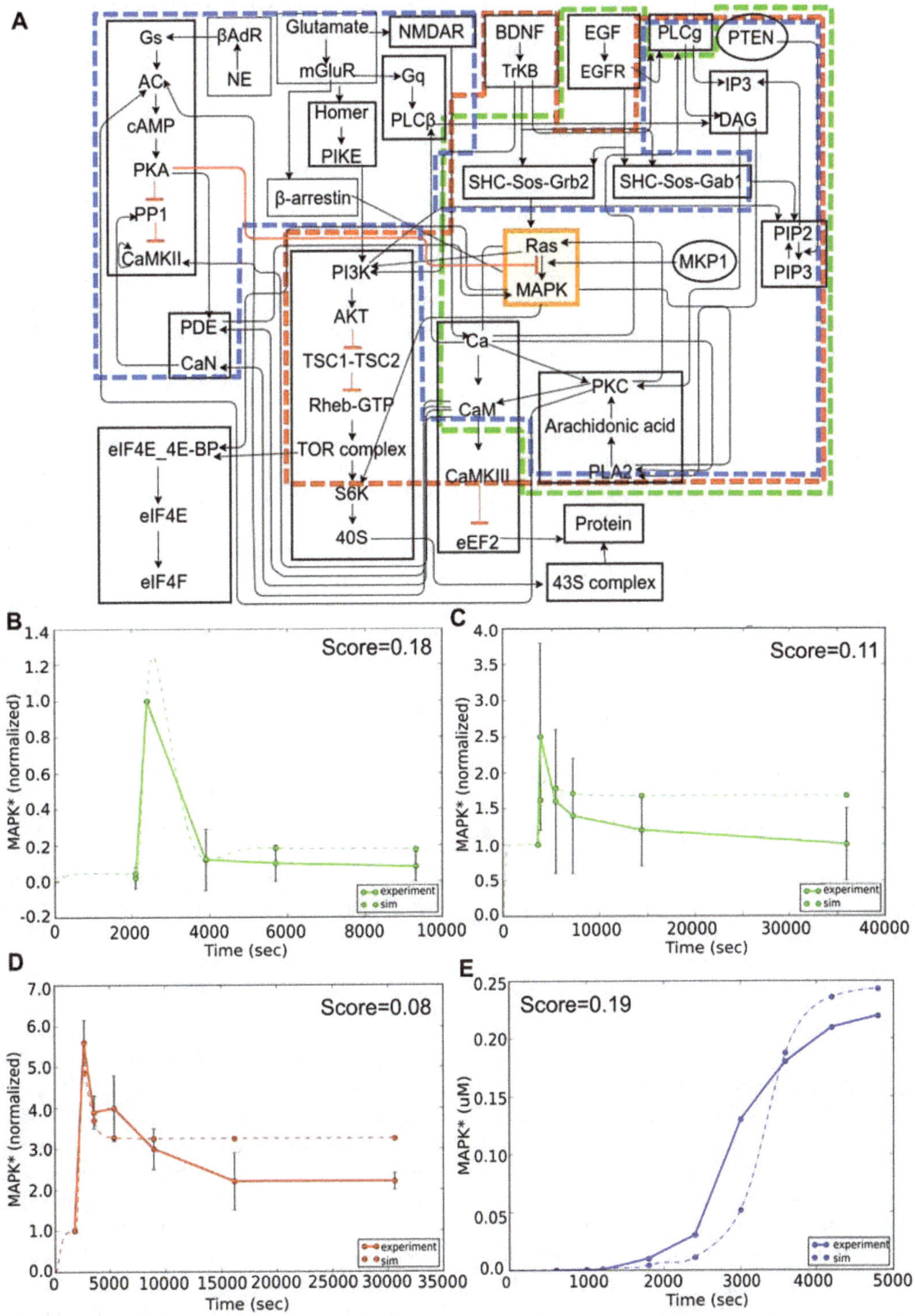

FIGURE 7 | Reproducibility example: multiple experimental inputs converging onto a common signaling pathway (MAPK). **(A)** Block diagram of composite model. Sub-models for the different inputs are indicated in green (epidermal growth factor, EGF), red (BDNF) and blue (Calcium). **(B)** Response to EGF stimulus is a transient activation of MAPK. Model (dashed green line) closely follows experimental curve (solid green line). **(C)** Response to EGF in similar preparation but lower dose. Note that the simulated peak response is higher than experiment in **(B)**, but lower in **(C)**, leading to difficulties in model fitting. **(D)** Response to BDNF stimulus is also a transient, but the time-course of MAPK signaling in this experiment is much longer than it was in panel **(B)**. **(E)** Response to an LTP-induction stimulus for calcium, consisting of three pulses separated by 600 s. Here the reference is an earlier simulation predicting sustained activation of MAPK. Remarkably, there is a reasonable match to the reference behavior in all three cases, despite the inputs converging onto the MAPK pathway through different signaling pathways, and the results drawn from very different data sources.

a sustained low response was preserved, but the time-courses and the intervening stages were quite different. Again, the model performed reasonably well in comparison to this experiment (**Figure 7D**). This was reassuring because it meant that the same core pathway generalized well for two completely different kinds of input. In these two experiments the stimulus and model system are the same, but there is a difference in dose. Even allowing for differences in effective dose, the simulation cannot fit both of these. As discussed above, the FindSim framework provides for a user-defined scoring scheme for each experiment, so that broader considerations can factor into how the user weights each experiment.

Finally, for Ca^{2+} input we asked if the model could replicate the qualitative behavior of sustained activity, that had been predicted in an earlier modeling study (Bhalla and Iyengar, 1999). Again, this activated a large number of distinct input stages but the core MAPK pathway was able to replicate the previous behavior of switching to a state of sustained high activity following three calcium pulses which corresponded to three tetanic stimuli used for LTP induction (**Figure 7E**). Overall, this exercise showed the efficacy of the FindSim framework in testing model reproducibility across quite different stimulus conditions.

DISCUSSION

We have developed FindSim, a framework for systematic, data-driven construction of large biologically detailed models of neuronal signaling. The key advances are: (1) A simulation pipeline that combines a database of structured experimental data with each model, to systematically generate scores of how well the model fits the entire dataset. (2) A way to systematically specify and extract small sub-parts of the full model upon which to carry out these simulated experiments. Together with the underlying Python-driven MOOSE simulation engine for multiscale models, this framework is an open, standards-driven, and scalable approach to developing reliable, large-scale models.

Big Models and Biological Problems

It is widely accepted that complex biological pathways benefit from structured modeling approaches to address the many routes by which signals flow between stimuli and physiological outcomes (Kitano, 2002; Hunter and Borg, 2003). This is particularly relevant for complex neurogenetic diseases such as autism, where mutations in key signaling components cause ramifying perturbations in many pathways. The complexity of this problem is exacerbated by cellular homeostasis mechanisms, which may lead to partial rescue of some symptoms, but not others. The expectation is that as models begin to incorporate the relevant range of pathways, these outcomes may be better understood. Further, such models would be excellent platforms upon which to conduct tests of possible pharmacological and other manipulations with the goal of suggesting treatments (Rajasethupathy et al., 2005).

Correctness of Big Models

A common criticism of big models, dating from the von Neumann tradition, is that they have so many parameters that the modeler could do anything (such as fit an elephant) with them. Here we first explain how the current model building pipeline counters this criticism. We then point to two ways in which the details embedded in a big model improve its testability and utility.

The modeling framework described in this study provides a systematic way to avoid the problems of multi-parameter models. Here we have formalized how multiple experiments map to different parts of the model. Further, this formalization facilitates parameterization, and testing, from individual reactions, to multi-pathway cascades. By testing the models at many scales of function, this approach is able to ensure not only that individual pathways work as observed, but that they work together in a manner consistent with experiment. This process has been adopted, albeit in a more free-form manner, for other large models (Bhalla and Iyengar, 1999; Karr et al., 2012).

There are two key positive aspects that large, detailed models bring to ascertaining correctness. The first is that there is a clear, usually one-to-one mapping between experimental entities (molecules, reactions) and their model counterparts. Thus, there is no ambiguity about what each readout represents. The second major positive of detail is that the curse of the abstract model—that it may abstract away essential functional detail—is avoided. A further, empirically noted corollary of having biologically detailed models is that they tend to partake of similar kinds of functional robustness as their biological counterparts (Morohashi et al., 2002). In biology this means that minor fluctuations in metabolism or protein distribution has little functional effect. In the model this brings the additional benefit that it tends to behave well even if the parameters are, inevitably, somewhat off. Thus, the methodology of the current study is designed to allow principled construction of large, detailed models that avoid the major drawbacks of such models, while benefiting from their advantages.

Big Data and Big Models

Our appreciation for biological complexity has risen steeply with the flood of large-scale data. As an example in neuronal signaling, we now know the identities of some 1500 postsynaptic proteins (Bayés et al., 2011), but our understanding of synaptic function has not kept pace with this explosion of data. Models have long been tools for understanding complex systems, as well as predicting their properties in health and disease (Kitano, 2002; Rajasethupathy et al., 2005). A systematic alignment of big data to developing big models is therefore highly desirable. One of the major problems with doing this is that a large fraction of current experiments is better at providing model *constraints* rather than model *parameters*. A model constraint is an observation that the model must satisfy, but it does not always yield easily usable data for improving the model. For improving models, one needs experiments that more directly provide parameters.

Automated parameter estimation and tuning is important for developing large, complex models. The current framework is designed to efficiently run many simulated experiments on a model, and this is of obvious utility for parameter estimation and tuning. This is a complex and well-studied topic (Chou and Voit, 2009; Geier et al., 2012; Sun et al., 2012) and is out of scope of the current report. A key feature of the FindSim framework is that every run computes a score of how well the model output fits the experiment. Effective scoring is itself closely linked to details of parameter optimization. Here we simply give the user freedom to specify arbitrary mathematical expressions for comparison of model output to experimental output, including error bars (example scoring formula in **Figure 5E**). This expression can also include less-tangible scaling factors based on the judgment of the team implementing the test, such as the reliability of the experimental approach, or whether the experimental system was a mouse or a rat.

Model constraints typically arise from remote input-output relationships. A peculiarity of biological signaling systems is that very long chains of elementary events, such as reactions, may link stimulus and response. For example, long-term potentiation (LTP), which is the staple of synaptic plasticity studies, is mechanistically separated from synaptic input patterns by at least the following steps: presynaptic calcium events, neurotransmitter release, synaptic channel opening, calcium influx, activation of kinase pathways, protein synthesis and receptor translocation (Bliss and Collingridge, 1993). Each of these steps may involve numerous biophysical events and chemical reactions. Yet at an observational level, LTP is reliable, easily measured, and well characterized. It is an excellent model constraint. From a modeling viewpoint, there are far more "good" experiments on LTP, than there are measurements of mechanisms of just one of its steps: dendritic protein synthesis. Big data is therefore of limited value for big models unless the experiments are designed to home in on, and parameterize, finer mechanistic steps. In the context of our modeling pipeline, experiments on small pathways are better for parameterization, including the use of optimization. Long-pathway experiments tell us what the overall model should do, but don't directly help us refine it. Thus, our data-model development framework defines the kinds of big data that are of most relevance to constructing reliable, big models.

Scalability

The current report describes the core concepts and implementation of a first level modelling and data organization effort for models of neuronal signaling. The approach is designed to be scalable both in the kinds of problems it can take on, and in the technical capabilities it brings to the table.

The current framework was designed around studies of autism spectrum disorders, with the technical aim of building sufficiently detailed models so as to be able to match up with the wide range of current data. Thus only a few models were initially envisioned: a control model, and a few with known disease-causing mutations. The approach is readily extended to many other neurodevelopmental and other diseases provided there are clear molecular signatures of the signaling deficit in each case.

An obvious further extension of the approach is to apply it to different cell-types, and in parallel to develop experiment libraries to parameterize them. In addition to neurons, it would be interesting to model glia, and then proceed to making models not just of individual neurons but small groupings of strongly coupled cells in neural tissue.

Scalability can also be envisaged as extending the experiment-model interplay to different physical processes. From the viewpoint of neuronal function, it is clearly important to also consider the domain of electrical activity of neurons. A few simulators (e.g., NEURON, MOOSE, STEPS) are now able to simultaneously model electrical and chemical signaling, but each has different ways to specify such multiscale models (Ray and Bhalla, 2008; Wils and De Schutter, 2009; McDougal et al., 2013). There are efforts to broaden model standards to include chemical as well as electrical signaling (Cannon et al., 2014). While the evolution of the FindSim framework to such models is beyond the scope of the current article, as proof of principle we illustrate the use of the FindSim format on the Hodgkin-Huxley model of an action potential[4]. This requires very minor extensions within the framework of a time-series experiment. We anticipate that an important direction for the FindSim framework will be to support multiscale experiments that synthesize electrophysiological stimuli with multiple signaling and physiological readouts.

A further aspect of scalability is the ability of this framework to host competing models, in the sense that models are hypotheses of neuronal signaling function. Here the value of the open experimental database becomes evident. Different groups can readily re-assign weights and scoring terms for different experiments, to develop models that better fit their interpretation of the experimental literature. The expectation is that such competing models would spur the execution of more definitive experiments to decide between the alternatives, and thus advance the field.

On the technical side, there are clear directions with respect to the evolution of the experiment specification format, including standards development for storing them in databases.

The current experiment specification is set up through a spreadsheet and stored in tab-separated value (tsv) format. Clearly a more flexible and powerful format would be desirable as we scale up to much larger models and datasets. We have considered extensions to the extant SED-ML standard (Waltemath et al., 2011) as one possible way to define the experiments. Another alternative may be JSON and its associated schema (Crockford, 2006). Each of these is also much better suited to being handled in a database. On the interface front it would be desirable to develop a browser-based graphical interface to the model/experiment building pipeline, where the runs may be hosted in the cloud. These all lend themselves to incorporation into the FindSim framework. In summary, the FindSim framework is a principled, scalable framework that lends itself to reproducibly integrating experiments with complex multiscale models of neuronal signaling systems.

The FindSim framework currently relies on human interactions between modelers and experimentalists for the "model mapping" (part 5 of the pipeline). This was a conscious

[4]https://github.com/BhallaLab/FindSim

choice on our part. This stage of the framework is an ideal place for encouraging interaction between human experts, since this is a stage that relies on expert judgment on what the various parts of a model and of an experiment mean. In terms of scalability, this may be a bottleneck. Indeed, other initiatives have aimed at automating similar processes (Cooper et al., 2011; Alm et al., 2015; Neal et al., 2015). It should be noted, however, that those automations depend on high-quality annotations. As such, they do not eliminate the need for human curation, it just happens at a different stage of the process (model/data annotation). Which of those two approaches is ultimately better scalable, and to what extent the expert annotation component can be automated, remains an interesting avenue for future research.

AUTHOR CONTRIBUTIONS

NV built the model, assembled the database of experimental conditions, designed the experiment interface and worked on the figures. GVHR worked on the code, designed the experiment interface and on the figures. MS examined existing model development projects, helped conceptualize the framework and wrote the article. UB worked on the code, designed the project and experiment interface and wrote the article.

FUNDING

GVHR was supported by the B-Life grant to UB from the Department of Biotechnology (DBT), Ministry of Science and Technology BT/PR12422/MED/31/287/2014. NV was supported by University Grants Commission (UGC)-ISF grant F.6-18/2014 (IC) to UB. UB is supported by National Centre for Biological Sciences, Tata Institute of Fundamental Research (NCBS-TIFR) and the J. C. Bose Fellowship SB/S2/JCB-023/2016.

ACKNOWLEDGMENTS

We acknowledge thoughtful discussions with Dagmar Waltemath, Jacob Snoep and Stuart Owen. We are also grateful to Aditi Bhattacharya and Richard Fitzpatrick for discussions on the framework and helping flesh out the requirements for data reporting.

REFERENCES

Alm, R., Waltemath, D., Wolfien, M., Wolkenhauer, O., and Henkel, R. (2015). Annotation-based feature extraction from sets of SBML models. *J. Biomed. Semantics* 6:20. doi: 10.1186/s13326-015-0014-4

Ashburner, M., Ball, C. A., Blake, J. A., Botstein, D., Butler, H., Cherry, J. M., et al. (2000). Gene ontology: tool for the unification of biology. The gene ontology consortium. *Nat. Genet.* 25, 25–29. doi: 10.1038/75556

Bayés, A., van de Lagemaat, L. N., Collins, M. O., Croning, M. D. R., Whittle, I. R., Choudhary, J. S., et al. (2011). Characterization of the proteome, diseases and evolution of the human postsynaptic density. *Nat. Neurosci.* 14, 19–21. doi: 10.1038/nn.2719

Beard, D. A., Britten, R., Cooling, M. T., Garny, A., Halstead, M. D. B., Hunter, P. J., et al. (2009). CellML metadata standards, associated tools and repositories. *Philos. Trans. A Math. Phys. Eng. Sci.* 367, 1845–1867. doi: 10.1098/rsta.2008.0310

Bhalla, U. S. (2002a). The chemical organization of signaling interactions. *Bioinformatics* 18, 855–863. doi: 10.1093/bioinformatics/18.6.855

Bhalla, U. S. (2002b). Use of kinetikit and GENESIS for modeling signaling pathways. *Methods Enzymol.* 345, 3–23. doi: 10.1016/s0076-6879(02) 45003-3

Bhalla, U. S., and Bower, J. M. (1993). Exploring parameter space in detailed single neuron models: simulations of the mitral and granule cells of the olfactory bulb. *J. Neurophysiol.* 69, 1948–1965. doi: 10.1152/jn.1993.69.6.1948

Bhalla, U. S., and Iyengar, R. (1999). Emergent properties of networks of biological signaling pathways. *Science* 283, 381–387. doi: 10.1126/science.283.5400.381

Bhalla, U. S., and Iyengar, R. (2001). Functional modules in biological signalling networks. *Novartis Found. Symp.* 239, 4–13; discussion 13–15, 45–51. doi: 10.1002/0470846674.ch2

Bliss, T. V., and Collingridge, G. L. (1993). A synaptic model of memory: long-term potentiation in the hippocampus. *Nature* 361, 31–39. doi: 10.1038/361031a0

Brazma, A., Hingamp, P., Quackenbush, J., Sherlock, G., Spellman, P., Stoeckert, C., et al. (2001). Minimum information about a microarray experiment (MIAME)-toward standards for microarray data. *Nat. Genet.* 29, 365–371. doi: 10.1038/ng1201-365

Brown, S.-A., Moraru, I. I., Schaff, J. C., and Loew, L. M. (2011). Virtual NEURON: a strategy for merged biochemical and electrophysiological modeling. *J. Comput. Neurosci.* 31, 385–400. doi: 10.1007/s10827-011-0317-0

Cannon, R. C., Gleeson, P., Crook, S., Ganapathy, G., Marin, B., Piasini, E., et al. (2014). LEMS: a language for expressing complex biological models in concise and hierarchical form and its use in underpinning NeuroML 2. *Front. Neuroinform.* 8:79. doi: 10.3389/fninf.2014.00079

Chou, I.-C., and Voit, E. O. (2009). Recent developments in parameter estimation and structure identification of biochemical and genomic systems. *Math. Biosci.* 219, 57–83. doi: 10.1016/j.mbs.2009.03.002

Cooper, J., Mirams, G. R., and Niederer, S. A. (2011). High-throughput functional curation of cellular electrophysiology models. *Prog. Biophys. Mol. Biol.* 107, 11–20. doi: 10.1016/j.pbiomolbio.2011.06.003

Crockford, D. (2006). The application/json Media Type for JavaScript Object Notation (JSON). Available online at: https://tools.ietf.org/html/rfc4627 [Accessed May 15, 2018].

De Schutter, E., and Bower, J. M. (1994). An active membrane model of the cerebellar Purkinje cell. I. Simulation of current clamps in slice. *J. Neurophysiol.* 71, 375–400. doi: 10.1152/jn.1994.71.1.375

Garcia, S., Guarino, D., Jaillet, F., Jennings, T. R., Pröpper, R., Rautenberg, P. L., et al. (2014). Neo: an object model for handling electrophysiology data in multiple formats. *Front. Neuroinformatics* 8:10. doi: 10.3389/fninf.2014.00010

Geier, F., Fengos, G., Felizzi, F., and Iber, D. (2012). Analyzing and constraining signaling networks: parameter estimation for the user. *Methods Mol. Biol.* 880, 23–39. doi: 10.1007/978-1-61779-833-7_2

Gleeson, P., Crook, S., Cannon, R. C., Hines, M. L., Billings, G. O., Farinella, M., et al. (2010). NeuroML: a language for describing data driven models of neurons and networks with a high degree of biological detail. *PLoS Comput. Biol.* 6:e1000815. doi: 10.1371/journal.pcbi.1000815

Gleeson, P., Silver, A., and Cantarelli, M. (2015). "Open source brain," in *Encyclopedia of Computational Neuroscience* (New York, NY: Springer.), 2153–2156.

Gouwens, N. W., Berg, J., Feng, D., Sorensen, S. A., Zeng, H., Hawrylycz, M. J., et al. (2018). Systematic generation of biophysically detailed models for diverse cortical neuron types. *Nat. Commun.* 9:710. doi: 10.1038/s41467-017-02718-3

HarshaRani, G. V., Vayttaden, S. J., and Bhalla, U. S. (2005). Electronic data sources for kinetic models of cell signaling. *J. Biochem. (Tokyo)* 137, 653–657. doi: 10.1093/jb/mvi083

Hayer, A., and Bhalla, U. S. (2005). Molecular switches at the synapse emerge from receptor and kinase traffic. *PLoS Comput. Biol.* 1, 137–154. doi: 10.1371/journal.pcbi.0010020

Heil, K. F., Wysocka, E., Sorokina, O., Kotaleski, J. H., Simpson, T. I., Armstrong, J. D., et al. (2018). Analysis of proteins in computational models of synaptic plasticity. *BioRxiv* [Preprint]. doi: 10.1101/254094

Hodgkin, A. L., and Huxley, A. F. (1952). A quantitative description of membrane current and its application to conduction and excitation in nerve. *J. Physiol.* 117, 500–544.

Hucka, M., Finney, A., Sauro, H. M., Bolouri, H., Doyle, J. C., Kitano, H., et al. (2003). The systems biology markup language (SBML): a medium for representation and exchange of biochemical network models. *Bioinformatics* 19, 524–531. doi: 10.1093/bioinformatics/btg015

Hucka, M., Nickerson, D. P., Bader, G. D., Bergmann, F. T., Cooper, J., Demir, E., et al. (2015). Promoting coordinated development of community-based information standards for modeling in biology: the COMBINE initiative. *Front. Bioeng. Biotechnol.* 3:19. doi: 10.3389/fbioe.2015.00019

Hunter, P. J., and Borg, T. K. (2003). Integration from proteins to organs: the physiome project. *Nat. Rev. Mol. Cell Biol.* 4, 237–243. doi: 10.1038/nrm1054

Jain, P., and Bhalla, U. S. (2009). Signaling logic of activity-triggered dendritic protein synthesis: an mTOR gate but not a feedback switch. *PLoS Comput. Biol.* 5:e1000287. doi: 10.1371/journal.pcbi.1000287

Ji, Y., Lu, Y., Yang, F., Shen, W., Tang, T. T.-T., Feng, L., et al. (2010). Acute and gradual increases in BDNF concentration elicit distinct signaling and functions in neurons. *Nat. Neurosci.* 13, 302–309. doi: 10.3410/f.3559973.3266072

Karr, J. R., Sanghvi, J. C., Macklin, D. N., Gutschow, M. V., Jacobs, J. M., Bolival, B., et al. (2012). A Whole-cell computational model predicts phenotype from genotype. *Cell* 150, 389–401. doi: 10.1016/j.cell.2012.05.044

Kent, W. J., Zweig, A. S., Barber, G., Hinrichs, A. S., and Karolchik, D. (2010). BigWig and BigBed: enabling browsing of large distributed datasets. *Bioinforma. Oxf. Engl.* 26, 2204–2207. doi: 10.1093/bioinformatics/btq351

Kim, M., Huang, T., Abel, T., and Blackwell, K. T. (2010). Temporal sensitivity of protein kinase a activation in late-phase long term potentiation. *PLoS Comput. Biol.* 6:e1000691. doi: 10.1371/journal.pcbi.1000691

Kitano, H. (2002). Systems biology: a brief overview. *Science* 295, 1662–1664. doi: 10.1126/science.1069492

Le Novère, N., Bornstein, B., Broicher, A., Courtot, M., Donizelli, M., Dharuri, H., et al. (2006). BioModels Database: a free, centralized database of curated, published, quantitative kinetic models of biochemical and cellular systems. *Nucleic Acids Res.* 34, D689–D691. doi: 10.1093/nar/gkj092

Li, L., Stefan, M. I., and Novère, N. L. (2012). Calcium input frequency, duration and Aamplitude differentially modulate the relative activation of calcineurin and CaMKII. *PLoS One* 7:e43810. doi: 10.1371/journal.pone.0043810

Lindskog, M., Kim, M., Wikström, M. A., Blackwell, K. T., and Kotaleski, J. H. (2006). Transient calcium and dopamine increase PKA activity and DARPP-32 phosphorylation. *PLoS Comput. Biol.* 2:e119. doi: 10.1371/journal.pcbi.0020119

Lisman, J. E. (1985). A mechanism for memory storage insensitive to molecular turnover: a bistable autophosphorylating kinase. *Proc. Natl. Acad. Sci. U S A* 82, 3055–3057. doi: 10.1073/pnas.82.9.3055

Manninen, T., Hituri, K., Kotaleski, J. H., Blackwell, K. T., and Linne, M.-L. (2010). Postsynaptic signal transduction models for long-term potentiation and depression. *Front. Comput. Neurosci.* 4:152. doi: 10.3389/fncom.2010.00152

Markram, H., Muller, E., Ramaswamy, S., Reimann, M. W., Abdellah, M., Sanchez, C. A., et al. (2015). Reconstruction and simulation of neocortical microcircuitry. *Cell* 163, 456–492. doi: 10.1016/j.cell.2015.09.029

Matiasz, N. J., Wood, J., Wang, W., Silva, A. J., and Hsu, W. (2017). Computer-aided experiment planning toward causal discovery in neuroscience. *Front. Neuroinform.* 11:12. doi: 10.3389/fninf.2017.00012

McDougal, R. A., Hines, M. L., and Lytton, W. W. (2013). Reaction-diffusion in the NEURON simulator. *Front. Neuroinformatics* 7:28. doi: 10.3389/fninf.2013.00028

Migliore, M., Morse, T. M., Davison, A. P., Marenco, L., Shepherd, G. M., and Hines, M. L. (2003). ModelDB: making models publicly accessible to support computational neuroscience. *Neuroinformatics* 1, 135–139. doi: 10.1385/ni:1:1:135

Morohashi, M., Winn, A. E., Borisuk, M. T., Bolouri, H., Doyle, J., and Kitano, H. (2002). Robustness as a measure of plausibility in models of biochemical networks. *J. Theor. Biol.* 216, 19–30. doi: 10.1006/jtbi.2002.2537

Narayanan, R., and Johnston, D. (2010). The h current is a candidate mechanism for regulating the sliding modification threshold in a BCM-like synaptic learning rule. *J. Neurophysiol.* 104, 1020–1033. doi: 10.1152/jn.01129.2009

Neal, M. L., Carlson, B. E., Thompson, C. T., James, R. C., Kim, K. G., Tran, K., et al. (2015). Semantics-based composition of integrated cardiomyocyte models motivated by real-world use cases. *PLoS One* 10:e0145621. doi: 10.1371/journal.pone.0145621

Rajasethupathy, P., Vayttaden, S. J., and Bhalla, U. S. (2005). Systems modeling: a pathway to drug discovery. *Curr. Opin. Chem. Biol.* 9, 400–406. doi: 10.1016/j.cbpa.2005.06.008

Ray, S., and Bhalla, U. S. (2008). PyMOOSE: Interoperable Scripting in Python for MOOSE. *Front. Neuroinform.* 2:6. doi: 10.3389/neuro.11.006.2008

Ray, S., Chintaluri, C., Bhalla, U. S., and Wójcik, D. K. (2016). NSDF: neuroscience simulation data format. *Neuroinformatics* 14, 147–167. doi: 10.1007/s12021-015-9282-5

Rübel, O., Dougherty, M., Prabhat, Denes, P., Conant, D., Chang, E. F., et al. (2016). Methods for specifying scientific data standards and modeling relationships with applications to neuroscience. *Front. Neuroinform.* 10:48. doi: 10.3389/fninf.2016.00048

Shouval, H. Z., Bear, M. F., and Cooper, L. N. (2002). A unified model of NMDA receptor-dependent bidirectional synaptic plasticity. *Proc. Natl. Acad. Sci. U. S. A.* 99, 10831–10836. doi: 10.1073/pnas.152343099

Silva, A. J., and Müller, K.-R. (2015). The need for novel informatics tools for integrating and planning research in molecular and cellular cognition. *Learn. Mem.* 22, 494–498. doi: 10.1101/lm.029355.112

Sivakumaran, S., Hariharaputran, S., Mishra, J., and Bhalla, U. S. (2003). The Database of Quantitative Cellular Signaling: management and analysis of chemical kinetic models of signaling networks. *Bioinformatics* 19, 408–415. doi: 10.1093/bioinformatics/btf860

Smolen, P., Baxter, D. A., and Byrne, J. H. (2006). A model of the roles of essential kinases in the induction and expression of late long-term potentiation. *Biophys. J.* 90, 2760–2775. doi: 10.1529/biophysj.105.072470

Stead, M., and Halford, J. J. (2016). Proposal for a standard format for neurophysiology data recording and exchange. *J. Clin. Neurophysiol.* 33, 403–413. doi: 10.1097/WNP.0000000000000257

Stefan, M. I., Edelstein, S. J., and Le Novère, N. (2008). An allosteric model of calmodulin explains differential activation of PP2B and CaMKII. *Proc. Natl. Acad. Sci. U S A* 105, 10768–10773. doi: 10.1073/pnas.0810309105

Stefan, M. I., Marshall, D. P., and Novère, N. L. (2012). Structural analysis and stochastic modelling suggest a mechanism for calmodulin trapping by CaMKII. *PLoS One* 7:e29406. doi: 10.1371/journal.pone.0029406

Stockton, D. B., and Santamaria, F. (2017). Integrating the allen brain institute cell types database into automated neuroscience workflow. *Neuroinformatics* 15, 333–342. doi: 10.1007/s12021-017-9337-x

Sun, J., Garibaldi, J. M., and Hodgman, C. (2012). Parameter estimation using meta-heuristics in systems biology: a comprehensive review. *IEEE/ACM Trans. Comput. Biol. Bioinform.* 9, 185–202. doi: 10.1109/tcbb.2011.63

Taylor, C. F., Hermjakob, H., Julian, R. K., Garavelli, J. S., Aebersold, R., and Apweiler, R. (2006). The work of the human proteome organisation's proteomics standards initiative (HUPO PSI). *OMICS* 10, 145–151. doi: 10.1089/omi.2006.10.145

Taylor, C. F., Paton, N. W., Lilley, K. S., Binz, P.-A., Julian, R. K., Jones, A. R., et al. (2007). The minimum information about a proteomics experiment (MIAPE). *Nat. Biotechnol.* 25, 887–893. doi: 10.1038/nbt1329

Teeters, J. L., Godfrey, K., Young, R., Dang, C., Friedsam, C., Wark, B., et al. (2015). Neurodata without borders: creating a common data format for neurophysiology. *Neuron* 88, 629–634. doi: 10.1016/j.neuron.2015.10.025

Teng, K. K., Lander, H., Fajardo, J. E., Hanafusa, H., Hempstead, B. L., and Birge, R. B. (1995). v-Crk modulation of growth factor-induced PC12 cell differentiation involves the Src homology 2 domain of v-Crk and sustained activation of the Ras/mitogen-activated protein kinase pathway. *J. Biol. Chem.* 270, 20677–20685. doi: 10.1074/jbc.270.35.20677

Waltemath, D., Adams, R., Bergmann, F. T., Hucka, M., Kolpakov, F., Miller, A. K., et al. (2011). Reproducible computational biology experiments with SED-ML--the simulation experiment description markup language. *BMC Syst. Biol.* 5:198. doi: 10.1186/1752-0509-5-198

Wils, S., and De Schutter, E. (2009). STEPS: modeling and simulating complex reaction-diffusion systems with python. *Front. Neuroinform.* 3:15. doi: 10.3389/neuro.11.015.2009

Wolstencroft, K., Krebs, O., Snoep, J. L., Stanford, N. J., Bacall, F., Golebiewski, M., et al. (2017). FAIRDOMHub: a repository and collaboration environment for sharing systems biology research. *Nucleic Acids Res.* 45, D404–D407. doi: 10.1093/nar/gkw1032

Wolstencroft, K., Owen, S., Horridge, M., Krebs, O., Mueller, W., Snoep, J. L., et al. (2011). RightField: embedding ontology annotation in spreadsheets. *Bioinformatics* 27, 2021–2022. doi: 10.1093/bioinformatics/btr312

4

Parameter Optimization Using Covariance Matrix Adaptation—Evolutionary Strategy (CMA-ES), an Approach to Investigate Differences in Channel Properties Between Neuron Subtypes

Zbigniew Jędrzejewski-Szmek[1†], *Karina P. Abrahao*[2], *Joanna Jędrzejewska-Szmek*[1†], *David M. Lovinger*[2] and *Kim T. Blackwell*[1,3*]

[1] Krasnow Institute of Advanced Study, George Mason University, Fairfax, VA, United States, [2] Laboratory for Integrative Neuroscience, Section on Synaptic Pharmacology, National Institute on Alcohol Abuse and Alcoholism, National Institutes of Health, Rockville, MD, United States, [3] Department of Bioengineering, Volgenau School of Engineering, George Mason University, Fairfax, VA, United States

***Correspondence:**
Kim T. Blackwell
kblackw1@gmu.edu

†Present Address:
Zbigniew Jędrzejewski-Szmek,
Red Hat Poland, Warsaw, Poland
Joanna Jędrzejewska-Szmek,
Department of Neurophysiology,
Nencki Institute of Experimental
Biology, Warsaw, Poland

Computational models in neuroscience can be used to predict causal relationships between biological mechanisms in neurons and networks, such as the effect of blocking an ion channel or synaptic connection on neuron activity. Since developing a biophysically realistic, single neuron model is exceedingly difficult, software has been developed for automatically adjusting parameters of computational neuronal models. The ideal optimization software should work with commonly used neural simulation software; thus, we present software which works with models specified in declarative format for the MOOSE simulator. Experimental data can be specified using one of two different file formats. The fitness function is customizable as a weighted combination of feature differences. The optimization itself uses the covariance matrix adaptation-evolutionary strategy, because it is robust in the face of local fluctuations of the fitness function, and deals well with a high-dimensional and discontinuous fitness landscape. We demonstrate the versatility of the software by creating several model examples of each of four types of neurons (two subtypes of spiny projection neurons and two subtypes of globus pallidus neurons) by tuning to current clamp data. Optimizations reached convergence within 1,600–4,000 model evaluations (200–500 generations × population size of 8). Analysis of the parameters of the best fitting models revealed differences between neuron subtypes, which are consistent with prior experimental results. Overall our results suggest that this easy-to-use, automatic approach for finding neuron channel parameters may be applied to current clamp recordings from neurons exhibiting different biochemical markers to help characterize ionic differences between other neuron subtypes.

Keywords: striatum, globus pallidus, MOOSE, neuronal model, biophysics, ion channels

INTRODUCTION

Computational models of neurons and networks are being used increasingly to test hypotheses regarding causation of biological mechanisms, e.g., ion channels, on neuron function. For example, the effect of blocking an ion channel on neuron activity (Tucker et al., 2012; Qian et al., 2014), the effect of a synaptic connection on network activity (Prinz et al., 2004; Damodaran et al., 2015), or the effect of morphology on neuron firing patterns (Schaefer et al., 2003; Meza et al., 2018) can be tested by computational models. Unlike in wet lab experiments, neither non-specific effects of drugs nor compensatory effects during development confound the results. Computational models also can be used to determine whether the observed differences in voltage trajectory (e.g., action potential width or firing rate) between neuron classes correspond to differences in ion channel conductances (Rumbell et al., 2016).

Whereas the simulation experiments (comparison of control and treatment models) are relatively simple, creation of the control model is exceedingly difficult. Developing a biophysically realistic, single neuron model requires equations describing ionic channel kinetics developed from voltage clamp data (Gurkiewicz and Korngreen, 2007; Taylor et al., 2009), cell morphology (Segev and London, 2000; Van Ooyen et al., 2002), and then ionic channel conductances are adjusted to match firing properties of the target neuron. The number of parameters and the non-linear interactions between ionic channels makes adjusting the parameters an extremely difficult problem. Furthermore, changes in current density of an outward current can be compensated by similar changes to inward current density or opposite changes to other outward currents (Marder and Goaillard, 2006). Thus, a single neuron class has numerous sets of parameters that produce the same observed physiology.

Several approaches have been developed recently for automatically adjusting parameters of computational neuronal models. Given the increase in computing power, the number of publications is increasing; thus, for brevity, we will mostly discuss the recent publications and refer the reader to a previous review of earlier publications (Van Geit et al., 2008). These methods vary not only in the search technique (i.e., the method of sampling the parameter space), but also in the fitness function used and the data used to fit the model. Perhaps the most successful approach is to fit a model to simulated data (Vanier and Bower, 1999; Brookings et al., 2014). The advantage of this approach is that a known solution exists. The disadvantage is that the goal of most parameter optimization is to fit electrophysiology data, which is a more difficult undertaking.

All optimization algorithms use one or more fitness functions (also called cost functions), which are measures of similarity between the model and the experiment. Comparing simulated and experimental voltage traces directly is a difficult problem, because a millisecond change in spike time, which misaligns the spikes, may produce a large difference in Euclidean distance between traces (though only a minor change in perceived similarity). A clever solution to this problem is to apply an adjustment in the simulation values, based on the difference between experimental and simulated values, to promote alignment of the traces (Abarbanel et al., 2009; Brookings et al., 2014). If multiple data traces are being fit, the similarity of each trace needs to be weighted to calculate an overall similarity value. A more common solution is to extract features of the voltage traces, such as spike width and firing rate, and then either combine them into a single objective (Holmes et al., 2006; Rumbell et al., 2016) or use a multi-objective optimization method (Druckmann et al., 2007; Hay et al., 2011; Rumbell et al., 2016; Neymotin et al., 2017). Feature extraction avoids the problem of spike alignment, but compounds the problem of how to weight the different features when combined into a single-objective.

Most of the modern search methods use variants of evolutionary algorithms (Vanier and Bower, 1999; Keren et al., 2005; Hendrickson et al., 2011b; Brookings et al., 2014; Martínez-Álvarez et al., 2016; Rumbell et al., 2016; Martínez-Cañada et al., 2017; Neymotin et al., 2017). The covariance matrix adaptation evolutionary strategy is a modern evolutionary algorithm that works quite well for large numbers of parameters (Hansen and Kern, 2004). CMA-ES combines an evolutionary approach with a model of the fitness landscape. In an evoluationary approach, a population of sample points (a sample point is the set of parameters that describe an individual model) is used to generate a new set of points to test, and the subset of points with the best fitness survives to the next generation. In CMA-ES the differences in average fitness between subsequent populations are used to evolve the center of the population toward the optimum. Moreover, knowledge about the interaction between parameters is iteratively gathered in a covariance matrix, which is used to allocate new sampling points so that points are close together in the directions which are well described and further apart in other directions. Because a derivative is never calculated, and just the ranking between solutions is used, this method is resilient to local fluctuations in the fitness landscape.

To simplify model creation, parameter tuning and reproducibility, the parameter optimization algorithm should work with models specified by a declarative model specification. Creation of neuronal models is a time consuming and error prone process, and model code all too often is written in a fashion that impedes reproducibility and extensibility (Gewaltig and Cannon, 2014). A declarative model specification, which separates the model parameters from the simulation itself, e.g., NeuroML (Gleeson et al., 2010; Cannon et al., 2014) or NineML (Raikov et al., 2011; Richmond et al., 2014) simplifies model development and enhances reproducibility. Furthermore, to enhance utility of a parameter optimization algorithm, setting up the optimization and specification of parameters to vary should be independent of the model specification itself.

We describe a versatile software tool, written in Python for the MOOSE simulator (Ray and Bhalla, 2008), for model creation and automatic parameter optimization that can be used by experimentalists and theoreticians alike to automatically fit a model to experimental traces for different neuron types without delving into simulator-specific details.

TABLE 1 | Types and subtypes of neurons used in the simulations.

Type	Subtypes	Names
Striatal Spiny Projecton (SP) neurons	Dopamine D1 receptor containing spiny projection neuron	D1-SPN
	Dopamine D2 receptor containing spiny projection neuron	D2-SPN
Globus Pallidus (GPe) neurons	Arkypallidal neuron	ArkyN
	Prototypical neuron	ProtoN

METHODS

Overview

We created multi-compartment, multi-conductance models of two neuron types. **Table 1** lists the two subtypes of neurons of the external globus pallidus (GPe): arkypallidal neuron (ArkyN) and prototypical neuron (ProtoN); and the two subtypes of striatal neurons: dopamine D1 receptor containing spiny projection neurons (D1-SPN) and dopamine D2 receptor containing spiny projection neurons (D2-SPN). To facilitate model development and inspection, we use a declarative parameter specification to create the models. Python scripts interpret the parameters to create and simulate the multi-compartmental, multi-ion channel model using the MOOSE simulator. For the parameter optimization, the simulated voltage response to current injection is compared to experimentally measured membrane potential using a feature-based fitness function. The parameters are optimized using the covariance matrix adaptation evolutionary strategy (https://github.com/CMA-ES/pycma).

Model Specification

To facilitate reproducibility, re-use and extension, the declarative model specification uses a modular format. The ion channel kinetics are specified in one file: (https://github.com/neurord/moose_nerp/blob/master/moose_nerp/d1d2/param_chan.py), e.g.,

```
# param_chan.py
from moose_nerp.prototypes.util import
  NamedDict
from moose_nerp.prototypes.chan_proto
  import (
    SSTauQuadraticChannelParams,
    AlphaBetaChannelParams,
    TauInfMinChannelParams,
    ChannelSettings,
    TypicalOneD)

qfactNaF = 2.5
Na_m_params = SSTauQuadraticChannelParams(
    SS_min = 0.0,
    SS_vdep = 1.0,
    SS_vhalf = -25e-3,
    SS_vslope = -10e-3,
    taumin = 0.1e-3/qfactNaF,
    tauVdep = 2.1025e-3/qfactNaF,
    tauVhalf = -62e-3,
    tauVslope = 8e-3)
Na_h_params = TauInfMinChannelParams(
    T_min = 2*0.2754e-3/qfactNaF,
    T_vdep = 2*1.2e-3/qfactNaF,
    T_vhalf = -42e-3,
    T_vslope = 3e-3,
    SS_min = 0.0,
    SS_vdep = 1.0,
    SS_vhalf = -60e-3,
    SS_vslope = 6e-3)
NaFparam = ChannelSettings(Xpow=3, Ypow=1,
  Zpow=0, Erev=50e-3, name='NaF')

KDr_X_params = AlphaBetaChannelParams(
    A_rate = 28.2,
    A_B = 0,
    A_C = 0.0,
    A_vhalf = 0,
    A_vslope = -12.5e-3,
    B_rate = 6.78,
    B_B = 0.0,
    B_C = 0.0,
    B_vhalf = 0.0,
    B_vslope = 33.5e-3)
KDr_Y_params = []
KDrparam = ChannelSettings(Xpow=1, Ypow=0,
  Zpow=0, Erev=-90e-3, name='KDr')

Channels = NamedDict(
'Channels',
    Krp = TypicalOneD(KDrparam, KDr_X_params
      , KDr_Y_params),
    NaF = TypicalOneD(NaFparam, Na_m_params,
       Na_h_params),
)
```

Both the morphology file (either standard GENESIS .p files or .swc files are supported by MOOSE) and conductances (in units of Siemens/m^2) are specified in a separate file (https://github.com/neurord/moose_nerp/blob/master/moose_nerp/d1d2/param_cond.py), e.g.,

```
# param_cond.py
from moose_nerp.prototypes.util import
  NamedDict

morph_file = {'D1':'MScell-Entire.p',
              'D2': 'MScell-Entire.p'}
NAME_SOMA='soma'

prox = (0, 26.1e-6) #units are meters
med = (26.1e-6, 50e-6)
dist = (50e-6, 1000e-6)

_D1 = NamedDict(
    'D1',
    KDr = {prox:150.963, med:70.25,
           dist:77.25},
```

```
    NaF = {prox:130e3, med:1894, dist:927},
)
_D2 = NamedDict(
    'D2',
    KDr = {prox:177.25, med:177.25, dist:27
      .25},
    NaF = {prox:150.0e3, med:2503, dist:1073
      },
)
Condset = NamedDict(
    'Condset',
    D1 = _D1,
    D2 = _D2,
)
```

Explicit spines, calcium dynamics, and synaptic channels are each optional and specified in separate files. Calcium dynamics can be specified either with a single time constant of decay or utilizing various mechanisms such as calcium buffers, pumps and diffusion. Model stimulation, creation of output elements and model simulation are clearly and explicitly separated from the model creation. Parameter specification files are imported in https://github.com/neurord/moose_nerp/blob/master/moose_nerp/d1d2/__init__.py:

```
# __init__.py
from .param_chan import (VMIN, VMAX, VDIVS,
           CAMIN, CAMAX, CADIVS,
           qfactNaF,
           Channels)
from .param_cond import (ghKluge,
           neurontypes,
           ConcOut, Temp,
           morph_file,
           Condset)

spineYN = False
synYN = False
calYN = True
```

Given these parameter files, the model creation and simulation procedures are implemented in __main__.py, e.g.:

```
# __main__.py
from moose_nerp.prototypes import
            (cell_proto,
            inject_func,
            standard_options)
from moose_nerp import d1d2
import moose

option_parser = standard_options
  .standard_options()
param_sim = option_parser.parse_args()

syn,neuron= cell_proto.neuronclasses(d1d2)
neuron_paths = {ntype:[neuron.path] for
(ntype, neuron) in neuron.items()}
pg = inject_func.setupinj(d1d2,
              param_sim.injection_delay,
              param_sim.injection_width,
              neuron_paths)
for injection_current in param_sim.
  injection_current:
  pg.firstLevel = injection_current
  moose.reinit()
  moose.start(param_sim.simtime) # this
    runs simulation for 'simtime'
```

We made the simplifying assumption that both subtypes of GPe neurons had similar kinetics and differed only in channel conductance, as previously suggested (Gunay et al., 2008). Similarly, both subtypes of SP neurons differed only in channel conductance. In contrast, channel kinetics of the GPe neurons differed from that of SP neurons. Models were simulated with PyMoose version 3.1.0 using the hsolve numerical solver. The complete model specification is available at https://github.com/neurord/moose_nerp/, with moose_nerp/d1d2 specifying the SP model parameters and moose_nerp/gp specifying the GPe model parameters.

Experimental Data

All animal handling and procedures were in accordance with the National Institutes of Health animal welfare guidelines and were approved by the George Mason University IACUC committee, or the National Institute on Alcohol Abuse and Alcoholism Animal Care and Use Committee. The experimental data used for the optimizations are part of the python package *waves*, available at https://github.com/neurord/waves. The data consists of recordings from identified external globus pallidus neurons and unidentified striatal spiny projection neurons. As the data was collected for other purposes, the current injection protocol was implemented only once per neuron.

Globus pallidus neuron data was obtained from recordings performed for a prior publication (Abrahao et al., 2017). Briefly, mouse coronal GPe slices, ages P23-P45, were prepared in sucrose cutting solution (in mM: 194 sucrose, 30 NaCl, 4.5 KCl, 26 $NaHCO_3$, 1.2 NaH_2PO_4, 10 D-glucose, 1 $MgCl_2$, and saturated with 95% O2/5% CO2). Slices were equilibrated for 30–40 min at 32°C in carbogen-bubbled aCSF (in mM: 124 NaCl, 4.5 KCl, 26 $NaHCO_3$, 1.2 NaH_2PO_4, 10 D-glucose, 1 $MgCl_2$, and 2 $CaCl_2$). Slices were then incubated at room temperature. Recordings were performed at 30–32°C using micropipettes (2–4 MΩ) filled with internal solution (in mM: 140 K-gluconate, 10 HEPES, 0.1 $CaCl_2$, 2 $MgCl_2$, 1 EGTA, 2 ATP-Mg, and 0.2 GTP-Na, pH 7.25, 300–305 mOsm. Neurons were visualized using an upright microscope (Scientifica, Uckfield, East Sussex, UK) with a LUMPlanFL N × 40/0.80 W objective (Olympus, Waltham, MA). Recordings were obtained using a Multiclamp 700 A amplifier, Digidata 1322 A digitizer and analyzed using pClamp 10.3 software (Molecular Devices, Sunnyvale, CA). A low-pass filter of 2 kHz and sampling frequency of 10 kHz were used. We used the spontaneous firing with no current injection during the 5th min of recording after breakthrough and the response to 1 s hyperpolarizing current injection (from −200 to −50 pA in 50 pA increments). Depolarizing current injection was not used since these neurons fire spontaneously. When recording in slices from wild-type C57BL/6J mice, 1% Neurobiotin (Vector Laboratories, Burlingame, CA) was added into the internal solution for *post hoc* immunocytochemistry of Parvalbumin (PV), a marker for fast spiking prototypical GPe neurons (ProtoN). Though the fast firing, PV+ neurons generally are considered prototypical neurons (four were used for the optimization), the low firing, PV− neurons (three were used for the optimization) are likely a mixture of arkypallidal and other neuron types. Nonetheless, for the purpose of evaluating subtype differences, we are labeling the three low firing, PV− neurons as ArkyN.

Spiny projection neuron data was collected in current clamp from dorso-lateral striatum of *ex vivo* brain slices of C57Bl6 male and female mice, ages P20–P28. Briefly, brain slices were extracted following decapitation of mice anesthetized with isoflurane. Brains were sliced using a VT1000S vibratome (Leica) in oxygenated ice-cold slicing solution (in mM: KCl 2.8, Dextrose 10, $NaHCO_3$ 26.2, NaH_2PO_4 1.25, $CaCl_2$ 0.5, Mg_2SO_4 7, Sucrose 210). Slices were incubated in aCSF (in mM: NaCl 126, NaH_2PO_4 1.25, KCl 2.8, $CaCl_2$, Mg_2SO_4 1, $NaHCO_3$ 26.2, Dextrose 11) for 30 min at 33°C, then removed to room temperature (21–24°C) for at least 90 more minutes before use. For whole cell recording, a single hemislice was transferred to a submersion recording chamber (ALA Science) gravity-perfused (at 1–2 ml/min) with oxygenated aCSF containing 50 μM picrotoxin (Tocris Bioscience). Temperature was maintained at 30–32°C (ALA Science) and was monitored with an external thermister. Pipettes were pulled from borosilicate glass on a laser pipette puller (Sutter P-2000) and fire-polished (Narishige MF-830) to a resistance of 3–7 MΩ. Pipettes were filled with a potassium based internal solution (in mM: K-gluconate 132, KCl 10, NaCl 8, HEPES 10, Mg-ATP 3.56, Na-GTP 0.38, Biocytin 0.77) for all recordings. Intracellular signals were collected in current clamp and filtered at 3 kHz using an Axon2B amplifier (Axon instruments), and sampled at 10–20 kHz using an ITC-16 (Instrutech) and Pulse v8.80 (HEKA Electronik). Series resistance (6–30 MΩ) was manually compensated. Voltage responses were collected using 400 ms hyperpolarizing current injection from −500 to −0 in 50 pA increments, and using 400 ms depolarizing current injections, starting from 100 or 200 pA increasing in 20 pA increments. Striatal neurons were identified as being SP neurons (as opposed to fast spiking or low-threshold-spiking interneurons) by their inward rectifier, shallow afterhyperpolarization (AHP), and long latency to fire an action potential in response to current injection. When recording from SP neurons identified using D1Cre- or D2Cre-GFP (green fluorescent protein), the D2Cre-GFP neurons have a lower rheobase current (Chan et al., 2012). Thus, for the purpose of evaluating subtype differences, SP neurons with a rheobase below 200 pA were considered D2-SPN (3 neurons used), and SP neurons with a rheobase above 300 pA were considered D1-SPN (3 neurons used).

Fitness Function

We compared multiple characteristics of spiking and non-spiking activity between simulation and experiment. The spiking characteristics include action potential (AP) time, width, height, number, AHP depth, AHP shape, and (for SP neurons) latency to spike in response to depolarizing current injection. Spike height is calculated with respect to the spike threshold, defined as the point where the membrane potential derivative exceeds 5% of the maximum. Spike height is the difference between spike threshold and the peak membrane potential, and spike width is full width at half height. The non-spiking characteristics include resting potential (both pre- and post-current injection), steady-state voltage response to current injection, time course of membrane potential (falling curve time constant), and rectification (sag caused by inward rectifier, which is the difference between steady state response and the minimum membrane potential deflection during negative current injection). Feature extraction functions are specified in https://github.com/neurord/ajustador/blob/master/ajustador/features.py, and they are combined into a fitness function in https://github.com/neurord/ajustador/blob/master/ajustador/fitnesses.py. To minimize simulation time, for each GPe neuron we used 2 hyperpolarizing traces and 1 trace with no current injection (which contained spontaneously generated action potentials); and for each SP neuron we used 1 hyperpolarizing and 3 depolarizing traces (one of which did not produce action potentials). The difference in feature values between model and data was normalized by dividing by the sum of the model and data response. This normalization converted the feature difference to a fractional, unitless difference. In their multi-objective normalization (Druckmann et al., 2007), divided by the standard deviation of the experimental data. Unfortunately this is not possible for us because our experimental data set is not large enough. We calculated a single fitness value from the weighted sum of the normalized feature differences. A user can further normalize the features by standard deviation by setting the weights equal to the multiplicative inverse of standard deviation, calculated either within neuron if multiple traces are collected or across neurons of a single type. For the simulations reported here, the weights on most features were equal to 1, with several exceptions to produce better fits visually (**Table 2** gives weight on each feature, and **Figure 2** illustrates experimental and simulated voltage traces for visual inspection of various features).

Parameter Optimization

In the optimization loop, the `ajustador.optimize.Optimizer` class is used as a wrapper for the actual fitting algorithm. Maximum conductances and passive electrical properties may be specified as parameters to vary. Each parameter is assigned an initial value and a permitted range of values (e.g., a minimum value of 0 prevents negative parameters). Appending _0, _1, or _2 to the channel name allows different conductances in the different neuron regions, corresponding to the regions specified in param_cond.py,

TABLE 2 | Weights on feature values to create fitness function.

Feature	D1-SPN and D2-SPN	ArkyN and ProtoN
Baseline pre	1	0
Baseline post	1	1
Rectification	0	2
Falling curve	1	1
Voltage response	1	1
Latency	1	0
Spike time	0	0.5
Spike width	1	1
Spike height	1	0.5
Spike count	1	1
AHP depth	1	1
AHP curve	4	1
Histogram	1	1

AHP curve was weighted higher for SPN to avoid the optimizer creating models with large, sharp AHPs. For the GPe models, spike height weight was reduced to avoid the optimizer producing an extreme mismatch in other features while trying to reduce spike height to the unusually small values observed experimentally. Spike time was reduced for both GPe and SPN models reflecting the high variability of this value between neurons of the same type. A weight of zero means to not use the feature, e.g., latency is not defined for a spontaneously spiking neuron. Features are further described in the online documentation (https://neurord.github.io/ajustador/features.html and https://neurord.github.io/ajustador/fitnesses.html). "histogram" is a root-mean-square of the difference between cumulative histograms of membrane potential-values in the two recordings.

otherwise the conductance in all neuron regions are made the same value. For the simulations reported, the initial values were conductances from a roughly hand-tuned model to start the optimization in an area that exhibits spiking behavior (Supplementary Figure 1, also available at https://github.com/neurord/ajustador/tree/master/FrontNeuroinf/FigSuppl_initialconditions.jpg). Each neuron of the same type started with the same initial value; thus any differences between neuron subtypes cannot be due to different initial conditions. The CMA-ES loop was started with a high initial estimate of variance, so that a diverse set of parameter values would be explored.

```
import ajustador as aju

P = ajustador.optimize.AjuParam
params = ajustador.optimize.ParamSet(
  P('RA',          12.004, min=0, max=100),
  P('RM',          9.427, min=0, max=10),
  P('CM',          0.03604, min=0, max=0.10),
  P('Cond_KDr',      14.5, min=0, max=100),
  P('Cond_NaF_0',    192000, min=0, max=1e6),
  P('Cond_NaF_1',    65300, min=0, max=1e6),
  P('Cond_NaF_2',     2500, min=0, max=1e6),
  P('morph_file', 'GP1_41comp.p', fixed=1),
  P('neuron_type', 'proto',        fixed=1),
  P('model',    'gp',         fixed=1))
```

The optimization object uses the specified parameter set, experimental traces, fitness function, and directory for storing the simulation results:

```
import gpedata_experimental as gpe

dataname='proto079'
exp_to_fit = gpe.data[dataname+'-2s'][[0,2,
  4]]

fitness = aju.fitnesses.combined_fitness(
                   'empty',
                    baseline =1,
                    rectification=2,
                    spike_width=1,
                    spike_latency=0,
                    spike_ahp=1
)
```

Experimental data can be specified using one of two different file formats: Igor binaries or comma separated values. The traces for the experiments are placed in a separate subdirectory, e.g., gpedata_experimental, and the class Param in the python package waves (https://github.com/neurord/waves) specifies the onset and offset time of the injection current, as well as the time frame for measuring baseline membrane potential and steady state depolarization. Since the data specification is a separate module, adding support for other file formats is straightforward.

It is also necessary to specify which type of model (GPe or SP neurons), which neuron subtype to optimize (e.g., for GPe either arkyN or protoN), and that the simulation is a MOOSE simulation:

```
ntype='proto'
modeltype='gp'

fit1 = aju.optimize.Fit(tmpdir,
             exp_to_fit,
             modeltype, ntype,
             fitness, params,
             _make_simulation=aju.optimize.
               MooseSimulation.make,
             _result_constructor=aju.
               optimize.
               MooseSimulationResult)
```

Functions in `ajustador.basic_simulation` are used by the parameter optimization to run the `MOOSE` simulation. They implement only the key model creation and simulation commands from __main__.py, thereby simplifying the interface between creation of neuron model and parameter optimization.

After the optimization is configured with this information, the optimization is performed for a specified number of generations, using a specified population size for each generation. The total number of model evaluations is the product of population size and generations. The simulations reported herein used the default population size of 8, but the user can specify other population sizes. Similarly, the user can specify the simulation seed to be used by the do_fit function:

```
generations=300
popsiz=8

fit1.load()

fit1.do_fit(generations, popsize=popsiz)
```

The python package ajustador is available at https://github.com/neurord/ajustador, and the scripts used to run the simulations are at https://github.com/neurord/ajustador/tree/master/FrontNeuroinf.

In many mathematical optimization scenarios, the calculation of the fitness of a single point (individual model) is quick, and the optimization loop is the important part. Here, as often in computational neuroscience, the simulation of each point is a lengthy process, requiring instantiation of the MOOSE interpreter, loading of the model, actual simulation, saving of the result to a file, and finally generating a fitness value from those results. The `Optimizer` class communicates with the implementation of CMA-ES to retrieve a set of points, perform simulations and calculate the fitness for all of them, feed the results back, so that the numerical algorithm can generate a new set of points to execute. Actual simulation is parallelized at a high level to speed up the whole process: although each individual simulation is single-threaded, during optimization multiple parameter combinations are evaluated together, and for each of those, multiple traces corresponding to different experimental conditions, e.g., different injection currents, need to be simulated. This means that we can take full advantage of available computational power by parallelizing at the level of whole simulations, one simulation per available processor core using a simple queue of jobs. We used Python's `multiprocessing` module (https://docs.python.org/3/library/multiprocessing.html) to schedule jobs on a single machine, and IPython's `ipyparallel` (https://ipyparallel.readthedocs.io/en/latest) on multiple machines in a local network. In both cases, the results were saved to disk to a directory with a file containing a copy of the simulation parameters, and files for the simulation results (typically, voltage traces over time). In the multi-machine case a network file system was used to access the storage area. Saving directly to disk provided a mechanism to introspect the running simulation and to retrieve the results for any previously-simulated parameter combination.

When the optimization is complete, the results include the set of parameters, the normalized feature differences, and the overall fitness value for each individual model. The fitness history is the plot of overall fitness value vs. model evaluations (each generation evaluates a population size of models).

To analyze whether parameters are predictive of different neuron subtypes, we used a two-step statistical analysis applied to the parameter values using SAS version 9.4. In step one, a stepwise discriminant analysis was performed (procedure STEPDISC), using the parameter values normalized by standard deviation (procedure STDIZE), to identify the parameters that could perform the best *linear* separation of the two neuron subtypes. In addition, we plotted one parameter value vs. a second parameter value, for all parameters, and inspected these graphs to visualize which parameters segregated and clustered the two neuron subtypes. In step two, a cluster analysis was performed using those variables identified in step one, to assess the extent to which the neuron subtypes segregated. Two methods of cluster analysis were performed. First the procedure CLUSTER was used to determine the optimum number of clusters. Then, the procedure FASTCLUS was used, on the data normalized with STDIZE and with the number of clusters determined by CLUSTER, to calculate the distance between clusters of same and different neuron subtypes. The procedure FREQ was appied to the output of the cluster analysis to generate the confusion matrices.

RESULTS

Declarative Model Specification

We created a python module called moose_nerp (moose neuron prototype) to simplify and standardize the creation and simulation of neuron models using the MOOSE software. The declarative framework facilitates reproducibility, re-use and extension of MOOSE models of neurons and networks. Each set of neuron models has a set of parameter files specifying (1) channel kinetics, (2) channel conductances and morphology, (3) synaptic channel parameters, (4) calcium mechanism parameters, and (5) spine parameters. Spines, synapses and calcium dynamics can be included or excluded with a simple parameter switch, e.g., calYN = True and spineYN = False. Parameter specifications for channel kinetics and conductances use similar organization, keywords and parameter types as NeuroML version2, facilitating conversion, whereas the parameters for calcium dynamics, such as buffer and pump specifications, do not yet have NeuroML version2 equivalents.

Two subtypes of each of two types of neuron models were created for use with the parameter optimization. Models of the two subtypes of neurons in the globus pallidus were developed, representing arkypallidal (low firing rate, PV−, ethanol sensitive) and prototypical (high firing rate, PV+, ethanol insensitive) by creating a set of parameter files. In addition, models of the two subtypes of striatal spiny projection neurons in the striatum were developed (called D1-SPN and D2-SPN, representing the direct pathway neurons that contain dopamine D1 receptors and the indirect pathway neurons that contain dopamine D2 receptors) by creating a second set of parameter files specifying channel kinetics, conductances, etc. Channel kinetics for the GPe neuron models were adapted from Hendrickson et al. (2011a); both arkyN and protoN neurons used the same channel kinetics and morphology. Channel kinetics for the SP neuron models were adapted from Jedrzejewska-Szmek et al. (2017); both D1-SPN and D2-SPN used the same morphology and channel kinetics. Both models used single time constant of decay for calcium dynamics, though calcium buffers, pumps and diffusion have been implemented in the SP neuron models and can be specified with a parameter switch.

Parameter Optimization Using CMA-ES

Parameter optimization was run on a 16-core Linux workstation with Intel® Xeon® CPU E5-2650 processors. Each of the four

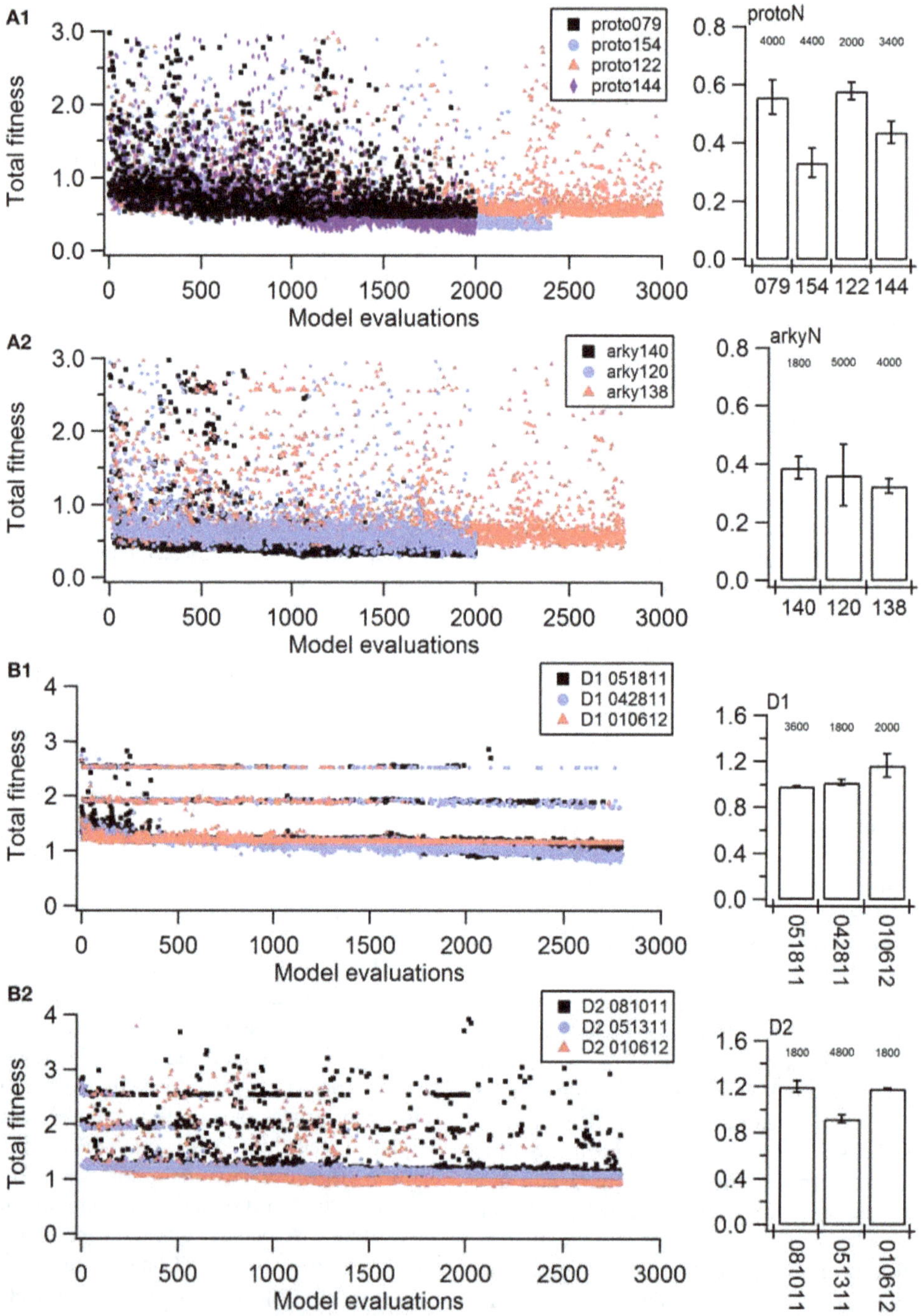

FIGURE 1 | Fitness history shows the fitness values rapidly reach good fits (within 1,000 model evaluations/sample points) and reaches an asymptote typically within 2,000 model evaluations/sample points). **(A)** Fitness vs. model evaluation for GPe neurons of **(A1)** prototypical type and **(A2)** arkypallidal type. **(B)** Fitness vs. model evaluation for SP neurons of **(B1)** D1 type and **(B2)** D2 type. Note that GPe neuron fitness values reached considerably lower values than SP neuron fitness values. Right panels show fitness vs. model evaluation for the 1st set of optimizations and left panels show the mean and standard deviation of the fitness values of the last 25 generations of the 2nd set of optimizations (which used a different random seed). The number above the bar gives the number of model evaluations to convergence for the 2nd set of optimizations.

neuron models was optimized to 3–4 sets of voltage traces, each set from a different, experimentally recorded neuron. For each recorded neuron, traces both with and without action potentials were utilized in a single optimization. Optimizations were run until the fitness value reached an asymptote, typically within 200–500 generations using a population size of 8

TABLE 3 | Characteristics of optimization simulations.

	SP	GPe
Number of compartments	189	41
Number of experimental traces used	4	3
Duration of trace	0.9 s	2 s
Simulation time*	12.4 ± 1.03 h per 1,000 models	8.5 ± 0.16 h per 1,000 models
Evaluations to convergence#	2,100 ± 500	3,514 ± 1,007
Evaluations till fitness value is within 5% of minimum	867 ± 1,185	2,482 ± 1,133

**Reported simulation time (mean and standard deviation) is for the second simulation seed. #Evaluations to convergence (mean and standard deviation) is for the second simulation seed; one of the GP simulations did not reach convergence within 5,000 model evaluations, yet reached a minimum fitness of 0.26.*

(**Figure 1**, **Table 3**). The convergence was determined from the change in mean fitness: the slope of the mean fitness across 25 generations must be <0.002 and the standard deviation of mean fitness across 25 generations must be less than 0.06 (implemented in https://github.com/neurord/ajustador/tree/master/ajustador/helpers/converge.py). For each optimization, all current injections are simulated in parallel. In general, each simulation job is submitted to a scheduler, and started when resources are available. The result is returned to the optimization algorithm when all requested points have been finished.

The parameter algorithm was able to find reasonable parameters for most of the data sets. We defined the feature funtions in a way that would give values on the order of one, so that when multiple features were combined with equal weights, all features could contribute significantly to the total. The optimizations were originally performed using equal weighting, and then repeated once or twice after visual comparison of simulations and experiments and adjusting the weights (**Table 2**) to de-emphasize spike time and improve the fit to shape of the AHP. **Figure 1** shows total fitness value vs. model evaluation for GPe neurons (A) and SP neurons (B). Most combined fitness values decreased to ~0.4 or less for the seven GPe neurons and to ~1.0 or less for the SP neurons. Simulations were repeated using a different random seed, with similar results: the change in minimum total fitness reached was 0.018 (6.4%) for GPe neurons and −0.041 (4.4%) for SP neurons.

Figure 2 shows an overlay of the model traces and experimental data for the optimizations in **Figure 1** to illustrate similarity between model and experiments. **Figures 2A,B** show optimizations of two different arkypallidal neurons from the external globus pallidus. For both neurons, the shape of the AHP and the amplitude of the sag match quite well. On the other hand, the fit to arky N 120 shows the difficulty in fitting to neurons with short action potentials (similar results are obtained with a spike height weight of 1.0). **Figure 2C** shows the fit to a prototypical neuron, which fires at a much faster rate than the arkypallidal neurons. The ability to match the shape of the AHPs is illustrated in **Figure 2C2** which expands the time scale of the plot. **Figures 2D,E** show optimizations of one D1-SPN and one D2-SPN. Again, AP characteristics and AHP shape fit quite well.

One motivation for using a multi-objective optimization is the observation that improvement in the fit of one feature often comes at the expense of another feature (Druckmann et al., 2007; Rumbell et al., 2016; Neymotin et al., 2017). To evaluate to what extent this trade-off occurs in these single objective optimizations, we evaluated the correlation between various feature functions for the 2.5% best fitting (lowest total fitness value) models (or the last 50 of the best fitting models if more than 2,000 evaluations were performed). The feature fitnesses and total fitness value for (mean over the 50 best models) for each data set is provided in **Tables 4A,B**. **Figures 3A–C, 4A–E** shows that very few trade-offs are evident between the features that comprise the fitness function. For the GPe neurons, spike height improves as spike width worsens, but this relationship does not hold for the SP neurons (**Figure 4E**). Several positive correlations are notable. An increase in AHP curve fitness is correlated with an increase in spike count fitness (**Figure 3C**), and an increase in voltage response fitness is correlated with an increase in spike time fitness (**Figure 3B**) for GPe neurons. For the SP neuron optimization, trade-offs are less apparent, and instead the charging curve fitness is positively correlated with the spike width fitness (**Figure 4A**), though negatively correlated with AHP curve (**Figure 4B**) fitness. In addition, the voltage response fitness is positively correlated with spike height fitness (**Figure 4C**). As the long latency to 1st spike in SP neurons is attributed to transient potassium currents, which also can produce large AHPs, we examined AHP curve vs. 1st spike latency (**Figure 4D**), but the correlation between these two features is quite small. Graphs of single features vs. total fitness (**Figures 3D–F, 4F–H**) demonstrate that most single features are either not correlated with the total fitness, or explain very little of the variance, e.g., voltage response for the GPe neurons (**Figure 3D**), and spike latency ($R = 0.05$) and spike count ($R = -0.31$) for SP neurons. A summary of all correlations is provided for GPe neurons in **Figure 3G**. The lack of correlation reflects that the total fitness is calculated from the combination of multiple features. An exception to this is the high correlation between AHP curve and total fitness for SP neurons, likely due to the high weight of this feature in the total fitness (**Figure 4H**). Curiously, in some cases feature fitness is negatively correlated with total fitness, such as spike width for both GPe neurons (**Figure 3F**) and SP neurons (**Figure 4F**), and charging curve for SP neurons (**Figure 4G**).This shows that strong fitting of a specific feature can result in a model that is weak when other features are considered, possibly because the model is not flexible enough to provide a good fit on all of those features.

Non-linear systems are often difficult to find parameters for because a unique set of parameters may not exist. Prior studies (Golowasch et al., 2002; Prinz et al., 2003a) have observed that higher outward conductances can be compensated by higher inward, or different potassium conductances can compensate for each other. To examine to what extent this occurs in our optimizations, we evaluated the correlation between the different conductances from the same best models as used above. **Figure 5** illustrates the conductances for the best GPe models and demonstrates several types of compensation. In the GPe neurons,

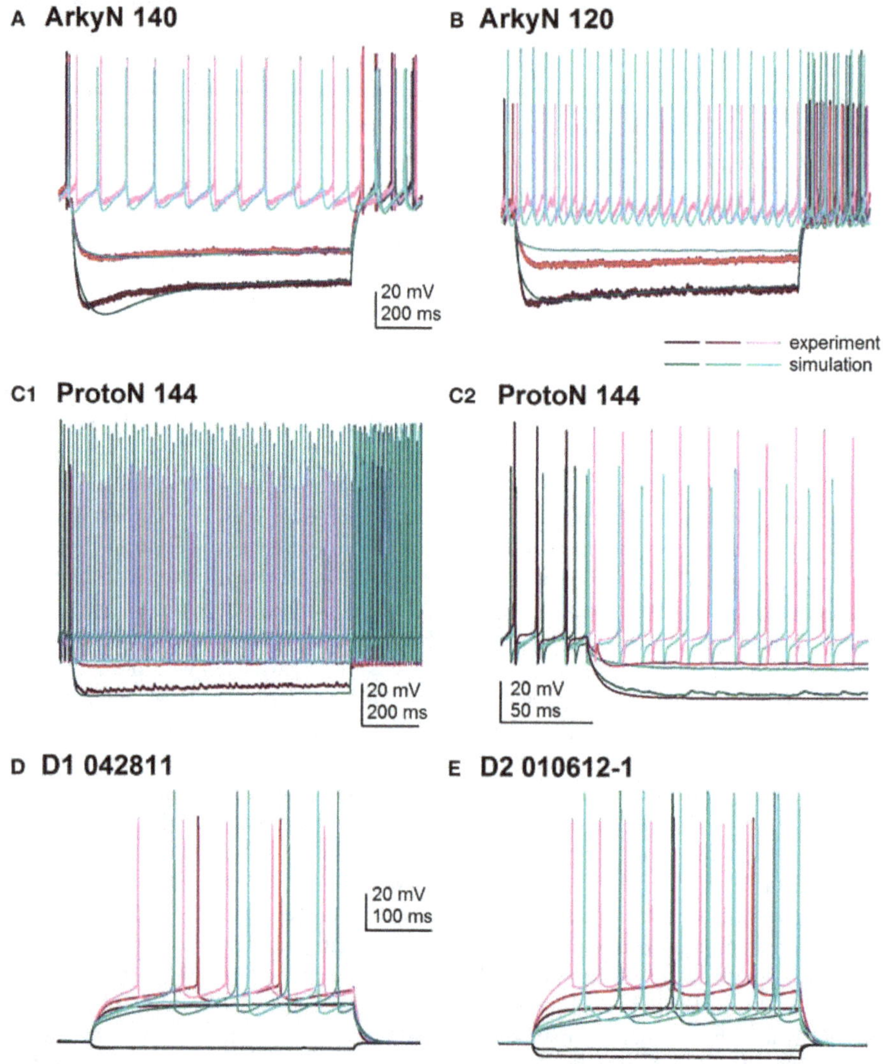

FIGURE 2 | Comparison of simulated and experimental traces. In all panels, simulations are in shades of turquoise and experimental data in shades of magenta. **(A)** Fit to arkypalidal cell #140 (minimum fitness = 0.29). Spike height, timing and AHP are all fit quite well. **(B)** Fit to arkypallidal cell #120 (minimum fitness = 0.29). This example shows the difficulty in fitting to spike height when spikes are shorter than usual. **(C)** Fit to protoypical cell #144 (minimum fitness = 0.25). C1 shows fit to entire 1 sec of current injection, whereas C2 zooms in to illustrate match to AHP shape. **(D)** Fit to D1R type of SP neuron (minimum fitness 0.78). **(E)** Fit to D2R type of SP neuron (minimum fitness 0.88). Both **(D,E)** show good fit to AP shape, AHP shape and long latency to fire.

an increase in the slow sodium current (Na_S) is compensated by a decrease in the fast sodium current (Na_F) in the axon (**Figure 5A**) or an increase in the KCNQ potassium current (**Figure 5B**). Similarly, an increase in the fast sodium current is compensated by an increase in the Kv3 potassium current (**Figure 5C**) or an increase in the fast transient potassium (KA_F) current (**Figure 5D**). There is a tradeoff between somatic and axonal transient potassium (KA_S) currents (**Figure 5E**). In contrast to these compensatory correlations, **Figure 5F** demonstrates a non-compensatory correlation: the dendritic KA_S current positively correlates with the dendritic Kv3 current. A similar range of correlations is apparent for the SP optimizations (**Figure 6**). **Figures 6A–C** shows inward currents compensating for outward currents. **Figure 6D** shows the slow transient potassium current (KA_S) compensating for the fast transient potassium current (KA_F) in the soma; whereas **Figures 6E,F** shows non-compensatory correlations: A correlated increase in two inward currents (**Figure 6E**), or a decrease in a calcium current correlated with an increase in a potassium current (**Figure 6F**).

Approach to Identifying Mechanisms Underlying Difference Between Cell Types

CMA outputs provide parameters for generating sets of good models instead of the parameters for the single best fit model. This has the advantage of providing sets of good models for performing simulation experiments and demonstrating robustness to parameter variations. In addition, the parameters

TABLE 4A | Mean feature fitnesses of the 50 best models for each of the globus pallidus neurons.

GPe	proto154F	proto144F	proto122F	proto079F	arky140F	arky138F	arky120F
Voltage response	0.367 ± 0.022	0.154 ± 0.085	0.289 ± 0.057	0.272 ± 0.081	0.240 ± 0.093	0.565 ± 0.076	0.273 ± 0.116
Baseline post	0.086 ± 0.034	0.093 ± 0.050	0.084 ± 0.047	0.125 ± 0.098	0.050 ± 0.036	0.066 ± 0.049	0.079 ± 0.055
Rectification	0.261 ± 0.107	0.324 ± 0.130	1.318 ± 0.015	0.705 ± 0.267	0.540 ± 0.037	0.853 ± 0.146	0.511 ± 0.241
Falling curve	0.222 ± 0.090	0.132 ± 0.074	0.298 ± 0.075	0.321 ± 0.173	0.227 ± 0.037	0.256 ± 0.113	0.155 ± 0.087
Spike time	0.058 ± 0.007	0.065 ± 0.038	0.075 ± 0.011	0.118 ± 0.015	0.052 ± 0.011	0.164 ± 0.015	0.087 ± 0.019
Spike width	0.450 ± 0.042	0.548 ± 0.028	0.325 ± 0.027	0.277 ± 0.077	0.455 ± 0.036	0.464 ± 0.089	0.278 ± 0.069
Spike height	0.075 ± 0.042	0.089 ± 0.042	0.332 ± 0.025	0.258 ± 0.089	0.077 ± 0.036	0.156 ± 0.065	0.287 ± 0.029
Spike count	0.144 ± 0.023	0.148 ± 0.047	0.121 ± 0.062	0.378 ± 0.121	0.103 ± 0.039	0.306 ± 0.087	0.326 ± 0.088
AHP amplitude	0.070 ± 0.033	0.112 ± 0.052	0.104 ± 0.047	0.115 ± 0.084	0.074 ± 0.035	0.104 ± 0.077	0.094 ± 0.083
AHP curve	0.693 ± 0.032	0.516 ± 0.022	0.534 ± 0.042	0.904 ± 0.046	0.616 ± 0.033	0.714 ± 0.032	0.712 ± 0.033
Histogram	0.299 ± 0.039	0.239 ± 0.092	0.329 ± 0.049	0.478 ± 0.110	0.146 ± 0.052	0.332 ± 0.096	0.271 ± 0.074
Total	0.316 ± 0.007	0.281 ± 0.015	0.484 ± 0.005	0.448 ± 0.026	0.310 ± 0.006	0.445 ± 0.016	0.348 ± 0.026

TABLE 4B | Mean feature fitnesses of the 50 best models for each of the striatal spiny projection neurons.

	D1_051811	D1_042811	D1_010612	D2_081011	D2_051311	D2_010612
Voltage response	0.996 ± 0.021	0.057 ± 0.032	0.228 ± 0.121	0.243 ± 0.121	0.414 ± 0.038	0.944 ± 0.025
Baseline pre	0.018 ± 0.001	0.072 ± 0.003	0.044 ± 0.007	0.110 ± 0.026	0.015 ± 0.001	0.073 ± 0.001
Baseline post	0.016 ± 0.001	0.057 ± 0.002	0.039 ± 0.008	0.004 ± 0.003	0.013 ± 0.001	0.061 ± 0.001
Falling curve	0.233 ± 0.039	0.058 ± 0.026	0.273 ± 0.084	0.393 ± 0.053	0.294 ± 0.111	0.076 ± 0.018
Spike width	0.253 ± 0.028	0.171 ± 0.022	0.055 ± 0.040	0.141 ± 0.030	0.040 ± 0.022	0.241 ± 0.016
Spike height	0.203 ± 0.008	0.096 ± 0.007	0.123 ± 0.005	0.187 ± 0.004	0.191 ± 0.010	0.191 ± 0.004
Spike latency	0.207 ± 0.017	0.311 ± 0.027	0.332 ± 0.086	0.339 ± 0.070	0.153 ± 0.017	0.313 ± 0.016
Spike count	1.077 ± 0.011	1.066 ± 0.001	1.021 ± 0.067	0.958 ± 0.044	0.946 ± 0.000	0.908 ± 0.004
AHP amplitude	0.187 ± 0.015	0.019 ± 0.013	0.342 ± 0.003	0.184 ± 0.014	0.256 ± 0.003	0.170 ± 0.013
AHP curve	2.434 ± 0.147	2.618 ± 0.062	3.750 ± 0.023	3.336 ± 0.032	3.437 ± 0.025	2.744 ± 0.019
Charging curve	0.147 ± 0.024	0.174 ± 0.025	0.056 ± 0.022	0.094 ± 0.026	0.058 ± 0.023	0.170 ± 0.030
Histogram	0.591 ± 0.011	0.075 ± 0.007	0.357 ± 0.019	0.392 ± 0.036	0.601 ± 0.010	0.441 ± 0.009
Total	0.851 ± 0.036	0.826 ± 0.016	1.142 ± 0.003	1.027 ± 0.0093	1.060 ± 0.006	0.899 ± 0.004

themselves can be analyzed to determine whether certain parameters are predictive of different cell types and capture the feature differences between neuron subtypes (**Table 5**). To address this latter question, we used a multi-step statistical analysis (discriminant analysis followed by cluster analysis) applied to the 50 best fitting models.

For the GPe neurons, graphical analysis revealed that capacitance (CM) and the large conductance, calcium dependent potassium current (BK) in soma and dendrite as the variables that best separate the data. The discriminant analysis similarly identified capacitance, but did not identify the BK conductance. Instead, it identified the slow transient potassium current (KA_S) in the soma. A plot of these parameter values (**Figures 7A,B**) demonstrate that the arkyN have either a higher somatic or dendritic BK conductance, and also have a higher capacitance. Inspection of the panels in **Figures 5, 7C,D** confirm that most of the other parameters do not separate the data by neuron class.

We performed a cluster analysis using these identified parameters (CM and either BK or KA_S). Because the BK conductance was elevated in either the soma or the dendrite, but not always both, we used the sum of the somatic and dendritic BK conductance as one of the variables. Two types of cluster analyses were performed. The first analysis used the SAS CLUSTER procedure, which performs a hierarchical cluster analysis without the need to specify either the number of clusters or the cluster size. This procedure provides a measure of the goodness of separation vs. number of clusters. Using the number of clusters suggested by the 1st cluster analysis, the second cluster analysis, which implements a disjoint cluster analysis using the SAS FASTCLUS procedure, then provides a measure of the distance between the clusters. This second procedure allowed quantification of the difference between neuron subtypes.

The disjoint cluster analysis using the 3 clusters suggested by the hierarchical cluster analysis correctly classifies all but two of the neuron parameter sets correctly (**Table 6**), regardless of whether BK or KA_S was used. This suggests that the parameters identified may represent subtype differences. The BK conductance in particular has already been demonstrated to differ between arkypallidal and prototypical GPe neurons. Because the parameter optimizations used the same morphology

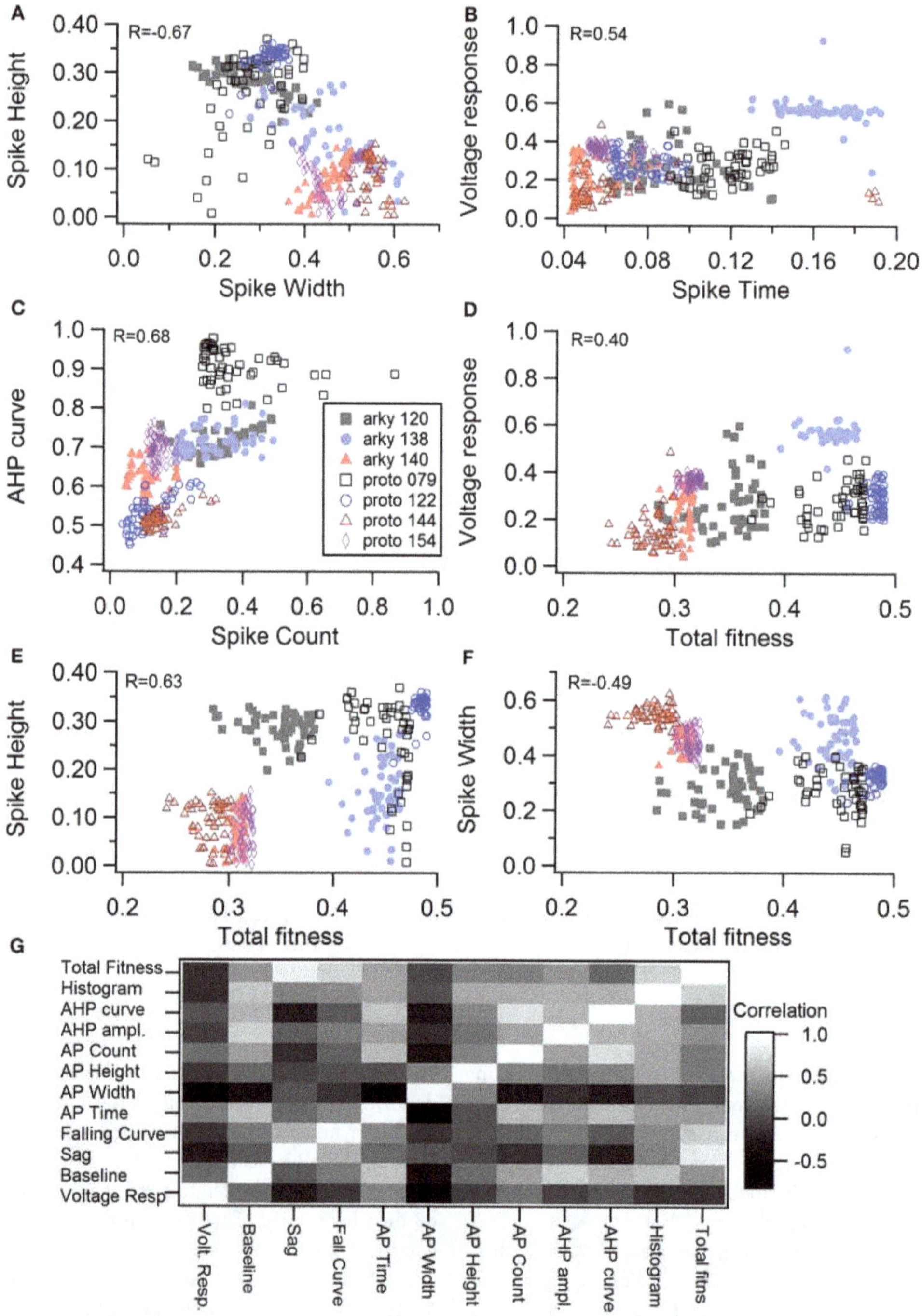

FIGURE 3 | Comparison of feature fitnesses for 50 best models for GPe neuron optimizations. **(A)** Spike height vs. spike width shows that improvements in spike height come at expense of worsening of spike width. In contrast to this trade-off, **(B)** steady state voltage response vs. spike time and **(C)** AHP curve vs. spike count show that two features can improve simultaneously. **(D–E)** contribution of voltage response **(D)**, spike height **(E)** and spike width **(F)** to the total fitness. Despite the significant positive correlation for two of the features, no one feature appears to control the fit. R is the Pearson's R correlation; all illustrated correlations are significant at $P < 0.0001$. Symbols corresponding to different neurons are the same in all panels and indicated in **C**. **(G)** Pairwise Pearson's R correlation between all features illustrated as image plot. AP: spike.

for arkyN and protoN, the difference in CM values suggests that the morphology of these two neurons differ, with arkypallidal neurons having either a larger number of dendrites or a greater number of spines. The greater conductance of the slow transient potassium channel may be producing the shallower AHPs in arkyN as compared to protoN (e.g., compare **Figure 2B** with **Figure 2C2**). The Euclidean distance between centroids of the two arkyN clusters (1.78) is smaller than the distance between

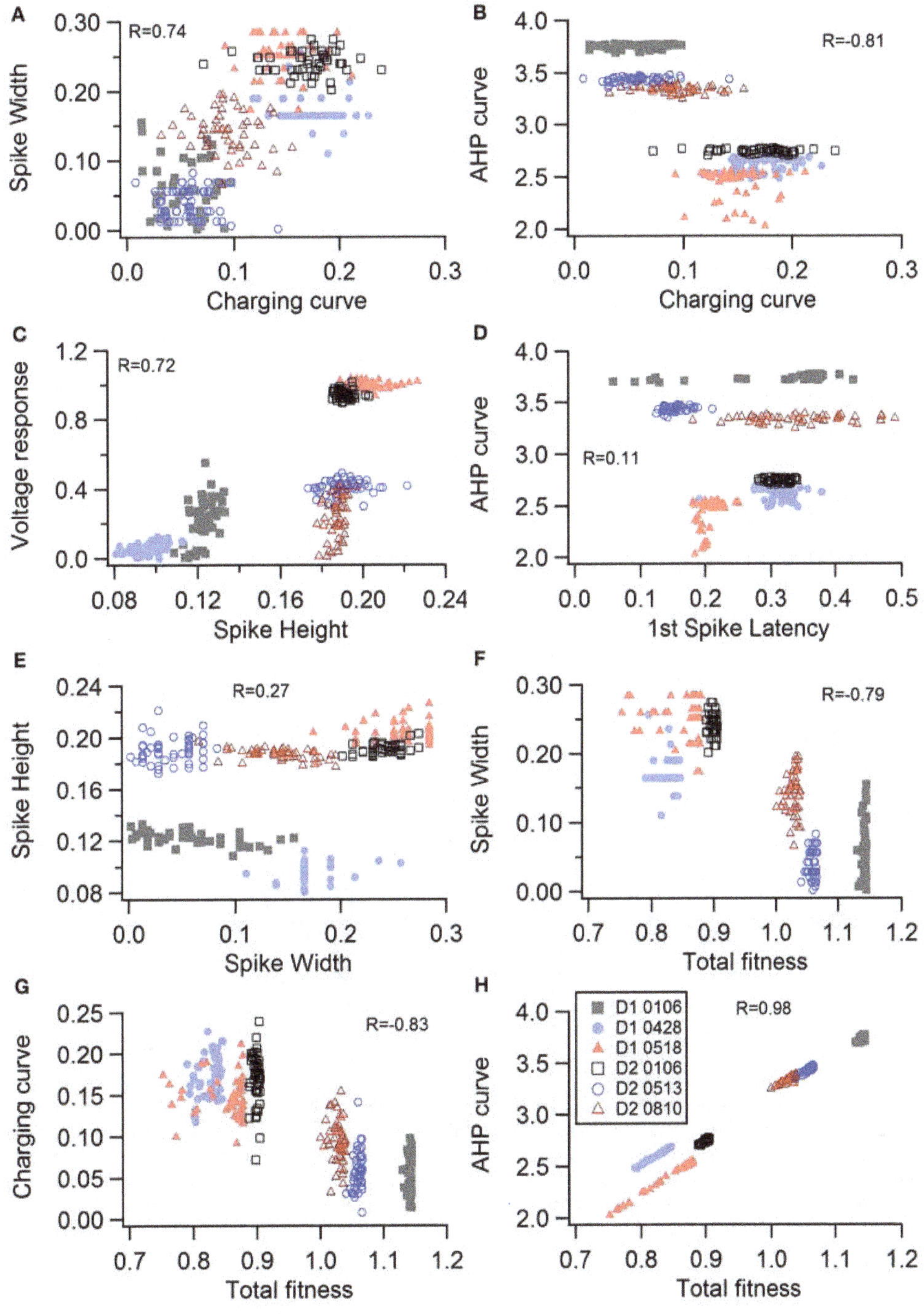

FIGURE 4 | Comparison of feature fitnesses for 50 best models for SP neuron optimizations. The positive correlations for **(A)** spike width vs. charging curve fitness and **(C)** voltage response vs. spike height show that two features can improve simultaneously. With some features, such as **(B)** AHP curve vs. charging curve fitness, there is a trade-off between these two features. **(D)** AHP curve is not correlated with 1st spike latency ($P = 0.052$). **(E)** Spike height vs. spike width does not appear to be correlated in the SP neurons, though reaching statistical significance ($P < 0.0001$). **(F–H)** Contribution of spike width **(F)**, charging curve **(G)**, and AHP curve **(H)** to the total fitness. Improvement in spike width is negatively correlated with total fitness. The strong correlation of AHP curve to total fitness is likely caused by strong weight on AHP curve in the fitness function. R is the Pearson's R correlation; Correlations above 0.7 are significant at $P < 0.0001$. Symbols corresponding to different neurons are the same in all panels and indicated in **H**.

centroids of the arkyN and protoN clusters (2.95 and 2.27). When the analysis was repeated on the best models from the second set of GPe optimizations, a similar KA_S conductance was identified, but instead of the CM or the BK conductance, KA_F, Na_F, and KDr were identified. The difference in these two sets of variables suggests that a larger set of optimizations is needed (with fewer

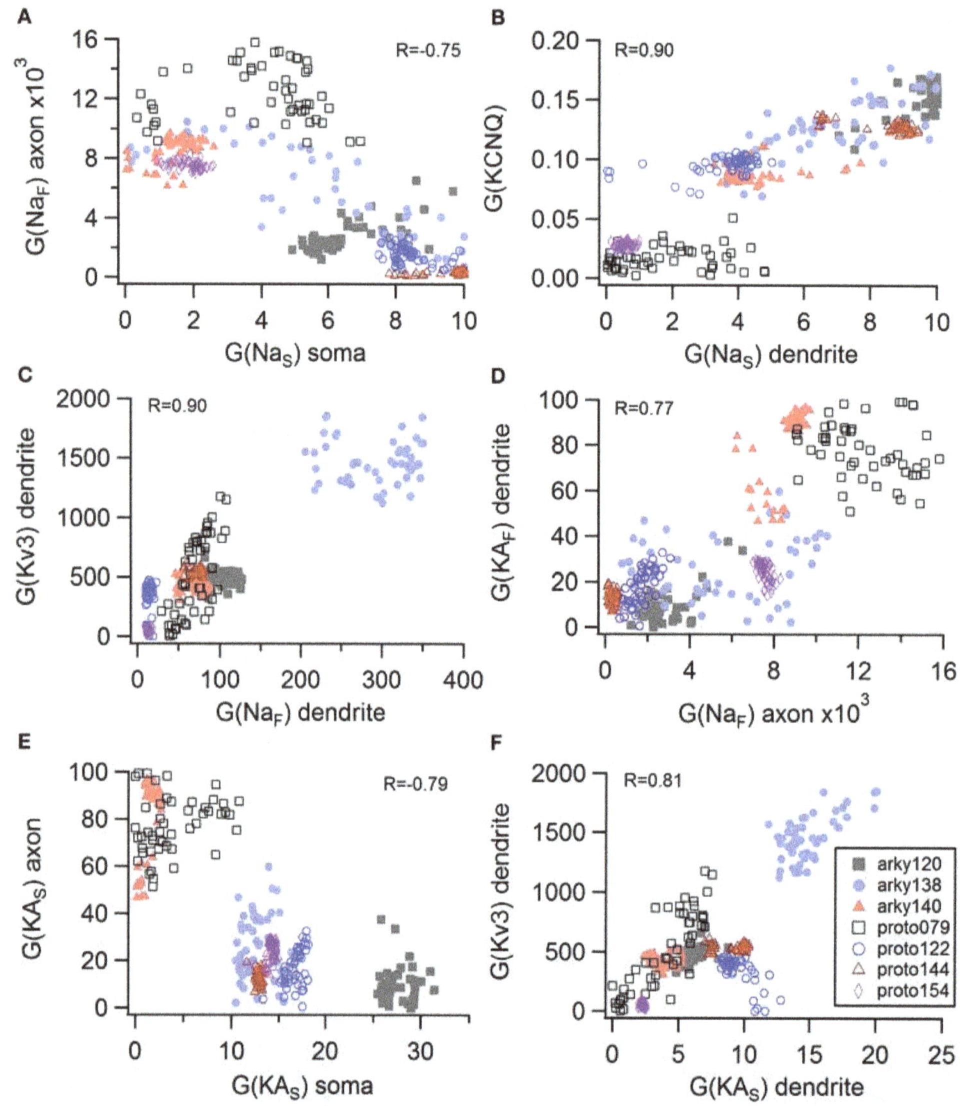

FIGURE 5 | Compensation and other correlations among channel conductances for GPe neurons. **(A)** A decrease in fast sodium conductance in the axon can be compensated by an increase in the slow sodium conductance in the soma. **(B–D)** An increase in conductance of various potassium channels can be compensated by an increase in sodium conductance. **(E)** An increase in the transient potassium current in the soma is correlated with a decrease in the axon. **(F)** A non-compensatory correlation: an increase in KA_S type of potassium conductance is associated with an increase in the Kv3 potassium conductance. R is the Pearson's R correlation; all illustrated correlations are significant at $P < 0.0001$. Symbols corresponding to different neurons are the same in all panels and indicated in **F**.

models per optimization) for accurate identification of differing channel conductances.

DISCUSSION

We created python code for automatic parameter optimization of single neuron models simulated using the MOOSE software. In order to facilitate development and reuse of multi-compartment, multi-conductance models, we used a declarative parameter specification to create the models, and then demonstrated its utility by creating two subtypes of two neuron types: striatal spiny projection neurons, and external globus pallidus neurons. We demonstrated the utility of the covariance matrix adaptation evolutionary strategy by tuning each model type to several sets of experimentally measured membrane potential responses to current injection. Each optimization required ~1 day of simulation time and only 1,600–4,000 evaluations, suggesting that a powerful supercomputer could be used to tune models to large data sets reasonably quickly. Statistical analysis of the resulting parameter sets revealed a small set of parameters that varied between neuron subtypes, indicating that this data-driven modeling approach would be a useful technique for identifying differences between neuron subtypes.

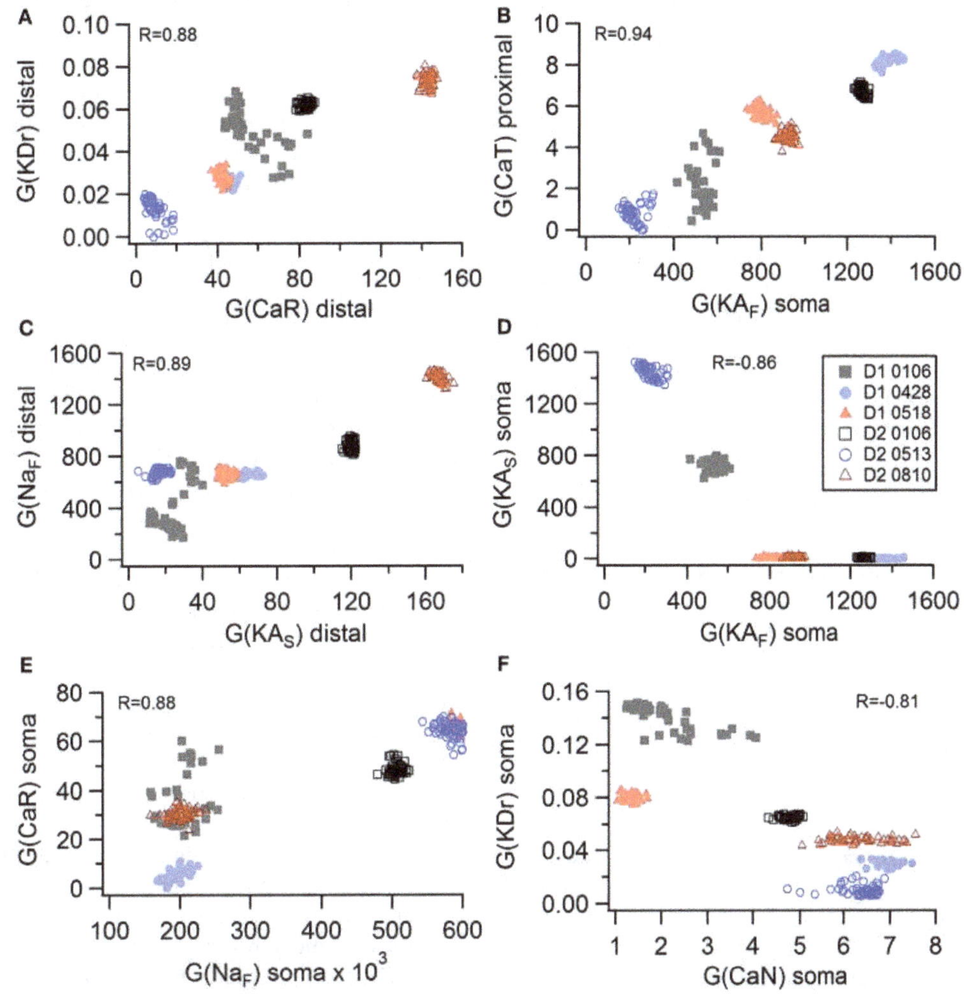

FIGURE 6 | Compensation and other correlations among channel conductances for SP neurons. **(A–C)** An increase in potassium channel conductance is compensated by an increase in inward channel conductance (sodium or calcium channels). **(D)** An increase in fast transient (KA_F) potassium channel conductance is compensated by a decrease in slow transient (KA_S) potassium channel conductance in in the soma. **(E,F)** Two non-compensatory correlations between channel conductances. **(E)** An increase in the fast sodium current in the soma is associated with an increase in the R type calcium channel (CaR) conductance. **(F)** An increase in delayed rectifier potasium channel is correlated with a decrease in N type calcium current in the soma. R is the Pearson's R correlation; all illustrated correlations are significant at $P < 0.0001$. Symbols corresponding to different neurons are the same in all panels and indicated in **E**.

The use of declarative model specification instead of procedural model specification is considered best practice in model development (Gewaltig and Cannon, 2014). A declarative model specification simplifies inspection of the model, and facilitates re-use and extension of the model. The most comprehensive declarative model specification language for multi-compartment, multi-channel models is NeuroML version 2 (Gleeson et al., 2010; Cannon et al., 2014). Its support by both MOOSE and NEURON would simplify exchange of models between simulators. One limitation with NeuroML is that the declarative specification for calcium dynamics is not yet developed; hence the difficulty in using the current NeuroML for our MOOSE models. Nonetheless, implementing a declarative parameter specification with organization and keywords similar to NeuroML will facilitate translation into NeuroML in the near future. A second key feature of our parameter optimization software is to have the optimization wrapped around existing models, similar to some existing optimization algorithms (Friedrich et al., 2014). An advantage of our optimization wrapper is that it keeps the declaration of the parameters and morphology declarative, in contrast to some other approaches (e.g., Brookings et al., 2014; Van Geit et al., 2016). In other words, the parameters for tuning are specified separately from the base model code, both for MOOSE models and for signaling pathway models that are specified and simulated in NeuroRD (https://github.com/neurord/neurord_fit). This approach eliminates the need either to re-specify the model using optimization specific annotations or to insert parameter ranges directly into the base model code.

TABLE 5 | Mean feature properties of data.

	arky (*N* = 3)	proto (*N* = 4)
AP count	33.67 ± 14.50	134.25 ± 38.66
Spike Height	0.0623 ± 0.0094	0.0675 ± 0.0100
Spike Width	0.00045 ± 0.00008	0.00028 ± 0.00008
Spike AHP	−0.0506 ± 0.0028	−0.0581 ± 0.0040
Baseline Vm	−0.0446 ± 0.0023	−0.0496 ± 0.0044
Rectification (at −200 pA)	0.00787 ± 0.00289	0.00298 ± 0.00299
deltaV (at −100 pA)	−0.0272 ± 0.0039	−0.0114 ± 0.0043
deltaV (at −200 pA)	−0.0430 ± 0.0068	−0.0229 ± 0.0029
Falling curve	0.0129 ± 0.0022	0.0072 ± 0.0014

Distinguishing features include number of action potentials, spike width, deltaV (input resistance), falling curve.

TABLE 6 | Confusion matrix for cluster analysis using CM and total BK conductance.

Cell	Cluster 1 (protoN)	Cluster 2 (arkyN)	Cluster 3 (arkyN)
Arky120	1*	48	1
Arky138	0	0	50
Arky140	0	50	0
Proto079	50	0	0
Proto122	50	0	0
Proto144	50	0	0
Proto154	50	0	0

*Note that labeling the clusters was performed post-hoc, based on the composition of the clusters. *Indicates the incorrectly classified parameter set.*

One limitation of our current optimization software is the inability to adjust half activation and time constants of channel gating for the ionic channels. An initial set of optimizations of the GPe neurons (results not shown) revealed that activation of the hyperpolarization activated cyclic-nucleotide gated (HCN) current in response to hyperpolarizing currents produced a "sag" that was much faster than observed experimentally. To improve this aspect of the fit, the time constant of one of the HCN currents was increased, and the optimizations illustrated all used this slower HCN channel. Given the number of ionic channels activated during action potentials, this hand-tuning approach is not practical for depolarization activated channels. The inability to tune channel characteristics may have contributed to the lower quality fits for the SP neurons. Currently, the software can adjust half activation of one of the channels; thus it will be straight forward to add the capability for all channels. Adding in these parameters should improve the ability to fit the model (Hendrickson et al., 2011b; Brookings et al., 2014; Neymotin et al., 2017), though it would double the number of parameters to tune.

CMA-ES was selected because it has properties which make it appropriate for fitting of complicated and slow-to-simulate models to experimental data: it is robust in the face of local fluctuations of the fitness function, deals well with a high-dimensional and discontinuous fitness landscape, and finally, is frugal with the number of required evaluations, especially compared to other evolutionary algorithms. CMA-ES has been applied to determine protein conformation (Bourquard et al., 2015), and parameters for spiking neuron models (Rossant et al., 2011). A benefit of this algorithm is its fast convergence time, even with large numbers of parameters. Though some parameter optimization algorithms suffer severe slowdowns when the number of parameters is increased, CMA-ES does not suffer from this problem until parameter numbers reach hundreds to thousands (Hansen and Kern, 2004; Hendrickson et al., 2011b; Friedrich et al., 2014; Neymotin et al., 2017). An approach to limit the number of parameters is to perform optimizations in several steps, such as optimizing the passive properties first and spiking activity second (Rumbell et al., 2016), optimizing parameters for proximal conductances to data collected from a neuron with the apical dendrite occluded (Bahl et al., 2012), or using data collected from somatic followed by dendritic recordings (Hay et al., 2011). Though this stepwise approach could facilitate parameter fitting using CMA-ES, avoiding a multi-step approach has the advantage of simplifying the model fitting procedure (conserving the work required from the scientist), and avoids the pitfall where various parameters are strongly correlated and the result of a multi-step fit differs from a single-step fit. Furthermore, fitting to passive properties can underestimate membrane resistance when channels have some activity at resting potential (Keren et al., 2009).

Several studies demonstrate that additional sources of data better constrain the fits. In other words, using measures at two spatial locations (Keren et al., 2009; Hay et al., 2011) or with pinched dendrite (Bahl et al., 2012) better constrains the data. Another data source is calcium dynamics, with simultaneous measures of calcium dynamics and electrical activity (Nevian and Sakmann, 2004; Day et al., 2008; Johenning et al., 2015; Ryu et al., 2017) providing dual contraints. When creating models of calcium dynamics, typically the buffer and pump properties (analogous to channel kinetics) are known (Lee et al., 2000), but pump density and buffer quantity are unknown and need to be adjusted (analogous to channel density). Given the ability of the software to model calcium dynamics, a logical extension would be to optimize to both electrical activity and calcium dynamics measurements. Adding in the calcium dynamics optimization includes reading in calcium imaging data and adapting the fitness function to calcium.

One of the difficult aspects of optimization is designing a fitness function that captures the perceived similarity between simulated and measured voltage traces (or calcium dynamics). One approach is to perform a point-by-point match to the voltage trace. This measure is problematic for neuron activity due to the narrow time window of spikes. A clever approach to avoid this problem has been implemented (Abarbanel et al., 2009; Brookings et al., 2014) and avoids sensitivity to the fitness functions selected. Unfortunately, the custom code to implement this approach is not written for an existing simulator; however, it would be interesting to incorporate that approach into a fitness function for use with MOOSE. A second approach is to use features of the data, such as spike time, width,

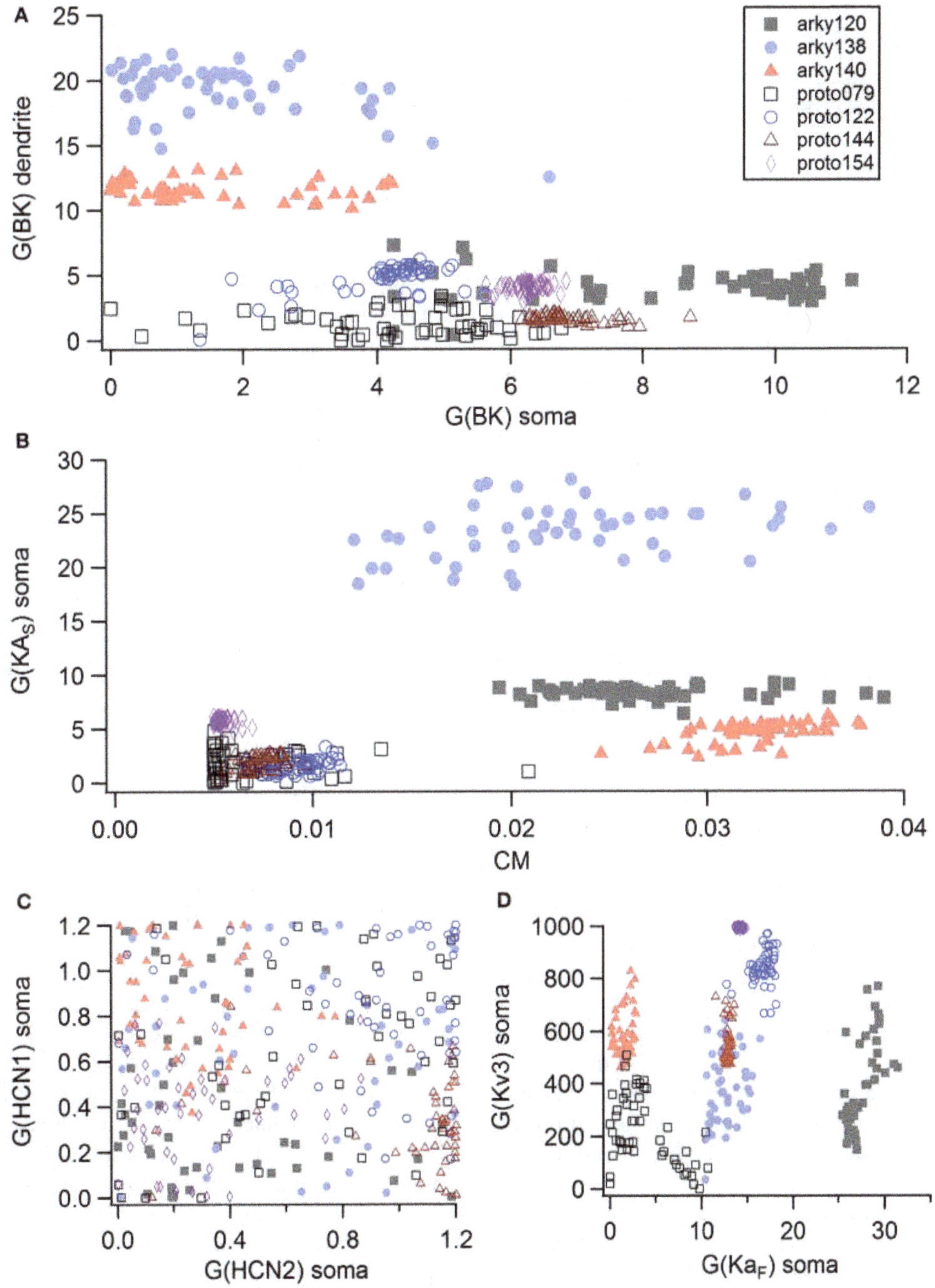

FIGURE 7 | A small number of parameters separate the two subtypes of GPe neurons. **(A)** The large conductance, calcium dependent potassium conductance (BK) in soma and dendrite are larger in arkyN than in protoN. **(B)** Capacitance (CM), and (to a lesser extent) the slow transient potassium channel conductance are greater in arkyN than in protoN **(C–D)** No systematic differences are observed in HCN conductance **(C)** or in Kv3 or KA_F **(D)** between arkyN and protoN. Symbols corresponding to different neurons are the same in all panels and indicated in **A**.

height, AHP shape as well as non-spiking features. The large number of features can be combined into a single feature, used individually in multi-objective optimization (Druckmann et al., 2007; Rumbell et al., 2016; Neymotin et al., 2017), or combined into one (or a few) combined features (Keren et al., 2009; Rumbell et al., 2016). One rationale for performing a multi-objective optimization is that an overall best match may not be possible; instead a multi-objective optimization provides a set of optimal solutions that represent the best trade-offs between conflicting objectives. Using multi-objective optimization also avoids the process of assigning weights to features, which by definition are to some extent arbitrary. Nevertheless, after obtaining the set of optimal solutions from a multi-objective optimization, finding one solution that achieves a good fit of all features may be difficult. We opted to combine multiple objectives (features) into a single fitness value, effectively preferring solutions that performed moderately well on all measures to those which were optimized toward some specific subset of features. Early explorations using multi-objective optimization yielded models that indeed fitted some features well, but at the same time were divergent enough in other characteristics that if observed experimentally, such neurons would be classified as a different type. For real neurons, natural variability exists between inviduals of the same type, and also between repeated measurements, yet the defining features are common to all neurons of a certain type. We feel that fitting very precisely to *some* characteristics of an invidual experimental measurement is less useful than fitting *all* features approximately.

An important concept utilized by multi-objective optimization is weighting the various feature fitnesses by variance across the data, under the assumption that more variable features should be less constrained. Weighting by variance (i.e., dividing by the standard deviation) also removes dimensionality from the data (e.g., dividing a difference of 10 mV by a standard deviation of 1 mV yields the dimensionless number of 10). This procedure allows fitness values of features with both small values (e.g., spike width measured in seconds) and large values (e.g., spike height measured in mV) to contribute meaningfully to the total fitness. Whereas the variance for the spike characteristics can be calculated within a neuron, a better variance estimate requires recordings of multiple trials or multiple neurons (Hendrickson et al., 2011b). Our algorithm removes dimensionality from the feature fitnesses by dividing the difference between data and simulations by the mean. The software also allows a weight to be specified, which could be (the inverse of) the variance between neurons. Clearly, another improvement to the software would be to add a module to calculate and use the variance between neurons either when current injection protocols are repeated several times or when multiple data sets are available.

A major concern with using parameter optimization to identify differences between neuron types is that unique parameter sets do not exist (Golowasch et al., 2002; Prinz et al., 2003b; Olypher and Calabrese, 2007; Hay et al., 2011). Instead there are multiple valid parameter sets with parameter co-variation, which hinders the ability to classify neurons based on these conductance parameters. Though CMA-ES takes into account these correlations during the optimization, CMA-ES does not find all parameter sets, since it continually seeks a (single) global minimum. In principal, CMA-ES could be initiated from different points in parameter space to find multiple local minima. Even with a single run of CMA-ES per neuron recording, analysis of the best parameter sets revealed several correlations between conductances when all models of a neuron subtype were considered. The most common correlations were compensatory, with increases in inward currents correlated with increases in outward currents, or increases in one type of potassium current correlated with a decrease in a different type of potassium current. Interestingly, most correlations were not observed for a single neuron, but were observed across the set of neurons, suggesting that differences in that set of conductances may represent natural variation within neuron subtypes (Taylor et al., 2009).

Optimization of several exemplars allowed us to evaluate differences between neuron subtypes. Experimentally, low frequency firing neurons of the globus pallidus, such as the arkypallidal neurons, show a slight increase of firing rate when the BK channel is blocked (Abrahao et al., 2017). In addition, ethanol (which directly targets the BK channel) does not affect the firing rate of high frequency firing, prototypical neurons of the globus pallidus; but does decrease the firing rate of low frequency GPe neurons by increasing the open probability of BK channels (Abrahao et al., 2017). These experimental data suggest that arkypallidal and prototypical neurons have different conductance of BK channels, as suggested by statistical analysis of the arkyN and protoN parameters. ArkyN and protoN neuron models also differed in transient potassium conductance, which has been reported experimentally (Hernández et al., 2015). The HCN channel also has been characterized in arkypallidal and prototypical neurons, with one report of a difference (Hernández et al., 2015) and one report of no difference (Mastro et al., 2014). Our observation of no difference in HCN currents between subtypes is consistent with the latter publication, but it is not inconsistent with the data from the former which shows that strong hyperpolarization is required to observe the greater sag ratio of PV− vs. PV+ neurons.

The optimization also reported that ArkyN had higher capacitance than ProtoN, a difference that is not supported experimentally. One possible cause of this discrepancy is the use of the same morphology for all GPe optimizations, since using a different morphology changes the fitted passive parameters (Holmes et al., 2006). The neurons from which electrophysiology data were obtained have not been reconstructed, precluding using the morphology that matches the data. In addition, the optimization may have (incorrectly) increased the ArkyN capacitance to produce shallow AHPs, to compensate for the present inability to adjust time constants and half activation values of the potassium currents. Note that the classification of arkypallidal vs. prototypical neurons is based on firing characteristics, with recent attempts to identify these neurons based on biochemical markers. There is broad agreement than PV+ neurons are prototypical, but PV− neurons can be prototypical cells, expressing Lhx6 (Mastro et al., 2014), or arkypallidal cells, expressing Npas1+ or FoxP2+ (Dodson et al., 2015; Hernández et al., 2015; Glajch et al., 2016). In fact, there are both similarities (HCN conductance) and differences (transient potassium current) between the Npas1+ and Lhx6+ neurons.

Future parameter optimization of morphlogically reconstructed neurons exhibiting these different markers may better determine ionic conductance differences among all these neuron types. Ideally, easy-to-use, automatic approaches for identifying neuron channel parameters may facilitate experiments used to characterize such differences.

AUTHOR CONTRIBUTIONS

ZJ-S: modeling and optimization software development, manuscript preparation; JJ-S: modeling software development, manuscript preparation; KA: GPe experiments, manuscript preparation; DL: GPe experiments, manuscript preparation; KB: SP experiments, modeling software development, model simulation and analysis, manuscript preparation.

FUNDING

This work was supported by the joint NIH-NSF CRCNS program through NIAAA grant R01DA03889 and NSF grant 1515686.

ACKNOWLEDGMENTS

Thanks to Rebekah Evans for collecting the SP experimental data.

REFERENCES

Abarbanel, H. D. I., Creveling, D. R., Farsian, R., and Kostuk, M. (2009). Dynamical state and parameter estimation. *SIAM J Appl. Dyn. Syst* 8, 1341–1381. doi: 10.1137/090749761

Abrahao, K. P., Chancey, J. H., Chan, C. S., and Lovinger, D. M. (2017). Ethanol-sensitive pacemaker neurons in the mouse external globus pallidus. *Neuropsychopharmacology* 42, 1070–1081. doi: 10.1038/npp.2016.251

Bahl, A., Stemmler, M. B., Herz, A. V., and Roth, A. (2012). Automated optimization of a reduced layer 5 pyramidal cell model based on experimental data. *J. Neurosci. Methods* 210, 22–34. doi: 10.1016/j.jneumeth.2012.04.006

Bourquard, T., Landomiel, F., Reiter, E., Crépieux, P., Ritchie, D. W., Azé, J., et al. (2015). Unraveling the molecular architecture of a G protein-coupled receptor/β-arrestin/Erk module complex. *Sci. Rep.* 5, 1–13. doi: 10.1038/srep10760

Brookings, T., Goeritz, M. L., and Marder, E. (2014). Automatic parameter estimation of multicompartmental neuron models via minimization of trace error with control adjustment. *J. Neurophysiol.* 112, 2332–2348. doi: 10.1152/jn.00007.2014

Cannon, R. C., Gleeson, P., Crook, S., Ganapathy, G., Marin, B., Piasini, E., et al. (2014). LEMS: a language for expressing complex biological models in concise and hierarchical form and its use in underpinning NeuroML 2. *Front. Neuroinform.* 8:79. doi: 10.3389/fninf.2014.00079

Chan, C. S., Peterson, J. D., Gertler, T. S., Glajch, K. E., Quintana, R. E., Cui, Q., et al. (2012). Strain-specific regulation of striatal phenotype in Drd2-eGFP BAC transgenic mice. *J.Neurosci.* 32, 9124–9132. doi: 10.1523/JNEUROSCI.0229-12.2012

Damodaran, S., Cressman, J. R., Jedrzejewski-Szmek, Z., and Blackwell, K. T. (2015). Desynchronization of fast-spiking interneurons reduces -band oscillations and imbalance in firing in the dopamine-depleted striatum. *J. Neurosci.* 35, 1149–1159. doi: 10.1523/JNEUROSCI.3490-14.2015

Day, M., Wokosin, D., Plotkin, J. L., Tian, X., and Surmeier, D. J. (2008). Differential excitability and modulation of striatal medium spiny neuron dendrites. *J. Neurosci.* 28, 11603–11614. doi: 10.1523/JNEUROSCI.1840-08.2008

Dodson, P. D., Larvin, J. T., Duffell, J. M., Garas, F. N., Doig, N. M., Kessaris, N., et al. (2015). Distinct developmental origins manifest in the specialized encoding of movement by adult neurons of the external globus pallidus. *Neuron* 86, 501–513. doi: 10.1016/j.neuron.2015.03.007

Druckmann, S., Banitt, Y., Gidon, A., Schürmann, F., Markram, H., and Segev, I. (2007). A novel multiple objective optimization framework for constraining conductance-based neuron models by experimental data. *Front. Neurosci.* 1, 7–18. doi: 10.3389/neuro.01.1.1.001.2007

Friedrich, P., Vella, M., Gulyás, A. I., Freund, T. F., and Káli, S. (2014). A flexible, interactive software tool for fitting the parameters of neuronal models. *Front. Neuroinform.* 8:63. doi: 10.3389/fninf.2014.00063

Gewaltig, M. O., and Cannon, R. (2014). Current practice in software development for computational neuroscience and how to improve it. *PLoS Comput. Biol.* 10:e1003376. doi: 10.1371/journal.pcbi.1003376

Glajch, K. E., Kelver, D. A., Hegeman, D. J., Cui, Q., Xenias, H. S., Augustine, E. C., et al. (2016). Npas1+ pallidal neurons target striatal projection neurons. *J. Neurosci.* 36, 5472–5488. doi: 10.1523/JNEUROSCI.1720-15.2016

Gleeson, P., Crook, S., Cannon, R. C., Hines, M. L., Billings, G. O., Farinella, M., et al. (2010). NeuroML: a language for describing data driven models of neurons and networks with a high degree of biological detail. *PLoS Comput. Biol.* 6:e1000815. doi: 10.1371/journal.pcbi.1000815

Golowasch, J., Goldman, M. S., Abbott, L. F., and Marder, E. (2002). Failure of averaging in the construction of a conductance-based neuron model. *J. Neurophysiol.* 87, 1129–1131. doi: 10.1152/jn.00412.2001

Günay, C., Edgerton, J. R., and Jaeger, D. (2008). Channel density distributions explain spiking variability in the globus pallidus: a combined physiology and computer simulation database approach. *J. Neurosci.* 28, 7476–7491. doi: 10.1523/JNEUROSCI.4198-07.2008

Gurkiewicz, M., and Korngreen, A. (2007). A numerical approach to ion channel modelling using whole-cell voltage-clamp recordings and a genetic algorithm. *PLoS Comput. Biol.* 3:e169. doi: 10.1371/journal.pcbi.0030169

Hansen, N., and Kern, S. (2004). Evaluating the CMA evolution strategy on multimodal test functions. *Parallel Probl. Solv. Nat. PPSN* 2004, 282–291. doi: 10.1007/978-3-540-30217-9_29

Hay, E., Hill, S., Schürmann, F., Markram, H., and Segev, I. (2011). Models of neocortical layer 5b pyramidal cells capturing a wide range of dendritic and perisomatic active properties. *PLoS Comput. Biol.* 7:e1002107. doi: 10.1371/journal.pcbi.1002107

Hendrickson, E. B., Edgerton, J. R., and Jaeger, D. (2011a). The capabilities and limitations of conductance-based compartmental neuron models with reduced branched or unbranched morphologies and active dendrites. *J.Comput. Neurosci.* 30, 301–321. doi: 10.1007/s10827-010-0258-z

Hendrickson, E. B., Edgerton, J. R., and Jaeger, D. (2011b). The use of automated parameter searches to improve ion channel kinetics for neural modeling. *J. Comput. Neurosci.* 31, 329–346. doi: 10.1007/s10827-010-0312-x

Hernández, V. M., Hegeman, D. J., Cui, Q., Kelver, D. A., Fiske, M. P., Glajch, K. E., et al. (2015). Parvalbumin+ neurons and Npas1+ neurons are distinct neuron classes in the mouse external globus pallidus. *J. Neurosci.* 35, 11830–11847. doi: 10.1523/JNEUROSCI.4672-14.2015

Holmes, W. R., Ambros-Ingerson, J., and Grover, L. M. (2006). Fitting experimental data to models that use morphological data from public databases. *J. Comput. Neurosci.* 20, 349–365. doi: 10.1007/s10827-006-7189-8

Jedrzejewska-Szmek, J., Damodaran, S., Dorman, D. B., Blackwell, K. T., et al. (2017). Calcium dynamics predict direction of synaptic plasticity in striatal spiny projection neurons. *Eur. J. Neurosci.* 45, 1044–1056. doi: 10.1111/ejn.13287

Johenning, F. W., Theis, A. K., Pannasch, U., Rückl, M., Rüdiger, S., and Schmitz, D. (2015). Ryanodine receptor activation induces long-term plasticity of spine calcium dynamics. *PLOS Biol.* 13:e1002181. doi: 10.1371/journal.pbio.1002181

Keren, N., Bar-Yehuda, D., and Korngreen, A. (2009). Experimentally guided modelling of dendritic excitability in rat neocortical pyramidal neurones. *J. Physiol* 587, 1413–1437. doi: 10.1113/jphysiol.2008.167130

Keren, N., Peled, N., and Korngreen, A. (2005). Constraining compartmental models using multiple voltage recordings and genetic algorithms. *J. Neurophysiol.* 94, 3730–3742. doi: 10.1152/jn.00408.2005

Lee, S. H., Schwaller, B., and Neher, E. (2000). Kinetics of Ca^{2+} binding to parvalbumin in bovine chromaffin cells: implications for $[Ca^{2+}]$ transients of neuronal dendrites. *J. Physiol.* 525(Pt 2), 419–432. doi: 10.1111/j.1469-7793.2000.t01-2-00419.x

Marder, E., and Goaillard, J. M. (2006). Variability, compensation and homeostasis in neuron and network function. *Nat. Rev. Neurosci.* 7, 563–574. doi: 10.1038/nrn1949

Martínez-Álvarez, A., Crespo-Cano, R., Díaz-Tahoces, A., Cuenca-Asensi, S., Ferrández Vicente, J. M., and Fernández, E. (2016). Automatic tuning of a retina model for a cortical visual neuroprosthesis using a multi-objective optimization genetic algorithm. *Int. J. Neural Syst.* 26:1650021. doi: 10.1142/S0129065716500210

Martínez-Cañada, P., Morillas, C., Plesser, H. E., Romero, S., and Pelayo, F. (2017). Genetic algorithm for optimization of models of the early stages in the visual system. *Neurocomputing* 250, 101–108. doi: 10.1016/j.neucom.2016.08.120

Mastro, K. J., Bouchard, R. S., Holt, H. A., and Gittis, A. H. (2014). Transgenic mouse lines subdivide external segment of the globus pallidus (GPe) neurons and reveal distinct GPe output pathways. *J. Neurosci.* 34, 2087–2099. doi: 10.1523/JNEUROSCI.4646-13.2014

Meza, R. C., López-Jury, L., Canavier, C. C., and Henny, P. (2018). Role of the axon initial segment in the control of spontaneous frequency of nigral dopaminergic neurons *in vivo*. *J. Neurosci.* 38, 733–744. doi: 10.1523/JNEUROSCI.1432-17.2017

Nevian, T., and Sakmann, B., (2004). Single spine Ca^{2+} signals evoked by coincident EPSPs and backpropagating action potentials in spiny stellate cells of layer 4 in the juvenile rat somatosensory barrel cortex. *J Neurosci.* 24, 1689–1699. doi: 10.1523/JNEUROSCI.3332-03.2004

Neymotin, S. A., Suter, B. A., Dura-Bernal, S., Shepherd, G. M., Migliore, M., and Lytton, W. W. (2017). Optimizing computer models of corticospinal neurons to replicate *in vitro* dynamics. *J. Neurophysiol.* 117, 148–162. doi: 10.1152/jn.00570.2016

Olypher, A. V., and Calabrese, R. L. (2007). Using constraints on neuronal activity to reveal compensatory changes in neuronal parameters. *J. Neurophysiol.* 98, 3749–3758. doi: 10.1152/jn.00842.2007

Prinz, A. A., Billimoria, C. P., and Marder, E. (2003a). Alternative to hand-tuning conductance-based models: construction and analysis of databases of model neurons. *J. Neurophysiol.* 90, 3998–4015. doi: 10.1152/jn.00641.2003

Prinz, A. A., Bucher, D., and Marder, E. (2004). Similar network activity from disparate circuit parameters. *Nat. Neurosci.* 7, 1345–1352. doi: 10.1038/nn1352

Prinz, A. A., Thirumalai, V., and Marder, E. (2003b). The functional consequences of changes in the strength and duration of synaptic inputs to oscillatory neurons. *J. Neurosci.* 23, 943–954. doi: 10.1523/JNEUROSCI.23-03-00943.2003

Qian, K., Yu, N., Tucker, K. R., Levitan, E. S., and Canavier, C. C. (2014). Mathematical analysis of depolarization block mediated by slow inactivation of fast sodium channels in midbrain dopamine neurons. *J. Neurophysiol.* 112, 2779–2790. doi: 10.1152/jn.00578.2014

Raikov, I., Cannon, R., Clewley, R., Cornelis, H., Davison, A., De Schutter, E., et al. (2011). NineML: the network interchange for neuroscience modeling language. *BMC Neurosci.* 12:P330. doi: 10.1186/1471-2202-12-S1-P330

Ray, S., and Bhalla, U. S. (2008). PyMOOSE: Interoperable Scripting in Python for MOOSE. *Front Neuroinformatics.* 2:6. doi: 10.3389/neuro.11.006.2008

Richmond, P., Cope, A., Gurney, K., and Allerton, D. J. (2014). From model specification to simulation of biologically constrained networks of spiking neurons. *Neuroinformatics* 12, 307–323. doi: 10.1007/s12021-013-9208-z

Rossant, C., Goodman, D. F., Fontaine, B., Platkiewicz, J., Magnusson, A. K., and Brette, R. (2011). Fitting neuron models to spike trains. *Front. Neurosci.* 5:9. doi: 10.3389/fnins.2011.00009

Rumbell, T. H., Draguljić, D., Yadav, A., Hof, P. R., Luebke, J. I., and Weaver, C. M. (2016). Automated evolutionary optimization of ion channel conductances and kinetics in models of young and aged rhesus monkey pyramidal neurons. *J. Comput. Neurosci.* 41, 65–90. doi: 10.1007/s10827-016-0605-9

Ryu, C., Jang, D. C., Jung, D., Kim, Y. G., Shim, H. G., Ryu, H. H., et al. (2017). STIM1 regulates somatic Ca^{2+} signals and intrinsic firing properties of cerebellar Purkinje neurons. *J. Neurosci.* 37, 8876–8894. doi: 10.1523/JNEUROSCI.3973-16.2017

Schaefer, A. T., Larkum, M. E., Sakmann, B., and Roth, A. (2003). Coincidence detection in pyramidal neurons is tuned by their dendritic branching pattern. *J. Neurophysiol.* 89, 3143–3154. doi: 10.1152/jn.00046.2003

Segev, I., and London, M. (2000). Untangling dendrites with quantitative models. *Science* 290, 744–750. doi: 10.1126/science.290.5492.744

Taylor, A. L., Goaillard, J. M., and Marder, E. (2009). How Multiple conductances determine electrophysiological properties in a multicompartment model. *J. Neurosci.* 29, 5573–5586. doi: 10.1523/JNEUROSCI.4438-08.2009

Tucker, K. R., Huertas, M. A., Horn, J. P., Canavier, C. C., and Levitan, E. S. (2012). Pacemaker rate and depolarization block in nigral dopamine neurons: a somatic sodium channel balancing act. *J. Neurosci.* 32, 14519–14531. doi: 10.1523/JNEUROSCI.1251-12.2012

Van Geit, W., De Schutter, E., and Achard, P. (2008). Automated neuron model optimization techniques: a review. *Biol. Cybern.* 99, 241–251. doi: 10.1007/s00422-008-0257-6

Van Geit, W., Gevaert, M., Chindemi, G., Rössert, C., Courcol, J.-D., Muller, E. B., et al. (2016). BluePyOpt: leveraging open source software and cloud infrastructure to optimise model parameters in neuroscience. *Front. Neuroinform.* 10:17. doi: 10.3389/fninf.2016.00017

Van Ooyen, A., Duijnhouwer, J., Remme, M. W., and Van Pelt, J. (2002). The effect of dendritic topology on firing patterns in model neurons. *Netw. Comput. Neural Syst.* 13, 311–325. doi: 10.1088/0954-898X/13/3/304

Vanier, M. C., and Bower, J. M. (1999). A comparative survey of automated parameter-search methods for compartmental neural models. *J. Comput. Neurosci.* 7, 149–171. doi: 10.1023/A:1008972005316

5

Credibility, Replicability and Reproducibility in Simulation for Biomedicine and Clinical Applications in Neuroscience

Lealem Mulugeta[1], Andrew Drach[2], Ahmet Erdemir[3], C. A. Hunt[4], Marc Horner[5], Joy P. Ku[6], Jerry G. Myers Jr.[7], Rajanikanth Vadigepalli[8] and William W. Lytton[9,10,11]**

[1] InSilico Labs LLC, Houston, TX, United States, [2] The Institute for Computational Engineering and Sciences, The University of Texas at Austin, Austin, TX, United States, [3] Department of Biomedical Engineering and Computational Biomodeling (CoBi) Core, Lerner Research Institute, Cleveland Clinic, Cleveland, OH, United States, [4] Department of Bioengineering and Therapeutic Sciences, University of California, San Francisco, San Francisco, CA, United States, [5] ANSYS, Inc., Evanston, IL, United States, [6] Department of Bioengineering, Stanford University, Stanford, CA, United States, [7] NASA Glenn Research Center, Cleveland, OH, United States, [8] Department of Pathology, Anatomy and Cell Biology, Daniel Baugh Institute for Functional Genomics and Computational Biology, Thomas Jefferson University, Philadelphia, PA, United States, [9] Department of Neurology, SUNY Downstate Medical Center, The State University of New York, New York, NY, United States, [10] Department of Physiology and Pharmacology, SUNY Downstate Medical Center, The State University of New York, New York, NY, United States, [11] Department of Neurology, Kings County Hospital Center, New York, NY, United States

***Correspondence:**
Lealem Mulugeta
lealem@insilico-labs.com
William W. Lytton
bill.lytton@downstate.edu

Modeling and simulation in computational neuroscience is currently a research enterprise to better understand neural systems. It is not yet directly applicable to the problems of patients with brain disease. To be used for clinical applications, there must not only be considerable progress in the field but also a concerted effort to use best practices in order to demonstrate model credibility to regulatory bodies, to clinics and hospitals, to doctors, and to patients. In doing this for neuroscience, we can learn lessons from long-standing practices in other areas of simulation (aircraft, computer chips), from software engineering, and from other biomedical disciplines. In this manuscript, we introduce some basic concepts that will be important in the development of credible clinical neuroscience models: reproducibility and replicability; verification and validation; model configuration; and procedures and processes for credible mechanistic multiscale modeling. We also discuss how garnering strong community involvement can promote model credibility. Finally, in addition to direct usage with patients, we note the potential for simulation usage in the area of Simulation-Based Medical Education, an area which to date has been primarily reliant on physical models (mannequins) and scenario-based simulations rather than on numerical simulations.

Keywords: computational neuroscience, verification and validation, model sharing, modeling and simulations, Simulation-Based Medical Education, multiscale modeling, personalized and precision medicine, mechanistic modeling

INTRODUCTION

One hallmark of science is reproducibility. An experiment that cannot be reproduced by others may result from statistical aberration, artifact, or fraud. Such an experiment is not credible. Therefore, reproducibility is the first stage to ensure the credibility of an experiment. However, reproducibility alone is not sufficient. For example, an *in vitro* experiment is performed to advance or aid the understanding of *in vivo* conditions. However, the applicability of *in vitro* results to the living tissue may be limited due to the artifact of isolation: a single cell or a tissue slice extracted from its environment will not function in precisely the way it functioned *in situ*. In medicine, animal models of a disease or treatment are frequently used, but may not be credible due to the many differences between the human and the monkey, rat, or another animal that may limit the transfer of findings from one species to another.

In the computational world, the credibility of a simulation, model or theory depends strongly on the projected model use. This is particularly true when translating a model from research usage to clinical usage. In research, innovation and exploration are desirable. Computer models are used to introduce or explore new hypotheses, ideally providing a new paradigm for experimentation. In this setting, the most important models may in some cases be the less credible ones – these are the models that stretch understanding by challenging the common view of how a particular system works, in order to offer a paradigm shift. Here, *prima facie* credibility is in the eye of the beholder, who is more likely representing the views of the community – the dominant paradigm.

In the clinical realm, by contrast, establishing credibility is of paramount importance. For pharmaceuticals, credibility is currently established through evidence-based medicine (EBM), ideally through double-blind trials with large numbers of patients. The downside of this statistical approach is that it necessarily aggregates a large number of disparate patients to achieve statistical significance. In some cases, this has resulted in tragedy, as a subgroup with particular genetics has a fatal response to a drug that is beneficial in the overall group (e.g., rofecoxib, brand-name Vioxx). As EBM gives way to precision medicine, pharmaceutical credibility will be established in each subgroup, or even at an individual level, to enhance safety. However, to establish pharmaceutical reliability for personalized medicine (precision with a subgroup of $n = 1$), a lack of comparator precludes the use of data-mining by definition. Simulations based on patient genetics and various levels of epigenetics up through brain connectomics will then be the only way to predict the response of an individual patient to a particular treatment. Such patient simulation would provide a prediction of the response of that patient's unique physiodynamics to a therapy. The credibility of such models will be essential.

In addition to pharmacotherapy, brain disease treatment also utilizes other therapeutic modalities, ranging from neurosurgery to the talk therapy of psychiatry and clinical psychology. While the latter will likely remain beyond the range of our modeling efforts, neurosurgery has already begun to benefit from modeling efforts to identify locations and pathways for epilepsy ablation surgery (Jirsa et al., 2017; Lytton, 2017; Proix et al., 2017). Another set of therapeutic approaches that are likely to benefit from modeling are the electrostimulation therapies that are finding increased use in both neurology and psychiatry, e.g., deep brain stimulation (DBS), transcranial magnetic stimulation (TMS), transcranial direct/alternating current stimulation (tDCS/tACS), and electroconvulsive therapy (ECT) (Kellner, 2012). Neurorehabilitation will also benefit from modeling to help identify procedures to encourage neuroplasticity at locations where change will have the greatest effect for relief of deficit.

In most respects, the issues of credibility, replicability, reproducibility for computational neuroscience simulation are comparable to those faced by researchers using simulation to study other organ systems. However, the complexity of the brain and several special features provide unique challenges. As with modeling of other organ systems, the relevant length scales range from molecular (angstrom) level up through tissue (centimeter) levels. Many experiments extend from the lowest to highest scales, for example evaluating performance on a memory task as a drug modifies ion channel activity at the molecular level. Compared to other organ systems, there is a particularly broad range of temporal scales of interest: 100 microseconds of sodium channel activation up to years of brain maturation and learning. In addition to physical scales of the central nervous system (CNS) itself, brain research includes further investigative levels of cognition, information, and behavior. An additional aspect of nervous system organization involves overlap between scales, which prevents encapsulation of one scale for inclusion in the higher scale. For example, spatiotemporal activity in apical dendrites of neocortical pyramidal cells (subcellular level) are co-extensive in both spatial and temporal scales with the scales of the local network (supracellular level).

In this paper, we will focus on the many issues of model credibility from a biomedical and clinical perspective. We will use *model* here forward to mean a mathematical model, primarily analyzed *in silico* via a *simulation*, which is the numerical instantiation of a mathematical model on a computer. We will identify explicitly in cases where we are discussing other types of models: verbal models, animal models, physical models, etc. Currently, there are still relatively few models of brain disease, and those remain in the research domain, rather than being practical clinical tools. Therefore, we are considering policy and practice for a future *clinical computational neuroscience*, based on the current uses of computational neuroscience in basic biomedical research, and on the clinical usage of simulations in other domains of medicine. In doing this, we will introduce some basic concepts that are important in the development of credible models: Reproducibility and Replicability; Verification and Validation.

REPRODUCIBILITY AND REPLICABILITY

Replicability, here subsuming repeatability, is the ability to achieve a fully identical result (Plesser, 2017). For example, in the case of neuronal network simulation, a simulation has been fully replicated when one can show that spike times, as well as all state variables (voltages, calcium levels), are identical to those in the original simulation. Replicability is a design desideratum in engineering when one wants to ensure that a system being distributed runs identically to a prototype system (Drummond, 2009; Crook et al., 2013; McDougal et al., 2016a).

Reproducibility, in contrast, is the ability of a simulation to be copied by others to provide a simulation that provides the same *results* (Crook et al., 2013; McDougal et al., 2016a). This will then depend on what one considers to be a result, which will reflect the purposes of the simulation and will involve some measures taken on the output. Taking again the case of the neuronal network simulation, a result might involve some direct statistical measures of spiking (e.g., population rates), perhaps complemented by the summary statistics provided by field potential spectra, likely ignoring state-variable trajectories or their statistics.

Replicability and reproducibility are inversely related. A turnkey system, provided on dedicated hardware or a dedicated virtual machine, will run identically every time and therefore be fully replicable. However, such a system will not be reproducible by outsiders, and may in some cases have been encrypted to make it difficult to reverse engineer. Generally, the higher level the representation is, the more readily other groups understand a simulation and reproduce the results, but the less likely it is that they obtain an identical result - lower replicability. Representations using equations - algebra, linear algebra, calculus - are identical worldwide and therefore can provide the greatest degree of reproducibility by any group anywhere. However, reproducing a simulation from equations is a laborious process, more difficult than reproducing from algorithms, which is, in turn, more laborious than reproducing from a declarative (e.g., XML) representation. A dedicated package in the domain which provides a declarative description of a simulation will be more easily ported than general mathematical declarative description for \dynamical systems. Even at the level of reproduction from software code, differences in numerical algorithms used in computer implementations will lead to somewhat different results.

Different software representations also provide different levels of difficulty in the task of reproducing a simulation by porting to another language. The major innovation in this respects has been the development and adoption of object-oriented languages such as Java and Python. In particular, the use of object inheritance allows the definition of a type (e.g., a cell) with a subsequent definition of particular subtypes, where each type has parameter differences that are easily found and can be clearly documented by provenance.

Some difficulties with precise replicability of simulations are common to many different simulation systems. In particular, a model that uses pseudo-random numbers will not replicate precisely if a different randomizer is used, if seeds are not provided, or if randomizers are not handled properly when going from serial to parallel implementations. One difficulty peculiar to neural simulation is related to the strong non-linearities (and numerical stiffness) associated with action potential spike thresholding. Spiking networks are sensitive to round-off error; a single time-step change in spike time will propagate to produce changes in the rest of the network (London et al., 2010).

In general, specific simulation programs have enhanced reproducibility by providing purpose-built software to solve the particular problems of the computational neuroscience domain. Typically, these packages couple ordinary differential equation (ODE) solvers for simulating individual neurons with an event-driven queuing system to manage spike event transmission to other neurons in neuronal networks. These facilities are provided by neuronal network simulators such as BRIAN (Goodman and Brette, 2008), PyNN (Davison et al., 2008), and NEST (Plesser et al., 2015), which allow spiking neurons to be connected in networks of varying size. It should be noted that these simulators are very different from the artificial neural networks used in deep learning, which do not implement spiking neurons. Some other packages also add the ability to do more detailed cellular simulation for the individual neurons by adding the partial differential equations (PDE) needed to simulate the internal chemophysiology that complements the electrophysiology of spiking - NEURON (Carnevale and Hines, 2006) and MOOSE (Dudani et al., 2009) provide this additional functionality. Many computational neuroscience simulations in are still carried out using general-purpose mathematical software, e.g., Matlab (The Mathworks, Inc., Natick, MA, United States); or by more general computer languages such as FORTRAN, C, or C++, limiting their reproducibility, reusability, and extensibility. However, it should also be noted that the popularity of software also plays a role. A language or package that is widely used will increase the number of people that can easily contribute to developing or utilizing the simulations.

Since computational neuroscience simulations are often very large, extensibility to high-performance computing (HPC) resources is also desirable and will enhance reproducibility. Some current simulator tools offer a direct path to these larger machines. NetPyNE, a declarative language built on top of NEURON, provides a general description of a network that can be run directly either on a serial processor or, via MPI (message passing interface), on an HPC resource (Lytton et al., 2016). The Neuroscience Gateway Portal provides a shared, NSF-supported graphical resource that simplifies HPC for a variety of simulators, including NetPyNE, NEURON, NEST, BRIAN, and others, avoiding the need for the user to know MPI usage (Carnevale et al., 2014).

Hypothetically, journal articles permit reproducibility using equations given in the Methods section. Often, however, full details are not provided due to the enormous complexity of information associated with many different cell types, and complex network connectivity (McDougal et al., 2016a). Furthermore, parameters and equations may be given for one figure, but not for all figures shown. Journal articles may also have typographical or omission errors. And even when the document is complete and entirely without error, errors are likely to creep in when reproduction is attempted, and the model is typed or scanned back into a computer. For all of these reasons, an electronic version of a model is more accurate and more immediately usable than a paper copy. Some journals, and many individual editors or reviewers, require software sharing as part of the publication process. However, some authors resist this mandate, desiring to retain exclusive access to their intellectual property.

Databases of models and parts of models have become important and have encouraged reproducibility in computational neuroscience (Gleeson et al., 2017). Additional value is added by utilizing formal model definitions such as ModelML, CellML, NeuroML, VCML, SBML (Hucka et al., 2003; Zhang et al., 2007; Lloyd et al., 2008; Moraru et al., 2008; Gleeson et al., 2010; Cannon et al., 2014). Major databases are being provided by the Human Brain Project, the Allen Brain Institute, the International Neuroinformatics Coordinating Facility, and others. Other databases include the NeuroMorpho.Org database of neuronal morphologies, the ModelDB database of computational neuroscience models (see this issue) in a variety of simulation packages and languages, and the Open Source Brain database for collaborative research (Gleeson et al., 2012, 2015; Gleeson et al., unpublished). We discuss these resources further in the section discussing the "Role of the Community."

A recent initiative to encourage reproducibility in science is the new *ReScience Journal* (rescience.github.io), which publishes papers that replicate prior computational studies. By hosting the journal on GitHub, new implementations are directly available alongside the paper, and alongside any ancillary materials identifying provenance or providing documentation. Recently, the classic Potjans-Diesmann cortical microcircuit model was ported from NEST to BRIAN, reproducing and confirming the primary results (Cordeiro et al., unpublished).

GOOD PRACTICES CONTRIBUTING TO SIMULATION CREDIBILITY

Verification and Validation (V&V)

Verification

Verification and validation (V&V) help users demonstrate the credibility of a computational model within the context of its intended use. This is accomplished by assessing the quantitative and qualitative aspects of the model that influence model credibility. The process of establishing the model's correctness and its capability to represent the real system is accomplished through the processes of verification, validation, uncertainty propagation, and sensitivity analysis. Of these, V&V represent the most well-known, and potentially confused, aspects of model assessment.

Computational models may be implemented using open-source or commercial (off-the-shelf) software, custom (in-house) code, or a combination of the two (modified off-the-shelf software). Verification assures that a computational model accurately represents the underlying mathematical equations and their solution on a specific code platform. Verification also emphasizes confirmation of parameter specification and the accurate translation of model data from model data sources into the model application. Full verification for all possible inputs is technically not possible due to the halting problem. Nonetheless, software implementation of model concepts should always include some level of code verification and, to the extent possible, follow best management practices and established quality-assurance processes. In the case of commonly used simulation packages, verification will be the responsibility of the platform developer and not of the user, but unanticipated usage can bring verification concerns back to the fore in particular cases.

Verification can be divided into two sequential steps: code verification and calculation verification. *Code verification*, initially performed by the software platform developer provides evidence that the numerical algorithms implemented in the code are faithful representations of the underlying physical or conceptual model of the phenomenon. Code verification should be repeated by the user in the case of novel usage of the simulator. Code verification establishes the reliability of the source code in representing the conceptual model, including relevant physics, for the problem. Ideally, benchmark problems with analytical solutions are employed to ensure that the computer code generates the correct solution at the specified order of accuracy. For example, a common reference in computational fluid dynamics (CFD) is laminar flow in a straight pipe with a circular cross-section, whose analytical solution is well-known (Bird et al., 1960; Stern et al., 2006). CFD modeling techniques are being used to provide insight into flow patterns and rupture-risk of cerebral artery aneurysms (Campo-Deaño et al., 2015; Chung and Cebral, 2015) and for interventional radiology planning (Babiker et al., 2013). Unfortunately, no analytic solutions are available for most computational neuroscience applications. Therefore, one is restricted to comparing results from one numerical approximation to that of another, without reference to any ground truth (Brette et al., 2007).

Next, *calculation verification* aims to estimate numerical and logical errors associated with the conceptual model implementation, i.e., the computational model representing the target application. Going back to the laminar pipe flow example, one would specify geometry, material properties, and loading conditions to match the problem at hand. This typically results in a problem that no longer has an analytical solution but must be solved numerically. Various aspects of the numerical representations, particularly discretization, are investigated and refined until the model is deemed to be accurate within a pre-specified tolerance. Upon completion of the calculation verification step, the developer has established (and should document) a bug-free implementation of the model concepts with reasonable parameter values.

One of aspect of verification that is often overlooked in the computational science community is the testing of model scripts and binary codes. Researchers tend to focus their attention on V&V in the context of overall program performance, but omit testing the functionality of individual software modules. Module verification can be implemented as a suite of tests which verify the functionality of individual functions and modules (unit tests) and their integration within the system (integration tests). It is common practice to automate the testing procedures using an automated testing framework to perform these tests after each version update.

Validation

Everyday vernacular often equates or confuses the terms "verification" and "validation." As described in the previous section, *verification* seeks to ensure the quality of the implementation of the conceptual model. Meanwhile, *validation* seeks to assess how well the conceptual model and its implementation on a specified code platform represent the real-world system for a defined application. More rigorously stated, validation is an assessment of the degree to which the model and simulation is an accurate representation of the response of the real system within the intended context of use. In this case, validation is a comparative process that defines a qualitative or quantitative measure of how the model differs from an appropriate experimental or other data source – the *referent*, generally a series of experiments in our context. Validation also helps to ensure that the computational model has *sufficient* rigor for the context of use, although a more rigorous or more precise model is not necessarily more credible.

The definition of an appropriate referent is a critical aspect of model validation. Ideally, a validation referent consists of data obtained from a system with high similarity to the system being modeled in an environment similar to that of the target system. In clinical computational neuroscience, this is often difficult since data is obtained from a rodent (not high similarity to human), and sometimes from a slice (environment not similar to *in vivo* situation). The data used should be considered to be high quality by the model end-user community, and should represent data not used in model development. This separates *design data* from *testing data* (also called fit vs. benchmark data, or calibration vs. validation data). Model limitations due to inadequacies of the validation referent should be communicated. Practitioners should also keep in mind that a model validation, or the understanding of the variability of the model in predicting real world response, is only valid in the area of the referents used in the validation process, as illustrated by the Validation Domain (**Figure 1**). The Application Domain may be larger than the Validation Domain; it establishes the range of input and output parameters relevant to the context of use of the computational model. As the application of the model deviates from the situational context described by the referent, the influence of the model validation information will also change.

In most cases, the more quantitative the comparison, the stronger the case that a model and simulation is contextually valid. Organizations such as the American Society of Mechanical Engineers have developed standards to guide the model practitioner in performing successful model validation activities for specific application domains[1]. These comparisons range from qualitative, graphical comparative measures to quantitative comparative measures relying on statistical analysis of referent and model variances, the latter obtained over a wide range of input parameter variation (Oberkampf and Roy, 2010). Ideally, the end-user community and regulatory agencies will play a role in assessing the adequacy of the validation based on the context of an expected application and the influence the model has on critical decision-making.

Aspects of Good Practice for Credibility

Software Aspects

The credibility of simulation results requires the reliability of simulation protocols and software tools. Good software practices include version control; clear, extensive documentation and testing; use of standard (thoroughly tested) software platforms; and use of standard algorithms for particular types of numerical solutions. It is also desirable to rely on existing industry standards and guidelines and to compare simulation results against competing implementations. To maintain the highest level of credibility, one would establish and follow these practices at every step of the development, verification, validation, and utilization of the simulation tools.

Version control is an approach for preserving model development and use histories, which can also be useful for tracing the provenance of model parameters and scope of applicability. There exists a large number of version control systems (VCS) which provide on-site, remote, or distributed solutions (e.g., Git, SVN, and Mercurial). In general terms, these systems provide tools for easy traceability of changes in individual files, attribution of modifications and updates to the responsible author, and versioning of specific snapshots of the complete system. Use of a VCS is recommended for both development (troubleshooting of bugs) as well as the day-to-day use of the modeling tools (monitoring of modeling progress).

Good documentation can be aided by the rigorous use of a detailed, dated electronic laboratory notebook (e-notebook). The e-notebook can provide automatic coordination with software versions and data output. E-notebooks are supported through various software packages, notably the Python Jupyter notebook and the Emacs org-mode notebook (Schulte and Davison, 2011; Stanisic et al., 2015; Kluyver et al., 2016). A major advantage over the traditional paper notebook is that the e-notebook can be directly integrated into simulation workflow, and will also provide direct pointers to simulation code, output, figures, data, parameter provenance, etc. This then allows later reviewers to identify all these links unambiguously. However, compared with a paper notebook, the e-notebook is at greater risk of falsification due to later rewriting. This risk can be reduced by including the e-notebook in the VCS, and can be eliminated by using blockchain technology (Furlanello et al., 2017). An e-notebook will also include informative records of model development and implemented assumptions; hypotheses and approaches to testing the hypotheses; model mark-up; detailed descriptions of the input and output formats; and simulation testing procedures. Going beyond the e-notebook, but also linked through it, the developer may add case studies, verification problems, and tutorials to ensure that other researchers and practitioners can learn to use the model.

It should be noted that even models developed following the aforementioned guidelines will have application bugs and usability issues. Thus, it is valuable to also cross-verify simulation results using alternative execution strategies and competing

[1] https://cstools.asme.org/csconnect/CommitteePages.cfm?Committee=100108782

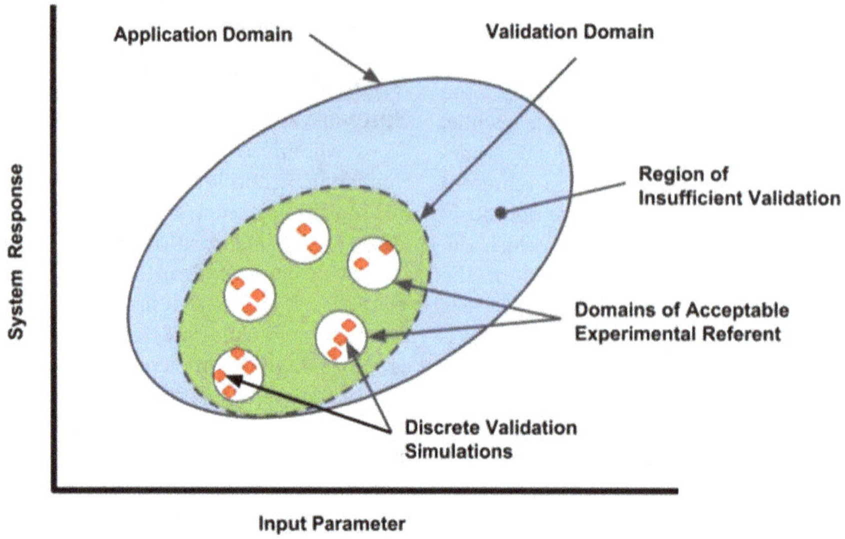

FIGURE 1 | Validation domain of a computational model for a range of input parameters and outputs (system responses). Red diamonds represent the validation set points, where comparisons between the computational model and applicable referents were conducted by discrete simulations performed in each referent sub-domain. The range of parameters evaluated establishes the Validation Domain (green ellipse), which will define the extent of the Application Domain (large blue ellipse) where model performance has established credibility. Applications of the model outside of the Application Domain lack validation and have lesser credibility.

model implementations – e.g., run a simulation using BRIAN and NEST (Cordeiro et al., unpublished) – to reduce the chance of obtaining spurious simulation results. In addition to the inter-model verification, simulation process should be governed by generally applicable or discipline-specific standard operating procedures, guidelines, and regulations.

Developing Credible Mechanism-Oriented Multiscale Models: Procedure and Process

In science, an explanation can be inductive, proceeding from repeated observation. Ideally, however, explanation precedes prediction, permitting deductive reasoning (Hunt et al., 2018). Simulation of a mechanistic multiscale model provides an explicit way of connecting a putative explanatory mechanism to a phenomenon of interest.

Credibility and reproducibility can be enhanced by taking note of the many factors and workflows required to build a credible simulation to be used in a clinical application. One of these, often overlooked, is the role of exploratory (non-credible) simulations in building credible simulations. We would argue that most of the simulations that have been done in computational neuroscience are exploratory, and that we can now begin winnowing and consolidating these to create credible simulations for clinical application.

Unfortunately, the problems in biology and particularly in neuroscience are characterized by (1) imprecise, limited measures – for example, EEG measures 6 cm of cortex at once (Nunez and Srinivasan, 2005); (2) complex observations whose relevance is sometimes unclear – there is no broad agreement on the relevance of particular bands of brain oscillations (Weiss and Mueller, 2012); (3) sparse, incommensurable and sometimes contradictory supporting information – for example, the difficulties of connecting microconnectomic (<1 mm; axon tracing, dual impalement, etc.) with macroconnectomic (1 cm; functional magnetic resonance imaging, fMRI) measures; and (4) high degree of uncertainty – parameter values obtained from brain slice work may differ from *in vivo* values. These limitations (left of ranges in **Figure 2**) contrast with the more solid information, concepts, observables and lower uncertainty associated with "classical" engineering of man-made devices such as computers, cars, and aircraft.

Model development is difficult, involving the need to consider and consolidate a large variety of factors from

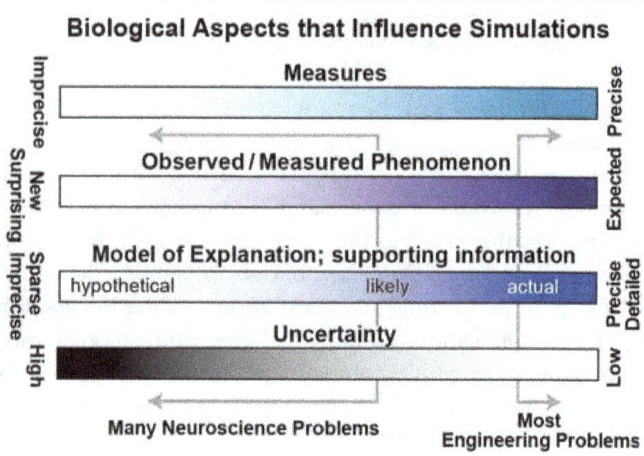

FIGURE 2 | Spectra to characterize biological aspects of interest. Classical engineering problems lie at the right side of each range, working with precise measures, strong expectations, detailed information and low uncertainty. Unfortunately, most neuroscience problems lie far to the left with weak measures, unclear phenomenology, sparse information and high uncertainty.

biology, engineering, mathematics, and design under the many constraints due to the limitations mentioned above. We have identified a set of procedures for the building of credible simulations, breaking out the many sub-workflows and processes involved (**Figure 3**). One can spend years building tools and running exploratory simulations that only lay the groundwork for future credible models. Nonetheless, it is important not to lose sight of the goal, which is to explain brain phenomenology at one or more levels of description: electrical rhythms, movement, behavior, cognition, etc.

The first task is to specify phenomena to be explained (**Figure 3b** – Observed Phenomenon). From this perspective, potentially relevant biological aspects are then organized together with relevant information and data into incipient explanations (**Figure 3c** – Descriptions and Explanations). In the computational neuroscience community, there are multiple perspectives regarding what information is to be considered relevant. For example, some argue that dendritic morphology and the details of ion channels are critical for understanding cortical networks (Amunts et al., 2017), while others consider that one need only consider simplified spiking cells (Diesmann et al., 1999; Potjans and Diesmann, 2014; Cain et al., 2016), and still others that it is best to work with high-level dynamical representations of populations (Shenoy et al., 2013) or mean-field theory (Robinson et al., 2002). Indeed all of these perspectives can be regarded as part of the explanatory modeling that will find its way into new concepts of (1) what is considered to be a relevant observation or measurement (**c** to **b** in **Figure 3**) and (2) what will be considered to be the form of an eventual causal explanation (**c** to **a**). Development of this incipient explanation will involve establishing mappings and drawing analogies between features of the explanation and particular measurements. These mappings and analogies may then be extended to provide working hypotheses and to actual preliminary biomimetic simulations for the eventual causal explanations.

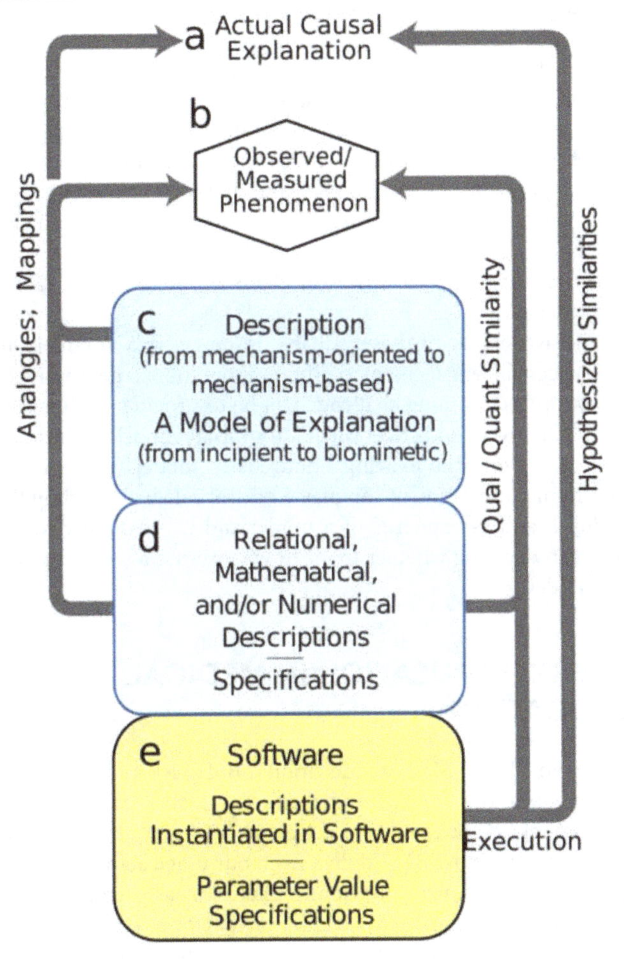

FIGURE 3 | Mechanistic multiscale modeling process. **(a)** Causal explanation to be discovered. **(b)** Observables of phenomena to be explained. **(c)** Process (workflow) to identify and organize related information into descriptions; this process will involve simulation. **(d)** Meta-modeling workflows required for defining the extent of the final model. **(e)** Credible simulation which matches target phenomenon within some tolerance.

A set of additional considerations (**Figure 3d** – Numerics and Specifications) provide the bridge from the exploratory activities (**Figure 3c** – Descriptions) to final credible models of (**Figure 3e** – Software). Although illustrated toward the bottom, these aspects of project formulation should be considered from the start as well. In computational neuroscience, potential use cases are still being developed and differ considerably across the four major clinical neuroscience specialties. Use cases, and data availability, will identify phenomena to be considered. For example, access to electroencephalography (EEG), but not electrocorticography, changes not only the type of software to be developed, but also the types of explanations to be sought. Use cases will also need to be organized based on expectations, separating near-term and long-term needs. New computational neuroscience users, use cases, and applications will arise in other specialties as they consider the innervation of other organs (Barth et al., 2017; Samineni et al., 2017; Vaseghi et al., 2017; Ross et al., 2018).

While identification of users and use cases remains relatively underdeveloped in computational neuroscience, the development of simulation tools is quite sophisticated. The need for multialgorithmic as well as multiphysics simulation has required that simulation platforms combine a variety of numerical and conceptual techniques: ODEs, PDEs, event-driven, graph theory, information theory, etc. Simulation techniques have been developed over more than a half-century, starting with the pioneering work of Hodgkin and Huxley (1952), Fitzhugh (1961), Rall (1962), and others. Today, we have a large variety of simulators with different strengths (Carnevale and Hines, 2006; Brette et al., 2007; Davison et al., 2008; Goodman and Brette, 2008; Bower and Beeman, 2012; Plesser et al., 2015; Tikidji-Hamburyan et al., 2017) that can be used individually or in combination, cf. MUSIC (Djurfeldt et al., 2010).

During the final stage of credible model development (**Figure 3e**), we demonstrate that the model provides the desired outputs to represent observations (**e** to **b**). A typical requirement is that simulation outputs agree with target phenomenon measurements within some tolerance. Since the simulation system will be multi-attribute and multiscale, it will at the very least begin providing mechanism-based, causal understanding across measures. To the extent that the model is truly biomimetic, direct mappings will exist to specific biological counterparts – voltages, spike times, field potential spectra, calcium levels, or others.

Although credible software appears to be the end of the road, actual practice will require that the resulting software system undergoes many rounds of verification, validation, refinement, and revision before even being released to users. From there, continued credibility requires continuing work on documentation, tutorials, courses, bug reports and bug fixes, requested front-end enhancements, and identified backend enhancements.

ROLE OF THE COMMUNITY

Community involvement is important to establish the credibility of the modeling and simulation process, and of the models themselves. The peer-review publication process serves as a traditional starting point for engaging the community. However, sharing of models, along with the data used to build and evaluate them, provides greater opportunities for the community to directly assess credibility. The role of sharing models and related resources has been acknowledged in the neurosciences community (McDougal et al., 2016a; Callahan et al., 2017). Related resources for sharing include documentation of the model (commonly provided in English) and implementation encoded in its original markup or code. With access to the model and its associated data and documentation, interested parties can then assess the reproducibility and replicability of the models and the simulation workflow first-hand. Further, reuse of the models and extensions of the modeling and simulation strategies for different applications can reveal previously unknown limitations. These various community contributions help build up the credibility of a model.

It is also important to note the value of cross-community fertilization to establish a common ground for credible modeling and simulation practices, to conform to and evolve standards that promote a unified understanding of model quality. Such standards enable individuals to easily exchange and reuse a given model on its own, or in combination with other models. Especially in multi-scale modeling, the ability to trust and build upon existing models can accelerate the development of these larger-scale efforts. Organizations such as the Committee on Credible Practice for Modeling and Simulation in Healthcare are leading efforts to establish such standards (Mulugeta and Erdemir, 2013).

Most community involvement in computational neuroscience has come through the establishment of databases and other resources that have encouraged submissions from the overall community of researchers. For example, the Scholarpedia resource established by Izhikevich and collaborators has hosted articles on computational neuroscience concepts and techniques that have been used to share concepts, modeling techniques, and information about particular modeling tools (Gewaltig and Diesmann, 2007; Wilson, 2008; Seidenstein et al., 2015). The Open Source Brain project provides a central location for collaborators working on modeling the nervous system of particular brain areas or of whole organisms, notably the OpenWorm project for modeling the full nematode nervous system (Szigeti et al., 2014). The Human Brain Project, an EU effort, has established a number of "Collaboratories," web-accessible platforms to curate models and conduct simulations, to encourage community involvement in coordinated projects (Amunts et al., 2017). One of these projects aims to identify the parameters underlying individual synaptic events recorded in voltage clamp experiments (Lupascu et al., 2016). The Allen Brain Institute, another large modeling and data collection center, shares all results with the community, even before publication. Most of the major simulator projects encourage contributions from the community to provide either simulator extensions or additional analytic tools. For example, the SenseLab project hosts a SimToolDB alongside ModelDB for sharing general simulation code (Nadkarni et al., 2002). ModelDB itself is a widely used resource which specifically solicits model contributions and then provides a starting point for many new modeling projects that are extensions or ports of existing models (Peterson et al., 1996; McDougal et al., 2016b).

The above databases are used to provide completed models that are designed to be stand-alone but can also be used as components of larger models. By contrast, detailed neuron morphologies and ion channel models are generally only used as starting points for other models to build models at higher scales. Examples of these databases include the NeuroMorpho.Org database of neuronal morphologies and the Channelpedia database of voltage-sensitive ion channels (Ascoli et al., 2007; Ranjan et al., 2011).

The availability of these valuable resources is a testament to the successful engagement of the computational neuroscience community. A coming challenge will be to provide mechanisms for the discovery and selection of appropriate models for defined contexts among the existing hundreds of models. Here again, community involvement can play a critical role by providing the feedback and assessments of a model and its credibility to aid others in deciding whether to, or how to, re-use a model or part of a model.

USE OF SIMULATION IN MEDICAL EDUCATION

Simulation-Based Medical Education (SBME) is rapidly growing, with applications for training medical students, and residents (Jones et al., 2015; Yamada et al., 2017). However, the use of the word *simulation* in SBME differs from our usage above. SBME is referring to *simulated reality*: paper exercises based on protocols; mannequins; re-enactments with live actors for physical exams or major disasters; detailed computer-based virtual reality training, similar to video games. Currently, even the most advanced mannequins and computer-generated simulations have very limited capacity to produce a realistic focal neurological deficit or combination of signs and symptoms. Design and implementation of SBME tools is especially challenging in brain disease due to the complexity of the brain, and the variety of its responses to insult (Chitkara et al., 2013; Ermak et al., 2013; Fuerch et al., 2015; Micieli et al., 2015; Konakondla et al., 2017). This complexity suggests that back-end multiscale modeling would be particularly valuable in SBME development for brain disease.

Mechanistic multi-scale modeling has been used in both pre-clinical and clinical education to explain disease causality. For example, a demyelination simulation, relevant to multiple sclerosis and Guillain-Barre syndrome, is available that demonstrates both the effects of demyelination on action potential propagation and the consequent increase in temperature sensitivity (Moore and Stuart, 2011). Although this model has not been linked directly to a hands-on SBME activity, it could be linked to a training activity for Nerve Conduction Studies. Another promising area of recent research interest is in the area of neurorobotics, where robotic arms have been linked to realistic biomimetic simulations in the context of neuroprosthetics (Dura-Bernal et al., 2014; Falotico et al., 2017). In the clinical neurosciences, epilepsy is one of the most successfully modeled disorders in neurology and neurosurgery (Lytton, 2008). Jirsa et al. (2017) have pioneered models of individual patients prior to epilepsy surgery - see Section "Personalized Medicine Simulation for Epilepsy.". These simulations could now be extended into training protocols for neurology and neurosurgery residents, offering an opportunity for melding educational simulation with computational neuroscience.

Current SBME efforts are focused on mannequins. A generic mannequin was used to train medical students to manage differential diagnoses and emergency procedures for status epilepticus and acute stroke (Ermak et al., 2013). The mannequin used was not capable of mimicking visible, or electrographic, signs of stroke or seizures. Instead, students were given chart data and simulation actors playing family member. Such simulations necessarily fall short on one aspect of effective implementation of SBME (Issenberg et al., 2005): the degree to which the simulation has a "real-life" feel.

In the future, life-like and highly immersive SBME will facilitate the learning of dangerous medical procedures, including emergencies and recovery from mistakes, in the way that is currently done with simulators used to train pilots, astronauts and flight controllers. Ideally, neurology and neurosurgery (and eventually psychiatry and physiatry) SBME systems will produce learned skills that are transferable to patient care. The predictive validity of the simulation could then be assessed by comparing performance measured under simulation conditions with corresponding measurements made on real patients (Konakondla et al., 2017). However, the skill level of a learner in the simulator should not be taken as a direct indication of real-life skill performance. In one example from flight training, a particular technique (full rudder), which served to "game" the simulator, resulted in a fatal accident due to tail separation when used in real life (Wrigley, 2013).

An example of SBME in neurosurgical training is the Neuro-Touch surgical training system developed by the National Research Council of Canada (Konakondla et al., 2017). The systems is built around a stereoscope with bimanual procedure tools that provide haptic feedback and a real-time computer-generated virtual tissue that responds to manipulation. As the surgeon is working through a surgical scenario, the simulator records metrics for detailed analysis to develop benchmarks for practitioners at different stages of training.

The Neurological Exam Rehearsal Virtual Environment (NERVE) virtual-patient SBME tool was developed to teach 1st- and 2nd-year medical students how to diagnose cranial nerve deficits (Reyes, 2016). Educational results were validated using questionnaires designed for virtual patient simulators (Huwendiek et al., 2014). An interesting future extension would be to provide an underlying simulator that would take account of the many complex neurological deficits found in patients due to the anatomical confluence of tracts in the brainstem. Such a simulator would be useful for neurology residents as well as for medical students.

To advance both the technologies and methodologies applied in SBME, the Society for Simulation in Healthcare (SSH) recently established the Healthcare Systems Modeling and Simulation Affinity Group. The Committee on Credible Practice of Modeling and Simulation in Healthcare (Mulugeta and Erdemir, 2013) has been collaborating with the SSH community by providing guidance on how to design and implement explicit multiscale computational models into traditional SBME systems. Additionally, the Congress of Neurological Surgeons has formed a Simulation Committee to create simulations for resident education (Konakondla et al., 2017). The US Food and Drug Administration (FDA) and the Association for the Study of Medical Education have also been working to publish standards and guidelines for regulatory submissions involving computational models and simulations for healthcare applications (Hariharan et al., 2017).

USE OF MODELING IN CLINICAL DOMAINS OF BRAIN DISEASE

Simulations in the clinical neuroscience domain have largely focused on accounting for the neural activity patterns underlying brain disease. Testing the predictions arising from the simulation is dependent on technological advances in neuromodulation, pharmacology, electrical stimulation, optogenetic stimulation, etc. Neuropharmacological treatment is systemic, with effects wherever receptors are found, often peripherally as well as centrally. Although targeted treatment with an implanted cannula is possible, it is not widely used clinically. By contrast, electrical stimulation can be highly targeted with a local placement of electrodes. Development of closed-loop systems and devices for brain stimulation (Dura-Bernal et al., 2015), are currently being used and show promise in treating a wide range of neurological diseases and disorders including Parkinson, depression, and other disorders (Johansen-Berg et al., 2008; Shils et al., 2008; Choi et al., 2015). Non-targeted electrostimulation using transcranial electrodes is also being widely used but remains controversial, and lacks precise clinical indications (Lefaucheur et al., 2014; Esmaeilpour et al., 2017; Huang et al., 2017; Lafon et al., 2017; Santos et al., 2017). Consideration is also being given to future use of optogenetic stimulation therapies that would offer still greater precision compared to electrical stimulation – targeting not only a particular area but a particular cell type or set of cell types within that area (Vierling-Claassen et al., 2010; Kerr et al., 2014; Samineni et al., 2017). All such stimulation protocols require identification of suitable, if not necessarily optimal, ranges of parameters, e.g., strength, duration, frequency, waveform, location, iterations, schedule, reference activity, etc. It is not generally feasible to evaluate this large and high-dimensional stimulus parameter space empirically through experimentation. Hence, stimulation development would benefit from the extensive explorations possible using simulation of the response of micro- and macro-scale neural circuits in the brain, potentially in patient-specific fashion.

Successful application of models in the clinical domain will in future depend on the use of credible practices to develop, evaluate, document and disseminate models and simulations, using the principles outlined above. Nonetheless, clinical applications will also always need to be verified and validated by in a clinical before being utilized. At present, studies have been done in the absence of standards for computational neuroscience models. The current manuscript is designed in part to continue the discussion about the development of such standards. Meanwhile, clinically relevant studies have been performed with varying degrees of adherence to engineering best-practices. Here, we briefly discuss two such studies, noting adherence to such practices and where investigators may have fallen short.

Simulation of Multi-Target Pharmacology

We first consider a mechanistic multiscale model of multi-target pharmacotherapy for disorders of cortical hyperexcitability (Neymotin et al., 2016). The study assessed hyperexcitability in an exploratory manner. They did not identify a single clinical context. Rather, they left the study open for exploration of cortical activation in both dystonia and seizures.

The multiscale model included molecular, cellular, and network scales, containing 1715 compartmental model neurons with multiple ion channels and intracellular molecular dynamics. Data used to develop the model was taken from a large number of sources including different species, different preparations (slice, cell culture, *in vivo, ex vivo*), different age animals, different states, different conditions. None of the data was taken from the clinical disorders in question due to limitations of human experimentation. As the model lacked a description of the motor output, the simulations could not be systematically evaluated in the context of dystonia. Beta activation in the cortex was used as a surrogate biomarker to evaluate whether simulations could account for activity patterns relevant to dystonia. However, as with many brain diseases, there is no established, clinically validated biomarker for dystonia. Additionally, the model lacked representations of spinal cord or limb, as well as many pharmacological parameters, particularly with respect to the role of neuromodulators (known unknown), brain states (less known unknown) and metabolic parameters.

The simulations were able to reproduce the target patterns of heightened cortical activity. The corresponding pathological parameter sets were identified by independent random variations in parameters. These simulations demonstrated degeneracy, meaning that there were many combinations of parameters that yielded the pathological syndrome. The primary result was that no individual parameter alteration could consistently distinguish between pathological and physiological dynamics. A support vector machine (SVM), a machine learning approach, separated the physiological from pathological patterns in different regions of high-dimensional space, suggesting multi-target routes from dystonic to physiological dynamics. This suggested the potential need for a multi-target drug-cocktail approach to intervening in dystonia.

Several aspects of best-practices were utilized in this study. Dissemination: The model was disseminated via publication and meeting presentations with the code made available via ModelDB resource (reference #189154). Documentation: Limited documentation was also made available at a level conforming to ModelDB requirements, consistent with practices accepted by the computational neuroscience community. Provenance: Due to the nature of the clinical domain, parameter provenance was partial; details of parameter sources were included in the paper. Replicability: Model replicability was tested by ModelDB curators, but was not tested directly by the manuscript reviewers. Reproducibility: There have not yet been any third-party studies reproducing the model. There are unexploited opportunities to compare the model with alternative implementations, for example by considering simpler modeling formalisms for single-neuron activity. The credibility of the simulations along with insights derived from the results would be enhanced by follow-on work that reproduces the simulations using similar or alternative implementations. Validation: The current lack of an adequate biomarker for dystonia limits the ability to validate this study in the future. Verification: The NEURON simulation platform was used in this study. It has been vetted both internally and in comparison to other simulators (Brette et al., 2007). Versioning: The Mercurial VCS was used to track parameter variations and match to corresponding simulations.

Personalized Medicine Simulation for Epilepsy

As a contrast to above examination of the credibility practices as applicable to a mechanistic multiscale model, we considered these issues in the context an individualized phenomenological model of seizure propagation by Proix et al. (2017), implemented using The Virtual Brain platform (Sanz-Leon et al., 2013). The study was aimed at demonstrating that patient-specific virtual brain models derived based on information from diffusion MRI technique have sufficient predictive power to improve diagnosis and surgery outcome in cases of drug-resistant epilepsy. Data from individual patient tractography and EEG was utilized to parameterize each individual model separately. The diffusion MRI-based connectivity observed between the parcellated brain regions in each individual was used to create patient-specific connectivity matrices that related distinct autonomous oscillators ("Epileptors") at each brain region. The resultant patient-specific virtual brain model was evaluated for its consistency in predicting seizure-like activity patterns in that patient.

Dissemination: The model and the results were disseminated as part of the published manuscript as well as through conference presentations and posters. Documentation: The platform is well documented. Internal documentation of individual models for use by neurosurgeons may be available but was not publically available, perhaps for reasons of patient confidentiality. Provenance: Provenance of connectivity data from individual patients was made clear. The Epileptor model is a phenomenological description of oscillatory patterns of activity in a bulk tissue (neural mass model); hence, there are no explicit parameters or variables that directly arise from specific molecular, cellular and metabolic pathways. Replicability: While the manuscript was peer-reviewed, it is not readily apparent if the model was tested directly in simulations by the manuscript reviewers. Reproducibility: Virtual Brain provides a particular dynamical formalism based on bulk activity. It would be interesting to see if alternative model formalisms that incorporate details at cellular scales would produce similar results. Validation: Alternative connectivity matrices and weightings were considered based on data from control subjects, shuffling the data, changing the weights while preserving the topology of the connectivity, and log-transformation. The authors demonstrated that prediction of seizure patterns was best when the patient-specific topology of the connectivity matrix was utilized. Verification: The study considered alternative models based on fast coupling, no time-scale separation, and a generic model that shows saddle-node bifurcation. Based on the simulations considering these alternative models, the authors concluded that weak coupling is necessary for the predictions on the recruited networks. The Virtual Brain platform has undergone considerable code testing over the years. Versioning: The platform is made available in a public repository using Git.

ACTIONABLE RECOMMENDATIONS AND CONCLUSIONS

The potential of modeling and simulation in clinical application and medical education are promising. However, this potential is mainly being tapped in the areas that are close to traditional engineering domains, such as CFD and stress analysis. For this reason areas of medicine that are related to blood flow, biomechanics and orthopedics have benefited most. By contrast, the brain has an idiosyncratic evolved set of mechanisms that are extremely difficult to reverse engineer and which draw on many areas of engineering, some of which have not been invented yet. Therefore, computational neuroscience remains primarily in the research domain, with only fragmented translations from computational neuroscience to clinical use or to medical education. As medical practice moves toward precision, and then personalized, healthcare, multiscale modeling will be necessary for simulating the individual patient's response to disease and treatment. To move toward this goal, we must cultivate credible modeling and simulation practices taken from traditional areas of engineering.

Model Configuration Management

Since many models will be built within the context of a simulation platform, we refer here to "Model configuration." However, all of these points apply *a fortiori* to models being built from scratch in a general-purpose programming language.

(1) Use *version control*: Git or Mercurial (hg) are preferred. GitHub can be used to host projects (Dabbish et al., 2012). In shared projects, version control establishes who is responsible for which pieces of code.

(2) Use an *electronic notebook* (e-notebook) with clear documentation of every stage of model development (including mistakes).

(3) Include *provenance* of parameters in e-notebook and via version control - parameters may be changed due to new experimental data, and it is valuable to have a clear record of when and why the change was made and what the consequence was for the model.

(4) Perform testing of model components: for example, demonstrate that the cell-types show proper firing characteristics before incorporating them into networks.

(5) Later in the process, develop a test suite for further testing. Ideally, model testing should be performed at every version update. A test suite can be linked to standard testing frameworks to automate this testing. Commonly used frameworks include Travis CI (Continuous Integration), Circle CI, Jenkins, and AppVeyor.

(6) Whenever possible, use reliable model development platforms such as NEST, BRIAN, NEURON, MOOSE, NENGO, PyNN, etc. This will increase the likelihood of accurate simulation and will enhance sharing. Similarly, model components should be taken from reliable databases of morphologies, channels and other components.

(7) Later in the process, encourage other groups to compare simulation results on alternative platforms or with different implementations.

Verify and Validate Models

(1) Simulation platform developers generally verify the adequacy of the numerical analysis. Some simulators offer alternative numerical solvers which can be tested to assess the qualitative similarity of results. For example, one problematic area is the handling of fixed and variable time steps for spike handling in networks (Lytton and Hines, 2005).

(2) Verify algorithms you develop. For example, when developing a neuronal network, make sure that the network design is correct before moving to actual simulation.

(3) Verify that the simulation is a reasonable implementation of the conceptual model, ideally by comparing a graphical output of basic phenomenology with target phenomena. It is tragically easy to move on to the analysis phase of the study without first looking at the raw output to make sure it is reasonable.

(4) Validate based on data from a real-world system. In some cases, it may be important to distinguish simulation results

from the same model for different situations, e.g., *in vitro* slice vs. *in vivo* background activation.
(5) Test robustness of a model to parameter changes to ascertain whether a particular result is only seen with a particular set of parameter choices.
(6) Document and propagate V&V testing processes and findings to the community.

Although all of these steps are valuable, it is important to understand that higher model fidelity and V&V rigor do not automatically translate to higher credibility.

Share Models and Data

(1) Submit models to shared databases such as ModelDB or via GitHub. Share widely – you can submit the same model to various databases, and submit components such as cells and ion channel definitions to component databases.
(2) Document thoroughly – the Methods section of a paper will provide an overall gloss but, typically, will not provide sufficient detail about software design and use. Comment code. Provide a README on how to launch the simulation.
(3) Disseminate – publish, of course, and present posters and talks to various audiences. In a multidisciplinary area such as computational neuroscience, the same model will say different things to different audiences – physiologists, anatomists, cognitive neuroscientists, neurologists, psychiatrists, other modelers.
(4) Join communities via organizations such as Society for Neuroscience (SFN), Computational and Systems Neuroscience (CoSyne), Organization for Computational Neuroscience (CNS).
(5) Obtain independent reviews of models. This is difficult and time-consuming but some grants are now providing funding explicitly to pay for consultants to review models (NIH, 2015).

Define Context of Use and Simulation Requirements

We distinguished above between *exploratory models*, done by an individual researcher in order to provide ideas and new hypotheses, and *context models*, purpose-built models for external users in a given environment, for example, clinical or medical education use. In the latter case, it is essential to be clear about who the users are and which usage patterns (sets of use cases) are to be targeted and which ones are to be excluded or to be left as part of longer-term goals. However, even exploratory models can benefit from these considerations, envisioning yourself, your team, and perhaps an experimental collaborator as users.

(1) Identify the *users*. Even if you are the only user at the beginning of the project, you will be sharing the model later, so you may want to take account of other users who are not as familiar with your domain. For clinical use, a clinical assistant for epilepsy would be different for neurosurgeons vs. neurologists.
(2) Identify the *context of use*. For example, will this model primarily be used to study dynamics, or will it be extended into information theory or will it be expected to perform a memory function, etc.
(3) Identify *intended uses*. You may have one intended use for yourself as a modeler to generate new theoretical hypotheses and another for your experimental colleague. In the context of an educational application, an SBME for medical students will be very different than an application for residents or continuing medical education.
(4) Attempt to identify *usage patterns* – it is often the case that underprepared users who have not read the manual use a program in unintended, and sometimes dangerous, ways. Platforms and programs can produce warnings when it detects that the user is trying to use unsuitable combinations of parameters, etc.

Translation of Computational Neuroscience Models for Clinical and Medical Education Use

In the preceding sections, we have given examples of particular clinical and educational/training scenarios that may be ripe for the introduction of simulation technology. Here we list both those already mentioned and others that have potential for future applications. This list is by no means complete.

(1) Education: Integration of modeling into mannequins and online virtual patients to reproduce neurological deficits in SBME. Initial versions of this would not require mechanistic multiscale modeling but could be done with phenomenological modeling. Future versions would incorporate mechanistic modeling to also incorporate the time-course of signs and symptoms (dynamics at multiple timescales).
(2) Training: Virtual reality simulators with haptic feedback for neurosurgery training.
(3) Personalized patient simulations to decide on surgery vs. interventional radiology (coiling) for aneurysms.
(4) Clinical decision making: Personalized patient simulations to decide on surgical approach for epilepsy surgery (Jirsa et al., 2017).
(5) Simulation for seizure prediction in Epilepsy Monitoring Unit (EMU).
(6) Personalized patient simulation to determine therapies for Parkinson disease to include combinations of surgical, electrical and pharmacological therapy (Grill and McIntyre, 2001; Hammond et al., 2007; Shils et al., 2008; Van Albada et al., 2009; Kerr et al., 2013; Holt and Netoff, 2017).
(7) Head, brain and neural modeling for understanding effects of different kinds of electrical stimulation including transcranial stimulation (Esmaeilpour et al., 2017; Huang et al., 2017; Lafon et al., 2017).
(8) Modeling vagal and peripheral nerve stimulation for treatment of systemic disorders (NIH SPARC program[2]).

[2]https://commonfund.nih.gov/sparc

(9) Psychiatry: identifying the varying roles of disorder in dopaminergic, glutamatergic, inhibitory and other deficits in schizophrenia to develop new multi-target therapies (Lisman et al., 2010).

(10) Neurorehabilitation (physiatry) Modeling the interface between neural and musculoskeletal models to treat spasticity or dystonia (van der Krogt et al., 2016).

AUTHOR CONTRIBUTIONS

LM and WL worked collaboratively to layout the contents of the manuscript, coordinate the team of co-authors, as well as edited the final draft of the manuscript. All of the co-authors drafted the specific section listed below beside their initials, as well as helped with the review and editing of the entire manuscript. LM: Abstract, Use of Simulation in Medical Education, and Actionable Recommendations and Conclusions, rewriting manuscript. AD: Software Aspects. AE and JK: Role of the Community. CH: Developing Credible Mechanism-Oriented Multiscale Models: Procedure and Process section. JM and MH: Verification and Validation (V&V). RV: Use of Modeling in Clinical Domains of Brain Disease. WL: Introduction, Reproducibility and Replicability, and Actionable Recommendations and Conclusions, rewriting manuscript.

FUNDING

This research was supported by NIH R01GM104139, R01EB024573, and USAMRMC W81XWH-15-1-0232 (AE); NIH R01 GM107340, U54 EB020405, P2C HD065690; USAMRMC W81XWH-15-1-0232 (JK); NIBIB U01 EB023224, NHLBI U01 HL133360, NIH OT2 OD023848 (RV); and NIH R01-EB022903, U01-EB017695, R01-MH086638, NYS DOH01-C32250GG-3450000 (WL).

ACKNOWLEDGMENTS

The authors would like to thank all members of the Committee on Credible Practice of Modeling & Simulation in Healthcare who have been dedicated to the advancement of the Committee's mission, but were not able to directly contribute to the development of this manuscript. The authors would also like to extend their sincerest gratitude to the Interagency Modeling and Analysis Group (IMAG), and the Multiscale Modeling Consortium (MSM) for enabling the Committee's work.

REFERENCES

Amunts, K., Ebell, C., Muller, J., Telefont, M., Knoll, A., and Lippert, T. (2017). The human brain project: creating a European research infrastructure to decode the human brain. *Neuron* 92, 574–581. doi: 10.1016/j.neuron.2016.10.046

Ascoli, G. A., Donohue, D. E., and Halavi, M. (2007). NeuroMorpho.Org: a central resource for neuronal morphologies. *J. Neurosci.* 27, 9247–9251. doi: 10.1523/JNEUROSCI.2055-07.2007

Babiker, M. H., Chong, B., Gonzalez, L. F., Cheema, S., and Frakes, D. H. (2013). Finite element modeling of embolic coil deployment: multifactor characterization of treatment effects on cerebral aneurysm hemodynamics. *J. Biomech.* 46, 2809–2816. doi: 10.1016/j.jbiomech.2013.08.021

Barth, B. B., Henriquez, C. S., Grill, W. M., and Shen, X. (2017). Electrical stimulation of gut motility guided by an in silico model. *J. Neural Eng.* 14:066010. doi: 10.1088/1741-2552/aa86c8

Bird, R. B., Stewart, W. E., and Lightfoot, E. N. (1960). Transport Phenomena, 1st Edn. Hoboken, NJ: John Wiley & Sons, 808.

Bower, J. M., and Beeman, D. (2012). *The Book of GENESIS: Exploring Realistic Neural Models with the GEneral NEural SImulation System*. Berlin: Springer Science & Business Media.

Brette, R., Rudolph, M., Carnevale, T., Hines, M., Beeman, D., Bower, J. M., et al. (2007). Simulation of networks of spiking neurons: a review of tools and strategies. *J. Comput. Neurosci.* 23, 349–398. doi: 10.1007/s10827-007-0038-6

Cain, N., Iyer, R., Koch, C., and Mihalas, S. (2016). The computational properties of a simplified cortical column model. *PLoS Comput. Biol.* 12:e1005045. doi: 10.1371/journal.pcbi.1005045

Callahan, A., Anderson, K. D., Beattie, M. S., Bixby, J. L., Ferguson, A. R., Fouad, K., et al. (2017). Developing a data sharing community for spinal cord injury research. *Exp. Neurol.* 295, 135–143. doi: 10.1016/j.expneurol.2017.05.012

Campo-Deaño, L., Oliveira, M. S. N., and Pinho, F. T. (2015). A review of computational hemodynamics in middle cerebral aneurysms and rheological models for blood flow. *Appl. Mech. Rev.* 67:030801. doi: 10.1115/1.4028946

Cannon, R. C., Gleeson, P., Crook, S., Ganapathy, G., Marin, B., Piasini, E., et al. (2014). LEMS: a language for expressing complex biological models in concise and hierarchical form and its use in underpinning NeuroML 2. *Front. Neuroinform.* 8:79. doi: 10.3389/fninf.2014.00079

Carnevale, T., and Hines, M. (2006). *The NEURON Book*. New York, NY: Cambridge University Press. doi: 10.1017/CBO9780511541612

Carnevale, T., Majumdar, A., Sivagnanam, S., Yoshimoto, K., Astakhov, V., Bandrowski, A., et al. (2014). The neuroscience gateway portal: high performance computing made easy. *BMC Neurosci.* 15(Suppl. 1):101. doi: 10.1186/1471-2202-15-S1-P101

Chitkara, R., Rajani, A. K., Oehlert, J. W., Lee, H. C., Epi, M. S., and Halamek, L. P. (2013). The accuracy of human senses in the detection of neonatal heart rate during standardized simulated resuscitation: implications for delivery of care, training and technology design. *Resuscitation* 84, 369–372. doi: 10.1016/j.resuscitation.2012.07.035

Choi, K. S., Riva-Posse, P., Gross, R. E., and Mayberg, H. S. (2015). Mapping the 'Depression Switch' during intraoperative testing of subcallosal cingulate deep brain stimulation. *JAMA Neurol.* 72, 1252–1260. doi: 10.1001/jamaneurol.2015.2564

Chung, B., and Cebral, J. R. (2015). CFD for evaluation and treatment planning of aneurysms: review of proposed clinical uses and their challenges. *Ann. Biomed. Eng.* 43, 122–138. doi: 10.1007/s10439-014-1093-6

Crook, S. M., Davison, A. P., and Plesser, H. E. (2013). "Learning from the past: approaches for reproducibility in computational neuroscience," in *20 Years of Computational Neuroscience*, ed. J. M. Bower (New York, NY: Springer), 73–102.

Dabbish, L., Stuart, C., Tsay, J., and Herbsleb, J. (2012). "Social coding in github: transparency and collaboration in an open software repository," in *Proceedings of the ACM 2012 Conference on Computer Supported Cooperative Work CSCW '12*, (New York, NY: ACM), 1277–1286. doi: 10.1145/2145204.2145396

Davison, A. P., Brüderle, D., Eppler, J., Kremkow, J., Muller, E., Pecevski, D., et al. (2008). PyNN: a common interface for neuronal network simulators. *Front. Neuroinform.* 2:11. doi: 10.3389/neuro.11.011.2008

Diesmann, M., Gewaltig, M. O., and Aertsen, A. (1999). Stable propagation of synchronous spiking in cortical neural networks. *Nature* 402, 529–533. doi: 10.1038/990101

Djurfeldt, M., Hjorth, J., Eppler, J. M., Dudani, N., Helias, M., Potjans, T. C., et al. (2010). Run-time interoperability between neuronal network simulators based on the MUSIC framework. *Neuroinformatics* 8, 43–60. doi: 10.1007/s12021-010-9064-z

Drummond, C. (2009). "Replicability is not reproducibility: nor is it good science," in *Proceedings of the Evaluation Methods for Machine Learning Workshop at the 26th ICML*, Montreal, QC.

Dudani, N., Ray, S., George, S., and Bhalla, U. S. (2009). Multiscale modeling and interoperability in MOOSE. *BMC Neurosci.* 10(Suppl. 1):54. doi: 10.1186/1471-2202-10-S1-P54

Dura-Bernal, S., Chadderdon, G. L., Neymotin, S. A., Francis, J. T., and Lytton, W. W. (2014). Towards a real-time interface between a biomimetic model of sensorimotor cortex and a robotic arm. *Patt. Recognit. Lett.* 36, 204–212. doi: 10.1016/j.patrec.2013.05.019

Dura-Bernal, S., Majumdar, A., Neymotin, S. A., Sivagnanam, S., Francis, J. T., and Lytton, W. W. (2015). "A dynamic data-driven approach to closed-loop neuroprosthetics based on multiscale biomimetic brain models," in *Proceedings of the IEEE Interanationl Conference on High Performance Computing 2015 Workshop: InfoSymbiotics/Dynamic Data Driven Applications Systems (DDDAS) for Smarter Systems*, (Bangalore: IEEE).

Ermak, D. M., Bower, D. W., Wood, J., Sinz, E. H., and Kothari, M. J. (2013). Incorporating simulation technology into a neurology clerkship. *J. Am. Osteopath. Assoc.* 113, 628–635. doi: 10.7556/jaoa.2013.024

Esmaeilpour, Z., Marangolo, P., Hampstead, B. M., Bestmann, S., Galletta, E., Knotkova, H., et al. (2017). Incomplete evidence that increasing current intensity of tDCS boosts outcomes. *Brain Stimul.* 11, 310–321. doi: 10.1016/j.brs.2017.12.002

Falotico, E., Vannucci, L., Ambrosano, A., Albanese, U., Ulbrich, S., Vasquez Tieck, J. C., et al. (2017). Connecting artificial brains to robots in a comprehensive simulation framework: the neurorobotics platform. *Front. Neurorobot.* 11:2. doi: 10.3389/fnbot.2017.00002

Fitzhugh, R. (1961). Impulses and physiological states in theoretical models of nerve membrane. *Biophys. J.* 1, 445–466. doi: 10.1016/S0006-3495(61)86902-6

Fuerch, J. H., Yamada, N. K., Coelho, P. R., Lee, H. C., and Halamek, L. P. (2015). Impact of a novel decision support tool on adherence to neonatal resuscitation program algorithm. *Resuscitation* 88, 52–56. doi: 10.1016/j.resuscitation.2014.12.016

Furlanello C., De Domenico, M., Jurman, G., and Bussola, N. (2017). Towards a scientific blockchain framework for reproducible data analysis. arXiv:1707.06552.

Gewaltig, M.-O., and Diesmann, M. (2007). NEST (NEural Simulation Tool). *Schol. J.* 2:1430. doi: 10.4249/scholarpedia.1430

Gleeson, P., Crook, S., Cannon, R. C., Hines, M. L., Billings, G. O., Farinella, M., et al. (2010). NeuroML: a language for describing data driven models of neurons and networks with a high degree of biological detail. *PLoS Comput. Biol.* 6:e1000815. doi: 10.1371/journal.pcbi.1000815

Gleeson, P., Davison, A. P., Silver, R. A., and Ascoli, G. A. (2017). A commitment to open source in neuroscience. *Neuron* 96, 964–965. doi: 10.1016/j.neuron.2017.10.013

Gleeson, P., Piasini, E., Crook, S., Cannon, R., Steuber, V., Jaeger, D., et al. (2012). The open source brain initiative: enabling collaborative modelling in computational neuroscience. *BMC Neurosci.* 13(Suppl. 1):7.

Gleeson, P., Silver, A., and Cantarelli, M. (2015). "Open source brain," in *Encyclopedia of Computational Neuroscience*, eds D. Jaeger and R. Jung (New York, NY: Springer), 2153–2156.

Goodman, D., and Brette, R. (2008). Brian: a simulator for spiking neural networks in python. *Front. Neuroinformat.* 2:5. doi: 10.3389/neuro.11.005.2008

Grill, W. M., and McIntyre, C. C. (2001). Extracellular excitation of central neurons: implications for the mechanisms of deep brain stimulation. *Thalamus Relat. Syst.* 1, 269–277. doi: 10.1017/S1472928801000255

Hammond, C., Bergman, H., and Brown, P. (2007). Pathological synchronization in Parkinson's disease: networks, models and treatments. *Trends Neurosci.* 30, 357–364. doi: 10.1016/j.tins.2007.05.004

Hariharan, P., D'Souza, G. A., Horner, M., Morrison, T. M., Malinauskas, R. A., and Myers, M. R. (2017). Use of the FDA nozzle model to illustrate validation techniques in computational fluid dynamics (CFD) simulations. *PLoS One* 12:e0178749. doi: 10.1371/journal.pone.0178749

Hodgkin, A. L., and Huxley, A. F. (1952). A quantitative description of membrane current and its application to conduction and excitation in nerve. *J. Physiol.* 117, 500–544. doi: 10.1113/jphysiol.1952.sp004764

Holt, A. B., and Netoff, T. I. (2017). Computational modeling to advance deep brain stimulation for the treatment of Parkinson's disease. *Drug Discov. Today Dis. Models* 19, 31–36. doi: 10.1016/j.ddmod.2017.02.006

Huang, Y., Liu, A. A., Lafon, B., Friedman, D., Dayan, M., Wang, X., et al. (2017). Measurements and models of electric fields in the in vivo human brain during transcranial electric stimulation. *Elife* 6:e18834. doi: 10.7554/eLife.18834

Hucka, M., Finney, A., Sauro, H. M., Bolouri, H., Doyle, J. C., Kitano, H., et al. (2003). The systems biology markup language (SBML): a medium for representation and exchange of biochemical network models. *Bioinformatics* 19, 524–531. doi: 10.1093/bioinformatics/btg015

Hunt, A. C., Erdemir, A., MacGabhann, F., Lytton, W. W., Sander, E. A., Transtrum, M. K., et al. (2018). The spectrum of mechanism-oriented models for explanations of biological phenomena. arXiv:1801.04909.

Huwendiek, S., De Leng, B. A., Kononowicz, A. A., Kunzmann, R., Muijtjens, A. M., Van Der Vleuten, C. P., et al. (2014). Exploring the validity and reliability of a questionnaire for evaluating virtual patient design with a special emphasis on fostering clinical reasoning. *Med. Teach.* doi: 10.3109/0142159X.2014.970622 [Epub ahead of print].

Issenberg, S. B., Mcgaghie, W. C., Petrusa, E. R., Lee Gordon, D., and Scalese, R. J. (2005). Features and uses of high-fidelity medical simulations that lead to effective learning: a BEME systematic review. *Med. Teach.* 27, 10–28. doi: 10.1080/01421590500046924

Jirsa, V. K., Proix, T., Perdikis, D., Woodman, M. M., Wang, H., Gonzalez-Martinez, J., et al. (2017). The virtual epileptic patient: individualized whole-brain models of epilepsy spread. *Neuroimage* 145, 377–388. doi: 10.1016/j.neuroimage.2016.04.049

Johansen-Berg, H., Gutman, D. A., Behrens, T. E. J., Matthews, P. M., Rushworth, M. F. S., Katz, E., et al. (2008). Anatomical connectivity of the subgenual cingulate region targeted with deep brain stimulation for treatment-resistant depression. *Cereb. Cortex* 18, 1374–1383. doi: 10.1093/cercor/bhm167

Jones, F., Passos-Neto, C. E., and Braghiroli, O. F. M. (2015). Simulation in medical education: brief history and methodology. *Princ. Pract. Clin. Res.* 1, 56–63.

Kellner, C. H. (2012). *Brain Stimulation in Psychiatry: ECT, DBS, TMS and Other Modalities*. Cambridge: Cambridge University Press. doi: 10.1017/CBO9780511736216

Kerr, C. C., O'Shea, D. J., Goo, W., Dura-Bernal, S., Francis, J. T., Diester, I., et al. (2014). Network-level effects of optogenetic stimulation in a computer model of macaque primary motor cortex. *BMC Neurosci.* 15(Suppl. 1):107. doi: 10.1186/1471-2202-15-S1-P107

Kerr, C. C., Van Albada, S. J., Neymotin, S. A., Chadderdon, G. L., Robinson, P. A., and Lytton, W. W. (2013). Cortical information flow in Parkinson's disease: a composite network/field model. *Front. Comput. Neurosci.* 7:39. doi: 10.3389/fncom.2013.00039

Kluyver, T., Ragan-Kelley, B., Pérez, F., Granger, B. E., Bussonnier, M., Frederic, J., et al. (2016). "Jupyter notebooks-a publishing format for reproducible computational workflows," in *20th International Conference on Electronic Publishing*, Amsterdam: IOS Press, 87–90.

Konakondla, S., Fong, R., and Schirmer, C. M. (2017). Simulation training in neurosurgery: advances in education and practice. *Adv. Med. Educ. Pract.* 8, 465–473. doi: 10.2147/AMEP.S113565

Lafon, B., Rahman, A., Bikson, M., and Parra, L. C. (2017). Direct current stimulation alters neuronal input/output function. *Brain Stimul.* 10, 36–45. doi: 10.1016/j.brs.2016.08.014

Lefaucheur, J.-P., André-Obadia, N., Antal, A., Ayache, S. S., Baeken, C., Benninger, D. H., et al. (2014). Evidence-based guidelines on the therapeutic use of repetitive transcranial magnetic stimulation (rTMS). *Clin. Neurophysiol.* 125, 2150–2206. doi: 10.1016/j.clinph.2014.05.021

Lisman, J. E., Pi, H. J., Zhang, Y., and Otmakhova, N. A. (2010). A thalamo-hippocampal-ventral tegmental area loop may produce the positive feedback that underlies the psychotic break in Schizophrenia. *Biol. Psychiatry* 68, 17–24. doi: 10.1016/j.biopsych.2010.04.007

Lloyd, C. M., Lawson, J. R., Hunter, P. J., and Nielsen, P. F. (2008). The CellML model repository. *Bioinformatics* 24, 2122–2123. doi: 10.1093/bioinformatics/btn390

London, M., Beeren, A. R. L., Häusser, M., and Latham, P. E. (2010). Sensitivity to perturbations in vivo implies high noise and suggests rate coding in cortex. *Nature* 466, 123–127. doi: 10.1038/nature09086

Lupascu, C. A., Morabito, A., Merenda, E., Marinelli, S., Marchetti, C., Migliore, R., et al. (2016). A general procedure to study subcellular models of transsynaptic signaling at inhibitory synapses. *Front. Neuroinform.* 10:23. doi: 10.3389/fninf.2016.00023

Lytton, W. W. (2008). Computer modelling of epilepsy. *Nat. Rev. Neurosci.* 9, 626–637. doi: 10.1038/nrn2416

Lytton, W. W. (2017). Computers, causality and cure in epilepsy. *Brain* 140, 516–526. doi: 10.1093/brain/awx018

Lytton, W. W., and Hines, M. L. (2005). Independent variable timestep integration of individual neurons for network simulations. *Neural Comput.* 17, 903–921. doi: 10.1162/0899766053429453

Lytton, W. W., Seidenstein, A., Dura-Bernal, S., Schurmann, F., McDougal, R. A., and Hines, M. L. (2016). Simulation neurotechnologies for advancing brain research: parallelizing large networks in NEURON. *Neural Comput.* 28, 2063–2090. doi: 10.1162/NECO_a_00876

McDougal, R. A., Bulanova, A. S., and Lytton, W. W. (2016a). Reproducibility in computational neuroscience models and simulations. *IEEE Trans. Biomed. Eng.* 63, 2021–2035. doi: 10.1109/TBME.2016.2539602

McDougal, R. A., Morse, T. M., Carnevale, T., Marenco, L., Wang, R., Migliore, M., et al. (2016b). Twenty years of ModelDB and beyond: building essential modeling tools for the future of neuroscience. *J. Comput. Neurosci.* 42, 1–10. doi: 10.1007/s10827-016-0623-7

Micieli, G., Cavallini, A., Santalucia, P., and Gensini, G. (2015). Simulation in neurology. *Neurol. Sci.* 36, 1967–1971. doi: 10.1007/s10072-015-2228-8

Moore, J. W., and Stuart, A. (2011). *Neurons in Action 2.* Oxford: Oxford University Press.

Moraru, I. I., Schaff, J. C., Slepchenko, B. M., Blinov, M. L., Morgan, F., Lakshminarayana, A., et al. (2008). Virtual cell modelling and simulation software environment. *IET Syst. Biol.* 2, 352–362. doi: 10.1049/iet-syb:20080102

Mulugeta, L., and Erdemir, A. (2013). "Committee on credible practice of modeling and simulation in healthcare," in *Proceedings of the ASME 2013 Conference on Frontiers in Medical Devices: Applications of Computer Modeling and Simulation, V001T10A015-V001T10A015,* (New York, NY: American Society of Mechanical Engineers). doi: 10.1115/FMD2013-16080

Nadkarni, P., Mirsky, J., Skoufos, E., Healy, M., Hines, M., Miller, P., et al. (2002). "Senselab: modeling heterogenous data on the nervous system," in *Bioinformatics: Databases and Systems*, ed. S. I. Letovsky (Boston, MA: Springer), 105–118. doi: 10.1007/0-306-46903-0_10

Neymotin, S. A., Dura-Bernal, S., Lakatos, P., Sanger, T. D., and Lytton, W. W. (2016). Multitarget multiscale simulation for pharmacological treatment of dystonia in motor cortex. *Front. Pharmacol.* 7:157. doi: 10.3389/fphar.2016.00157

NIH (2015). *PAR-15-085: Predictive Multiscale Models for Biomedical, Biological, Behavioral, Environmental and Clinical Research (U01)." Department of Health and Human Services.* Available at: http://grants.nih.gov/grants/guide/pa-files/PAR-15-085.html [accessed January 8, 2015].

Nunez, P. L., and Srinivasan, R. (2005). *Electric Fields of the Brain: The Neurophysics of EEG*, 2nd Edn. New York, NY: Oxford University Press.

Oberkampf, W. L., and Roy, C. J. (2010). *Verification and Validation in Scientific Computing.* Cambridge: Cambridge University Press. doi: 10.1017/CBO9780511760396

Peterson, B. E., Healy, M. D., Nadkarni, P. M., Miller, P. L., and Shepherd, G. M. (1996). ModelDB: an environment for running and storing computational models and their results applied to neuroscience. *J. Am. Med. Inform. Assoc.* 3, 389–398. doi: 10.1136/jamia.1996.97084512

Plesser, H., Diesmann, M., Marc-Oliver, G., and Morrison, A. (2015). "NEST: the neural simulation tool," in *Encyclopedia of Computational Neuroscience*, eds D. Jaeger and R. Jung (New York, NY: Springer), 1849–1852.

Plesser, H. E. (2017). Reproducibility vs. Replicability: a brief history of a confused terminology. *Front. Neuroinform.* 11:76. doi: 10.3389/fninf.2017.00076

Potjans, T. C., and Diesmann, M. (2014). The cell-type specific cortical microcircuit: relating structure and activity in a full-scale spiking network model. *Cereb. Cortex* 24, 785–806. doi: 10.1093/cercor/bhs358

Proix, T., Bartolomei, F., Guye, M., and Jirsa, V. K. (2017). Individual brain structure and modeling predict seizure propagation. *Brain* 140, 651–654. doi: 10.1093/brain/awx004

Rall, W. (1962). Electrophysiology of a dendritic neuron model. *Biophys. J.* 2, 145–167. doi: 10.1016/S0006-3495(62)86953-7

Ranjan, R., Khazen, G., Gambazzi, L., Ramaswamy, S., Hill, S. L., Schürmann, F., et al. (2011). Channelpedia: an integrative and interactive database for ion channels. *Front. Neuroinform.* 5:36. doi: 10.3389/fninf.2011.00036

Reyes, R. (2016). *An Empirical Evaluation of an Instrument to Determine the Relationship Between Second-Year Medical Students' Perceptions of NERVE VP Design Effectiveness and Students' Ability to Learn and Transfer Skills from NERVE.* Orlando, FL: University of Central Florida.

Robinson, P. A., Rennie, C. J., and Rowe, D. L. (2002). Dynamics of large-scale brain activity in normal arousal states and epileptic seizures. *Phys. Rev. E Stat. Nonlin. Soft Matter Phys.* 65, 041924. doi: 10.1103/PhysRevE.65.041924

Ross, S. E., Ouyang, Z., Rajagopalan, S., and Bruns, T. M. (2018). Evaluation of decoding algorithms for estimating bladder pressure from dorsal root ganglia neural recordings. *Ann. Biomed. Eng.* 46, 233–246. doi: 10.1007/s10439-017-1966-6

Samineni, V. K., Mickle, A. D., Yoon, J., Grajales-Reyes, J. G., Pullen, M. Y., Crawford, K. E., et al. (2017). Optogenetic silencing of nociceptive primary afferents reduces evoked and ongoing bladder pain. *Sci. Rep.* 7:15865. doi: 10.1038/s41598-017-16129-3

Santos, M. D. D., Cavenaghi, V. B., Mac-Kay, A. P. M. G., Serafim, V., Venturi, A., Truong, D. Q., et al. (2017). Non-invasive brain stimulation and computational models in post-stroke aphasic patients: single session of transcranial magnetic stimulation and transcranial direct current stimulation. A Randomized Clinical Trial. *Sao Paulo Med. J.* 135, 475–480. doi: 10.1590/1516-3180.2016.0194060617

Sanz-Leon, P., Knock, S., Woodman, M., Domide, L., Mersmann, J., McIntosh, A., et al. (2013). The virtual brain: a simulator of primate brain network dynamics. *Front. Neuroinform.* 7:10. doi: 10.3389/fninf.2013.00010

Schulte, E., and Davison, D. (2011). Active documents with org-mode. *Comput. Sci. Eng.* 13, 66–73. doi: 10.1109/MCSE.2011.41

Seidenstein, A. H., Barone, F. C., and Lytton, W. W. (2015). Computer modeling of ischemic stroke. *Scholarpedia J.* 10:32015. doi: 10.4249/scholarpedia.32015

Shenoy, K. V., Sahani, M., and Churchland, M. M. (2013). Cortical control of arm movements: a dynamical systems perspective. *Annu. Rev. Neurosci.* 36, 337–359. doi: 10.1146/annurev-neuro-062111-150509

Shils, J. L., Mei, L. Z., and Arle, J. E. (2008). Modeling parkinsonian circuitry and the DBS electrode. II. Evaluation of a computer simulation model of the basal ganglia with and without subthalamic nucleus stimulation. *Stereotact. Funct. Neurosurg.* 86, 16–29. doi: 10.1159/000108585

Stanisic, L., Legrand, A., and Danjean, V. (2015). An effective git and org-mode based workflow for reproducible research. *ACM SIGOPS Operat. Syst. Rev.* 49, 61–70. doi: 10.1145/2723872.2723881

Stern, F., Wilson, R., and Shao, J. (2006). Quantitative V&V of CFD simulations and certification of CFD codes. *Int. J. Numer. Methods Fluids* 50, 1335–1355. doi: 10.1002/fld.1090

Szigeti, B., Gleeson, P., Vella, M., Khayrulin, S., Palyanov, A., Hokanson, J., et al. (2014). OpenWorm: an open-science approach to modeling caenorhabditis elegans. *Front. Comput. Neurosci.* 8:137. doi: 10.3389/fncom.2014.00137

Tikidji-Hamburyan, R. A., Narayana, V., Bozkus, Z., and El-Ghazawi, T. A. (2017). Software for brain network simulations: a comparative study. *Front. Neuroinform.* 11:46. doi: 10.3389/fninf.2017.00046

Van Albada, S. J., Gray, R. T., Drysdale, P. M., and Robinson, P. A. (2009). Mean-field modeling of the basal ganglia-thalamocortical system. II: dynamics of parkinsonian oscillations. *J. Theor. Biol.* 257, 664–688. doi: 10.1016/j.jtbi.2008.12.013

van der Krogt, M. M., Bar-On, L., Kindt, T., Desloovere, K., and Harlaar, J. (2016). Neuro-musculoskeletal simulation of instrumented contracture and spasticity assessment in children with cerebral palsy. *J. Neuroeng. Rehabil.* 13:64. doi: 10.1186/s12984-016-0170-5

Vaseghi, M., Salavatian, S., Rajendran, P. S., Yagishita, D., Woodward, W. R., Hamon, D., et al. (2017). Parasympathetic dysfunction and antiarrhythmic effect of vagal nerve stimulation following myocardial infarction. *JCI Insight* 2:e86715. doi: 10.1172/jci.insight.86715

Vierling-Claassen, D., Cardin, J. A., Moore, C. I., and Jones, S. R. (2010). Computational modeling of distinct neocortical oscillations driven by cell-type selective optogenetic drive: separable resonant circuits controlled by low-threshold spiking and fast-spiking interneurons. *Front. Hum. Neurosci.* 4:198. doi: 10.3389/fnhum.2010.00198

Weiss, S., and Mueller, H. M. (2012). Too many betas do not spoil the broth': the role of beta brain oscillations in language processing. *Front. Psychol.* 3:201. doi: 10.3389/fpsyg.2012.00201

Wilson, C. (2008). Up and down states. *Scholarpedia J.* 3:1410. doi: 10.4249/scholarpedia.1410

Wrigley, S. (ed.). (2013). "Negative training: when the simulator lies," in *Why Planes Crash Case Files: 2001*. Mannheim: Fear of Landing.

Yamada, N. K., Fuerch, J. H., and Halamek, L. P. (2017). Simulation-based patient-specific multidisciplinary team training in preparation for the resuscitation and stabilization of conjoined twins. *Am. J. Perinatol.* 34, 621–626. doi: 10.1055/s-0036-1593808

Zhang, C., Bakshi, A., and Prasanna, V. K. (2007). "ModelML: a markup language for automatic model synthesis," in *Proceedings of the IEEE International Conference on Information Reuse and Integration 2007* (Las Vegas, IL: IEEE), doi: 10.1109/iri.2007.4296640

6

Intra- and Inter-Scanner Reliability of Voxel-Wise Whole-Brain Analytic Metrics for Resting State fMRI

Na Zhao[1,2], Li-Xia Yuan[3], Xi-Ze Jia[1,2], Xu-Feng Zhou[1,2], Xin-Ping Deng[1,2], Hong-Jian He[3], Jianhui Zhong[3], Jue Wang[1,2] and Yu-Feng Zang[1,2]**

[1] Center for Cognition and Brain Disorders, Institutes of Psychological Sciences, Hangzhou Normal University, Hangzhou, China, [2] Zhejiang Key Laboratory for Research in Assessment of Cognitive Impairments, Hangzhou, China, [3] Center for Brain Imaging Science and Technology, Key Laboratory for Biomedical Engineering of Ministry of Education, College of Biomedical Engineering and Instrumental Science, Zhejiang University, Hangzhou, China

***Correspondence:**
Jue Wang
juefirst@163.com
Yu-Feng Zang
zangyf@hznu.edu.cn

As the multi-center studies with resting-state functional magnetic resonance imaging (RS-fMRI) have been more and more applied to neuropsychiatric studies, both intra- and inter-scanner reliability of RS-fMRI are becoming increasingly important. The amplitude of low frequency fluctuation (ALFF), regional homogeneity (ReHo), and degree centrality (DC) are 3 main RS-fMRI metrics in a way of voxel-wise whole-brain (VWWB) analysis. Although the intra-scanner reliability (i.e., test-retest reliability) of these metrics has been widely investigated, few studies has investigated their inter-scanner reliability. In the current study, 21 healthy young subjects were enrolled and scanned with blood oxygenation level dependent (BOLD) RS-fMRI in 3 visits (V1 – V3), with V1 and V2 scanned on a GE MR750 scanner and V3 on a Siemens Prisma. RS-fMRI data were collected under two conditions, eyes open (EO) and eyes closed (EC), each lasting 8 minutes. We firstly evaluated the intra- and inter-scanner reliability of ALFF, ReHo, and DC. Secondly, we measured systematic difference between two scanning visits of the same scanner as well as between two scanners. Thirdly, to account for the potential difference of intra- and inter-scanner local magnetic field inhomogeneity, we measured the difference of relative BOLD signal intensity to the mean BOLD signal intensity of the whole brain between each pair of visits. Last, we used percent amplitude of fluctuation (PerAF) to correct the difference induced by relative BOLD signal intensity. The inter-scanner reliability was much worse than intra-scanner reliability; Among the VWWB metrics, DC showed the worst (both for intra-scanner and inter-scanner comparisons). PerAF showed similar intra-scanner reliability with ALFF and the best reliability among all the 4 metrics. PerAF reduced the influence of BOLD signal intensity and hence increase the inter-scanner reliability of ALFF. For multi-center studies, inter-scanner reliability should be taken into account.

Keywords: inter-scanner reliability, intra-scanner reliability, ALFF, PerAF, ReHo, voxel-wise whole-brain analysis

INTRODUCTION

With its advantages of being non-invasive, fairly good spatial as well as temporal resolution, and very similar design across studies, resting-state functional magnetic resonance imaging (RS-fMRI) of blood oxygenation level dependent (BOLD) technique is promising for clinical research to reveal abnormal spontaneous brain activity. Therefore, intra- and inter-scanner reliability is essential in RS-fMRI studies.

In recent years, the intra-scanner reliability (i.e., test-retest reliability) of many metrics in RS-fMRI has been investigated, such as the amplitude of low frequency fluctuations (ALFF) (Zuo et al., 2010a; Li et al., 2012; Zuo and Xing, 2014; Somandepalli et al., 2015; Zou et al., 2015), regional homogeneity (ReHo) (Li et al., 2012; Zuo et al., 2013; Somandepalli et al., 2015), seed-based functional connectivity (FC) (Shehzad et al., 2009; Patriat et al., 2013; Pannunzi et al., 2017), group-level dual regression independent component analysis (drICA) (Zuo et al., 2010b), voxel-mirrored homotopic connectivity (VMHC) (Zuo et al., 2010c), graph theory (Wang et al., 2011; Braun et al., 2012; Tomasi and Volkow, 2014; Andellini et al., 2015; Aurich et al., 2015). Generally, most of these metrics showed moderate to high intra-scanner reliability.

While many studies have investigated the intra-scanner reliability of RS-fMRI metrics, only one article, to the best of our knowledge, studied the inter-scanner reliability of BOLD RS-fMRI. Jann and colleagues scanned BOLD RS-fMRI data on two same type of scanners (3T Siemens TIM Trio) with identical scanning parameters (Jann et al., 2015). They identified five networks with ICA and computed voxel-wise intra-class correlation (ICC) coefficient within each network. The authors found moderate to high inter-scanner reliability. One limitation for ICA is that only a limited number networks are analyzed. In practice, to map the inter-scanner reliability of every voxel in the whole brain, i.e., "voxel-wise whole-brain" (VWWB) analysis, is needed.

Amplitude of low frequency fluctuation, ReHo, and degree centrality (DC) are three most commonly used methods of VWWB analysis (Zang et al., 2015). The intra-scanner reliability or test-retest reliability of the three metrics have been widely investigated (Zuo et al., 2010a; Li et al., 2012; Liao et al., 2013). However, the inter-scanner reliability of the three metrics has not been thoroughly studied yet. Therefore, the main purpose of the current study was to systematically measure the intra- and inter-scanner reliability of the 3 RS-fMRI metrics. Lower reliability might be due to either random variance or systematic difference. To investigate potential systematic difference between each pair of visits, we performed paired t-tests. Furthermore, since magnetic field inhomogeneity between different scanners could lead to the difference of relative BOLD signal intensity (i.e., voxel-level intensity relative to the mean intensity of the whole brain), so we also aimed to investigate to what extent the inter-scanner reliability was influenced by the difference of relative BOLD signal intensity between scanners.

According to the algorithms deriving the three metrics, the relative BOLD signal intensity will affect the three metrics differently. ReHo value and DC value are standardized at voxel-level, i.e., voxel-level ReHo value is from 0 to 1 and DC value of each voxel is $-1 \sim +1$. Therefore, ReHo and DC value may not be substantially dependent on the BOLD signal intensity. But, as shown in our previous study (Jia et al., 2017), voxel-level ALFF absolute value is highly dependent on the BOLD signal intensity. Existing solutions include dividing ALFF of each voxel by the global mean ALFF of the whole brain, namely mALFF in the REST software (Song et al., 2011), Z-standardization (minus mean and then divided by the standard deviation of the whole brain) (Yan et al., 2013), and so on. Magnetic field inhomogeneity will affect the mALFF value in the corresponding areas. Therefore, in our previous study, we proposed PerAF, i.e., percent amplitude of fluctuation as a contrast to mean BOLD signal of a single time series, as standardization procedure within a time series (Jia et al., 2017). PerAF could be further standardized by global mean PerAF, i.e., mPerAF (Jia et al., 2017). In the current study, we hypothesized that mPerAF would increase the inter-scanner reliability.

MATERIALS AND METHODS

Participants

Twenty-one healthy participants (21.8 ± 1.8 years old, 11 females) with no history of neurological or psychiatric disorders were recruited. The present study was approved by the Ethics Committee of the Center for Cognition and Brain Disorders (CCBD) at Hangzhou Normal University (HZNU). Written informed consent was obtained from each subject prior to participation.

Data Acquisition

All subjects were scanned 3 times, with the first two visits (V1, V2, approximately 2 weeks apart) on one GE 3T scanner (MR-750, GE Medical Systems, Milwaukee, WI), located at the CCBD of HZNU. The third visit (V3, about 8 months after V2) was on a Siemens 3T scanner (Prisma, Siemens Healthineers Erlangen, Germany), located at the center for Brain Imaging Science and Technology of Zhejiang University (ZJU). All the raw data will be publicly accessed at https://www.nitrc.org/.

For scans on GE scanner, a gradient echo echo-planar imaging (EPI) pulse sequence was used for BOLD images with following parameters: repetition time (TR) = 2000 ms; echo time (TE) = 30 ms; flip angle (FA) = 90°; 43 slices with interleaved acquisition; matrix = 64 × 64; field of view (FOV) = 220 mm; acquisition voxel size = 3.44 mm × 3.44 mm × 3.20 mm. Moreover, a high resolution T1 anatomical scan was scanned for the spatial normalization (176 sagittal slices, thickness = 1 mm, TR = 8.1 ms, TE = 3.1 ms, FA = 8°, FOV = 250 mm).

For scans on Siemens scanner, the BOLD EPI parameters including TR, TE, FA, slice number, acquisition matrix, and FOV were the same as those obtained from the GE. A high resolution T1 anatomical image was also scanned (176 sagittal slices, thickness = 1 mm, TR = 1800ms, TE = 2.28 ms, FA = 8°, FOV = 250 mm).

For each visit, all the participants underwent two 8-min RS-fMRI sessions, during which they were asked to relax with either EO or EC, not to think of anything in particular, and not to fall asleep. The order of the two sessions was counter-balanced across subjects. To minimize head movement, straps and foam pads were used to fix the head comfortably during scanning.

Data Preprocessing

Analysis of the RS-fMRI data was performed using DPABI 4.3 toolbox (DPABI_V2.3[1]) (Yan et al., 2016), and Resting-State fMRI Data Analysis Toolkit (RESTplus1.1[2]). The preprocessing included the following procedures: (1) removal of the first 10 volumes; (2) slice timing correction; (3) head motion correction; (4) coregistration of T1 image to the averaged EPI image; (5) spatial normalization to standard Montreal Neurological Institute (MNI) space using "Dartel +segment"; (6) regression of head motion effects with the Friston-24 parameter model. All the subject's head motion were lower than our criteria of 2 mm and 2°. Additionally, regression of head motion, white matter (WM) and cerebrospinal fluid (CSF) was also performed, and the results were presented in the **Supplementary Material**; (7) removal of linear trends.

mALFF Calculation

Before ALFF calculation, spatial smoothing (Gaussian kernel of full-width half maximum, FWHM = 6 mm) was performed. Then, with the Fast Fourier Transform (FFT), the time courses of RS-fMRI signal were converted to frequency domain. The averaged square root across a frequency band of 0.01 - 0.08 Hz was calculated as ALFF (Zang et al., 2007). For standardization purpose, ALFF of each voxel was divided by the global mean ALFF, and a mALFF map was obtained.

mPerAF Calculation

PerAF refers to the percentage of BOLD fluctuation relative to the mean BOLD signal intensity (Jia et al., 2017) of a given time series. After spatial smoothing (Gaussian kernel of full-width half maximum, FWHM = 6 mm) and a band-pass filtering (0.01 - 0.08 Hz), PerAF was calculated. We calculated PerAF as follows (Jia et al., 2017):

$$\text{PerAF} = \frac{1}{n}\sum_{i=1}^{n}\left|\frac{X_i - \mu}{\mu}\right| \times 100\% \quad (1)$$

$$\mu = \frac{1}{n}\sum_{i=1}^{n} X_i \quad (2)$$

where, X_i is the BOLD signal intensity of the *ith* time points, n is the total number of time points of a given time series, and μ is the mean intensity of that time series.

Finally, PerAF of each voxel was divided by the global mean PerAF with the Resting-State fMRI Data Analysis Toolkit (RESTplus1.1, see text footnote 2). Hence, a mPerAF map was obtained.

mReHo Calculation

Before ReHo calculation, band-pass filtering (0.01 - 0.08 Hz) was performed. ReHo was calculated by using Kendall coefficient of concordance (KCC) as the following formula (Zang et al., 2004):

$$w = \frac{\sum_{i=1}^{n}(R_i)^2 - n\left(\bar{R}_i\right)^2}{\frac{1}{12}K^2\left(n^3 - n\right)} \quad (3)$$

[1]http://rfmri.org/dpabi

[2]http://www.restfmri.net

where w is the KCC (ranged from 0–1) of given 27 nearest neighboring voxels was assigned to the center voxel. K is the number neighboring voxels (here, K = 27,including the center voxel), $\bar{R}_i$ is the mean rank across nearest neighbors (27 voxels) at the *ith* time point, n is the total number of time points of the time series. For standardization purpose, each voxel's ReHo value was divided by the global mean ReHo, and hence a mReHo map was obtained. Spatial smoothing (FWHM = 6 mm) was performed after the ReHo calculation.

mDC Calculation

Before DC calculation, band-pass filtering (0.01 - 0.08 Hz) was performed. DC represents the functional strength of a given voxel with all voxels in the brain. We calculated the Pearson correlation of the time series of a given voxel with that of each voxel in the whole brain. It should be noted that a previous study has shown that binary DC and weighted DC were highly similar (Liao et al., 2013). Then binary Pearson correlation coefficient was used with a threshold of 0.25. Then the summed value was assigned to that given voxel. Voxel-wise whole-brain DC map was obtained. For standardization purpose, each voxel's DC was divided by the global mean DC, then a mDC map was obtained (Zuo et al., 2012). Then, spatial smoothing was performed (FWHM = 6 mm).

Relative BOLD Signal Intensity

Relative BOLD signal intensity in the current study was the voxel-level signal intensity relative to the mean signal intensity of the whole brain. After normalization, the BOLD signal intensity of each voxel in the mean EPI image (over 230 time points) was divided by the global mean BOLD signal intensity of that image. Hence, a relative BOLD signal intensity image was obtained.

Intra-Class Correlation Coefficient (ICCs)

The intra-scanner (i.e., V1 vs. V2) and inter-scanner (i.e., V1 vs. V3 and V2 vs. V3) reliability of the metrics including of mALFF, mReHo, mDC, and mPerAF were estimated using ICC for EO and EC, respectively, in a way of VWWB analysis according to the following equation (Shrout and Fleiss, 1979):

$$\text{ICC} = \frac{MSb - MSw}{MSb + (K-1)\,MSw} \quad (4)$$

where, MSb represents between-subject effect, MSw represents within-subject effect, and K is the number of sessions.

To view the regions with moderate or higher reliability, a threshold of ICC > = 0.4 was used to generate ICC maps. Further, a histogram of all voxels of each ICC map was plotted to visually compare the intra- or inter-scanner reliability among metrics and between EO and EC conditions. In addition, the ICC was again calculated while regressing out head motion, WM and CSF. The results with regression were very similar with the results of without regression (see the **Supplementary Material**).

Paired *t*-Test Between Each Pair of Visits

To investigate the difference of each pair of visits, we performed paired *t*-test on mALFF, mReHo, mDC, mPerAF, and relative BOLD signal intensity maps (i.e., voxel-level intensity relative

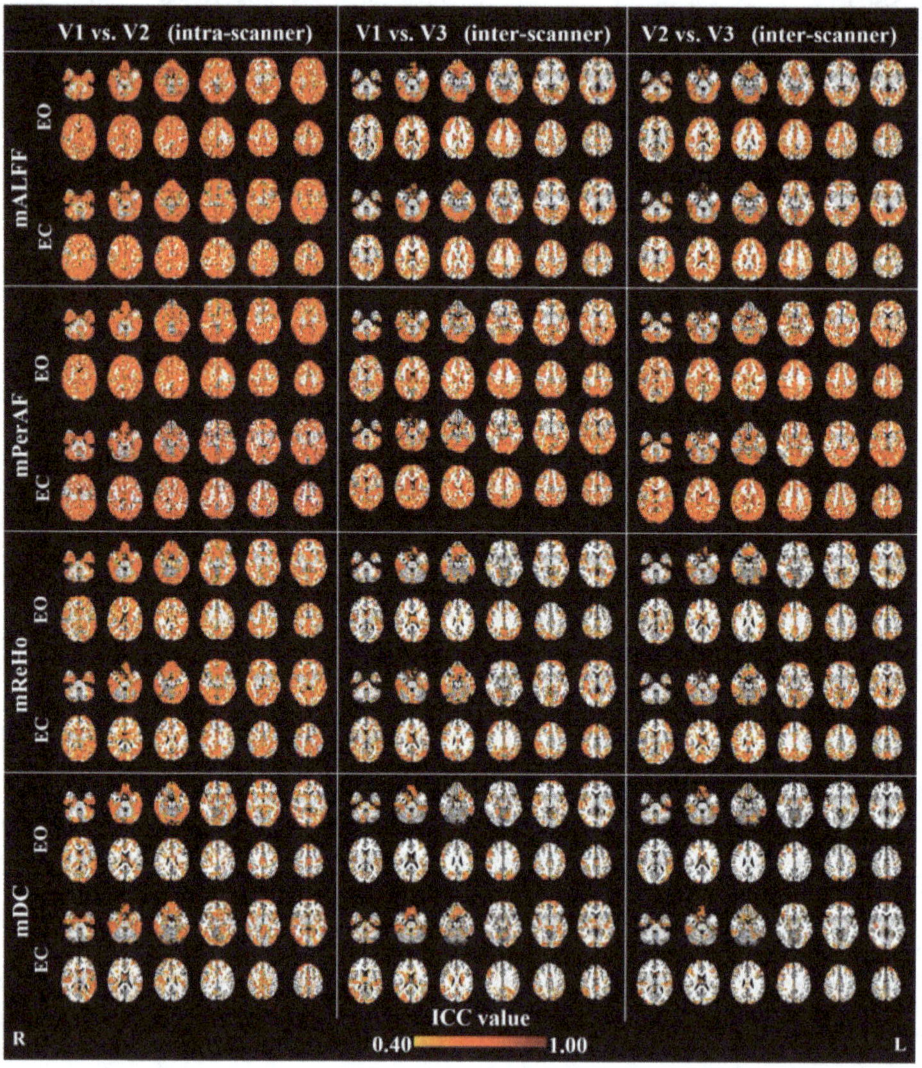

FIGURE 1 | The intra- and inter-scanner reliability of mALFF, mPerAF, mReHo and mDC of eyes open (EO) and eyes closed (EC). The Z coordinates were from −36 to +52 with a step of 8 mm. ICC: intra-class correlation. V: visit.

to the mean intensity of the whole brain). In addition, to account for confounding effects, head motion, WM and CSF were regressed out in the preprocessing stage. Further, sex, age, and interval days between each pair of visits were taken as covariates when performing paired t-tests. The results with regression were very similar with the results of without regression (see the **Supplementary Material**). It should be noted that the purpose of the paired t-test was to find potential differences. Therefore, a voxel level $p < 0.05$ was used without multiple comparison correction.

RESULTS

Intra- and Inter-Scanner Reliability

Maps of intra- and inter-scanner reliability of the VWWB metrics were shown in **Figure 1**. The reliability histograms were shown in **Figures 2, 3**. The number of voxels with ICC > = 0.4 for each metric in each condition was shown in **Table 1**. Overall, the intra-scanner reliability was higher than the inter-scanner reliability of all the 4 VWWB metrics under both EO and EC conditions. Moreover, gray matter showed higher both intra- and inter-scanner reliability than the WM for all the 4 VWWB metrics (**Figure 1**).

Summarized comparisons of reliability were as follows:

(I) Intra-scanner reliability > inter-scanner reliability (for all metrics) (**Figure 2** and **Table 1**);
(II) Intra-scanner reliability: mPerAF ≈ mALFF > mReHo > mDC (**Figure 2** and **Table 1**);
(III) Inter-scanner reliability: mPerAF > mALFF > mReHo > mDC (**Figure 2** and **Table 1**);
(IV) EO ≈ EC (all metrics) (**Figure 3** and **Table 1**).

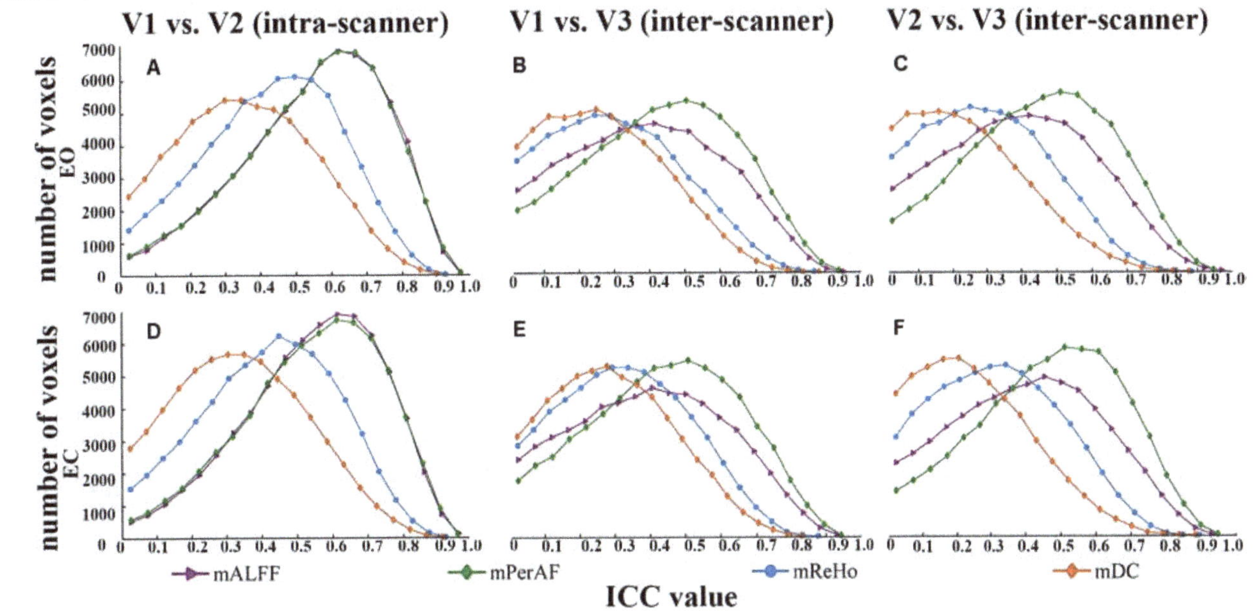

FIGURE 2 | The comparison of reliability histogram among metrics of EO and EC. Intra-scanner reliability: **(A,D)**; Inter-scanner reliability: **(B,C,E,F)**. ICC: intra-class correlation. V: visit.

Intra- and Inter-Scanner Difference

The inter-scanner difference appears larger than the intra-scanner difference for all the four metrics (**Figure 4**).

As for the intra-scanner difference of mALFF under EO, a few clusters in the right hemisphere showed significant lower mALFF for V1 than V2 (**Figure 4**). As for the inter-scanner difference, V1 and V2 showed significantly higher mALFF than V3 in large part of the inferior and anterior brain regions, while showed significantly lower mALFF than V3 in large part of superior and posterior brain regions. By visual inspection, the inter-scanner difference patterns were similar for V1-V3 and V2-V3 under both EO and EC (**Figure 4**). The relative BOLD signal intensity (i.e., voxel-level intensity relative to the mean intensity of the whole brain) in some brain areas also showed significant intra-scanner difference (**Figure 4**). Specifically, the right hemisphere of V1 showed lower relative BOLD signal intensity than V2, while the left hemisphere showed higher relative BOLD signal intensity for V1 than V2, under both EO and EC (**Figure 4**).

Notably, as shown in **Figure 4**, the inter-scanner differences of the relative BOLD signal intensity were very similar with that of inter-scanner mALFF differences (V1 vs. V3 and V2 vs. V3), but not with that of mReHo or mDC.

DISCUSSION

Reliability of Metrics

The results of moderate to high intra-scanner reliability (i.e., test-retest reliability) of mALFF, mPerAF, mReHo, and mDC were consistent with previous studies (Zuo et al., 2010c, 2012, 2013; Li et al., 2012; Somandepalli et al., 2015; Jia et al., 2017). Zuo and Xing (2014) systematically investigated the test-retest reliability (i.e., intra-scanner reliability) of ALFF, ReHo and DC. They found that DC displayed the worst reliability, being consistent with our findings. As for comparison between ALFF and ReHo, Zuo and Xing found slightly better test-retest reliability of ReHo than ALFF, while Somandepalli and colleagues found that the reliability of ALFF was slightly greater than ReHo (Somandepalli et al., 2015). We also found slightly better reliability of ALFF than ReHo. In summary, ALFF and ReHo shows similar reliability, while both ALFF and ReHo shows much higher reliability than DC.

Our previous study had suggested that the number of voxels with ICC > 0.5 of mPerAF were slightly larger than that of mALFF (number of voxels for short-term reliability: 46336 vs. 44089 voxels; long-term reliability: 31248 vs. 30866 voxels) (Jia et al., 2017). In the current study, we found that the mALFF was similar to mPerAF in intra-scanner reliability, but mPerAF was better than mALFF in inter-scanner reliability (**Figure 2** and **Table 1**). For standardization purpose, ALFF was usually divided by the mean ALFF of the entire brain, i.e., mALFF (Zang et al., 2007). Such standardization procedure seemed work well for different scanning sessions in the same scanner. However, as shown in **Figure 4**, the relative BOLD signal, i.e., the mean BOLD signal divided by that of the entire brain, was significantly different between the Siemens and GE scanners. The spatial pattern of mALFF difference between the two scanners was very similar with the spatial pattern of relative BOLD signal difference (**Figure 4**). As compared with mALFF, mPerAF has two stages of standardization (Jia et al., 2017). The first stage is percent amplitude of fluctuation at single voxel or signal time series level. The second stage is similar as that of mALFF, i.e., divided by the mean PerAF of the entire brain. While the intra-scanner reliability was almost the same for mALFF and mPerAF,

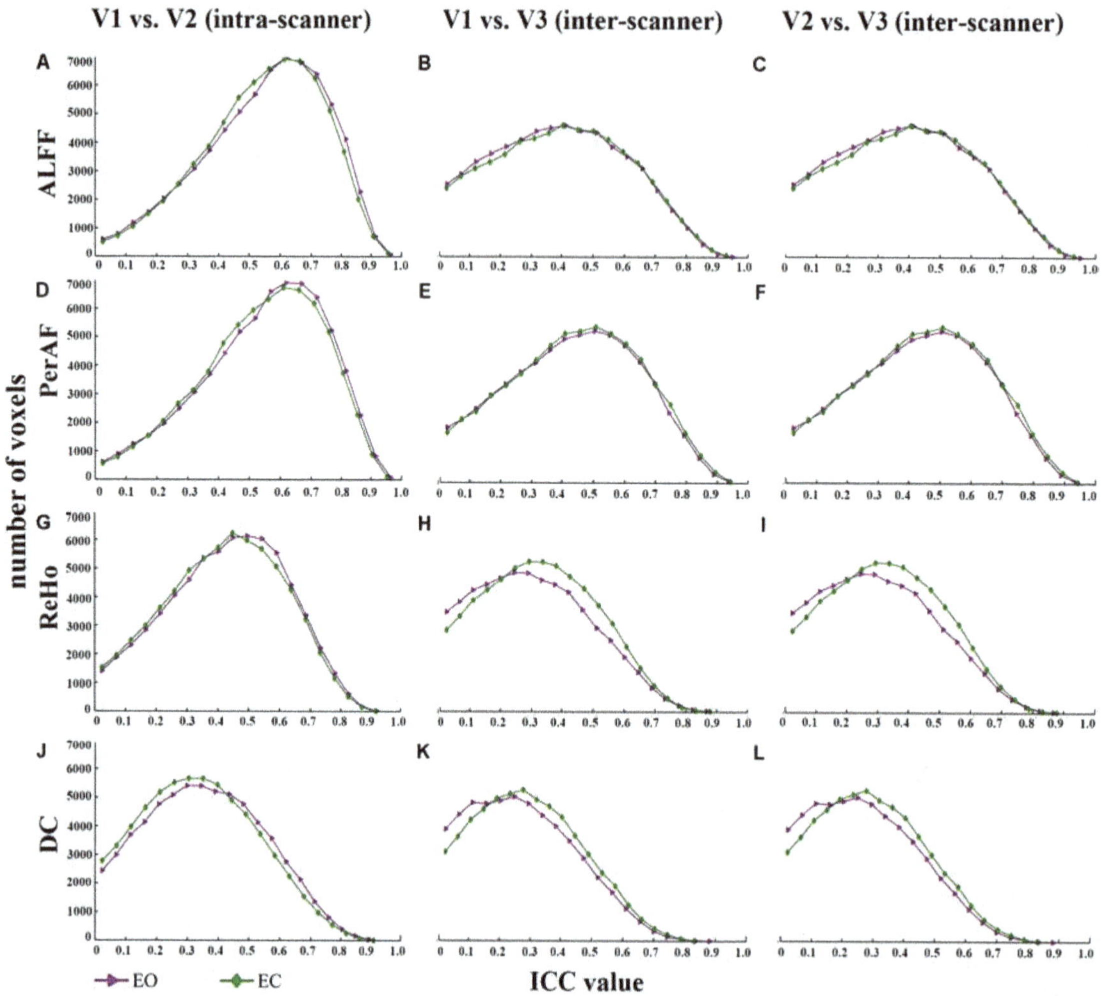

FIGURE 3 | The comparison of reliability histogram between EO and EC. Intra-scanner reliability: **(A,D,G,J)**; Inter-scanner reliability: **(B,C,E,F,H,I,K,L)**. ICC: intra-class correlation. V: visit.

TABLE 1 | The number of voxels with ICC > = 0.4 (with head motion regression).

		The number of voxels with ICC > = 0.4 (with head motion regression)		
		V1 vs. V2 (intra-scanner)	**V1 vs. V3 (inter-scanner)**	**V2 vs. V3 (inter-scanner)**
mALFF	EO	53992	28553	29057
	EC	53946	29917	31105
mPerAF	EO	53896	37072	39002
	EC	42670	38421	42158
mReHo	EO	39018	18157	17058
	EC	37366	21867	20422
mDC	EO	26763	13311	9608
	EC	24030	16410	10541

ICC: intra-class correlation. EO: eyes open. EC: eyes closed. V: visit.

the inter-scanner reliability of mPerAF was slightly higher than mALFF. By simulation, it was shown that the ALFF was affected by the mean value of BOLD signal intensity, but PerAF was not (Jia et al., 2017). The relative BOLD signal intensity of the two visits on the same scanner was very similar, however, was very different for the two visits on two different scanners. The better inter-scanner reliability of mPerAF over mALFF suggests that mPerAF could calibrate the variation brought by the difference of relative BOLD signal intensity of different scanners.

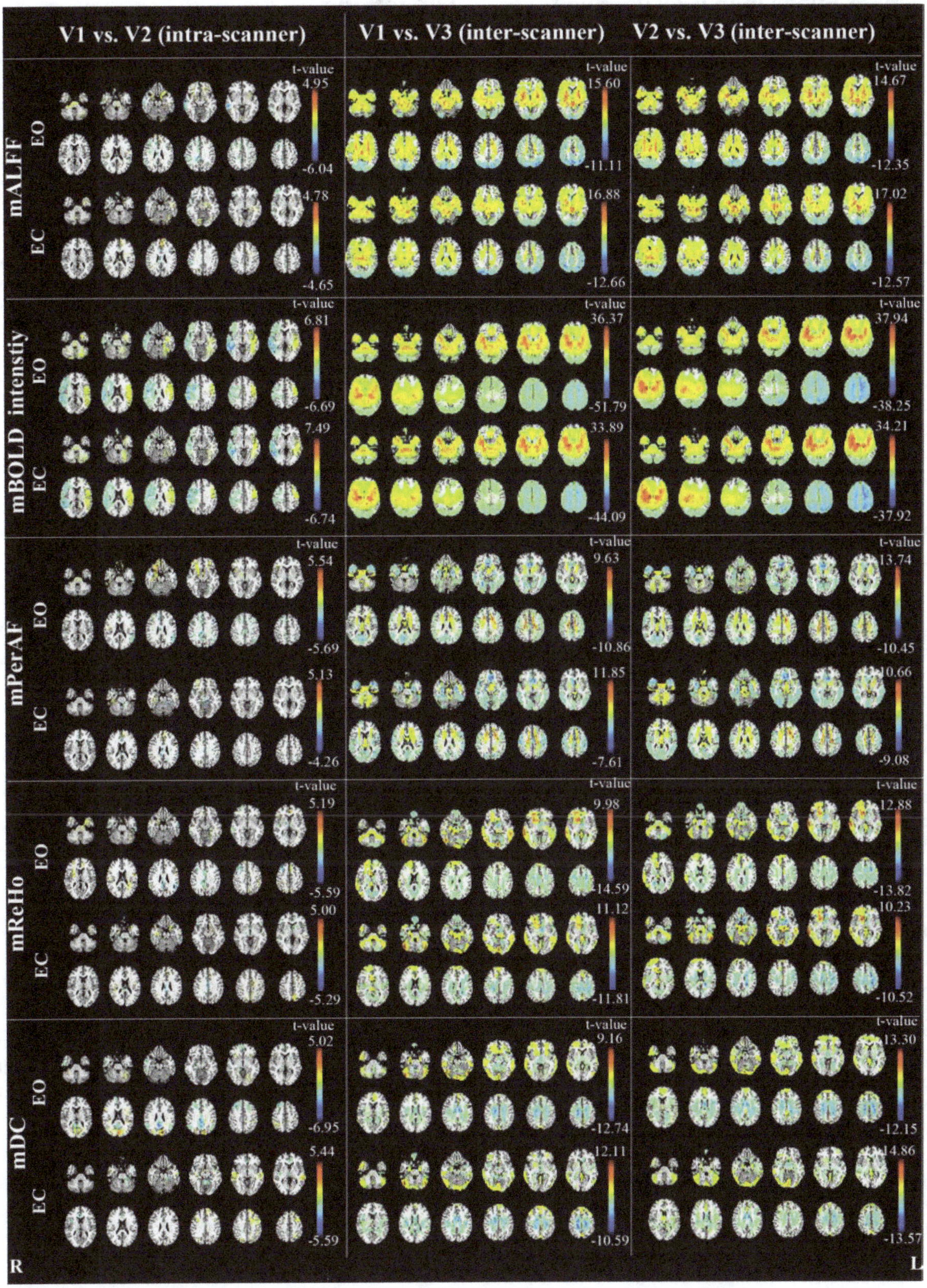

FIGURE 4 | The intra- and inter-scanner difference of mALFF, mPerAF, mReHo and mDC of EO and EC ($p < 0.05$, uncorrected). The Z coordinates were from −36 to +52 with a step of 8 mm. V: visit.

Reliability of Eyes Open (EO) vs. Eyes Closed (EC) Conditions

In RS-fMRI studies, EO, EC, and EO with fixation (EO-F) are three widely used awake conditions. Although Fox and colleagues reported that the FC pattern of the default mode network (DMN) was very similar across the three conditions (Fox et al., 2005), Yan et al. (2009) found that the local activity (including ALFF) and the FC were significantly different among the three conditions in the DMN as well as in the sensorimotor cortex and visual cortex. The difference between EO and EO-F was not as big as the difference between EO and EC with or without fixation (Yan et al., 2009). Therefore, similar to a few previous studies (Liu et al., 2013; Yuan et al., 2014; Zou et al., 2015), the current study included only EO and EC conditions but did not include EO-F condition. However, Patriat and colleagues investigated the test-retest reliability of the three conditions and concluded that, overall, EO-F had the highest test-retest reliability of FC (Patriat et al., 2013). It should be noted that Patriat and colleagues only investigated networks with significant connectivity, but not the whole brain. Future study should pay attention on the test-retest reliability of the VWWB metrics, i.e., mALFF, mPerAF, mReHo, and mDC of RS-fMRI with all three conditions (EO, EC, and EO-F). But it should keep in mind that EO-F is, at least as compared with EO and EC, a certain task condition. It requires the participant to cooperate as much as possible during scanning. While such cooperation might be easily achievable for young adult volunteers, it might be a cognitive burden for other participants, especially patients. Therefore, for a patient study, it should be cautious to use only EO-F as the RS-fMRI scanning condition.

As for the comparison of test-retest reliability between EO and EC, Zou and colleagues reported that EO showed slightly higher test-retest reliability than EC for mALFF (Zou et al., 2015). In the current study, we found that EO and EC showed very similar reliability, both for intra-scanner (i.e., test-retest) and inter-scanner comparisons.

ICC vs. Paired *t*-Test

Most reliability studies of RS-fMRI have utilized ICC. But lower ICC could be due to both random variance and systematic variance. Therefore, we performed paired t-test between each pair of two visits. As expected, we found very significant between-scanner differences for all metrics. The brain regions showing significant between-scanner differences were largely overlapped with the brain regions showing lower inter-scanner reliability, especially in the WM. Such systematic difference was the most prominent for mALFF. As discussed in the section of "4.1. Reliability of metrics", it might be due to the computational limitation of mALFF. To some extent, mPerAF reduced such systematic difference. We therefore recommend mPerAF over mALFF in future studies.

We found small systematic difference by intra-scanner paired *t*-test for mALFF, mPeAF, mReHo, and mDC. The areas showing lower ICC did not show significant difference by the paired *t*-test. It means the lower ICC in these areas might be due to random variance between the two visits on the same scanner.

Limitations

There were a few limitations. First, because we intended to investigate both intra- and inter-scanner reliability, the order of the two visits of inter-scanner reliability was unable to be randomized. If a study aims to investigate only the inter-scanner reliability, the order of the two visits should be counter-balanced. Second, the current study only investigated VWWB metrics of RS-fMRI. Future studies should also investigate the inter-scanner reliability of other metrics. Third, in order to keep consistent among metrics in our study, we used the same standardization procedure of "dividing global mean value" for all metrics. However, it has been reported that the standardization procedure could affect the test-retest reliability of ALFF, ReHo, and DC differently (Yan et al., 2013). Therefore, the standardization procedure should be further investigated.

CONCLUSION

The inter-scanner reliability was much lower than intra-scanner reliability. For all the 4 metrics of RS-fMRI, mDC showed the lowest intra- and inter-scanner reliability. mPerAF showed similar intra-scanner reliability as mALFF, but showed increased inter-scanner reliability over mALFF. We thus recommend using mPerAF for future studies. Measurements under eyes open and eyes closed conditions showed very similar reliability. Paired *t*-test may provide additional information for studies on either intra-scanner or inter-scanner reliability.

AUTHOR CONTRIBUTIONS

NZ, JW, and Y-FZ analyzed the data and wrote the paper. L-XY collected and processed the data. X-ZJ, X-FZ, and X-PD processed the data. JZ and H-JH collected the data. All authors designed the experiments.

FUNDING

This work was supported by the Natural Science Foundation of China (Nos. 81520108016, 81661148045, 81701776, and 31471084) and Y-FZ was partly supported by "Qian Jiang Distinguished Professor" program.

ACKNOWLEDGMENTS

We are grateful to Dong-Qiang Liu and Yuan-Yuan Li for the help of the data collection.

REFERENCES

Andellini, M., Cannatà, V., Gazzellini, S., Bernardi, B., and Napolitano, A. (2015). Test-retest reliability of graph metrics of resting state MRI functional brain networks: a review. *J. Neurosci. Methods* 253, 183–192. doi: 10.1016/j.jneumeth.2015.05.020

Aurich, N. K., Filho, J. O. A., da Silva, A. M. M., and Franco, A. R. (2015). Evaluating the reliability of different preprocessing steps to estimate graph theoretical measures in resting state fMRI data. *Front. Neurosci.* 9:48. doi: 10.3389/fnins.2015.00048

Braun, U., Plichta, M. M., Esslinger, C., Sauer, C., Haddad, L., Grimm, O., et al. (2012). Test-retest reliability of resting-state connectivity network characteristics using fMRI and graph theoretical measures. *NeuroImage* 59, 1404–1412. doi: 10.1016/j.neuroimage.2011.08.044

Fox, M. D., Snyder, A. Z., Vincent, J. L., Corbetta, M., Van Essen, D. C., and Raichle, M. E. (2005). From the cover: the human brain is intrinsically organized into dynamic, anticorrelated functional networks. *Proc. Natl. Acad. Sci. U.S.A.* 102, 9673–9678. doi: 10.1073/pnas.0504136102

Jann, K., Gee, D. G., Kilroy, E., Schwab, S., Smith, R. X., Cannon, T. D., et al. (2015). Functional connectivity in BOLD and CBF data: SIMILARITY and reliability of resting brain networks. *NeuroImage* 106, 111–122. doi: 10.1016/j.neuroimage.2014.11.028

Jia, X. Z., Ji, G. J., Liao, W., Lv, Y. T., Wang, J., Wang, Z., et al. (2017). Percent amplitude of fluctuation: a simple measure for resting-state fMRI signal at single voxel level. *bioRxiv* [Preprint]. doi: 10.1101/214098

Li, Z., Kadivar, A., Pluta, J., Dunlop, J., and Wang, Z. (2012). Test-retest stability analysis of resting brain activity revealed by BOLD fMRI. *J. Magn. Res. Imag.* 36, 334–354. doi: 10.1016/j.biotechadv.2011.08.021.Secreted

Liao, X., Xia, M., Xu, T., Dai, Z., Cao, X., Niu, H., et al. (2013). Functional brain hubs and their test-retest reliability: a multiband resting-state functional MRI study. *NeuroImage* 83, 969–982. doi: 10.1016/j.neuroimage.2013.07.058

Liu, D., Dong, Z., Zuo, X., Wang, J., and Zang, Y. (2013). Eyes-open/eyes-closed dataset sharing for reproducibility evaluation of resting state fMRI data analysis methods. *Neuroinformatics* 11, 469–476. doi: 10.1007/s12021-013-9187-0

Pannunzi, M., Hindriks, R., Bettinardi, R. G., Wenger, E., Lisofsky, N., Martensson, J., et al. (2017). Resting-state fMRI correlations: from link-wise unreliability to whole brain stability. *NeuroImage* 157, 250–262. doi: 10.1016/j.neuroimage.2017.06.006

Patriat, R., Molloy, E. K., Meier, T. B., Kirk, G. R., Nair, V. A., Meyerand, M. E., et al. (2013). The effect of resting condition on resting-state fMRI reliability and consistency: a comparison between resting with eyes open, closed, and fixated. *NeuroImage* 78, 463–473. doi: 10.1016/j.neuroimage.2013.04.013

Shehzad, Z., Kelly, A. M. C., Reiss, P. T., Gee, D. G., Gotimer, K., Uddin, L. Q., et al. (2009). The resting brain: unconstrained yet reliable. *Cereb. Cortex* 19, 2209–2229. doi: 10.1093/cercor/bhn256

Shrout, P. E., and Fleiss, J. L. (1979). Intraclass correlations: uses in assessing rater reliability. *Psychol. Bull.* 86, 420–428. doi: 10.1037/0033-2909.86.2.420

Somandepalli, K., Kelly, C., Reiss, P. T., Zuo, X. N., Craddock, R. C., Yan, C. G., et al. (2015). Short-term test-retest reliability of resting state fMRI metrics in children with and without attention-deficit/hyperactivity disorder. *Dev. Cognit. Neurosci.* 15, 83–93. doi: 10.1016/j.dcn.2015.08.003

Song, X. W., Dong, Z. Y., Long, X. Y., Li, S. F., Zuo, X. N., Zhu, C.-Z., et al. (2011). REST: a Toolkit for resting-state functional magnetic resonance imaging data processing. *PLoS One* 6:e25031. doi: 10.1371/journal.pone.0025031

Tomasi, D., and Volkow, N. D. (2014). Mapping small-world properties through development in the human brain: disruption in schizophrenia. *PLoS One* 9:e96176. doi: 10.1371/journal.pone.0096176

Wang, J.-H., Zuo, X.-N., Gohel, S., Milham, M. P., Biswal, B. B., and He, Y. (2011). Graph theoretical analysis of functional brain networks: test-retest evaluation on short- and long-term resting-state functional MRI data. *PLoS One* 6:e21976. doi: 10.1371/journal.pone.0021976

Yan, C., Liu, D., He, Y., Zou, Q., Zhu, C., Zuo, X., et al. (2009). Spontaneous brain activity in the default mode network is sensitive to different resting-state conditions with limited cognitive load. *PLoS One* 4:e5743. doi: 10.1371/journal.pone.0005743

Yan, C. G., Craddock, R. C., Zuo, X. N., Zang, Y. F., and Milham, M. P. (2013). Standardizing the intrinsic brain: Towards robust measurement of inter-individual variation in 1000 functional connectomes. *NeuroImage* 80, 246–262. doi: 10.1016/j.neuroimage.2013.04.081

Yan, C. G., Wang, X., Di, Zuo, X. N., and Zang, Y. F. (2016). DPABI: data processing & analysis for (resting-state) brain imaging. *Neuroinformatics* 14, 339–351. doi: 10.1007/s12021-016-9299-4

Yuan, B. K., Wang, J., Zang, Y. F., and Liu, D. Q. (2014). Amplitude differences in high-frequency fMRI signals between eyes open and eyes closed resting states. *Front. Hum. Neurosci.* 8:503. doi: 10.3389/fnhum.2014.00503

Zang, Y., Jiang, T., Lu, Y., He, Y., and Tian, L. (2004). Regional homogeneity approach to fMRI data analysis. *Neuroimage* 22, 394–400. doi: 10.1016/j.neuroimage.2003.12.030

Zang, Y. F., He, Y., Zhu, C. Z., Cao, Q. J., Sui, M. Q., Liang, M., et al. (2007). Altered baseline brain activity in children with ADHD revealed by resting-state functional MRI. *Brain Dev.* 29, 83–91. doi: 10.1016/j.braindev.2006.07.002

Zang, Y. F., Zuo, X. N., Milham, M., and Hallett, M. (2015). Toward a meta-analytic synthesis of the resting-state fMRI literature for clinical populations. *BioMed Res. Int.* 2015, 3–5. doi: 10.1155/2015/435265

Zou, Q., Miao, X., Liu, D., Wang, D. J. J., Zhuo, Y., and Gao, J. H. (2015). Reliability comparison of spontaneous brain activities between BOLD and CBF contrasts in eyes-open and eyes-closed resting states. *NeuroImage* 121, 91–105. doi: 10.1016/j.neuroimage.2015.07.044

Zuo, X. N., Di Martino, A., Kelly, C., Shehzad, Z. E., Gee, D. G., Klein, D. F., et al. (2010a). The oscillating brain: complex and reliable. *NeuroImage* 49, 1432–1445. doi: 10.1016/j.neuroimage.2009.09.037

Zuo, X. N., Ehmke, R., Mennes, M., Imperati, D., Castellanos, F. X., Sporns, O., et al. (2012). Network centrality in the human functional connectome. *Cereb. Cortex* 22, 1862–1875. doi: 10.1093/cercor/bhr269

Zuo, X. N., Kelly, C., Adelstein, J. S., Klein, D. F., Castellanos, F. X., and Milham, M. P. (2010b). Reliable intrinsic connectivity networks: test-retest evaluation using ICA and dual regression approach. *NeuroImage* 49, 2163–2177. doi: 10.1016/j.neuroimage.2009.10.080

Zuo, X. N., Kelly, C., Di Martino, A., Mennes, M., Margulies, D. S., Bangaru, S., et al. (2010c). Growing together and growing apart: regional and sex differences in the lifespan developmental trajectories of functional homotopy. *J. Neurosci.* 30, 15034–15043. doi: 10.1523/JNEUROSCI.2612-10.2010

Zuo, X. N., and Xing, X. X. (2014). Test-retest reliabilities of resting-state FMRI measurements in human brain functional connectomics: a systems neuroscience perspective. *Neurosci. Biobehav. Rev.* 45, 100–118. doi: 10.1016/j.neubiorev.2014.05.009

Zuo, X. N., Xu, T., Jiang, L., Yang, Z., Cao, X. Y., He, Y., et al. (2013). Toward reliable characterization of functional homogeneity in the human brain: preprocessing, scan duration, imaging resolution and computational space. *NeuroImage* 65, 374–386. doi: 10.1016/j.neuroimage.2012.10.017

7

Toward Rigorous Parameterization of Underconstrained Neural Network Models Through Interactive Visualization and Steering of Connectivity Generation

Christian Nowke [1†], Sandra Diaz-Pier [2*†], Benjamin Weyers [1], Bernd Hentschel [1], Abigail Morrison [2,3,4], Torsten W. Kuhlen [1] and Alexander Peyser [2]*

[1] Visual Computing Institute, RWTH Aachen University, JARA-HPC, Aachen, Germany, [2] SimLab Neuroscience, Jülich Supercomputing Centre (JSC), Institute for Advanced Simulation, JARA, Forschungszentrum Jülich GmbH, Jülich, Germany, [3] Institute of Neuroscience and Medicine, Institute for Advanced Simulation, JARA Institute Brain Structure-Function Relationships, Forschungszentrum Jülich GmbH, Jülich, Germany, [4] Institute of Cognitive Neuroscience, Faculty of Psychology, Ruhr-University Bochum, Bochum, Germany

***Correspondence:**
Christian Nowke
cnowke@gmail.com
Sandra Diaz-Pier
s.diaz@fz-juelich.de

† These authors have contributed equally to this work.

Simulation models in many scientific fields can have non-unique solutions or unique solutions which can be difficult to find. Moreover, in evolving systems, unique final state solutions can be reached by multiple different trajectories. Neuroscience is no exception. Often, neural network models are subject to parameter fitting to obtain desirable output comparable to experimental data. Parameter fitting without sufficient constraints and a systematic exploration of the possible solution space can lead to conclusions valid only around local minima or around non-minima. To address this issue, we have developed an interactive tool for visualizing and steering parameters in neural network simulation models. In this work, we focus particularly on connectivity generation, since finding suitable connectivity configurations for neural network models constitutes a complex parameter search scenario. The development of the tool has been guided by several use cases—the tool allows researchers to steer the parameters of the connectivity generation during the simulation, thus quickly growing networks composed of multiple populations with a targeted mean activity. The flexibility of the software allows scientists to explore other connectivity and neuron variables apart from the ones presented as use cases. With this tool, we enable an interactive exploration of parameter spaces and a better understanding of neural network models and grapple with the crucial problem of non-unique network solutions and trajectories. In addition, we observe a reduction in turn around times for the assessment of these models, due to interactive visualization while the simulation is computed.

Keywords: simulation and modeling, neural networks, structural plasticity, interactive systems, high performance computing, visualization software

INTRODUCTION AND RELATED WORK

Neuronal models and neural mass models, usually based on coupled systems of differential equations, contain many degrees of freedom which determine the dynamics of the system. In a neural network, these models are interconnected and the strength of the interactions between elements can also change through time.

Since biological evidence to specify a complete set of parameters for a neural network model is often incomplete, conflicting, or measured to an insufficient level of certainty, parameter fitting is typically required to obtain outputs comparable to experimental results (see for example, López-Cuevas et al., 2015; Schuecker et al., 2015; Zaytsev et al., 2015; Schirner et al., 2016). And even *if* we had infinite experimental data available, Cubitt et al. (2012) have shown that, regardless of how much experimental data is acquired for a general system, the inverse problem of extracting dynamical equations from experimental data is intractable: "extracting dynamical equations from experimental data is NP hard." This implies that in neural networks, the problem of finding the exact free parameters for a simulation leading to results matching experimental measurements cannot be solved in polynomial time, at least under the current understanding of computational complexity.

However, we can explore the parameter space with forward simulations in order to discover the system's characteristic behaviors and thus limit the search space to a computationally tractable sub-problem in an educated manner. The definition of these subspaces can then be the basis for robust—and non-arbitrary—parameter determination (in other words, mathematically valid performance function minimization). In fact, given the known mathematical characteristics of the dynamics of neuronal and neural mass networks, investigators should characterize the solution spaces of sufficiently complex networks and models before selecting what they propose are statistically diagnostic simulation trajectories. In practice, this rarely happens, even though parameter fitting without sufficient constraints and a rigorous exploration of the possible solution space can lead to conclusions valid only around local minima or around non-minima. Researchers frequently stay within arbitrary regions in the parameter space which show interesting behaviors, leaving other regions unexplored.

Visual parameter space exploration has been successfully applied in several key scientific areas, as detailed by Sedlmair et al. (2014). Combined with interactive simulation steering, the time for obtaining optimal parameter space solutions can be significantly reduced (Matković et al., 2008, 2014). Whitlock et al. (2011) present an integration of VisIt (Childs et al., 2005), a flexible end-user visualization system, into existing simulation codes. This approach enables *in situ* processing of large datasets while adding visual analysis capabilities at simulation runtime. A similar approach has been suggested by Fabian et al. (2011) for ParaView (Henderson, 2004).

Coordinated multiple views (CMVs) as proposed by North and Shneiderman (1997) and Wang Baldonado et al. (2000) can assist in visual parameter space exploration. CMVs are a category of visualization systems that use two or more distinct views to support the investigation of a single conceptual entity. For example, a CMV system can display a 3D rendering of a building (the conceptual entity) alongside a top-down view of its schematics—whenever a room is selected within the schematic overview, the 3D rendering will highlight the room's location. Roberts (2007) shows that CMVs support exploratory data analysis by offering interaction with representations of the same data while emphasizing different details. Ryu et al. (2003) present CMV systems that have been successfully utilized to uncover complex relationships by enabling users to relate different data modalities and scales, and assisting researchers in context switches, comparative tasks, and supplementary analysis techniques. Additional examples of such systems are presented by North and Shneiderman (2000), Boukhelifa and Rodgers (2003), and Weaver (2004).

Visual exploration of neural network connectivity, e.g., by displaying spatial connectivity data in 3D renderings, has previously been employed by scientists to better understand and validate models as well as to support theories regarding the networks' topological organization (Migliore et al., 2014; Roy et al., 2014). The infinite solution space of suitable connectivity paths and end configurations for neural networks makes fully automatic parameter fitting "hard," since it involves satisfying multiple contradictory objectives and qualitative assessment of complex data, as explained by Sedlmair et al. (2014). Kammara et al. (2016) conclude that for multi-objective optimization problems, visualization of the optimization space and trajectories permits more efficient and transparent human supervision of optimization process properties, e.g., diversity and neighborhood relations of solution qualities. They also point their work toward interactive exploration of complex spaces which allows expert knowledge and intuition to quickly explore suitable locations in the parameter space.

To address efficient but rigorous parameter space exploration, we have developed an interactive tool for visualizing and steering parameters in neural network simulation models. In this work, we focus particularly on the generation of connectivity, since finding suitable connectivity configurations for neural network models constitutes a complex parameter search scenario. The generation of local connectivity is achieved using structural plasticity in NEST (Bos et al., 2015) following simple homeostatic rules described in Butz and van Ooyen (2013). We specify the problem from the control theory perspective, as variations in the structure system control the transition in its dynamics from an initial to a final state following a defined trajectory. The tool allows researchers to steer the parameters of the structural plasticity during the simulation, thus quickly growing networks composed of multiple populations with individually targeted mean activities. The flexibility of the software allows the exploration of other connectivity and neuron variables apart from those presented as use cases. We use CMVs to interactively plot firing rates and connectivity properties of populations while the simulation is performed. Moreover, simulation steering is realized by providing interactive capabilities to influence simulation parameters on the fly.

We have developed this tool based on two use cases where visual exploration is key for obtaining insights into non-unique dynamics and solutions. The first use case focuses on the generation of connectivity in a simple two population network. Here we show how the generation of connectivity to a desired level of average activity in the network can be achieved by taking multiple trajectories with different biological significance. The second use case is inspired by a whole brain simulation described in Deco et al. (2013), where the exploration of non-unique connectivity solutions is desired to understand the behavior of the model.

Applying this approach, an intractable inverse problem can be reduced to a tractable subspace, and the requirements for statistically valid analyses can be determined. Visualization can simplify a complex parameter search scenario, helping in the development of mathematically robust descriptions amenable to further automated investigation of characteristic solution ensembles. Observing the evolution of connectivity, especially in cases where several biologically meaningful paths may lead to the same solutions, can be useful for a better understanding of development, learning and brain repair. This work is a first step toward developing new analytic and computational solutions to specific inverse problems in neuronal and neural mass networks. Our software platform promotes rigorous analysis of complex network models and supports well-informed selection of parameters for simulation.

This paper is structured as follows: first, we present an introduction to generic dynamic neural network models from a control theory perspective. Next, we describe connectivity construction and its effects on the dynamics of the system. Then, the development process and design of the steering and visualization tool is detailed. The fifth section describes the results of using the steering tool in two different use cases. Finally, we discuss our results and present open questions and future work.

GENERAL FORM OF NETWORK DYNAMICS

Let a neural network be defined by a set of ordinary differential equations in which $x_1(t), x_2(t)...x_n(t)$ are state variables of the system at time t. We assume that neurons in this model can be either in an active or quiescent state. The master equation of a neural network has been derived and explained in Cowan (1991) and Ohira and Cowan (1993). This equation provides a mathematical description of the evolution of stochastic neural networks in the form of a Liouvillian:

$$L = \alpha \sum_{i=1}^{N} (\Delta_{+i} - 1)\, \Delta_{-i} + \sum_{i=1}^{N} (\Delta_{-i} - 1)\, \Delta_{+i}\, \phi \left(\frac{1}{n_i} \sum_{j=1}^{N} \omega_{ij} x_j \right) \tag{1}$$

where α is the decay function after a neuron has spiked, Δ_{+i} and Δ_{-i} are the raising and lowering operators which take a neuron i to and from an activation state, n_i is the number of connections to neuron i, N is the total number of neurons in the network, ϕ is the activation rate function which depends on the neuron model and ω_{ij} is the strength of the connection between neuron i and j. Synaptic growth and connectivity variations in neural networks further increase the complexity of the system. In the case of variable connectivity, the network master equation is transformed into:

$$\begin{aligned} L = {} & \alpha \sum_{i=1}^{N} (\Delta_{+i} - 1)\, \Delta_{-i} \\ & + \sum_{i=1}^{N} (\Delta_{-i} - 1)\, \Delta_{+i}\, \phi \left(\frac{1}{n_i(u(t))} \sum_{j=1}^{N} \omega_{ij}(u(t))\, x_j \right) \end{aligned} \tag{2}$$

where both ω_{ij} and n_i depend on the control signal u coming from the synaptic and structural plasticity algorithms at time t. We introduce this formulation to expose variables $u(t)$ in the system, which can be controlled. We are interested in modifying these signals in order to induce changes in the network and thus achieve a target dynamic profile. However, it is worth noting that our approach is also applicable to non-stochastic neural networks.

Control Theory for Network State Trajectories

Both synaptic and structural plasticity can be seen as biological controllers in a multi-objective optimization problem. Under this view, the system gradually creates and destroys connections between neurons, or modifies the strength of existing synapses (control), to achieve a transition from one initial state to a final steady (or even homeostatic) state. This final state can be a previously known activity state which has been altered, as in repair after a lesion, or a new activity state to be achieved, as is the case in learning. Thus, the evolving connectivity problem can be mathematically expressed in terms of control theory as defined in Kirk (2012).

In our case, the control signals refer to the variations in the connectivity of the network while the states refer to the dynamics of the network. The state equations take the form of:

$$\dot{\mathbf{x}} = \mathbf{a}(\mathbf{x}(t), \mathbf{u}(t), t) \tag{3}$$

where $\mathbf{u}$ is the history of control signals during the interval $[t_0, t_f]$, and the state trajectory denoted by $\mathbf{x}$ is the history of state values during the same time interval. A control history which satisfies the constraints of the system (in this case, experimental parameters of neurons and synapses) during the time interval of interest is called an "admissible control." On the other hand, an "admissible trajectory" is a state trajectory which satisfies the constraints of the state variables through the whole period of interest. The final state of the system is then required to lie in a specific region, defined as the target set, of the $n+1$-dimensional state-time space.

By applying the control signal $\mathbf{u}(t)$ from t_0 to t_f, the system will evolve from its initial state x_0 following some trajectory to a final state x_f. The "performance" of this trajectory is the difference between a desired and the obtained measure for a heuristic involving the dynamics of the system. In our case, the performance function is given by the homeostatic rules the system must follow. To reach a defined target activity regime, we cannot know *a priori* whether an optimal admissible control exists, which leads the system through an admissible trajectory for a given performance function. It may be impossible to find such a control history, and even if it exists, it may not be unique or numerically stable.

The optimization problem posed seeks a global minimum for one or more admissible trajectories of the system. For the class of neural networks described by the dynamical equations above, the problem of finding the exact control signals or free parameters for a simulation leading to experimental results cannot be solved in polynomial time. However, it may still be possible to confirm solutions in polynomial time.

CONNECTIVITY GENERATION IN NEURAL NETWORKS

Previous research by Sporns et al. (2005) has found that the assembly of anatomical connections among neurons, also known as the connectome, plays a fundamental role in explaining the high-level activities of the brain. However, the exact relationship between anatomical links and the functions performed by the brain has aspects that remains unclear. An attempt to model biologically realistic circuits immediately runs into the problem that the structure of the brain has yet to be comprehensively characterized. Existing connectomic datasets are incomplete or contain large uncertainties (Bakker et al., 2012). Conversely, information about the average electrical activity in specific brain regions is easier to acquire either directly, e.g., electroencephalogram, extracellular electrode recordings of spiking activity and local field potential, or indirectly, e.g., functional magnetic resonance imaging and optogenetics/calcium imaging.

Variations in the physical elements, which constitute a neural network, can be modeled using synaptic and structural plasticity. Structural plasticity, a model of the dynamic creation and deletion of synapses in a neural network, is desirable from two main perspectives. The primary purpose is to study the neurobiological phenomenon of morphological transformations that a neuron or set of neurons undergoes through time, leading to the creation or deletion of synapses. This phenomenon is part of brain development, learning and repair. However, a promising secondary role suggested by Diaz-Pier et al. (2016) is the automatic generation of neuron-to-neuron synapses to compensate for gaps in experimental connectivity data. Using structural plasticity, a network can autonomously generate synapses to achieve a stable desired profile of electrical activity, a measure that is experimentally more accessible than detailed connectivity data. By progressively and slowly changing the connections between neurons in the network and the weight of these connections for all regions, the structural plasticity algorithm is able to find stable configurations within the desired firing rate profile.

The structural plasticity implementation in NEST is based on the model proposed by Butz and van Ooyen (2013) and described in detail by Diaz-Pier et al. (2016). In this plasticity framework, neurons have contact points called synaptic elements which increase or decrease in number according to simple homeostatic rules. When new synaptic elements become available, they can be used to create new synapses. If the contact points are eliminated, the synapses formed earlier are destroyed. Homeostatic rules applied to the synaptic elements are intended to take the mean electrical activity to a desired state.

A Gaussian curve (**Figure 1**) is an example of a homeostatic rule describing the growth rate of connection points for neurons. The original model by Butz and van Ooyen (2013) uses intracellular calcium concentration as a proxy for the mean firing rate. In this paper's examples, we will use a variation directly referencing the mean firing rate as our homeostatic rule.

The parameters defining the growth and decay of synapses are the minimum firing rate η required to generate synaptic elements (or destroy them, depending on sign of ν), the value ν of the growth rate curve when the firing rate is $(\varepsilon - \eta)/2$, and the target firing rate ε. Modifying these values alters the way connectivity is created and destroyed in the network.

Thus, to calculate the number of synaptic elements per second (dn/dt) to create (or remove, if negative), we use:

$$\frac{\mathrm{d}n}{\mathrm{d}t} = \nu\ \mathrm{H}[\lambda - \eta]\left[2\ \mathrm{pow}_2\left(-\left[2\frac{\lambda - \eta}{\epsilon - \eta} - 1\right]^2\right) - 1\right] \tag{4}$$

where $\mathrm{pow}_2\, x$ is the power function 2^x and $\mathrm{H}[x]$ is the Heaviside step function equal to 0 when $x < 0$, otherwise 1. Equation (4) is equivalent to the Gaussian used in Diaz-Pier et al. (2016) after directly replacing the calcium concentration with the firing rate λ. In this paper's simulations, this form is not biologically motivated, but is a homeostatic meta-rule being used to numerically solve for networks consistent with fixed firing rates.

The firing rate λ at time t used in Equation (4) is calculated by low-pass filtering spike train data by convolving that data with an exponential decay kernel (Park et al., 2013): the current firing rate λ is increased by $1/\tau$ spikes/s for each spike and decays exponentially with a time constant $\tau = 10$ s between firing times. Thus,

$$\tau\frac{\mathrm{d}\lambda}{\mathrm{d}t} = -\lambda + \sum_{t^f}\delta\left(t - t^f\right) \tag{5}$$

where t^f are the firing times of the neuron and δ is the Dirac delta function. This calculation is internal to NEST and independent of our tool. When the convolution technique isn't suitable, an alternate mean firing rate can be computed using a user-defined window size applied to binned spike trains.

As discussed in the previous section, synaptic and structural connectivity can be seen as multi-objective optimization algorithms which take the network from an initial state to a final state where *something has been learned* or *a new activity pattern has been enabled.* Partial information about the connectivity can be combined with information about average activity in

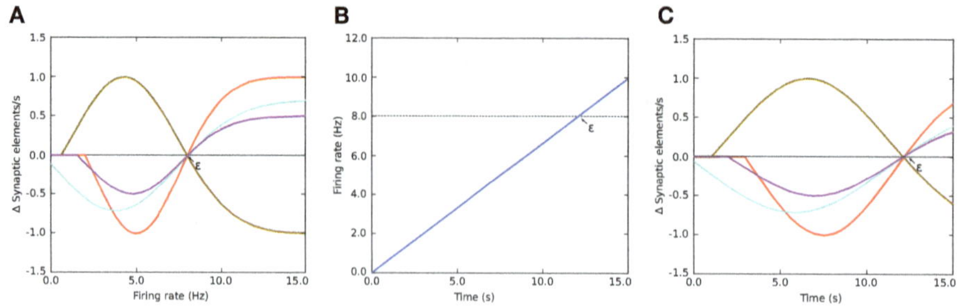

FIGURE 1 | (A) Example of growth rate curves determining the rate of creation or deletion of synaptic elements in the structural plasticity model. The parameters which define the shape of the curve are two firing rates, the minimal firing rate for creating/deleting synaptic elements η and the target firing rate ϵ, and the growth rate ν which is the value of the curve in synaptic elements/s when the firing rate $\lambda = (\epsilon - \eta)/2$. The red, cyan and purple curves have a negative value of ν which implies that synaptic elements will be deleted when the current firing rate is less than the target rate. These curves are therefore suitable for inhibitory synapses. Conversely, synaptic elements will be created when the current firing rate exceeds the target. The brown curve has a positive ν which works in the opposite way. All curves display different values of η; in particular, the cyan curve has a negative value of η. In these cases, all curves have a target firing rate ϵ of 8 Hz. It is important to note the slope of each curve close to the target firing rate ε; this slope is critical for the stability of the optimization algorithm. **(B)** Firing rate externally imposed on sample systems with Gaussian growth curves shown in **(A,C)** the resulting evolution of synaptic growth rate through time due to the firing rate changes depicted in **(B)**. See **Figure 5B** for an equivalent Gaussian growth curve for the two-population example in this paper, and the resulting free (not driven) dynamics in **Figures 5C–E**.

the system to initialize models of structural plasticity filling the gaps in the constraints of the system. However, finding suitable connectivity configurations and generation trajectories for neural network models is non-trivial, which is exacerbated by the nature of experimental data. The known experimental data often fails to sufficiently constrain the model to parameter subspaces that can be completely explored with reasonable resources within reasonable time frames.

Enabling structural plasticity for a single population to reach a targeted activity level is usually unproblematic, fast, and relatively insensitive to the choice of parameters such as ν and η. However, a big challenge arises when structural plasticity is involved simultaneously on several interconnected populations with differing levels of activity. Even small changes in the connectivity of each population will impact the activity of all others to which it is connected, leading to a propagated destabilization. Another parameter which has a great impact on stability is the update interval at which synapses can be deleted or created. As in any control system, the delay between a control change and the response of the system strongly determines the capability of the controller to keep the system in a stable region.

In Diaz-Pier et al. (2016), the simulations were performed statically, meaning no steering was possible during runtime. Due to the large combination of parameters to be controlled and variables to be observed during the search process, brute-force parameter search based on static simulation proved to be insufficient to obtain stable states. The selection of adequate parameters to define and constrain the growth of network connectivity, especially for multi-population or coupled networks, is not trivial since some values might lead to unstable setups. Therefore, modifying the characteristics of the growth behavior (ν and η see **Figure 1**) for each population and the update interval *during simulation* becomes crucial for finding a suitable stable state for multi-population networks. We use the terms "population" and "region" interchangeably to refer to groups of neurons. The term chosen depends on the use case. In general, a region contains one or more populations while populations specify groups of neurons of the same type. Connectivity exists both within and between populations and regions. All types of connectivity can be subject to plasticity or remain fixed after setup. The software can be modified to take into account any number of populations per region, arbitrary types of neurons, and any number of regions. The user can also specify different types of connections between the same populations and apply various structural plasticity rules to each of them. The user can choose between a variety of connectivity modalities in NEST, ranging from one-to-one, all-to-all, fixed in-degree, fixed out-degree, fixed total number of connections, and pairwise Bernoulli. However, structural plasticity support is only currently implemented for one-to-one and all-to-all connectivity. Other modalities can be used, but structural plasticity will not affect these connections.

In the context of a simulation with evolving connectivity, the dynamic nature of the parameter search workflow derived from the two use cases presented later requires:

- **W1:** The simultaneous analysis of several changing variables by an expert.
- **W2:** Comparing the level of activity of several populations simultaneously.
- **W3:** Changing simulation parameters at any moment in each population of the network.
- **W4:** Snapshotting a time point in the simulation and storing the connectivity state.
- **W5:** Loading a previously stored connectivity state.

This workflow can potentially be assisted with an interactive tool enabling scientists to explore and steer such simulations within the space of possible trajectories. To achieve this goal, a scientist needs interactive feedback on the number of connections and the level of electrical activity in all populations.

IN SITU VISUALIZATION AND STEERING OF CONNECTIVITY GENERATION

To enable navigation through the connectivity generation parameter space, we developed a tool enabling interactive steering and visualization. The development was driven by the need to rapidly reach stable configurations of connectivity in multiple tightly connected populations. We then extended the tool to support further use cases which are presented later. The tool allows for the visualization of trajectories that the system undergoes during simulation by showing the changes in the observable states of the network (specifically the activity and connection properties of the network). In addition, this tool allows for the modification of the control signals for the generation of connectivity, i.e., the plasticity algorithm's parameters.

The developed tool realizes a CMV system by applying principles of event-driven architectures as presented in Abram and Treinish (1995), Michelson (2006), and Nowke et al. (2015). The development of the tool was organized into four stages: first, the simulation script was modified to retrieve electrical activity and connectivity values; second, the visualization components and user interfaces were developed; third, processing of parameter changes from the user interface was added; and finally, the simulation script was optimized to run on supercomputers.

In the first step, we started by reproducing the plots from the non-interactive analysis workflow used in the second use case. This initial design phase revealed the following visualization requirements (**R1–R5**), followed by the requirements for simulation steering (**R6–R10**). These requirements hold for all presented use cases:

R1: Deal with at least $2 \times N$ representations of time series data (electrical activity and connectivity), where N is the number of populations in the simulation.

R2: Interactively plot the firing rate for selected populations. The firing rate from the last simulation step should be displayed as soon as its computation concludes.

R3: Interactively plot connections for each population. As for the firing rate, the latest total connections per population should be displayed.

R4: Enable the selection and filtering of populations for plotting and further investigation. The means to select and filter populations of interest must be provided.

R5: Have a well defined way to distinguish populations in the plot. Since multiple populations can be selected for comparison, visual clutter needs to be avoided.

R6: The user interface must allow for the modification of each population's growth rate ν and apply each value in the simulation.

R7: The user interface must allow for the modification of a population's minimum electrical activity η and transfer the new value to the simulation engine.

R8: The user interface must allow for the modification of the update interval and transfer its change to the simulator.

R9: Control the NEST simulation from within a graphical user interface. Provide the means to start or stop the simulation, trigger the saving and loading of a network state, and allow convenient access to the visualizations.

R10: Enable loading and saving of the current network state (connections and user controlled parameters).

Requirements **R1–R5** cover the parameter search workflow **W1** and **W2**. **R6–R10** target **W3–W5**. Based on these requirements, we developed the software architecture as depicted in **Figure 2**. Each box in this figure we term a service. Services and the simulation engine NEST exclusively communicate via events. Communication via events allows us to treat each visualization as an independent loosely-coupled service. One benefit of this approach is that all services are independent of each other, facilitating the production of small reusable software components that are easy to maintain and can be reused in different contexts.

Event-communication is realized with the "*nett*" messaging framework (see Supplementary Material), which is an open source C++ network library facilitating data transfer between application boundaries based on the publish and subscribe pattern. To enable communication between applications, *nett* provides *slots*. A slot is an unidirectional communication channel strictly typed to an event. Slots exist in two flavors: out-slots for publishing events and in-slots for subscribing to these. Consequently, subscribing slots can be connected to several publishers emitting the same event. An event is defined via a customizable schema, describing the fundamental data types the event is composed of. Moreover, *nett* provides Python bindings, making it possible to communicate between Python, i.e., the visualization implementations, and C++ applications, i.e., NEST.

Streaming simulation results from NEST is already possible with the MUSIC interface (Djurfeldt et al., 2010). However, MUSIC is specifically built for transferring large arrays of structured data in parallel with a certain step size and with a focus on latency. It is tailored to multi-scale coupling and large data

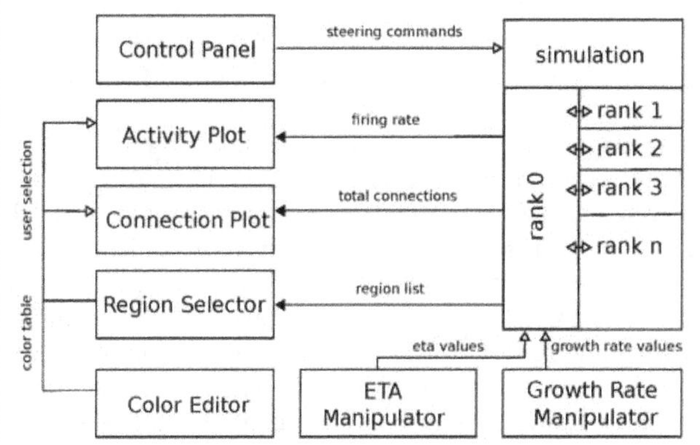

FIGURE 2 | Overview of the system architecture: boxes denote individual services. Black arrows mark communication from the simulation engine to the visualization front-ends. Vice versa, white arrows indicate event-flow from the visualization services to the simulation engine. Ranks indicate individual MPI processes responsible for the parallel computation of the neural network. The "ETA" (η) and "growth rate" (ν) manipulators control the respective variables from **Figure 1**.

transfer. In comparison, *nett* focuses on arbitrary serialization of data through tiny pipes and is based on a publish-and-subscribe communication mechanism. In addition, it is intended for point-to-point continuous streaming and is event-driven in comparison to the pull-driven communication regime by MUSIC. Furthermore, *nett* offers routing discovery while MUSIC relies an a static configuration on startup. In summary, *nett* is tailored to concise and light data transport and easy to integrate data streaming from C++ or Python codes.

The rest of this section will outline the required simulation instrumentation and the visualization services in more detail.

Simulation Instrumentation

Interactive steering relies on a bidirectional communication between the visualization and steering interfaces to a simulator. In our setup, activity levels and connectivity from populations computed by NEST are transferred via event communication over a network connection to the visualizations, where users can modify parameters of the simulation model, which in turn are fed back to the simulator. The values of interest are the firing rate of each population which serves as a proxy for electrical activity and a population's total connections formed due to connectivity generation. These are the observable states of the network. Steering parameters are the minimum firing rate η and the growth rate ν of each population, the update interval for the connectivity generation, and finally, basic commands to NEST such as ending or resetting the simulation, and storing or loading the current network state.

To retrieve firing rates and total connections, instrumentation of the simulation script is required. To this end, the simulation acquires the latest firing rates and total connections of each population in each iteration and publishes these as events. Then, parameter changes from the graphical steering interfaces, asynchronously retrieved during the model's computation, are applied and the next iteration is continued.

To adapt a NEST simulation to a different use case, the first step consists of determining what data needs to be transferred from or to the simulation. The next step consists of creating an event definition schema for the data to be transferred if one is not yet present. Then, slots for communicating this data definition can be created: out-slots for publishing data and in-slots to retrieve it. Once slots are created, in-slots need to be connected to their corresponding out-slots. Any in-slot should be used in a thread to asynchronously retrieve data without blocking the computation of the simulation. Once an event is received by a slot, its data needs to be applied in the next iteration of the simulation. In a complementary fashion, out-slots send the simulation results for each iteration by retrieving values of interest from the simulation and filling the slot's event and sending it. The same methodology is used for visualizations or graphical user interfaces which are use case specific.

Visualization System Overview

The visualization system consists of six services fulfilling the above listed requirements. A demonstration video of the tool can be found in Supplementary Material (see video **Movie 1**). In the following, we outline each service and its responsibility in the workflow.

Control Panel

The *Control Panel* is the central place to provide convenience functionality, i.e., to start the simulation, all visualization services, steering interfaces, the *Color Editor*, and *Region Selector* (see **Figure 3**). It serves as an entry point for users to start the investigation of structural plasticity. The user interface facilitates changing the update interval (**R8**) and allows the simulation to be paused or restarted (**R9**). In addition, it provides a graphical interface for loading and saving the network state (**R10**).

Region Selector

The *Region Selector* is a graphical interface displaying a list of all populations in the simulation (see **Figure 3**, rightmost element). These populations are defined by the network modeler in the simulation script as part of the instrumentation process. This is detailed in the instrumentation manual in Supplementary Material. The list provides the means to select populations of interest whose connectivity and firing rates should be plotted (**R4**). To this end, the *Region Selector* retrieves the number of populations from the simulation (see **Figure 2**). The user can then select multiple populations by clicking on them. All connected visualizations are linked with the current selections; thus it can be used to synchronize all tools for filtering data and in this way populations of interest can be focused (**R4**). The *Region Selector* can also be used to inspect individual populations of interest. By double clicking on a population in the list, an additional *Activity Plot* and *Connectivity Plot* is created plotting only the selected population of interest. This functionality can be used on multiple populations, independently of selections performed later on and facilitates the pairwise comparison of populations.

Activity Plot

The assessment of the simulation results is based on the inspection of a population's firing rate. The *Activity Plot* is an interactive service that plots the firing rates of populations selected in the region selector (**R1**). It is used to visualize the trajectories that the network traverses in terms of its functional states. To this end, it connects to the region selector and listens for incoming selection events (**R4**). To display the firing rate (**R2**), the service directly connects to the simulation to retrieve the last iteration result. Interactive zooming and panning capabilities allow the scientist to focus on details on demand, following the "information seeking" mantra postulated by Shneiderman (1996). Interactive zooming can be used to zoom into a specific time interval and assess the depicted curve in more detail. Panning allows the user to move the selected time interval of interest, effectively moving the curve to the left or right. The information seeking mantra states that users should be able to get an overview first, then zoom and filter the data, and finally query details on demand. Furthermore, axes can be independently scaled or their data range confined. In the *Activity Plot's* initial configuration, which can be modified by the user, both axes will be scaled in such a way that all retrieved firing rate

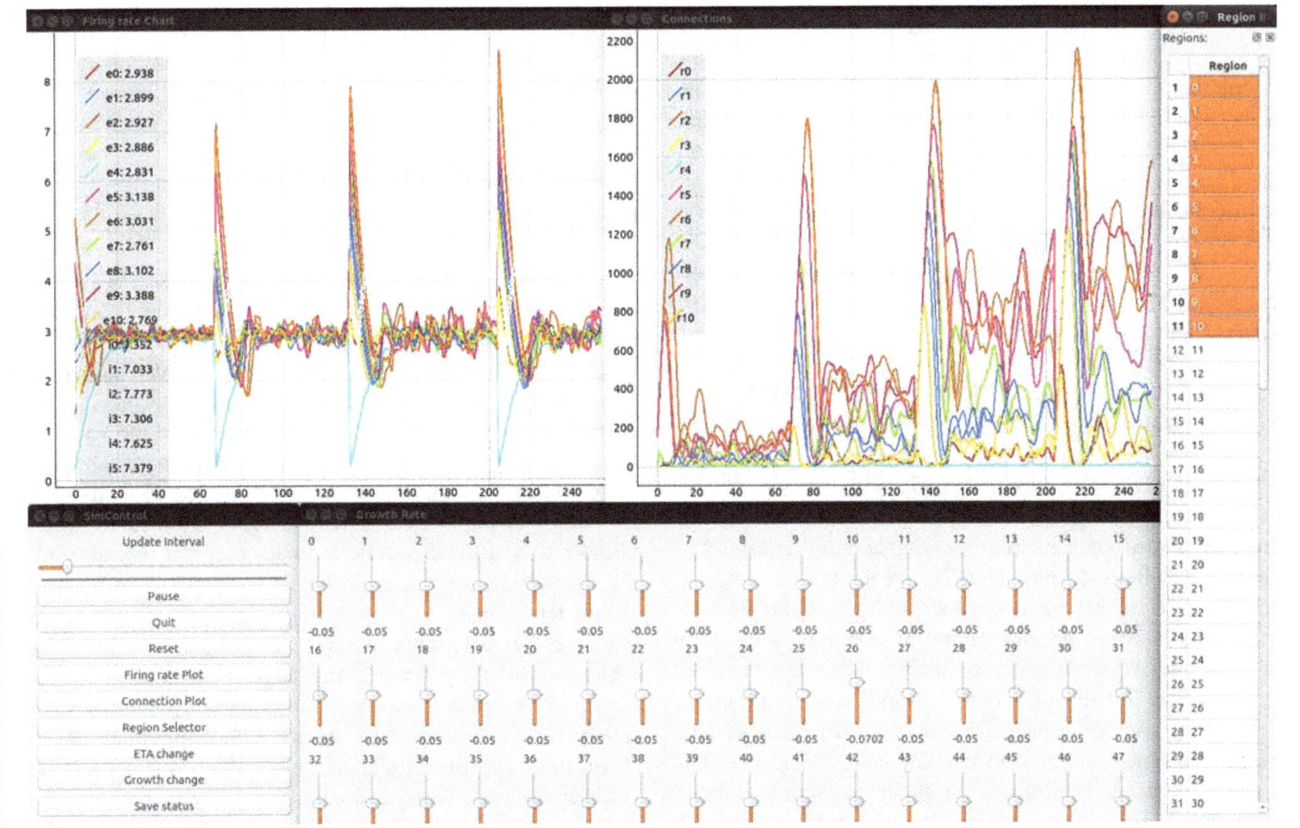

FIGURE 3 | Firing rate in spikes/s of simulated brain regions **(Upper left)** and total connections **(Upper right)** are retrieved while a NEST simulation is performed. Time is measured in number update intervals. The steering interfaces (*Control Panel* and growth rate manipulation; bottom left and center) allow interactive parameter space exploration which is synchronized with the current simulation. The growth rate (in Δ synaptic elements/ms) for each region can be controlled using the corresponding slider. The region selector (far right) provides the means to filter the brain regions of interest depicted in the plots. The legends provided in each plot denote the current selection from the region selector along with the color used to identify the corresponding curve. Specifically in the example shown, the labels *e0* - *e10* and *i0* - *i5* identify the average firing rate for excitatory and inhibitory populations in network regions 0-10 accordingly. Labels *r0* - *r10* identify total outgoing connections from network regions 0–10. Please refer to section 5.2 for more details on the network model used in this example. Please refer to the video **Movie 1** in Supplementary Material, for a detailed explanation of the tool's interface.

values are visible. The tool also allows the user to export the plot as a figure. To distinguish multiple curves, a color table can be defined via the *Color Editor* (**R5**), as discussed below. A legend in the upper left corner relates the selected populations to the depicted curves shown in **Figure 3** in the upper left window. In addition, it shows the latest firing rate next to each population's legend label. The legends can be changed by the user of the tool. In this work we use the label *e* and *i* to identify excitatory and inhibitory populations and a number to identify the region they belong to. Individual *Activity Plots* can be used in conjunction with the region selector by specifying a population of interest. Therefore, multiple plots can be used for comparison tasks (**R1**). In this setup, the visualization ignores user input and is fixed to the initial selection.

Connectivity Plot

The *Connectivity Plot* (see **Figure 3**, upper right window) displays the total number of connections for a population in accordance with **R3**. Since structural plasticity is responsible for a change in the total connections depending on the population's firing rate, the plot is the primary means to verify the structural plasticity model. It shows the trajectories of the network in terms of its structure. This visualization is connected to the region selector and thus enables filtering of the populations to be displayed (**R4**). Analogously to the *Activity Plot*, it is linked to the *Color Editor*. Whenever attributes like color, line-style-drawing, or thickness are changed, these values are applied. The legends can be changed by the user of the tool. In this work we use the label *r* and a number to identify the total connectivity values for an specific region. Like the *Activity Plot* service, it offers interactive zooming and panning functionality. Likewise, axes are automatically scaled such that all retrieved connectivity values are depicted. In addition, plots can be exported as figures for publication purposes or the tracking of results.

Color Editor

The *Color Editor* provides a graphical user interface that mediates the customization of color, line drawing style, and line thickness for each population's firing rate and connectivity plots. Whenever the user changes an entry, a "color changed" event is emitted and processed by the *Activity Plots* and *Connectivity Plots.* In addition, the color table is saved to disk for later reuse. Its primary use is to help in distinguishing curves within the plotting visualizations (**R5**). The *Color Editor* enables the customization of the depicted firing rate and connectivity curves in the plot. Here, users can select a color for a population's inhibitory (I) and excitatory (E) population by clicking on the corresponding list entry. In addition, line drawing style and thickness can be controlled. The population's name is equal to its specified counterpart in the simulation.

Manipulation of Structural Plasticity Parameters

The user interfaces for η and ν are the primary means of steering the simulation for the parameter space exploration (**R6** and **R7**). This interface allows for the modification of the control signals, enabling the structural plasticity algorithm to take the system from its current state to a desired final state (see **Figure 3**, bottom center). Both steering interfaces are designed as separate standalone services that can be started within the *Control Panel.* The η and ν services provide graphical user interfaces, each presenting one slider for each population. Their influence on the creation or deletion of synapses is indicated in **Figure 1**. Each slider is named according to the population's label and shows the current value used in the simulation. Whenever the user changes a value by adjusting the slider, an event is emitted which is subsequently processed and applied by the simulation in its next iteration step. The upper and lower limits for the control parameters can be defined inside the scripts for each controller interface. Please refer to the instrumentation manual in Supplementary Material, for more details.

Loading and Saving Network States

To re-use previously found connectivity patterns in neighboring points of the parameter space, we implemented a save and load functionality (**R10**). The current values for η and ν are saved for each population as well as the connectivity update interval. All current connections between all neurons are also saved. These connections are defined by a source neuron, a target neuron and the synapse model which links them. Finally, the total number of connections for each population are exported to a file which can be used in the next phase of the simulation loop.

To re-use a previously created snapshot, we first load the types of all synaptic elements for each population. When using the structural plasticity framework in NEST, the first step consists of defining the plastic synapses. This requires the specification of a synapse model as well as the definition of pre- and post-synaptic elements between which a synapse can be created. The growth curves for these synaptic elements are reconstructed using the stored values for η and ν. Then the synaptic elements are registered in the structural plasticity framework and the update interval is set for the simulation. This is performed by using the set status functions of NEST through PyNEST/CyNEST (Eppler et al., 2009; Zaytsev and Morrison, 2014). Finally, all connections are recreated, marking them as non-static links which can be modified by the structural plasticity algorithm. In this way, a new network with differing global parameters such as global coupling or inhibitory strength can start from a partial solution and arrive at the target activity values more quickly. For more details about the implementation of the structural plasticity framework please refer to Diaz-Pier et al. (2016). This functionality can be triggered from the *Control Panel.*

RESULTS

In this section, we present the results obtained from two use cases in connectivity generation. For the first use case, the results of running structural plasticity simulations before the interactive visualization tool was developed were previously reported in Diaz-Pier et al.(2016, **Figure 5**, section 3.3.1). **Figure 4** (from this current paper) shows the equivalent output for the second use case, reflecting the previous visualization approach. Due to the large number of unlabeled curves, the inability to focus on data for particular populations and the lack of interactivity with the visualization, using this static approach makes it very difficult for the user to identify the evolution of connectivity in relation to parameter changes. Moreover, a new simulation run is required whenever any parameter needs to be changed. Even when some regions have easily reached the target activity of 3 spikes/s, for some set-ups it is extremely challenging to identify suitable trajectories that lead to stable solutions for all populations.

In this type of simulation, the system is constrained by connectivity data and desired activity levels obtained from experimental measurements. However, these constraints still allow the system to reach non-physiological states such as saturating at high firing rates (see **Figure 4**). Moreover, the system may follow several trajectories to reach these implausible states, indicating that the system is under-constrained. On the other hand, there are many admissible trajectories which take the system to biologically plausible states. Biologically meaningful trajectories should be identified by heuristics, expert knowledge, and further experimental measurements gained through a deeper understanding of the parameter space to which the neural circuit is subject. At first glance, it is not clear how to explore the parameter space in these complex systems, as the large number of variables and long simulation times make it unfeasible to find stable populations through a brute force approach, and no heuristic is available to reduce the dimensionality. Without expert knowledge in a closed loop setup, admissible trajectories are fundamentally hard to find.

In the following sections, we demonstrate the challenges of parameterizing network models and the potential for an interactive visualization and steering tool, such as the one we propose, to address them. All experiments have been implemented with NEST 2.10.0 (Bos et al., 2015) and its Python language bindings which are described in Eppler et al. (2009); Zaytsev and Morrison (2014). The complete NEST scripts used in this work can be found in a GitHub repository. For more details, please see Supplementary Material.

Two Population Model

In this use case, we create a model with two populations of point neurons, one excitatory and one inhibitory as

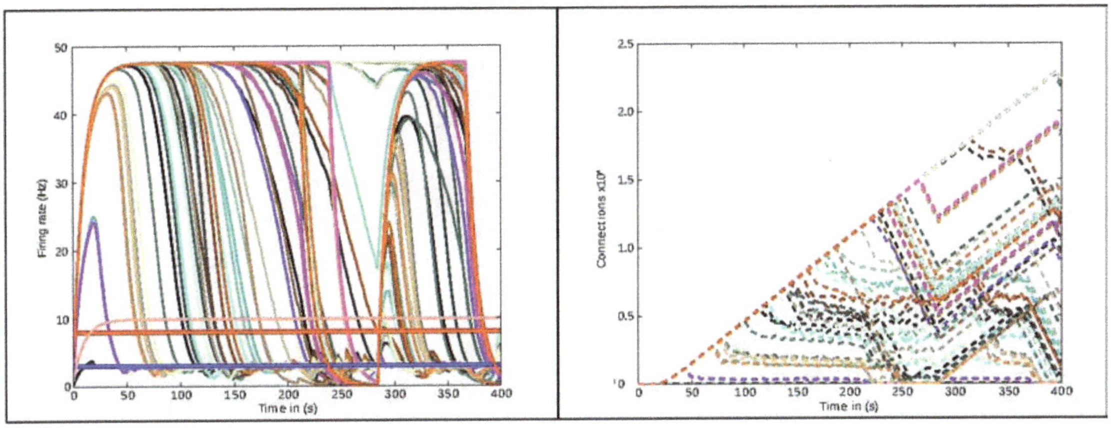

FIGURE 4 | Previous method of visualizing simulations: visualization of the simulation as performed before the presented tool was developed. The figure shows the evolution of the average firing rate for each region (solid curves) and numbers of outgoing connections (dashed curves) from each region using structural plasticity in a non-interactive (static) experiment. Each color represents a different population. In this static approach, a large number of independent simulator runs are performed over a predetermined, non-interactive parameter space and then displayed with *ad hoc* scripts. Mapping the non-physiological solutions with saturated firing rates onto regions of the parameter spaces is highly non-trivial (compare approach with **Figure 3**).

TABLE 1 | Network parameters for the first and second use cases.

Parameter	Value
Capacitance of the membrane C_m	0.25 nF
Resting potential V_L	−65 mV
Threshold membrane potential V_{thr}	−50 mV
Reset membrane potential V_{res}	−65 mV
Refractory time τ_{ref}	2 ms
Growth rate excitatory synaptic elements	0.0001 elements/ms
Growth rate inhibitory synaptic elements	0.0004 elements/ms

shown in **Figure 5A**. The whole network contains 1,000 leaky integrate-and-fire neurons with exponential-shaped post-synaptic currents, of which 80% belong to the excitatory population and the rest to the inhibitory population. Parameters for the point neurons are listed in **Table 1**. All neurons receive independent background excitatory Poisson noise at a rate of 10 kHz. At the beginning of the simulation, no connections between neurons are present. The system is allowed to create both excitatory and inhibitory connections (red and blue dashed arrows, respectively, in **Figure 5A**), using the structural plasticity framework in NEST. The weights for the created synapses are 1 and −1 respectively. The evolution of the firing rate (**Figure 5C**) and the growth of connections (**Figure 5C**) is regulated by two homeostatic rules defined by Gaussian curves, as shown in **Figure 5D**. The target average activity of the inhibitory population is set to 20 Hz while the target average activity in the excitatory population is set to 5 Hz. **Figure 5C** shows the evolution of the growth rate for excitatory synaptic elements in both populations during a simulation. These dynamics originate from the fixed firing rate curves shown in **Figure 5B**. The structural plasticity algorithm uses that relation at every simulation step to decide how many connections to create or delete.

The evolution of the connectivity generation can be guided by modifying the growth rate and shape of the Gaussian curve linked to each type of connection. **Figures 5D,E** show an example of this process. In this use case, an interesting feature to observe using the visualization and steering tool is the path to the solution. With the configurations used here, one can see how allowing faster growth of inhibition triggers an overshoot in the generation of excitatory connection to compensate. As a result, a rewiring of the system is obtained. These paths to the solution can be linked to onsets of critical periods in learning and healing or by external stimulation (Hensch, 2005). By regulating the speed of the creation of connections in the system, scientists can explore different paths to solution where the relationship between excitation and inhibition changes through time.

Figure 6 shows the evolution of growth rate (synaptic elements/s), firing rate (Hz) and connectivity (total number of connections) for six examples of the multiple trajectories and connectivity configurations that the network can show. All examples start with an initial growth rate of 0.0001 synaptic elements/ms. **Figure 6A** shows a smooth growth similar to **Figure 5**, but where the control signals have been modified to reduce the overshoot in the inhibitory population. That is done by reducing the initial growth rate to 0.00005 at iteration 8 (mark a.1). **Figure 6B** shows an example of a simulation where the control signals for growth start with aggressive growth values, producing a constant oscillatory behavior. That is achieved by changing the growth rate from 0.0001 to 0.0010 at iteration 38 (mark b.1) and then to 0.0030 at iteration 80 (mark b.2). Following these signals, the connectivity update interval is increased to 500 ms (from the standard length of 100 ms), which produces a big oscillation, triggering a rewiring of the network (mark b.3). Finally, growth is reduced to a slower pace, which helps the system settle at a stable state. This reduction is achieved

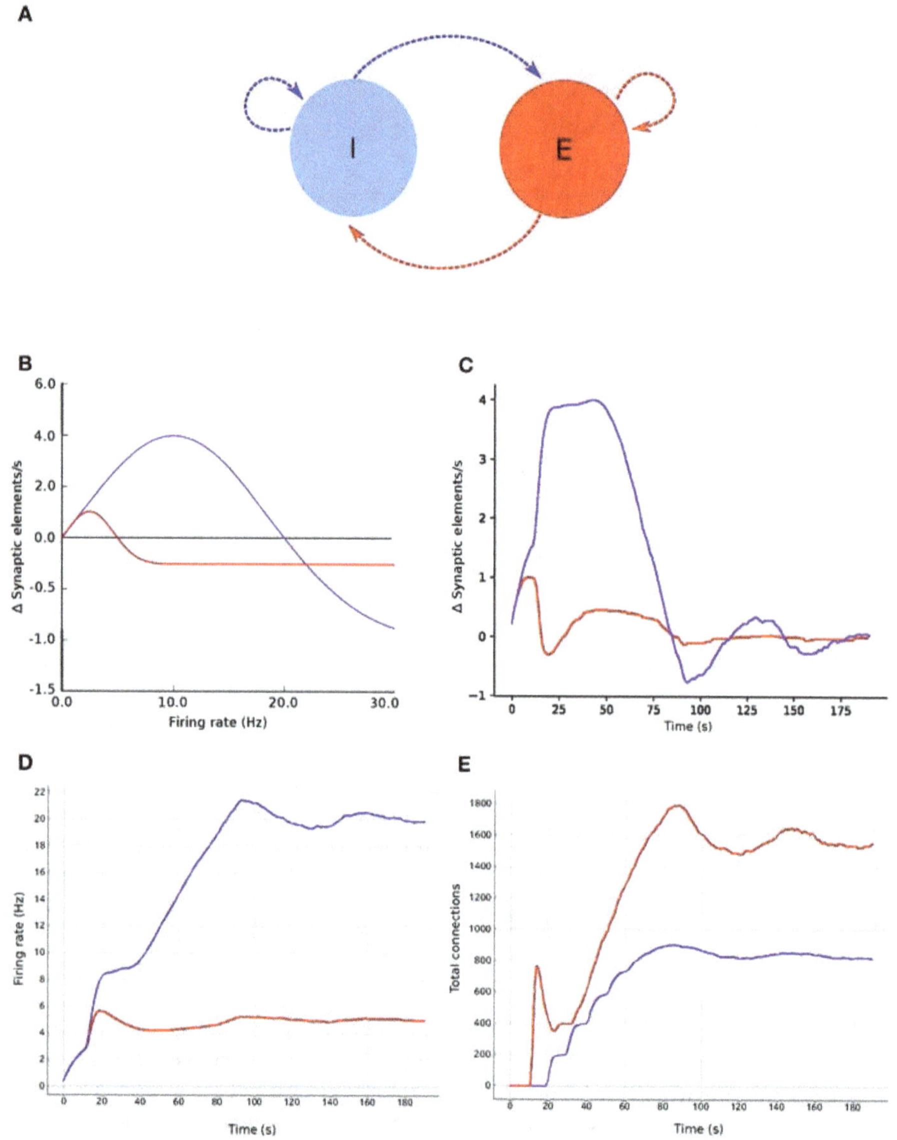

FIGURE 5 | Evolution of firing rate and connectivity for the two population example: **(A)** abstract view of the model consisting of two populations, one excitatory (red) and one inhibitory (blue) with respectively excitatory connections (red arrows) and inhibitory connections (blue arrows), both controlled by structural plasticity; **(B)** Gaussian growth curves mapping current firing rate to growth rates (see **Figure 1**); **(C)** growth rate dynamics; **(D)** evolution of the firing rate; and **(E)** evolution of the total number of connections during the simulation. Colors in **(B–E)** are as in **(A)**.

by setting the growth rate to 0.00005 at update 161 (mark b.4). The final connectivity is very similar to the one reached in **Figure 5**. This example shows a different trajectory which reaches the same final state.

Figure 6C illustrates very fast initial growth by changing the growth to 0.004 at iteration 46 (mark c.1). Then, a sharp reduction in growth when the system oscillates near the target firing rate. The growth rate is changed to 0.0018 at iteration 98 and further down to 0.0007 at iteration 103 (marks c.2 and c.3 accordingly). **Figure 6D** shows a case which seems stable in terms of activity, but is unstable in terms of connectivity, as it exhibits a constant race between excitation and inhibition in the connectivity to maintain the target activity. The growth rate is set to 0.001 at iteration 24 (mark d.1), to 0.0056 at iteration 52 (mark d.2) and to 0.0020 at iteration 78 (mark d.3). **Figure 6E** shows a trajectory which is not biologically meaningful. This network has been built only from excitatory connections by modulating the growth of connections very carefully around the target activity. Here, we have defined a growth curve that does not allow the creation of inhibitory connections unless the activity is above the desired firing rate. Finally, in **Figure 6F**, we see a trajectory which is not admissible (not biologically meaningful) because the network is taken to an artificially high firing rates before it settles back to its target. At iteration 17, the growth rate is set to 0.002

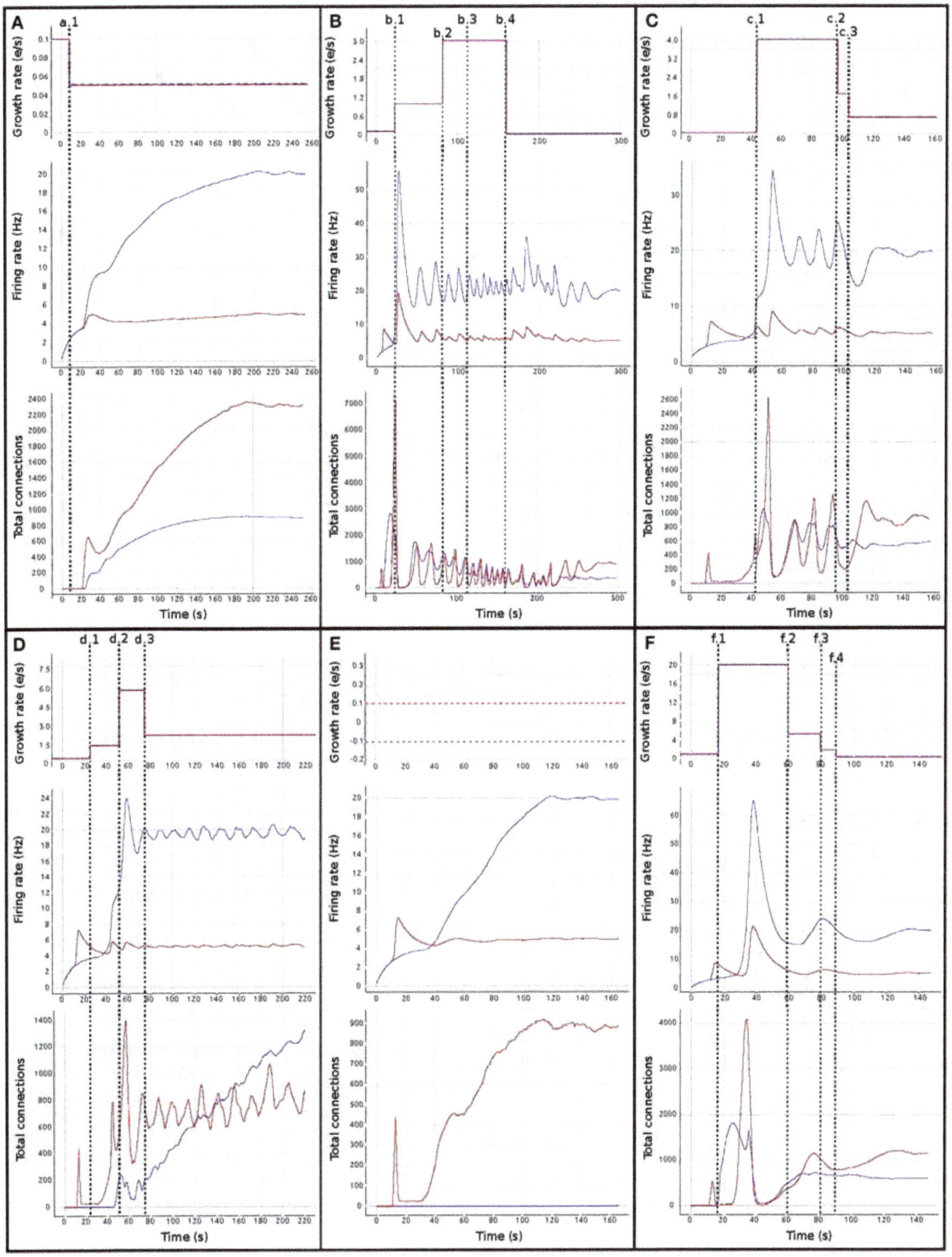

FIGURE 6 | Evolution of growth rate (Top), firing rate (Middle), and outgoing connections (Bottom) for six different trajectories **(A–F)** in the two population model use case, excitatory (red) and inhibitory (blue). Vertical dashed lines correspond to manual changes using the graphic interface to the growth rate (top curves) or update interval (at b.3) control variables. All other simulation parameters are held constant for all runs, including initial growth rate. Please see the main text for a discussion of the features of each set of trajectories.

(mark f.1) and then slowly reduced to 0.00056 at iteration 60, to 0.0002 at iteration 80 and finally to 0.00005 at iteration 90 (marks f.2, f.3, and f.4 accordingly). This graph shows how a network can traverse biologically inadmissible trajectories and still reach the target activity.

These results show that several instantiations of the same system using different dynamics lead to the same target activity but different connectivity patterns. Visualization and steering is fundamental for producing, observing, studying and cataloging these behaviors in the network. See Bahuguna et al. (2017) for an example of the same phenomenon exhibited in a more complex network. Thus using target activity as a tuning parameter without this kind of exploration leads to selecting one of these network connectivity states arbitrarily. The resulting model may not be representative of the kinds of networks that produce this activity, or of the target system to be modeled.

In other words, the target activity does not uniquely identify a network, or even a contiguous volume of parameter space, but is the property of a distribution of distinct networks distinguished by parameters that are not the direct targets of research—this class of inverse problem is degenerate. The network structure may be critically path-dependent, dependent upon parameters which are stochastic sequences (external control variables) or even dependent upon numerically unstable parameter functions. Simple networks such as the one shown in this example are frequently used in computational neuroscience but rarely with consideration to the careful characterization of the parameter spaces. Thus, in the absence of analytical methods to identify alternative solutions in the parameter space, steered visualization is a highly effective method for producing, observing, comparing and cataloging network configurations.

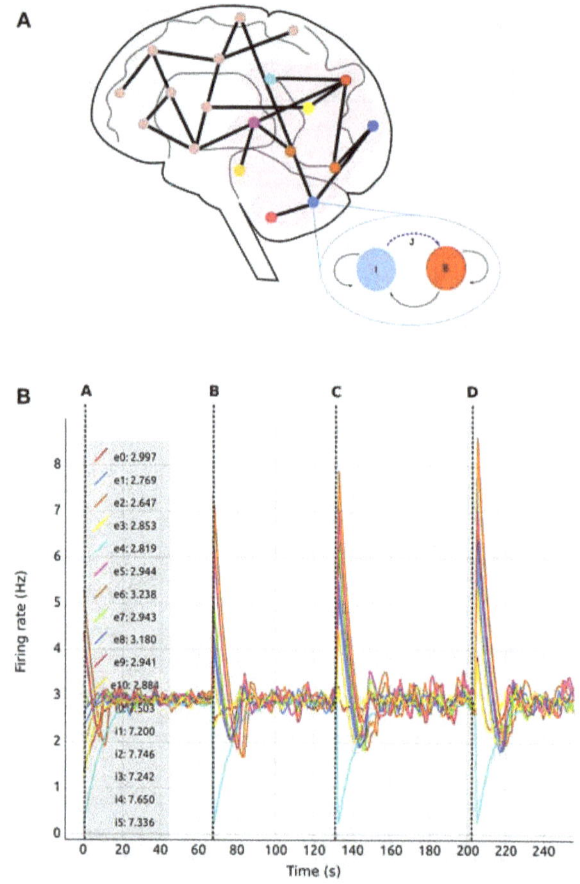

FIGURE 7 | Use case 1 inspired by Deco et al. (2014) whole brain model. (A) Abstract representation of the whole brain model including 68 regions. A subset of the regions is selected (pink area). The zoom-in view of one of the regions shows the abstract model of each region, consisting of two populations, one excitatory (red) and one inhibitory (blue). Inhibitory connections to excitatory neurons in the same region (blue dashed arrow labeled *J*) are subject to structural plasticity. **(B)** *Activity Plot* (see section 4.2.3) of selected regions (0–10) as a function of biological time. Regions are numbered from 0 to 67. Tags *eX* and *iX* identify curves for excitatory and inhibitory populations in the *Xth* region. A legend (upper left) indicates the current selection. The number following the colon after the tag is the region's firing rate during the last simulation step. Vertical dashed lines separate sections of the simulation with differing values of the global connectivity coupling (see section 5) , G = (A) 0.5; (B) 1.0; (C) 1.5; (D) 2.0. The vertical dashed lines are superimposed on this plot and are not part of the *Activity Plot* service. Increases to the global coupling parameter lead to an increase in the strength of the connections between regions. The firing rate spikes initially as a response to this change; in response, structural plasticity modifies connectivity according to the homeostatic rules until the firing rate stabilizes again closer to the target firing rate.

Whole Brain Simulation

This use case is inspired by a previous study by Deco et al. (2014). The experiment consists of a whole brain simulation using 68 interconnected brain regions, each of which represented by a spiking network containing 200 conductance-based leaky integrate-and-fire neurons, as illustrated in **Figure 7A**. The original work by Deco et al. (2014) uses a Dynamic Mean Field Model (DMFM) originally developed in Wong and Wang (2006).

The coupled non-linear stochastic equations of the DMFM describe the behavior of mean-field neuronal regions and their influence on each other:

$$\begin{aligned} \dot{\mathbf{s}} &= \mathbf{s}/\tau_s + (1-\mathbf{s})\gamma H(\mathbf{x}) + \sigma \boldsymbol{\nu}(t) \\ H(\mathbf{x}) &= (a\mathbf{x} - b)/\Big(1 - \exp\big(-d(a\mathbf{x} - b)\big)\Big) \\ \mathbf{x} &= wJ_N\mathbf{s} + GJ_N\mathbf{C}\mathbf{s} + I_0 \end{aligned} \tag{6}$$

where H represents the population firing rate function; $\mathbf{s}$ is the vector representing the average gating variable for each region; a, b, d, and σ are scaling parameters; γ and τ_s are kinetic parameters; $\boldsymbol{\nu}$ is the stochastic input vector; w is the local excitatory recurrence; J_N is the synaptic coupling; G is the general coupling factor; $\mathbf{C}$ is the connectivity matrix; I_0 is the effective external current; and $\mathbf{x}$ is the state variable vector for the regions. This model is applied in Deco et al. (2013) to describe a system dominated at the measured time frame by NMDA gating, while AMPA and GABA gating are neglected as "fast" variables. For a complete description and analysis of the model, see Wong and Wang (2006) and Deco et al. (2014).

Here, we apply a mapping from the DMFM to a network of point neurons. In our simulation, each region contains two populations, one excitatory (80% of the total neurons in the region) and one inhibitory (20%). In this case, neurons in NEST do not represent biological neurons but processing units whose mathematical description at population level is equivalent to the elements which comprise the DMFM. The initial parameters used to set up the network are taken from Deco et al. (2013) and detailed in **Table 2**. For a complete explanation of the model and its motivation, see Deco et al. (2013) and Wong and Wang (2006).

Recurrent excitatory connections have a strength of 1.4 pA, while recurrent inhibitory connections have a weight of -1.0 pA. Each neuron per region initially receives 160 excitatory connections from the local excitatory population. Only inhibitory connections are created during the simulation (blue dashed arrow tagged J in the region zoom in of **Figure 7A**) since we are only interested in substituting the feedback inhibition control algorithm described by Deco et al. (2014). The inter-regional connectivity (black lines between regions in **Figure 7A**) is specified from structural data obtained by DTI, which results in a connectivity matrix C, but further regulated by the general coupling parameter G, a multiplicative factor. This enables the linear modification of the strength of the connections without altering the ratio of connectivity among regions. Thus, the total weight of the connections between regions is equal to $G \cdot C$ pA. Each connection between regions is made between a single representative neuron in each excitatory population. Connections between regions are only excitatory. Additionally, all neurons receive independent background input from a Poisson generator producing spike trains with a rate of 11.9 kHz.

We followed the procedure described by Deco et al. (2014) through the generation of synaptic activity, substituting the feedback inhibition control used in that paper with our interactive exploration method. The strength of the background input was tuned to achieve a firing rate of 3 spikes/s for the excitatory population and 8 spikes/s for the inhibitory population when regions were isolated (without inter-region connections). In Deco et al. (2014), an iterative tuning strategy was used to determine the intra-region inhibition for the DMFMs required to produce an activity profile consistent with experimental observations. The key insight inspiring our approach is that finding the intra-region inhibition can be mapped on to determining the number of inhibitory connections required to produce the same activity pattern in a multi-area spiking neuronal network. Finding the right amount of inhibition per region which satisfies all the dependencies is still a hard multi-objective optimization problem, especially if the space cannot be interactively explored. This is demonstrated in **Figure 4**, which shows the result of simulating one static parameter setup for the connectivity generation programmatically.

TABLE 2 | Network parameters taken from Deco et al. (2013) for each region.

Parameter	Excitatory neurons	Inhibitory neurons
Number of neurons N_r	160	40
Capacitance of the membrane C_m	0.5 nF	0.2 nF
Membrane leak conductance g_m	25 ns	20 ns
Resting potential V_L	−70 mV	−70 mV
Threshold membrane potential V_{thr}	−50 mV	−50 mV
Reset membrane potential V_{res}	−55 mV	−55 mV
Refractory time τ_{ref}	2 ms	1 ms

In this setup, the tool was used with different values for the inter-region global coupling factor G. A complete view of the visualization and steering tool for this use case is shown in **Figure 3**. By using the tool, we detected that as G grows, it becomes more difficult to bring all regions to the desired activity state, and the standard deviation of the average firing rate increases as well. G has this impact because any change in one region due to G has a strong impact on all other regions dynamically reacting to the change in G. This effect is visible in **Figures 7**, **8**, where the time it takes for all regions to stabilize increases as the value of G grows.

We are also able to detect which regions are more crucial for stability, since they have a higher inter-connectivity to other regions. **Figure 9** shows a comparison of the evolution of the firing rate and outgoing connections of four regions. Each peak shows an increment in the global coupling value G by 0.5, starting from a base value of 0.5. Regions 25 and 63 show large oscillations due to their high connectivity with multiple other regions. Conversely, regions 0 and 10 rapidly reach a stable state even for high values of G. This capacity for detailed inspection allows the researcher to verify that all regions reach the desired average activity while the simulation is running, and thus drastically decreases turn-around times to research this behavior.

The search algorithms proposed in Deco et al. (2014) and Schirner et al. (2016) are based on an update pattern which (in the same terms as the algorithms used in this work) can be described by a fixed step update around the target activity, as shown in **Figure 10**. The effectiveness of a fixed search approach in the connectivity parameter space depends mainly on two factors. First, the effectiveness is dependent on the size of the correlation step. If the step is too small, it will take too long to reach the target activity if the initial conditions are not close to the solution. If the step is too large, the system will oscillate because the corrections are too coarse. Second, the effectiveness is dependent on the accuracy. The speed to find a solution is inversely proportional to the desired accuracy. The correction step should also be smaller than the accuracy, otherwise the system may oscillate indefinitely around the final target state without ever reaching a state with the desired accuracy. In summary, the ability of the search algorithm to find a solution depends on the initial conditions, the size of the update step and the desired accuracy. Our proposed approach allows the size of the update step and the speed with which changes take place to be adapted during simulation. This solves the problem of the dependency between step and accuracy and also allows the system to potentially find a solution from a broader range of initial conditions due to the capacity to increase the resolution of the search as the target state is approached.

In addition to the advantages in speed and use of computational resources which our expert-steered approach confers over brute force parameter search (and which may, in fact, be computationally intractable), the process of steering allows the researcher more insight into the system. Whereas

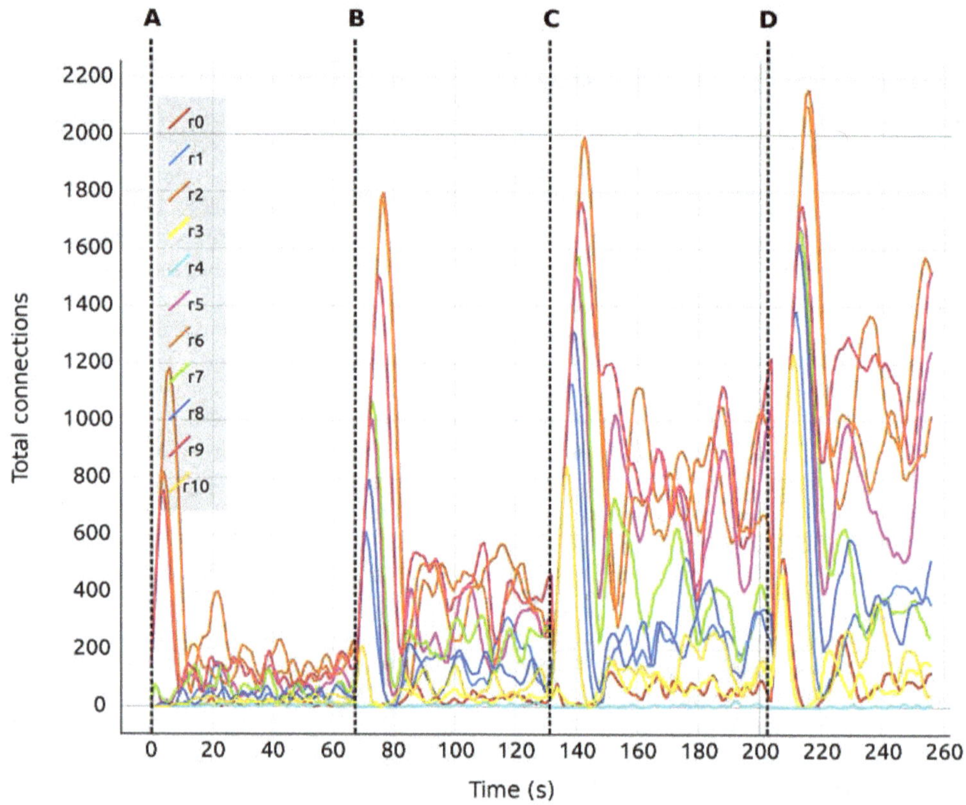

FIGURE 8 | Total number of connections for selected regions (0–10) as a function of biological time. Colors are synchronized between this plot and the *Color Editor*. Vertical dashed lines separate sections of the simulation with differing values of the global connectivity coupling (see section 5), G = (A) 0.5; (B) 1.0; (C) 1.5; (D) 2.0. Regions are coupled and numbered from 0 to 67. Tag *rX* identifies the curve for the total number of connections corresponding to the *Xth* region.

in the first use case, the primary finding was that multiple connectivity configurations can result in the same activity profile, in the second use case we are able to identify which regions are most critical for the overall network stability, as illustrated in **Figure 9**. Thus, interactive visualization can support the researcher in sensitivity analysis, which is essential for understanding the main driving parameters of the model and for making better inferences about the relations between parameters and function. As with the multiple configurations observed in the first use case, it is rare to encounter a network modeling study in computational neuroscience where a sensitivity analysis has been carried out (but see Bos et al., 2016 for a counter example).

Usage of the Tool

In this section, we summarize the main steps required to use the tool to take the system from its initial state to a final connectivity setup where the target mean activity values are achieved. A step-by-step tutorial video of carrying out parameter exploration on a network using our tool is provided in Supplementary Material (**Movies 1, 2**). In the following, we make reference to the requirements listed in section 4. The first step during the simulation steering is to determine which regions have one or more of the following characteristics (**R2–R5**):

- the electrical activity is far from the target activity, and there is no tendency of the system to correct for this error (or the correction is too slow);
- the electrical activity oscillates around the target activity and the oscillations are of equal or higher amplitude in each cycle;
- or the number of connections does not converge even though electrical activity is around the target activity.

This is achieved using the visualization tool by observing the firing rate and connectivity plots. **Figure 7** shows the evolution of the firing rate for the first ten regions of the brain model. **Figure 8** shows the changes in connectivity which are guided by the homeostatic growth rules defined for the structural plasticity algorithm. Each curve in the plot is uniquely identified by color and linked to a population or region, thus enabling the assessment of the three above listed characteristics. Reaching the targeted stable state is indicated when all firing rate curves converge to the target activities while the connection curves flatten to horizontal lines. This allows the user to simply and effectively identify which regions deviate from the target state and to correct the structural parameters according to the following criteria:

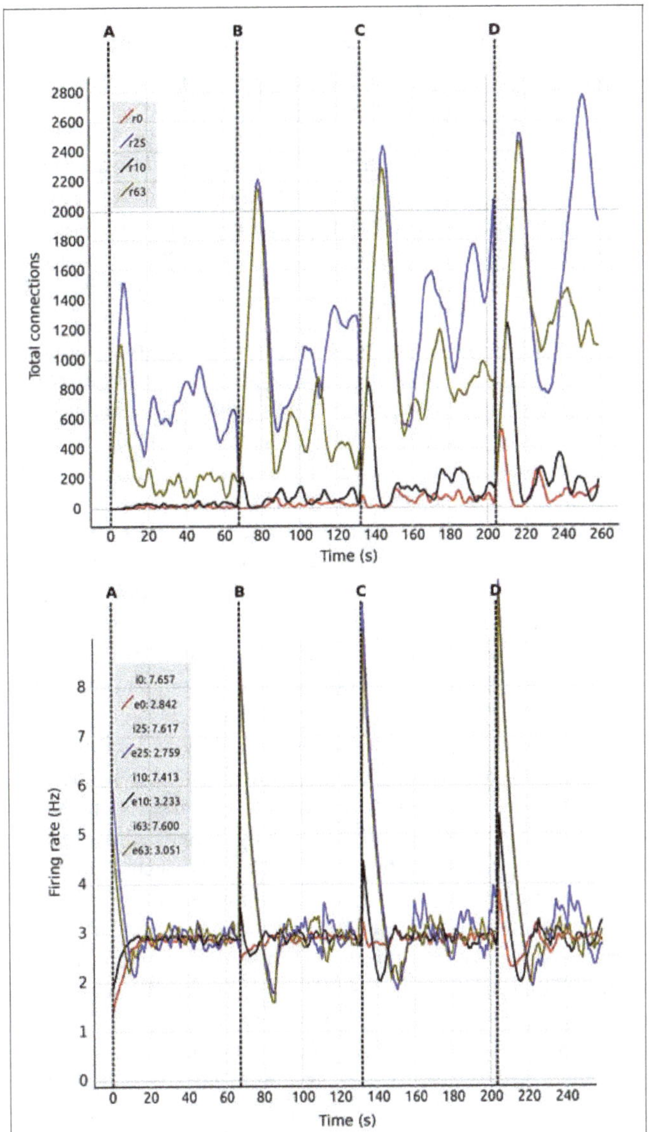

FIGURE 9 | Number of connections **(Top)** and firing rate **(Bottom)** shown in comparison of four regions (0, 10, 25, 63). Vertical dashed lines separate sections of the simulation with differing values of the global connectivity coupling, $G =$ (A) 0.5; (B) 1.0; (C) 1.5; (D) 2.0. Regions are numbered from 0 to 67. Tags *eX* and *iX* identify curves for excitatory and inhibitory populations in the *Xth* region. The number at the side of the tags denotes the current value of the average firing rate for each region.

- If the actual electrical activity is far away from the target activity, the growth rate ν for that region should be increased (**R6**).
- If the actual electrical activity oscillates around the target activity, the growth rate ν for that region should be decreased in small increments and the value of η should be reduced to decrease the rate of change in the number of created and deleted synaptic elements around the target point ε (**R6–R7**).
- If the number of connections does not converge, highly interconnected regions should be identified and the growth rate ν should be modified down in all of them (**R7**). In this case, the update interval can also be modified to a smaller value to have a faster response of the control changes in the connectivity (**R8**). A shorter update interval allows better and smoother control, but impacts the performance of the simulation.

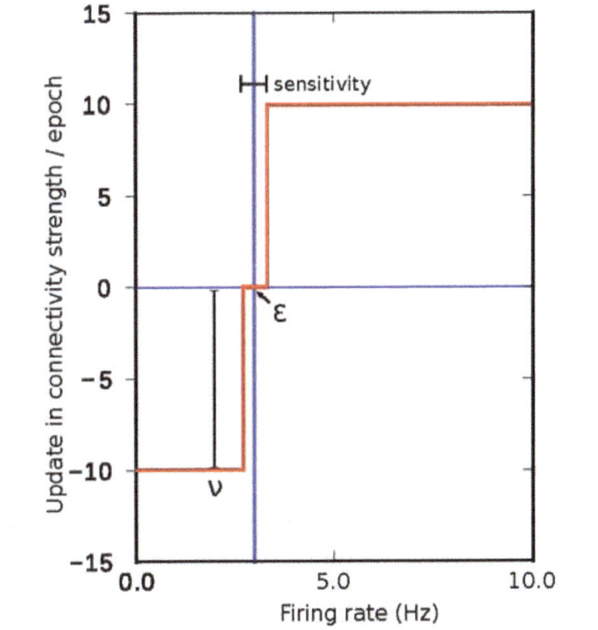

FIGURE 10 | Connectivity update rule employed in the algorithms proposed in Deco et al. (2014) and Schirner et al. (2016), where a fixed value is added or subtracted iteratively to the inner inhibitory connectivity until convergence to the desired firing rate is achieved in each simulated region.

The resulting network state can be saved and used later as a starting point for other parameter combinations, thereby minimizing the need for further computations using similar values of the global coupling term (**R9–R10**).

Implementing Further Use Cases

Using an event-driven architecture, our framework provides a convenient way for domain scientists to extend the tool to their needs. This tool can be used with any neuron and any synapse model in NEST, except for gap junctions. By using the scripts provided in the Supplementary Material (versions for all use cases discussed in this manuscript) as templates, the user can easily change the neuron and synapse model to explore the impact of these variations. An instrumentation manual which specifies the steps required to integrate the tool with other network models implemented in NEST can be found as part of the Supplementary Material. The instrumentation manual provides instructions based on examples for NEST, but the tool can be adapted to other simulators providing a Python interface by replacing the corresponding functionality. However, if the simulator does not provide an interface to Python, instrumentation will require

TABLE 3 | Estimation on the complexity to adapt the *nett* messaging framework to different steering and visualization use cases.

Challenge	Solution	Complexity
Change network topology	Change number of populations	Simple
Increase the size of the network	Increase the number of neurons in the simulation script	Simple
Retrieve additional parameter	Create new event definition	Medium
Add a new model parameter	Create new event definition	Medium
Connect different simulators with Python interface	Create new event definition for the specific simulation values	Medium-hard
No Python / C++ environment	None	Hard

substantial development effort by the user. **Table 3** provides estimates for the complexity of adapting the *nett* messaging library to different use cases. The complete tool and the underlying messaging framework is open source (for further details, see Supplementary Material).

Simulating on a Supercomputer

To leverage the power of supercomputers to reduce turn-around times for parameter space exploration, the simulation scripts can be adapted to use MPI. In this section, we show an example of adapting the whole brain simulation use case described in section 5.2 to supercomputers. To ensure that each process is in sync with all steering commands, one process (rank 0) serves as master. Only this master process establishes a connection to the visualization front-ends and processes their steering events. Then parameter synchronization is conducted via synchronization barriers with the remaining compute nodes. The master process is responsible for gathering the electrical activities and total connections from all other compute nodes to finally send these to the visualization front-ends.

After all the simulations had been parallelized, we adapted the tool to cope with the supercomputing environment. A challenge of the current usage conditions of most supercomputing environments is their batch-mode operation where users submit jobs which are granted compute time after a possibly long delay; interactive supercomputing is still a work in progress as outlined in Lippert and Orth (2014). Since our tool relies on a network connection to NEST, the IP-address of the compute-node running the simulator is unknown *a priori*. To circumvent this issue, we rely on the supercomputer's global file system: when the simulation is granted compute time, the node's IP-address is obtained and written to disk. Subsequently, all visualization services use this configuration file and connect to the given address. However, one limitation of this approach is the need to start the simulation first.

Since the visualization tools are independent of the network topology and size, the scaling impact of the network's performance can be measured while neglecting the communication overhead. To simulate a larger number of populations with a larger number of neurons, it is crucial to use supercomputers. To this end, we deployed the tool to the JURECA supercomputer at the Jülich Super Computing Centre. JURECA has 260 compute nodes with Intel Xeon E5 − 2680 v3 Haswell CPUs with 2×12 cores per CPU, 128 GB of RAM per node and runs CentOS 7. To assess the speed-up obtained using this machine, we used the third use case's setup and measured the execution times for 50 updates of connectivity in the network, with an update interval of 100 ms. Using a full node on JURECA, we were able to obtain a 2.94-fold speed-up compared to the workstation setup, which uses 8 Intel Core i7 − 4710MQ CPUs @ 2.50 GHz and 16 GB of RAM running on Ubuntu 16.10.

Figure 11 shows a strong scaling test for different numbers of neurons per population. Simulation scalability increases with the number of neurons per population—particularly for 8, 000 neurons per population (a total of 544, 000 neurons in the network). This is due to the network size and spike distribution overhead; larger networks benefit more from the larger number of compute-nodes and overcomes the inter-process communication and intra-process spike distribution overhead up to the point that the global number of spikes dominates performance (for a current discussion, see Jordan et al., 2018). In addition, the number of synapses increases quadratically with the number of neurons per population, which highly impacts the scalability of the simulation.

On the other hand, visualization scalability is dominated by the data gathering step at every update interval. For the case of large networks like the 8, 000 neuron network, the impact of the data gathering step can be reduced by gathering information from only a portion of the network. A well selected statistical sample would provide enough information about the ensemble behavior of the populations while benefiting performance. The current paradigm for the tool funnels data from a large number of compute backends to a single frontend visualizer. In order to scale with increasing numbers of backend nodes for massive supercomputing, a more complex data flow and analysis framework will be needed, such as a multi-node reduction stage to reduce the impedance between the backends and frontend, as well as reducing the load on the fronted. A generalized software framework for such infrastructure to couple visualization with supercomputing at scale is, to our knowledge, currently not available, and is a work in progress.

DISCUSSION AND CONCLUSION

In this paper, we have introduced a visualization and steering tool for the interactive analysis of connectivity generation in NEST. To show its applicability, we have presented two use cases where the tool was used to visualize and steer populations of point spiking neurons to reach a desired target activity level. Our results indicate that by interactively exploring the parameter space and possible trajectories, scientists can gain a better understanding of the system and concentrate on regions of biological interest, as compared to a blind brute force exploration. The improvements over brute force exploration are due to the effects of changes in specific parameters in the network which can be visualized and states outside the admissible regions which can be identified and

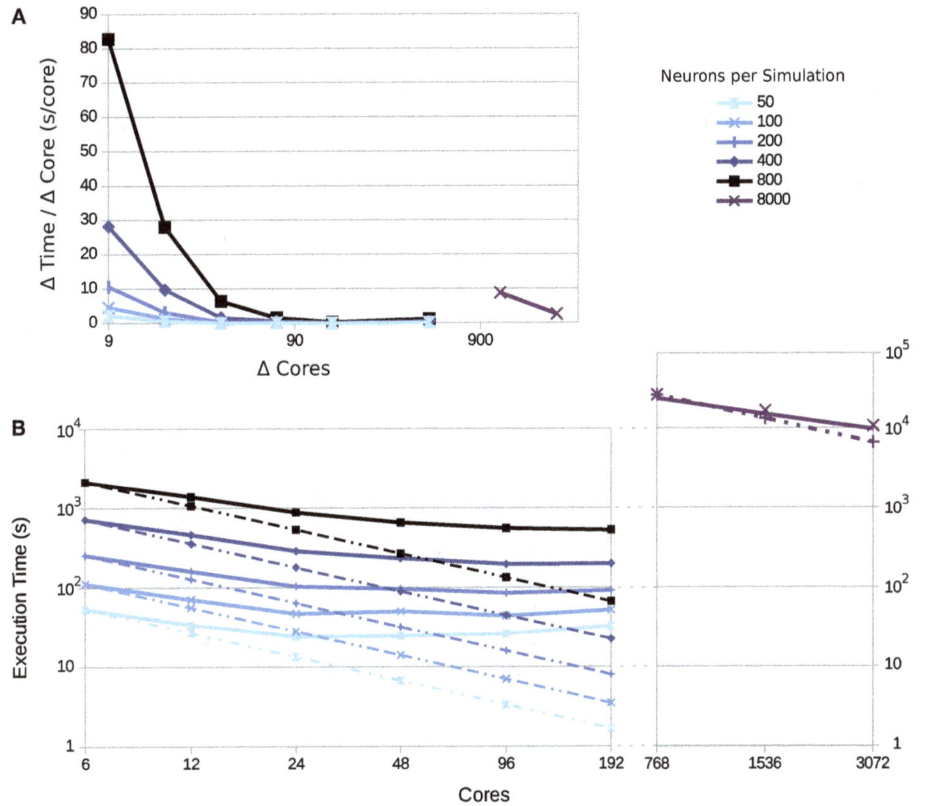

FIGURE 11 | Execution time as a function of the number of compute nodes for varying numbers of neurons per population: 50, 100, 200, 400, 800, and 8, 000; curves shaded from light to dark. Dotted lines indicate ideal scaling, while solid lines represent experimental results. **(A)** The change in time consumed per core added. Each point is the difference in the execution time divided by the difference in cores for consecutive points in **(B)**; points are placed at the midpoint between the source measurements. **(B)** The execution time for each simulation as the number of cores are varied; for the simulation with 8, 000 neurons per populations, measurements were made only for 768–3,072 cores, since fewer cores leads to excessive time demands. The simulated biological time was 5 s using an update interval of 100 ms.

excluded from further simulation. These improvements lead to a reduction in computational resources and an educated definition of interesting parameters, states and trajectories.

In this work, we have presented results using the interactive steering and visualization tool for two use cases where a desired firing rate was set by the modeler at the beginning of the simulation. We have used firing rate calculations produced internally in NEST to guide the generation of connectivity. This method for computing the mean firing rate can impact the performance of the control system since controllability depends on the delay between measuring an observable and producing a response. However, the tool is independent of this calculation and other techniques, such as spike train binning, can be used instead to increase the controllability. Calculation of firing rates on streams of spike trains might become computationally intensive with increasing network size. Future implementation of other techniques to increase the data gathering speed will lower delays and allow other spike processing techniques to be efficiently implemented as alternatives to the convolution approach.

The use cases presented were selected for their differing degrees of complexity in terms of connectivity and network definition. In the simple use case, different connectivity configurations lead to the same activity profiles even when some of the trajectories are biologically inadmissible. With our approach, the user can concentrate on exploring only those configurations which are of interest in answering the scientific question posed. In **Figure 6**, we show different trajectories produced using structural plasticity following homeostatic rules to fit the system to a firing rate profile. Even the non-biological parameters of the optimizing algorithm itself have an impact on the final configuration of the network. For example, if one performs a gradient descent to optimize the activity profile of a network, the results will be sensitive to any arbitrary choice of initial states of the populations and connectivity. With our tool we can characterize the distribution of representative models and results.

In the second use case, our tool also enables a sensitivity analysis of the system by visualizing the effect that changes in the connectivity have on the dynamics of the full system. Thus, the user can draw better conclusions about the relationships between the controllable parameters, in this case connectivity, and the observables of the system, in this case the firing rate of each population. We can see the relative sensitivity of the system to the biologically relevant parameters (connectivity) and the non biological parameters of the optimization algorithm. Our tool can provide more insight into how different types of synapses are created or modified in the neural circuit to give rise to different features in the dynamics of the system.

As we have discussed in this paper, a brute force exploration of the parameters of a network can easily become a computationally intractable problem. Choosing a single random configuration or even only a small sample of configurations from the whole space without a proper characterization of their distribution is unlikely to lead to a statistically valid distribution of the results. Interactive visualization is a way to move toward statistically validated conclusions as it allows an assessment of the essential features of the system, ultimately leading to automated sampling.

While the resulting connectivity patterns are not necessarily unique, our approach enables exploration and assessment of these solutions and their paths. The main contribution of this approach is the use of interactive visualization and parameter control techniques. These techniques allow the system to be controlled and stabilized within a physiological configuration space by an expert. When increasing the number of neurons and populations, the number of parameters to tune increases, resulting in an ever harder-to-reach stable state. Thus, interactive visualization becomes even more important. The knowledge gained through interactive exploration can lead to the development of automated tools assisting in the parameter space exploration.

Using this approach, we can reduce the turn-around times of exploring different connectivity configurations in comparison to simulating all possible parameter configurations and assess reasonable configurations in a later phase. The speed-up achieved by this exploration is mainly due to four factors. First, it is not necessary to simulate the system for long times iteratively; instead, the modifications are performed on demand. Second, partial solutions can be reused for different global parameter combinations, resulting in the reduction of total computational costs. Third, the user can visualize the behavior of the system's observables with respect to individual parameters, allowing the user to isolate regions of interest and form a better understanding. Finally, we can study the transition points in the activity of the networks, which are produced by the underlying connectivity variations, and interact with the tuning algorithms by visualizing their impact.

As stated before, the connectivity solutions and paths to solutions for the presented use cases are not unique, rendering a knowledgeable exploration process crucial. Thus, the interactive analysis process can help the user accomplish the following:

1. Form an understanding of the implication of different parameter setups for each network model.
2. Validate the models.
3. Define biologically meaningful populations of interest for the simulation.
4. Derive measures for the automatic or semi-automatic assessment of the models' behavior leading to automated tools guiding the exploration process.

While the generation of connectivity based on empirical constraints for the dynamic system or experimental data inherently leads to non-unique solutions and especially solutions which are physiologically implausible, the ability to identify and explore subsets of the solution space is valuable to form an understanding of the dynamic nature of these systems.

In this work, we have formalized the effects of dynamic connectivity of a network in terms of control theory. We take into account that the network starts at an initial state and is taken to a final state through the introduction of control signals which alter the connectivity of the network. In this case, control of the synapse creation and deletion is induced by the structural plasticity algorithm. The eigenvalues of the Liouvillian of the network are thus modified with these signals through the evolution of the simulation and the state of the neurons in the network is changed. Visualization shows the immediate effects of the control signals in the system. The results shown in section 5.1 exemplify how even a simple network can traverse different admissible trajectories (**Figures 6A–E**) using different elements from the set of all possible controls. We show how the unconstrained system can traverse an inadmissible trajectory (**Figure 6F**) or end in states outside of the admissible set (**Figure 6D**). We have also seen how inadmissible control signals are still able to give rise to admissible trajectories and final states (**Figure 6E**).

We adapted the tool to scale with supercomputers allowing larger networks to be simulated and finer simulation stepping to be used, thus achieving more accurate results. This way, researchers can explore the manifold solutions and paths of connectivity satisfying average activity targets in a variety of neural network models. Our tool gathers data from the simulation at specific intervals, which impacts the performance as the networks become larger. Continuously streaming data from of the simulation by using, for example, MUSIC (Djurfeldt et al., 2010) or the NEST I/O backends can reduce this bottleneck and allow greater flexibility in the network size.

In summary, our interactive tool provides the means to visualize and steer connectivity generation of a running NEST simulation to stabilize complex non-linear systems. The applied concepts of the tool are generalizable and extensible to other types of systems with similarly large degrees of freedom. Adapting and exploring further model parameters, e.g., synaptic weights and delays, background input frequency, and variation in weights of spike-timing-dependent plasticity synapses is possible. Our implementation is open to the public (see Supplementary Material).

In the future, we would like to explore further techniques to track already explored parameter spaces, to develop semi-automatic systems to guide researchers in tracking manifold solution spaces and to extend the tool to support further use cases. Currently, the saved state refers only to the connectivity and last values of all variables at the time of saving. We are working to provide a visualization that shows parameter changes for reproducing all trajectories. For the moment, the loading features are limited and the subject of future work. In addition, we are adding support for machine learning algorithms coupled with the interactive exploration for various network variables beyond connectivity. Our goal is to to detect oscillations and other troubling behavior in the network using machine learning and then to correct this behavior by use of the controllers. Other target control measures such as power-spectrum shape and inter-population correlations may be interesting as complex control variables in the context of machine learning. The modularity of the software, primarily derived from applying an event driven design, allows for such additions in a non-intrusive manner.

Linking the time axes of the activity and connection plots to allow for coordinated zooming is currently not supported but would be a useful extension to the analysis workflow. A visualization of changes in the network's eigenvalues as connectivity evolves is also subject to future work. The creation of additional plots for further variables is simple and can be achieved by adapting the scripts used in the presented use cases (see Supplementary Material). Connecting another visualization application to the NEST simulator is in principle feasible but requires adapting the visualizer to our communication protocol.

We argue that it is crucial to explore the distribution of paths to solutions instead of focusing on just *a* possible solution satisfying a set of constraints. To develop this understanding, interactive exploration of dynamic systems is a key tool for developing mathematical intuition, and thus for deriving mathematically robust descriptions. These descriptions are then amenable to further automated investigation of characteristic solution ensembles.

AUTHOR CONTRIBUTIONS

CN and SD-P have contributed equally to this paper. CN developed the interactive steering tool and the framework. In addition, he designed the data flow for steering the main structural plasticity parameters. SD-P, AP, and AM defined the use cases. SD-P evaluated the results and compared the process of parameter navigation with and without the steering tool. AP provided the high performance computing knowledge to port and optimize the code for supercomputing usage. BW, BH, and TK provided scientific guidance on the visualization tool. AM provided neuroscientific guidance and assessed the usability of the tool for generalized use cases. CN, SD-P, AM, and AP wrote the paper.

FUNDING

The authors would like to acknowledge the support by the Excellence Initiative of the German federal and state governments, the Jülich Aachen Research Alliance—High-Performance Computing, the Helmholtz Association through the portfolio theme Supercomputing and Modeling for the Human Brain (SMHB) and the Initiative and Networking Fund. In addition, this project has received funding from the European Union's Horizon 2020 Research and Innovation Programme under grant agreement No 720270 (HBP SGA1) and No 785907 (HBP SGA2). Finally, this project has received funding from the German Federal Ministry of Education and Research ("D-USA Verbund: Mechanistische Zusammenhänge zwischen Struktur und funktioneller Dynamik im menschlichen Gehirn," project no. 01GQ1504B). Responsibility for the content of this publication belongs to the authors.

SUPPLEMENTARY MATERIAL

Movie 1 | Introduction to the interactive steering and visualization tool.

Movie 2 | Using the interactive steering and visualization tool in a specific use case for structural plasticity in NEST.

Presentation 1 | Instrumentation manual.

We have included two videos as Supplemental Material that demonstrate our visualization tool. The first video presents its basic structuring and functionality. The second one discusses one use case for structural plasticity and explains how the tool can help in the assessment of the simulation. Moreover, we have included an instrumentation manual describing the general process for modifying simulation scripts in order to use the tool.

The *nett* messaging framework can be downloaded at https://devhub.vr.rwth-aachen.de/VR-Group/nett.git, and https://devhub.vr.rwth-aachen.de/VR-Group/nett-python.git. The NEST structural plasticity framework can be found at https://github.com/sdiazpier/nest-simulator.git, branch `sp_rate` and tag `sp_viz_rate`.

The visualization tool, simulation scripts for both use cases, and a user manual to build the code can be found at https://github.com/sdiazpier/isv_neuroscience. In addition to the use cases discussed in this work, a script showing the instrumentation of the cortical microcircuit model (Potjans and Diesmann, 2014) is also provided in the aforementioned git repository.

REFERENCES

Abram, G., and Treinish, L. (1995). "An extended data-flow architecture for data analysis and visualization," in *Proceedings of the 6th Conference on Visualization'95* (Washington, DC: IEEE Computer Society), 263.

Bahuguna, J., Tetzlaff, T., Kumar, A., Hellgren Kotaleski, J., and Morrison, A. (2017). Homologous basal ganglia network models in physiological and parkinsonian conditions. *Front. Comput. Neurosci.* 11:79. doi: 10.3389/fncom.2017.00079

Bakker, R., Wachtler, T., and Diesmann, M. (2012). Cocomac 2.0 and the future of tract-tracing databases. *Front. Neuroinform.* 6:30. doi: 10.3389/fninf.2012.00030

Bos, H., Diesmann, M., and Helias, M. (2016). Identifying anatomical origins of coexisting oscillations in the cortical microcircuit. *PLoS Comput. Biol.* 12:e1005132. doi: 10.1371/journal.pcbi.1005132

Bos, H., Morrison, A., Peyser, A., Hahne, J., Helias, M., Kunkel, S., et al. (2015). NEST 2.10.0.

Boukhelifa, N., and Rodgers, P. J. (2003). A model and software system for coordinated and multiple views in exploratory visualization. *Inform. Visuali.* 2, 258–269. doi: 10.1057/palgrave.ivs.9500057

Butz, M., and van Ooyen, A. (2013). A simple rule for dendritic spine and axonal bouton formation can account for cortical reorganization after focal retinal lesions. *PLoS Comput. Biol.* 9:e1003259. doi: 10.1371/journal.pcbi.1003259

Childs, H., Brugger, E. S., Bonnell, K. S., Meredith, J. S., Miller, M., Whitlock, B. J., et al. (2005). "A contract-based system for large data visualization," in *Proceedings of IEEE Visualization 2005* (Minneapolis, MN), 190–198.

Cowan, J. D. (1991). "Stochastic neurodynamics," in *Advances in Neural Information Processing Systems* (Denver, CO), 62–69.

Cubitt, T. S., Eisert, J., and Wolf, M. M. (2012). Extracting dynamical equations from experimental data is NP hard. *Phys. Rev. Lett.* 108:120503. doi: 10.1103/PhysRevLett.108.120503

Deco, G., Ponce-Alvarez, A., Hagmann, P., Romani, G. L., Mantini, D., and Corbetta, M. (2014). How local excitation–inhibition ratio impacts the whole brain dynamics. *J. Neurosci.* 34, 7886–7898. doi: 10.1523/JNEUROSCI.5068-13.2014

Deco, G., Ponce-Alvarez, A., Mantini, D., Romani, G. L., Hagmann, P., and Corbetta, M. (2013). Resting-state functional connectivity emerges from structurally and dynamically shaped slow linear fluctuations. *J. Neurosci.* 33, 11239–11252. doi: 10.1523/JNEUROSCI.1091-13.2013

Diaz-Pier, S., Naveau, M., Butz-Ostendorf, M., and Morrison, A. (2016). Automatic generation of connectivity for large-scale neuronal network models through structural plasticity. *Front. Neuroanat.* 10:57. doi: 10.3389/fnana.2016.00057

Djurfeldt, M., Hjorth, J., Eppler, J. M., Dudani, N., Helias, M., Potjans, T. C., et al. (2010). Run-time interoperability between neuronal network simulators based on the music framework. *Neuroinformatics* 8, 43–60. doi: 10.1007/s12021-010-9064-z

Eppler, J. M., Helias, M., Muller, E., Diesmann, M., and Gewaltig, M.-O. (2009). PyNEST: a convenient interface to the NEST simulator. *Front. Neuroinform.* 2:12. doi: 10.3389/neuro.11.012.2008

Fabian, N., Moreland, K., Thompson, D., Bauer, A. C., Marion, P., Geveci, B., et al. (2011). "The paraview coprocessing library: a scalable, general purpose *in situ* visualization library," in *LDAV*, eds D. Rogers and C. T. Silva (Providence, Rl: IEEE), 89–96.

Henderson, A. (2004). *The ParaView Guide: A Parallel Visualization Application.* Clifton Park, NY: Kitware.

Hensch, T. K. (2005). Critical period plasticity in local cortical circuits. *Nat. Rev. Neurosci.* 6, 877–888. doi: 10.1038/nrn1787

Jordan, J., Ippen, T., Helias, M., Kitayama, I., Sato, M., Igarashi, J., et al. (2018). Extremely scalable spiking neuronal network simulation code: from laptops to exascale computers. *Front. Neuroinform.* 12:2. doi: 10.3389/fninf.2018.00002

Kammara, A. C., Palanichamy, L., and König, A. (2016). Multi-objective optimization and visualization for analog design automation. *Complex Intell. Syst.* 2, 251–267. doi: 10.1007/s40747-016-0027-3

Kirk, D. (2012). *Optimal Control Theory: An Introduction.* Dover Books on Electrical Engineering. Mineola, NY: Dover Publications.

Lippert, T., and Orth, B. (2014). *Supercomputing Infrastructure for Simulations of the Human Brain.* Cham: Springer International Publishing.

López-Cuevas, A., Castillo-Toledo, B., Medina-Ceja, L., and Ventura-Mejía, C. (2015). State and parameter estimation of a neural mass model from electrophysiological signals during the status epilepticus. *NeuroImage* 113, 374–386. doi: 10.1016/j.neuroimage.2015.02.059

Matković, K., Gračanin, D., Jelović, M., and Hauser, H. (2008). Interactive visual steering-rapid visual prototyping of a common rail injection system. *IEEE Trans. Visual. Comput. Graph.* 14, 1699–1706. doi: 10.1109/TVCG.2008.145

Matković, K., Gračanin, D., Splechtna, R., Jelović, M., Stehno, B., Hauser, H., et al. (2014). Visual analytics for complex engineering systems: hybrid visual steering of simulation ensembles. *IEEE Trans. Visual. Comput. Graph.* 20, 1803–1812. doi: 10.1109/TVCG.2014.2346744

Michelson, B. M. (2006). Event-driven architecture overview. *Patricia Seybold Group* 2:12. doi: 10.1571/bda2-2-06cc

Migliore, M., Cavarretta, F., Hines, M. L., and Shepherd, G. M. (2014). Distributed organization of a brain microcircuit analyzed by three-dimensional modeling: the olfactory bulb. *Front. Comput. Neurosci.* 8:50. doi: 10.3389/fncom.2014.00050

North, C., and Shneiderman, B. (1997). *A Taxonomy of Multiple Window Coordination Technical Research Report.* College Park, MD: Institute for Systems Research. Available online at: http://hdl.handle.net/1903/5892

North, C., and Shneiderman, B. (2000). "Snap-together visualization: a user interface for coordinating visualizations via relational schemata," in *Proceedings of the Working Conference on Advanced Visual Interfaces, AVI '00* (New York, NY: ACM), 128–135.

Nowke, C., Zielasko, D., Weyers, B., Hentschel, B., Peyser, A., and Kuhlen, T. (2015). Integrating visualizations into modeling NEST simulations. *Front. Neuroinform.* 9:29. doi: 10.3389/fninf.2015.00029

Ohira, T., and Cowan, J. D. (1993). Master-equation approach to stochastic neurodynamics. *Phys. Rev. E* 48:2259. doi: 10.1103/PhysRevE.48.2259

Park, I. M., Seth, S., Paiva, A. R. C., Li, L., and Principe, J. C. (2013). Kernel methods on spike train space for neuroscience: a tutorial. *IEEE Signal Process. Mag.* 30, 149–160. doi: 10.1109/MSP.2013.2251072

Potjans, T. C., and Diesmann, M. (2014). The cell-type specific cortical microcircuit: relating structure and activity in a full-scale spiking network model. *Cereb. Cortex* 24, 785–806. doi: 10.1093/cercor/bhs358

Roberts, J. C. (2007). "State of the art: coordinated & multiple views in exploratory visualization," in *Fifth International Conference on Coordinated and Multiple Views in Exploratory Visualization (CMV 2007)* (Zurich), 61–71.

Roy, D., Sigala, R., Breakspear, M., McIntosh, A. R., Jirsa, V. K., Deco, G., et al. (2014). Using the virtual brain to reveal the role of oscillations and plasticity in shaping brain's dynamical landscape. *Brain Connect.* 4, 791–811. doi: 10.1089/brain.2014.0252

Ryu, Y. S., Yost, B., Convertino, G., Chen, J., and North, C. (2003). Exploring cognitive strategies for integrating multiple-view visualizations. *Proc. Hum. Fact. Ergonom. Soc. Annu. Meeting* 47, 591–595. doi: 10.1177/154193120304700371

Schirner, M., McIntosh, A. R., Jirsa, V., Deco, G., and Ritter, P. (2016). Bridging multiple scales in the human brain using computational modelling. bioRxiv. doi: 10.1101/085548

Schuecker, J., Schmidt, M., van Albada, S. J., Diesmann, M., and Helias, M. (2015). Fundamental activity constraints lead to specific interpretations of the connectome. arXiv:1509.03162.

Sedlmair, M., Heinzl, C., Bruckner, S., Piringer, H., and Möller, T. (2014). Visual parameter space analysis: a conceptual framework. *IEEE Trans. Visual. Comput. Graph.* 20, 2161–2170. doi: 10.1109/TVCG.2014.2346321

Shneiderman, B. (1996). "The eyes have it: a task by data type taxonomy for information visualizations," in *Proceedings 1996 IEEE Symposium on Visual Languages* (San Francisco, CA), 336–343. doi: 10.1109/VL.1996.545307

Sporns, O., Tononi, G., and Kötter, R. (2005). The human connectome: a structural description of the human brain. *PLoS Comput. Biol.* 1:e42. doi: 10.1371/journal.pcbi.0010042

Wang Baldonado, M. Q., Woodruff, A., and Kuchinsky, A. (2000). "Guidelines for using multiple views in information visualization," in *Proceedings of the Working Conference on Advanced Visual Interfaces - AVI '00* (New York, NY), 110–119.

Weaver, C. (2004). "Building highly-coordinated visualizations in Improvise," in *IEEE Symposium on Information Visualization, 2004* (Austin, TX: IEEE Computer Society), 159–166.

Whitlock, B., Favre, J. M., and Meredith, J. S. (2011). "Parallel *in situ* coupling of simulation with a fully featured visualization system," in *EGPGV* (Bangor), 101–109.

Wong, K.-F., and Wang, X.-J. (2006). A recurrent network mechanism of time integration in perceptual decisions. *J. Neurosci.* 26, 1314–1328. doi: 10.1523/JNEUROSCI.3733-05.2006

Zaytsev, Y. V., and Morrison, A. (2014). CyNEST: a maintainable Cython-based interface for the NEST simulator. *Front. Neuroinform.* 8:23. doi: 10.3389/fninf.2014.00023

Zaytsev, Y. V., Morrison, A., and Deger, M. (2015). Reconstruction of recurrent synaptic connectivity of thousands of neurons from simulated spiking activity. *J. Comput. Neurosci.* 39, 77–103. doi: 10.1007/s10827-015-0565-5

8

Rigorous Neural Network Simulations: A Model Substantiation Methodology for Increasing the Correctness of Simulation Results in the Absence of Experimental Validation Data

Guido Trensch [1], Robin Gutzen [2], Inga Blundell [2], Michael Denker [2] and Abigail Morrison [1,2,3]*

[1] Simulation Lab Neuroscience, Jülich Supercomputing Centre, Institute for Advanced Simulation, JARA, Jülich Research Centre, Jülich, Germany, [2] Institute of Neuroscience and Medicine (INM-6) and Institute for Advanced Simulation (IAS-6) and JARA Institute Brain Structure-Function Relationships (INM-10), Jülich Research Centre, Jülich, Germany, [3] Faculty of Psychology, Institute of Cognitive Neuroscience, Ruhr-University Bochum, Bochum, Germany

***Correspondence:**
Guido Trensch
g.trensch@fz-juelich.de

The reproduction and replication of scientific results is an indispensable aspect of good scientific practice, enabling previous studies to be built upon and increasing our level of confidence in them. However, reproducibility and replicability are not sufficient: an incorrect result will be accurately reproduced if the same incorrect methods are used. For the field of simulations of complex neural networks, the causes of incorrect results vary from insufficient model implementations and data analysis methods, deficiencies in workmanship (e.g., simulation planning, setup, and execution) to errors induced by hardware constraints (e.g., limitations in numerical precision). In order to build credibility, methods such as verification and validation have been developed, but they are not yet well-established in the field of neural network modeling and simulation, partly due to ambiguity concerning the terminology. In this manuscript, we propose a terminology for model verification and validation in the field of neural network modeling and simulation. We outline a rigorous workflow derived from model verification and validation methodologies for increasing model credibility when it is not possible to validate against experimental data. We compare a published minimal spiking network model capable of exhibiting the development of polychronous groups, to its reproduction on the SpiNNaker neuromorphic system, where we consider the dynamics of several selected network states. As a result, by following a formalized process, we show that numerical accuracy is critically important, and even small deviations in the dynamics of individual neurons are expressed in the dynamics at network level.

Keywords: reproducibility, verification and validation, model validation, SpiNNaker, fixed-point numeric, spiking network models

1. INTRODUCTION

Even for domain experts, it is often difficult to judge the correctness of the results derived from a neural network simulation. The factors that determine the correctness of the simulation outcome are manifold and often beyond the control of the modeler. It is therefore of great importance to develop formalized processes and methods, i.e., a systematic approach, to build credibility. This applies not only to the modeling, implementation, and simulation tasks performed in a particular study, but also to their reproduction in a different setting. Although appropriate methods exist, such as verification and validation methodologies, they are not yet well-established in the field of neural network modeling and simulation. One reason may lie in the rapid rate of development of new neuron and synapse models, impeding the development of common verification and validation methods, another is likely to be that the field has yet to absorb knowledge of these methodologies from fields in which they are common practice. This latter point is exacerbated by partly contradicting terminology around these areas.

In this study, we propose a reasonable adaptation of the existing terminology for model verification and validation and apply it to the field of neural network modeling and simulation. We introduce the concept of *model verification and substantiation* and apply it to the issue of reproducibility on a worked example. Specifically, we quantitatively compare a minimal spiking network model capable of exhibiting the development of polychronous groups, as described in Izhikevich (2006), to its reproduction on the SpiNNaker (a contraction of Spiking Neural Network Architecture) neuromorphic system (Furber et al., 2013). The Izhikevich (2006) study is highly cited as an account of how spike patterns emerge from network dynamics, and contains a number of non-standard features in its conceptual and implementational choices that make it a particularly illustrative example for the verification process. The choice of a network reproduction implemented on SpiNNaker as a target for comparison is motivated by the fact that SpiNNaker is subject to rather different constraints from typical simulation platforms, in particular the restriction to fixed-point arithmetic, and so demonstrates interestingly different verification problems. With this process we demonstrate the value of software engineering methodologies, such as refactoring, for verification tasks.

Moreover, this study contributes to a question that is intensively debated in the neuromorphic community: how do hardware constraints on numerical precision affect individual neuron dynamics and, thus, the results obtained from a neural network simulation? We compare the neuronal and network dynamics between the original and the SpiNNaker implementation, and our results show that numerical accuracy is critically important; even small deviations in the dynamics of individual neurons are expressed in the dynamics at network level.

This study arose within a collaboration using the same initial study to examine different aspects of rigor and reproducibility in spiking neural network simulations, which we describe briefly here to motivate the scope of the current study. Firstly, a frequent source of errors in a neural network simulation is unsuitable choices of numerics for solving the system of ordinary differential equations underlying the selected neuron model. In section 3.4.2 we focus on the issues of time step and data type; the question of which solver to use is addressed in Blundell et al. (2018b), who present a stand-alone toolbox to analyze the system of equations and automatically select an appropriate solver for it. Secondly, a key aspect of our study is the reproduction of the network described in Izhikevich (2006) on SpiNNaker, as described in sections 3.1.2 and 3.4.1. The difficulties of creating such a reproduction are comprehensively examined by Pauli et al. (2018). Their investigation of the features of source code that support or diminish the reproducibility of a network model is based on reproducing the Izhikevich (2006) study in the NEST simulator (Gewaltig and Diesmann, 2007). In addition to developing a checklist for authors and reviewers of network models, they demonstrate that the reported results are extremely sensitive to implementation details. Finally, in order to determine whether two simulations are producing results of acceptable similarity, we employ a statistical analysis of spiking activity. This is summarized in section 3.2.2; the complete description and derivation of this analysis can be found in our companion paper (Gutzen et al., 2018).

2. TERMINOLOGY

2.1. Reproducibility and Replicability

Reproducibility and replicability are indispensable aspects of good scientific practice. Unfortunately, the terms are defined in incompatible ways across and even within fields.

In psychology, for example, *reproducibility* may mean completely re-doing an experiment, whereas *replicability* refers to independent studies that yield similar results (Patil et al., 2016). For computational experiments, where the outcome is usually deterministic[1], *reproducibility* is understood as obtaining the same results by a different experimental setup conducted by a different team (Association for Computing Machinery, 2016; see also Plesser, 2018). Although attempts were made to help resolve the ambiguity in the terminology by explicitly labeling the terms or by attempting to inventory the terminology across disciplines (Barba, 2018), the problem persists. Plesser (2018) gives a brief history of this confusion.

In this study, we follow the definitions suggested by the *Association for Computing Machinery* (Association for Computing Machinery, 2016):

> **Replicability** *(Different team, same experimental setup) The measurement can be obtained with stated precision by a different team using the same measurement procedure, the same measuring system, under the same operating conditions, in the same or a different location on multiple trials. For computational experiments, this means that an independent group can obtain the same result using the authors own artifacts.*

[1]In analog neuromorphic systems the outcome is not only determined by the initial conditions. Chip fabrication tolerances and thermal noise add a stochastic component.

Reproducibility *(Different team, different experimental setup) The measurement can be obtained with stated precision by a different team, a different measuring system, in a different location on multiple trials. For computational experiments, this means that an independent group can obtain the same result using artifacts which they develop completely independently.*

To be more specific about the terminology of reproducibility, in this study we aim for *results reproducibility* (Goodman et al., 2016; see also Plesser, 2018).

Results reproducibility *Obtaining the same results from the conduct of an independent study whose procedures are as closely matched to the original experiment as possible.*

2.2. Model Verification and Validation

The critical question for all modeling tasks is whether the model provides a sufficiently accurate representation of the system being studied. Evaluating the results of a modeling effort is a non-trivial exercise which requires a rigorous validation process.

The term *validation*, or more generally *verification and validation* also require a precise definition, as they have different meanings in different contexts. In software engineering, for example, verification and validation is the objective assessment of products and processes throughout the life cycle. Its purpose is to help the development organization build quality into the system (Bourque and Fairley, 2014). With respect to the development of computerized models, verification and validation are processes that accumulate evidence of a model's correctness or accuracy for a specific scenario (Thacker et al., 2004).

As a cornerstone for establishing credibility of computer simulations, the Society for Computer Simulation (SCS) formulated a standard set of terminology intended to facilitate effective communication between model builders and model users (Schlesinger et al., 1979). This early definition is very general and often does not do justice to a particular modeling domain. Therefore, domain specific adaptations to the terminology can be found, but having fundamentally the same meanings. For the field of neural network modeling and simulation we propose the terminology shown in **Figure 1B**, amended from Thacker et al. (2004). While Thacker et al. (2004) uses the terms *reality of interest*, *conceptual model*, and *computerized model*, we prefer the terms *system of interest*, *mathematical model*, and *executable model*. The terms are more explicit and better express the underlying intent. In particular, due to the empirical challenges of neurobiology, spiking neural network models are often not based on a specific biological network that could be considered "reality" and from which ground truth behavior can be recorded, in contrast to, for example, the air flow around a wing. The term "system of interest" recognizes that the process of verification and validation can also be applied to systems without concrete physical counterparts.

The essence of the introduced terminology is the division of the modeling process into three major elements as illustrated in **Figures 1A,B**.

Reality or **system of interest** is an *"entity, situation, or system which has been selected for analysis."* The conceptual or **mathematical model** is defined as a *"verbal description, equations, governing relationships, or natural laws that purport to describe reality or the system of interest"* and can be understood as the precise description of the modeler's intention (Schlesinger et al., 1979). The formulation of the conceptual or mathematical model is derived in a process called **analysis and modeling** and its applicability is motivated in a process termed qualification or **confirmation**. However, the conceptual or mathematical model by itself is not able to simulate the system of interest. By means of applying software engineering and development efforts, it has to be implemented as a computerized or **executable model**.

By separating the understanding of a model into a mathematical and an executable model, this terminology also illustrates the difference between verification and validation.

Verification describes the process of ensuring that the mathematical model is appropriately represented by the executable model, and improving this fit.

Model verification is the assessment of a model implementation. Neural network models are mathematical models that are written down in source code as numerical algorithms. Therefore, it is useful to define two indispensable assessment activities:

Source code verification tasks confirm that the functionality it implements works as intended.
Calculation verification tasks assess the level of error that arises from various sources of error in numerical simulations as well as to identify and remove them (Thacker et al., 2004).

This process mainly involves the quantification and minimization of errors introduced by the performed calculations. Only when the executable model is verified it can be reasonably validated.

The **validation** process evaluates the consistency of the predictive simulation outcome with the system of interest.

The validation process aims at the agreement between experimental data that defines the *ground truth* for the system of interest and the simulation outcomes. This evaluation needs to take into consideration the domain of intended application of the mathematical model as well as its expected level of agreement, since any model is an abstraction of the system of interest and only intended to match to a certain degree and for certain prescribed conditions.

2.3. Model Verification and Substantiation: Model Assessment in the Absence of Experimental Data

For neural network simulations, the ground truth of the system of interest can be provided by empirical measurements of activity data, for example single unit and multi-unit activity gathered by means of electrophysiological recordings. However, there are a number of reasons why this data may prove inadequate for validation. Firstly, depending on the

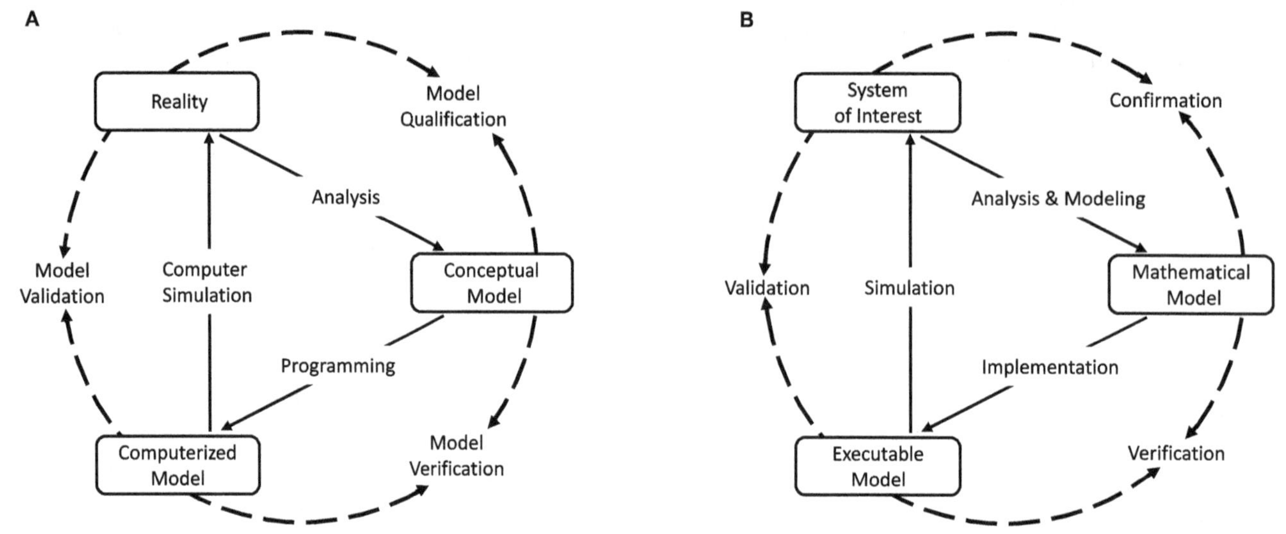

FIGURE 1 | Interrelationship of the basic elements for modeling and simulation. In order to be able to apply the terminology, introduced by Schlesinger et al. (1979) for modeling and simulation processes **(A)**, to numerical models for neural network simulations, a less generic terminology is more expedient. We propose the terminology shown in **(B)** which we have adapted slightly from Thacker et al. (2004). While Thacker et al. (2004) uses the terms *reality of interest*, *conceptual model*, and *computerized model*, we prefer the terms *system of interest*, *mathematical model*, and *executable model* as they better express the underlying intent. The model distinguishes between modeling and simulation activities (black solid arrows), and assessment activities (red dashed arrows).

specification of the system of interest, such data can be scarce. Secondly, even for comparatively accessible areas and assuming perfect preprocessing (e.g., spike sorting), single cell recordings represent a massive undersampling of the network activity. Thirdly, for a large range of computational neuroscientific models, the phenomenon of interest cannot be measured in a biological preparation: for example, any model relying on the plasticity of synapses within a network.

Consequently, for many neuronal network models, the most that the modeler can do with the available experimental data is to check for consistency, rather than validate in the strong sense. Thus, we are left with an incomplete assessment process. However, circumstantial evidence to increase the credibility of a model can be acquired by comparing models and their implementations against each other with respect to consistency (Thacker et al., 2004; Martis, 2006). Such a technique can be meaningful in accumulating evidence of a model's plausibility and correctness even if none of the models is a *"validated model"* that may act as a reliable reference.

To avoid ambiguity with the existing model verification and validation terminology, we propose the term ***"substantiation."***

> **Substantiation** describes the process of evaluating and quantifying the level of agreement of two executable models.

Model verification and substantiation are then processes that accumulate *circumstantial evidence* of a model's correctness or accuracy by a quantitative comparison of the simulation outcomes from validated or non-validated model implementations. The interrelationship of the modeling, simulation, and assessment activities are shown in **Figure 2**. To this end, the modeler has to define reasonable acceptance criteria that define the limits within which the process can be executed. In this study, we will demonstrate the usefulness of such an approach.

2.4. Application of Terminology to Neural Network Modeling and Simulation

Applying the given terminology to the domain of neural network modeling and simulations, we will use the terms as follows. *Replication* means using the author's own model, which may consist of the model source code, scripts for network generation and simulation execution as well as additional software components in a particular version (e.g., if a specific simulation software is used). A replication should aim for bit-identicality. Although computers are deterministic, this is not always feasible, for example, if the seed of the pseudorandom number generator has not been recorded, or the generated trajectory of pseudorandom numbers is dependent on the software version or the underlying hardware. Beyond this, replicable models should have the property of delivering exactly the same result in successive simulations on the same hardware. When using random number generators, this entails setting a seed.

A *reproduction* (or specifically, *results reproduction*) is then the re-implementation of the model in a different framework, e.g., expressing a model as a stand-alone script using neural simulation tools, such as NEURON (Hines and Carnevale, 1997), Brian (Goodman and Brette, 2008), NEST (Gewaltig and Diesmann, 2007), or the SpiNNaker neuromorphic system (Furber et al., 2013), and getting statistically the same results.

Applying the terminology defined in this section, one can say: in this study, we replicate a published model and create a reproduction of the model on the SpiNNaker neuromorphic system. In an iterative process of model substantiation, we arrive

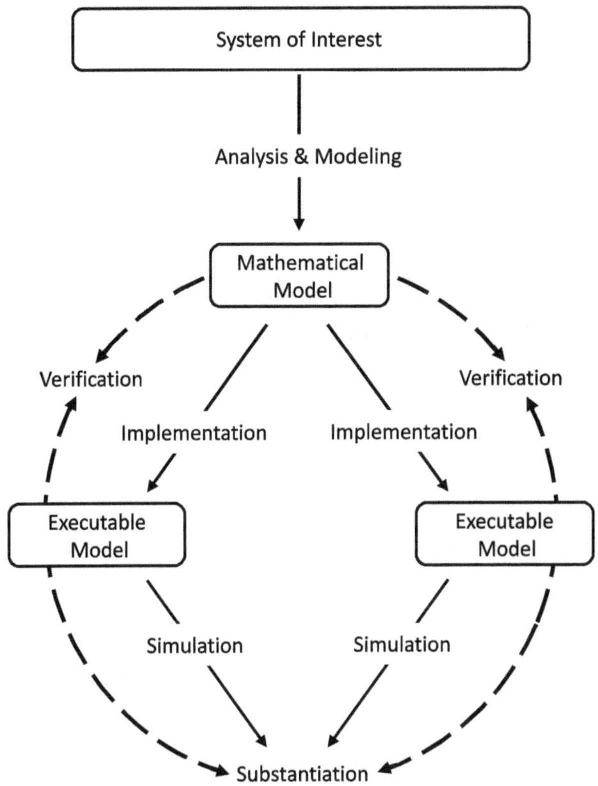

FIGURE 2 | Model verification and substantiation workflow. The workflow shown can be thought of as the combination of two separate model verification and validation processes (**Figure 1**) without the backward reference to the system of interest, i.e., the validation of the model. In this concept, the consistency of the simulation outcomes of two executable models that share the same system of interest and mathematical model is evaluated, in an assessment activity we term *"substantiation."* Modeling and simulation activities are indicated by black solid arrows, whereas assessment activities are indicated by red dashed arrows.

at the point that both executable models are verified, and in good agreement with one another.

3. MODEL VERIFICATION AND SUBSTANTIATION OF THE IZHIKEVICH POLYCHRONIZATION MODEL: THE REPRODUCTION OF SELECTED NETWORK STATES ON SPINNAKER

3.1. Definition of the Model Verification and Substantiation Methodology Entities

For the purposes of demonstrating a rigorous model verification and substantiation methodology, we define as our *system of interest* the mammalian cortex. A mathematical and executable model of this system was proposed by Izhikevich (2006), who demonstrated that this model exhibits the development of polychronous groups. The mathematical model is described in detail in section 3.1.1, the corresponding executable model, referred to in the following as the *C model*, constitutes one target of the verification and substantiation process illustrated in **Figure 2**. For the other target, we reproduce the mathematical model on the SpiNNaker neuromorphic system (Furber et al., 2013); the resultant executable model is referred to as the *SpiNNaker model* (see section 3.1.2).

3.1.1. Mathematical Model

3.1.1.1. Network topology

The network connectivity is illustrated in **Figure 3**. A population of 800 excitatory neurons makes random connections to itself and to a population of 200 inhibitory neurons using a fixed out-degree of 100. Excitatory synaptic connections are initially set to a strength of $w_{ij} = 6.0$ and a conduction delay D_{ij} drawn from a uniform integer distribution such that $D_{ij} \in [1, 2, \ldots, 20]$ ms. The inhibitory population is connected with the same out-degree to the excitatory population only, forming connections with a fixed synaptic strength and delay, $w_{ij} = -5.0, D_{ij} = 1$ ms.

3.1.1.2. Component dynamics

Each neuron in the network is described by the simple neuron model presented in Izhikevich (2003), which can reproduce a variety of experimentally observed firing statistics:

$$\dot{v} = 0.04v^2 + 5v + 140 - u + I \tag{1}$$

$$\dot{u} = a(bv - u) \tag{2}$$

$$\text{if } v \geq 30 \text{ mV, then} \begin{cases} v \leftarrow c \\ u \leftarrow u + d \end{cases} . \tag{3}$$

Equations (1)–(3) describe the time evolution of the membrane voltage $v(t)$ and the threshold dynamic variable $u(t)$ of a single neuron. For the polychronization model, excitatory neurons are parameterized to show regular-spiking: $(a, , b, c, d) = (0.02, 0.2, -65.0, 8.0)$, and inhibitory neurons are parameterized to exhibit fast-spiking: $(a, b, c, d) = (0.1, 0.2, -65.0, 2.0)$.

The excitatory connections are plastic and evolve according to an additive spike-timing-dependent plasticity (STDP) rule:

$$w \leftarrow \begin{cases} w + A_+ \cdot \exp(-\Delta t/\tau_+) & : \Delta t \geq 0 \\ w - A_- \cdot \exp(\Delta t/\tau_-) & : \Delta t < 0 \end{cases} \tag{4}$$

where $\tau_+ = \tau_- = 20$ ms, $A_+ = 0.1$ mV, $A_- = 0.12$ mV, and Δt is the difference in time between the last post-synaptic and pre-synaptic spikes, i.e., positive on occurrence of a post-synaptic spike and negative on occurrence of a pre-synaptic spike. However, the rule has an unusual variant: synaptic weight changes are buffered for one biological second and then the weight matrix is updated for all plastic synapses simultaneously. Thus, synaptic weights are constant for long periods, causing the network dynamics to break down into epochs.

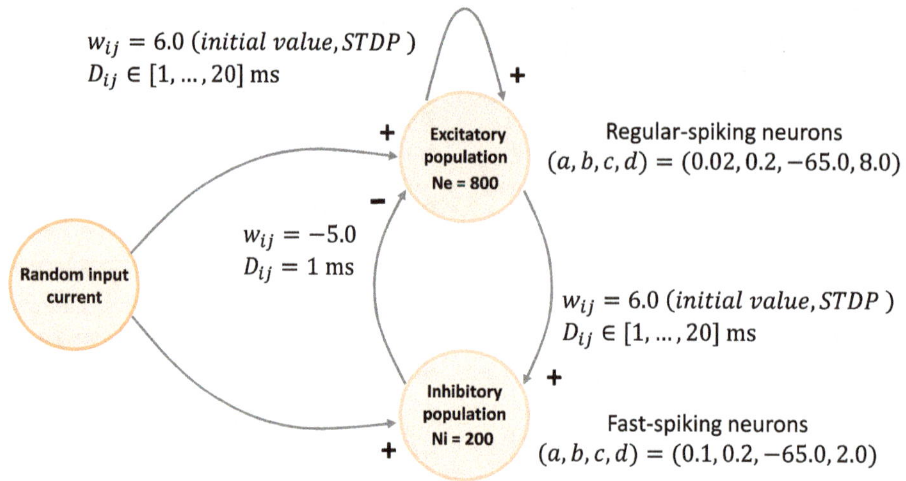

FIGURE 3 | Network architecture. The minimal spiking network exhibiting polychronization as decribed in Izhikevich (2006). The input to the network is a constant current of $I_{ext} = 20$ pA into a single neuron, which is randomly selected in each simulation time-step. Please see section 3.1.1 for a detailed description of the mathematical model.

3.1.2. Executable Models

3.1.2.1. C model

The original network model and its analysis form a stand-alone application. Several implementations are available for download from the author's website[2]: a MATLAB implementation (*spnet.m*) and two versions of a C/C++ implementation (*spnet.cpp, poly_spnet.cpp*). They differ slightly in algorithms and functionality and thus do not exhibit bit-identical behavior. All implementations use a grid-based simulation paradigm with a resolution of 1 ms. Threshold detection according to Equation (3) is performed only at the grid points. For numerical integration of the ODE system consisting of the Equations (1) and (2) a Forward Euler method is used. From the two available versions of the C/C++ implementation we selected the computationally more precise variant *poly_spnet.cpp* that makes use of double precision data types and also implements the analysis, i.e., algorithms for detecting polychronous groups.

3.1.2.2. SpiNNaker model

The SpiNNaker neuromorphic system is a massively parallel multi-core computing system designed to provide a real-time simulation platform for large neural networks (Furber et al., 2013). The largest available system is a half-million core machine[3]. The real-time capability is achieved at an simulation resolution of $h = 1$ ms using a grid-based simulation paradigm. This is analog to the integration scheme and simulation paradigm used in the original C model implementation. For our study, we use a SpiNN-3 development board that houses 4 SpiNNaker chips, each containing 18 ARM968 processing cores (Temple, 2011a). For simulation control and cross-development, the SpiNN-3 board must be connected to a host system, which then communicates with the board via Ethernet-based UDP packets (Temple, 2011b). The SpiNNaker software stack (Rowley et al., 2017b) supports the implementation of neural network simulations in PyNN[4]. In addition, it offers several neuron and synapse models as well as a template that enables user to develop custom neuron and synapse models using the event-driven programming model employed by SpiNNaker kernel (Rowley et al., 2017a), available for download from the SpiNNaker repository on GitHub[5]. The SpiNNaker model used in this study was developed from scratch, making use of this template to produce the various Izhikevich neuron model implementations presented in this manuscript.

3.2. Definition of the Model Substantiation Assessment

In the absence of specific biological data to define the ground truth for the system of interest, we are left with the simulation outcomes of the two executable models. Here, we consider the dynamics of five selected network states in the C model. The dynamics is assessed by applying statistical analysis methods to the spike train activity data (see section 3.2.2). For an in-depth treatment of the analysis methods used for comparison, see the companion study (Gutzen et al., 2018). Note that we do not use the emergence of polychronous groups or their statistics to define the ground truth, as this turns out to be rather sensitive to details not only of the mathematical model, but also of the implementational choices used to generate the executable model. For a comprehensive investigation of this aspect, see Pauli et al. (2018).

[2]https://www.izhikevich.org/publications/spnet.htm
[3]http://apt.cs.manchester.ac.uk/projects/SpiNNaker/project/Access/
[4]PyNN is a common interface for neural network simulators (Davison et al., 2009).
[5]https://github.com/SpiNNakerManchester/sPyNNaker8NewModelTemplate

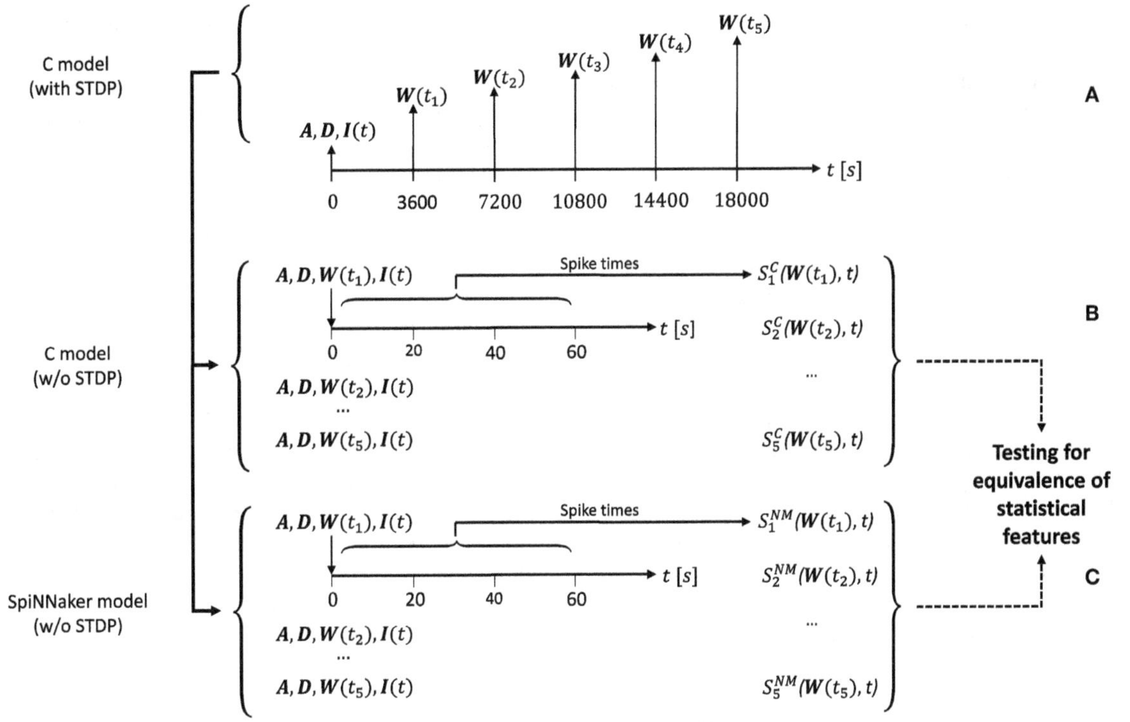

FIGURE 4 | The experimental set-up for the simulations. **(A)** To create the reference data, the C model is executed (with STDP) and the connectivity matrix $\boldsymbol{A}$ and delay matrix $\boldsymbol{D}$ are saved. Then five times are selected, for which the weight matrix $W(t_i)$ is recorded. Along with the input stimulus to the network $I(t)$, these matrices determine five network states for later comparison. These initial conditions are then set for an implementation of the C model **(B)** and for the SpiNNaker model **(C)**, both without STDP. This results in the network spiking activity recordings $S_i^C(W(t_i), t)$ and $S_i^{NM}(W(t_i), t)$ for five simulation runs for the C model and the SpiNNaker model, respectively.

3.2.1. Experimental Set-Up

In order to generate the network activity data for the comparison tasks carried out in the model substantiation process, we perform the following steps, illustrated in **Figure 4**.

First, for a given realization (i.e., an implementation and selection of a random seed) for the C model, we execute the model for a duration[6] of 5 h. During this time we select five times $t_i, i = (1, 2, \ldots, 5)$ (here: after 1, 2, 3, 4, and 5 h), at which we save the weight matrix $\boldsymbol{W}(t_i)$, containing the current strength of each synapse according to the STDP rule described in section 3.1.1. In addition, we save the connectivity matrix $\boldsymbol{A}$, the delay matrix $\boldsymbol{D}$ and the first 60 s' worth of the random series of neurons to which an additional stimulus is provided, $\boldsymbol{I}(t)$. This procedure is illustrated in **Figure 4A**.

In a second step, we switch STDP off in the C model. In five consecutive simulation runs, we initialize the network with $\boldsymbol{A}, \boldsymbol{D}, \boldsymbol{I}$, and the respective $\boldsymbol{W}(t_i)$, and record the resultant spiking activity $S_i^C(\boldsymbol{W}(t_i), t)$ over 60 s, as illustrated in **Figure 4B**. These activity recordings define five dynamic states of the network at different stages of its evolution, constituting the reference data (i.e., fulfilling the role that ground truth data plays in a classical model validation assessment).

[6]This refers to the simulated time and not to the run time of the simulation.

Finally, we repeat the second step using the SpiNNaker model (see **Figure 4C**), resulting in corresponding network activity recordings $S_i^{NM}(\boldsymbol{W}(t_i), t)$. To perform the model substantiation assessment, the spiking data S_i^C and S_i^{NM} are analyzed and compared as described in section 3.2.2.

Note that although the parameters and properties of the polychronization model remain untouched, model implementations do change in successive iterations of the verification and substantiation process as described below; consequently, so do the reference data.

3.2.2. Analysis of Network Spiking Activity

Besides a verification on the level of the dynamics of an individual neuron, we assess the degree of similarity between the different implementations of the Izhikevich polychronization model on the descriptive level of the population dynamics (cf. also, Gutzen et al., 2018). As issues such as the choice of 32/64-bit architecture, floating-point/fixed-point arithmetic, compiler options influencing the evaluation order of expressions or the choice of pseudorandom numbers and the corresponding seed should not be considered part of the mathematical model, it is legitimate and expected that different implementations will not yield an exact spike-by-spike correspondence (but see Pauli et al., 2018 for a counterexample). We therefore resort to testing for equivalence of statistical features extracted from the population dynamics. These tests are conducted in an automated, formal framework that conducts statistical analysis of parallel spike trains using the standardized implementations found in the *Electrophysiology Analysis Toolkit*[7] (Elephant, RRID:SCR_003833) as its backend. We stress the importance of using a common tool to extract the statistical features for both simulation outcomes in the substantiation procedure in order to prevent distortions in the substantiation outcome due to discrepancies in the implementations of the substantiation procedure itself. In addition, making use of methods provided by such open-source projects greatly contributes to the correctness and replicability of the results.

When choosing the measures by which to compare the network activity, it is essential to assess diverse aspects of the dynamics. Besides widely used standard measures to characterize the statistical features of spike trains or the correlation between pairs of spike trains, this may also include additional measures that reflect more specific features of the network model (e.g., spatio-temporal patterns). Here, we apply tests that compare distributions of three statistical measures extracted from the population dynamics: the average firing rates, the local coefficient of variation as a measure of spike time regularity (Shinomoto et al., 2003), and the pairwise correlation coefficients between all pairs of parallel spike trains (bin width: 2 ms). They can be regarded as forming a hierarchical order and evaluate different aspects of the network dynamics: rates consider the number of observed spikes, whilst ignoring their temporal structure; the local coefficient of variation considers the serial correlations inherent in a spike train, whilst ignoring the relationship between spike trains; the cross correlation considers coordination across neurons.

It should be noted that, as shown later in this study, this conceptual hierarchy does not imply a hierarchy of failure, i.e., a correspondence on the highest level (here: cross correlation) does not automatically imply correspondence of the other measures. Therefore, it is imperative to independently evaluate each statistical property. We evaluate the similarity of the distributions of these measures between simulations using the effect size (Cohen's d), i.e., the normalized difference between the means of the distributions (Cohen, 1988). In addition to the substantiation tests selected for the current study, more intricate comparisons can evaluate the correlation structure and dynamical features of the network activity in greater detail, outlined in our companion study (Gutzen et al., 2018).

3.3. Definition of the Model Verification and Substantiation Workflow

As stated above, model substantiation evaluates the level of agreement between executable models and their implementations, but is not conclusive whether the model itself is correct, i.e., an appropriate description of an underlying biological reality. It is therefore out of scope of this study to evaluate any neuroscientific aspects of the model described in Izhikevich (2006).

Derived from the concept of model verification and substantiation (**Figure 2**), the workflow in **Figure 5** depicts a condensed illustration of the activities performed in this study. We execute the workflow several times whilst subjecting the C and SpiNNaker model implementations to various implementation and verification activities. The latter can be divided into two categories: source code verification and calculation verification.

The purpose of source code verification is to confirm that the functionality it implements works as intended (Thacker et al., 2004). Unlike commercially developed production software, scientific source code is used to draw scientific conclusions and, thus, it should act as an available reference (Benureau and Rougier, 2017).

The purpose of calculation verification is to assess the level of error that arise from various sources of error in numerical simulations as well as to identify and remove them. The types of errors that can be identified and removed by calculation verification are, e.g., errors caused by inadequate discretization and insufficient grid refinement as well as errors by finite precision arithmetic. Insufficient grid refinement is typically the largest contributor to error in calculation verification assessment (Thacker et al., 2004).

3.4. Application of the Method

The model verification and substantiation process we describe in this study required three iteration cycles, named Iteration I, II, and III, until an acceptable agreement was achieved. **Figure 6** shows a complete and detailed breakdown of the activities, which were shown in more general form in **Figure 5**.

In the following, we describe for each iteration the verification activities that identified issues with the executable models, and the consequent adaptations to the C and SpiNNaker model implementations. The substantiation activity performed at the end of each iteration is marked in **Figure 6** with I, II, and III, respectively; the results for each one are given in **Figure 7**. A full description of these and further substantiation activities is provided in our companion study (Gutzen et al., 2018).

In order to be able to reproduce the findings of this work and our companion study (Gutzen et al., 2018), all source code and simulation data is available online. The model source codes, simulation scripts and the codes used in the verification activities are available on GitHub[8] (doi: 10.5281/zenodo.1435831). The simulation data and scripts used for the quantitative comparisons of statistical measures in the substantiation task can be found on GIN[9].

3.4.1. Iteration I

In the first iteration, our main focus is source code verification. For the C model, this takes the form of assessing and improving source code quality, whereas for the SpiNNaker model implementation we carry out functional testing.

[7] http://neuralensemble.org/elephant

[8] https://github.com/gtrensch/RigorousNeuralNetworkSimulations

[9] https://web.gin.g-node.org/INM-6/network_validation

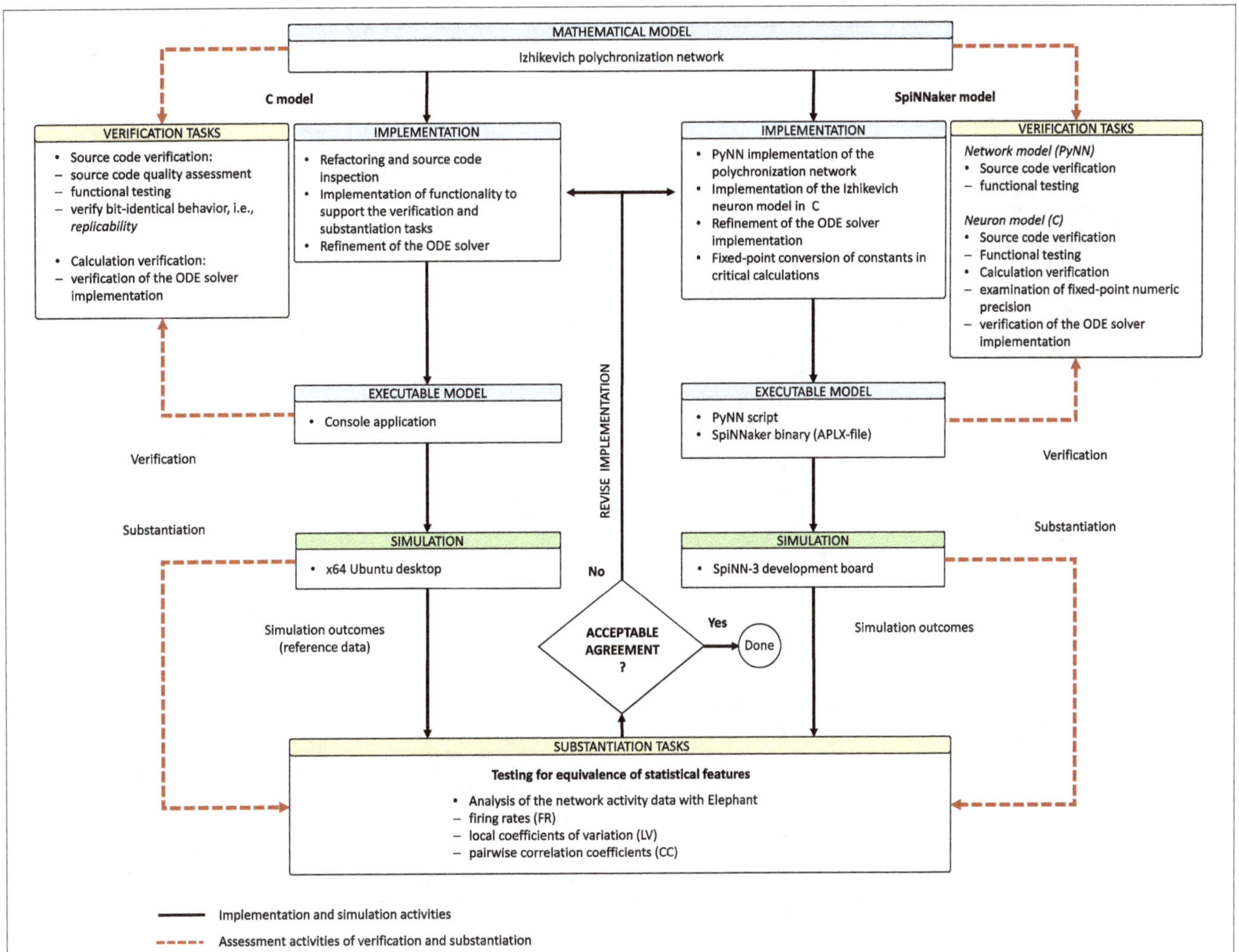

FIGURE 5 | Model verification and substantiation workflow as it was conducted. The figure depicts in a condensed form the instantiation of the model verification and substantiation workflow (**Figure 2**) introduced in section 2.3 and carried out in this study.

3.4.1.1. C model

The *poly_spnet.cpp* source code hides the algorithms—which seem to be derived from MATLAB programming paradigms—behind hard-to-read source code. To improve the readability, understand the algorithms, and find potential programming and implementation errors, we subjected the source code to a refactoring[10] and code inspection task.

We fully reworked the source code by following clean code heuristics (Martin and Coplien, 2009). Code sections concerned with the analysis and not part of the model itself were removed from the source code, kept separately and were only used for functional testing. Whilst going through this iterative refactoring and code inspection process, we made sure that the model remained bit-identical after every iteration, i.e., ensuring replicability (see section 2).

In order to support the experimental setup and make the substantiation activities possible, we added functionality that allows network states to be saved and reloaded. For producing the network activity data for use in substantiation, i.e., the quantitative comparisons of statistical measures, we also switched off STDP (see also section 3.2.1). For convenient functional testing and debugging purposes, the implementation was adapted to allow the polychronization model to be down-scaled to a 20 neuron test network. This size was selected to be small enough for convenient manual debugging, whilst large enough to exhibit spiking behavior and have a non-trivial connectivity matrix.

Performing the refactoring task not only helped understand the C model implementation and algorithms, which is essential, it also laid the foundation for the implementation of the SpiNNaker model.

[10]Refactoring—a software engineering method from the area of software maintenance—is source code transformation which reorganizes a program without changing its behavior. It improves the software structure and the readability, and so avoids the structural deterioration that naturally occurs when software is changed Sommerville, 2015.

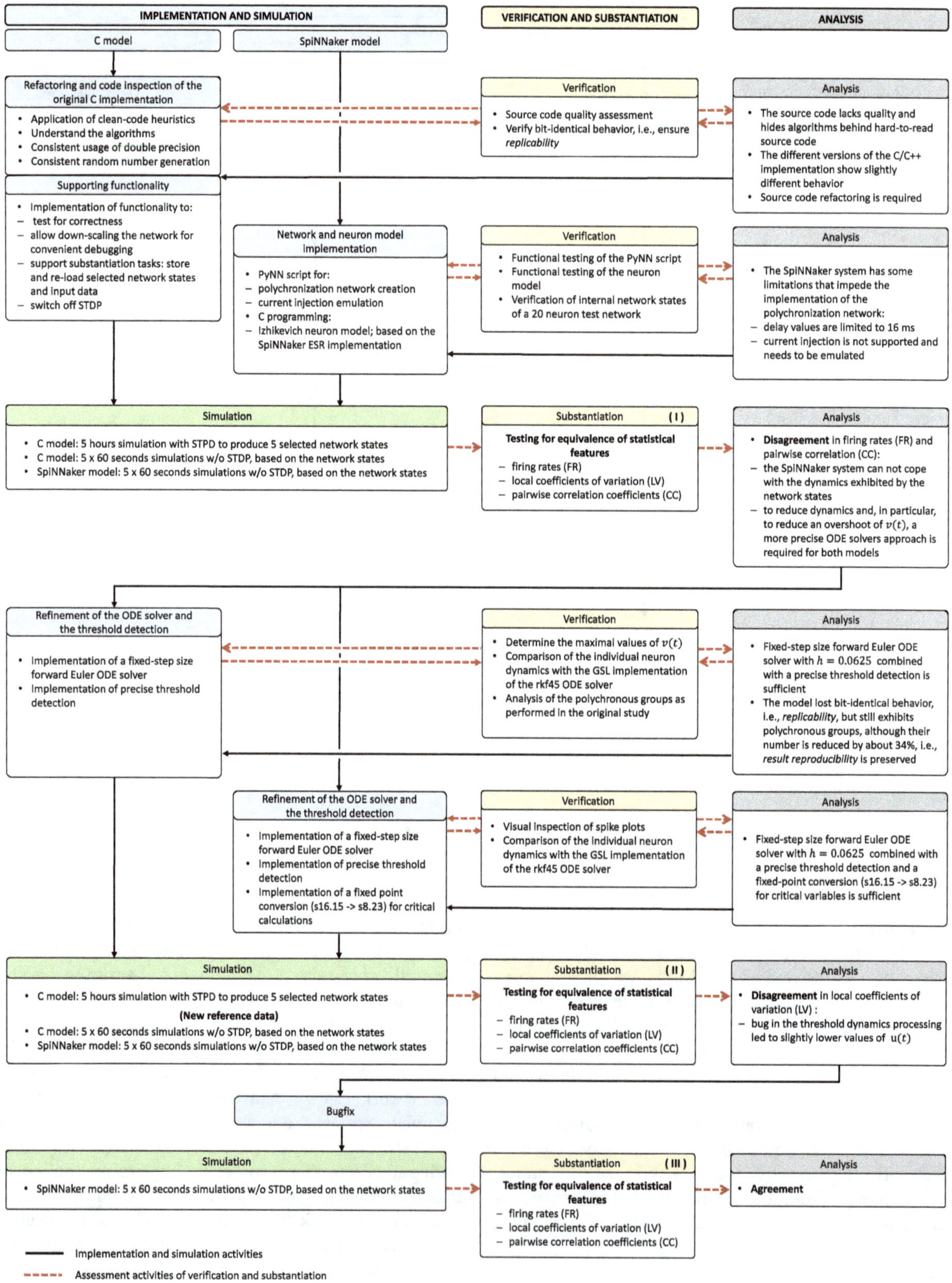

FIGURE 6 | Model verification and substantiation iterations and activities conducted. The activities carried out as part of the model verification and substantiation process, which we briefly outlined in **Figure 5**, can be further broken down to a more detailed view. The diagram represents this iterative process in a linear fashion, where three iterations have been conducted. The model substantiation activity performed at the end of each iteration is marked with I, II, and III, which corresponds to the results summary shown in **Figure 7**.

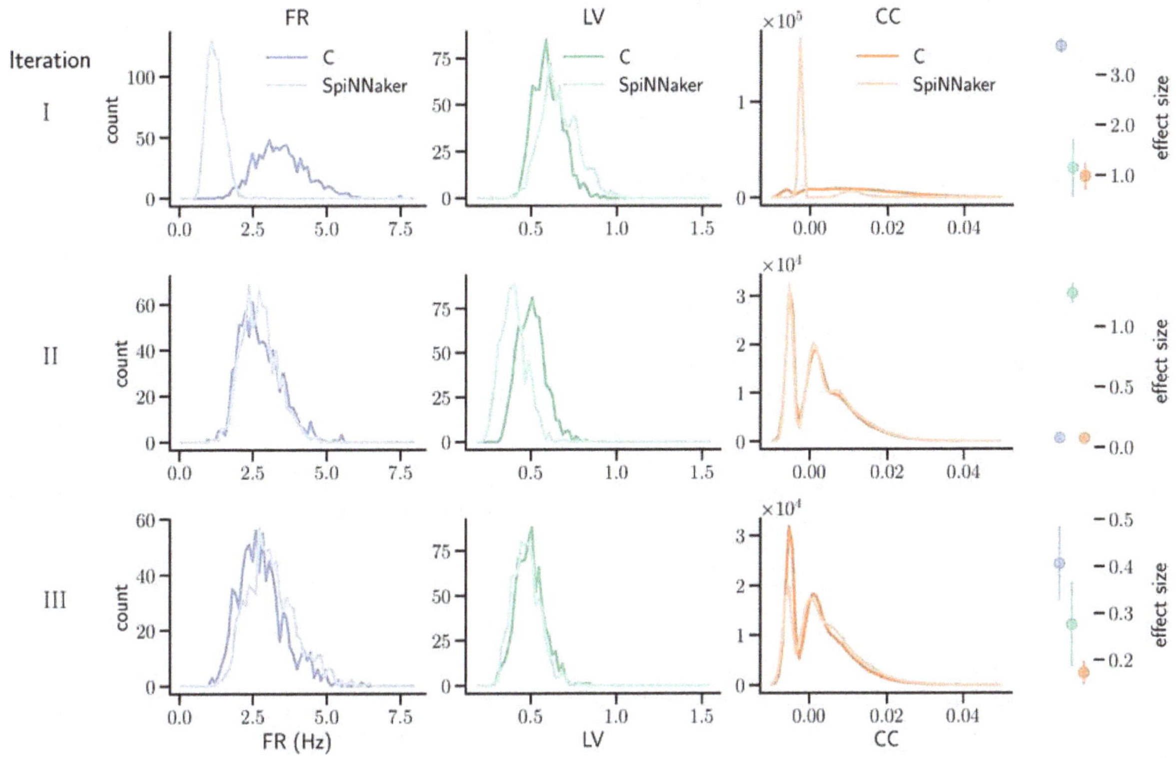

FIGURE 7 | Model substantiation assessment based on spike data analysis. Histograms (70 bins each) of the three characteristic measures computed from 60 s of network activity after the fifth hour of simulation: Left, firing rates (FR); middle, local coefficients of variation (LV); right, pairwise correlation coefficients (CC). For FR and LV, each neuron enters the histogram, for CC each neuron pair. Results are shown for three iterations (rows) of the substantiation process of the C model (dark colors) and SpiNNaker model (light colors), cf. **Figure 6**. On the far right, the difference between the respective distributions is quantified by the effect size: the graph shows the mean and standard deviation effect size calculated for each of the five network states (after 1, 2, 3, 4, and 5 h of simulation).

3.4.1.2. SpiNNaker model

For the initial iteration of the SpiNNaker model, we used the Explicit Solver Reduction (ESR) implementation of the Izhikevich model provided by the SpiNNaker software stack (Hopkins and Furber, 2015). For network creation, simulation control and execution as well as for functional testing, we developed PyNN scripts that allowed us to conveniently perform the simulation, the verification tasks, and substantiation activities. Additional development work was required to circumvent a few restrictions of the SpiNNaker system and its software stack, namely:

The SpiNNaker framework does not allow external current injection: During each 1 ms simulation time-step, an external current of $I_{\text{ext}} = 20$ pA is injected into a randomly selected neuron. This current injection is emulated by two spike source arrays forming one-to-one connections to the two populations of the polychronization network. Those connections use static synapses, translating an external spike event into an injected current.

The amount of data that needs to be held on the SpiNN-3 board during simulation may become too large for 60 s simulation time: To limit the amount of data, we divided a single simulation run into 60 cycles. At the end of each cycle, the simulation is halted for data exchange, and then resumed.

We used three approaches to functionally test the PyNN scripts and to verify the implementation of the neuron model:

Manual low level debugging on the SpiNNaker system to verify the correctness of state variables, program flow and algorithms: The SpiNNaker system offers a low level command line debugging tool called *ybug* and the SpiNNaker kernel also allows log information to be sent to an internal i/o-buffer. The buffer is read at simulation termination and accessible with *ybug*. We used this basic debugging technique to verify the internal states of the neuron model, the correctness of injected current values as well as to verify the correctness of the program flow of the algorithms that we implemented.

Verification of the neuron dynamics using a PyNN test script applying an external constant current to individual neurons and recording the state variables: We recorded the dynamics of individual neurons resulting from an injected constant current and compared the data with the results obtained from a stand-alone C console application that implements the same algorithms.

Functional testing with a small (20 neuron) version of the polychronization network: We used a down-scaled version of the polychronization network (16 excitatory and

4 inhibitory neurons) to verify the functional correctness of the simulation setup. As the connectivity matrix was derived from simulations of the C model, it further served for testing the functionality added to support the activities carried out during the substantiation process, e.g., the export of the connectivity matrix created by simulation runs of the C model and its import into the SpiNNaker simulation.

3.4.1.3. Substantiation

We simulated the models to generate the data for the quantitative comparisons of the statistical measures, as described in sections 3.2.1 and 3.2.2, respectively. The results are summarized in the top row of **Figure 7**. This reveals a substantial mismatch, most dominantly visible in the distribution of the firing rates (FR) and the pairwise correlation coefficients (CC). This mismatch, as quantified by the effect size, is consistently observed for all five reference network states. Therefore, we conclude that the models do not show an acceptable agreement and the substantiation assessment failed at the end of Iteration I. Although the effect size is a very simple measure which only takes into account the means and standard deviations of the distributions, it provides an intuitive quantification of differences which is unbiased by the sample size. However, since the effect size can not detect discrepancies in the distribution shape, a visual inspection is essential and additional comparison methods, such as hypothesis tests, may be needed. In **Figure 7** we only show the measures computed from 60 s of network activity after the fifth hour. For a visual inspection of the computed measures from the network states after 1, 2, 3, 4, and 5 h of simulation, see **Figures S1–S5** in the **Supplementary Material**.

3.4.2. Iteration II

The substantial discrepancies revealed by the model substantiation assessment performed in Iteration I suggests that there are numerical errors in one or both of the executable models. In the second iteration, we therefore focus on calculation verification. To this end, monitoring functionality was included to record the minimal, maximal, and average values of the model state variables. We find that the largest contributors to error are the choice of solver for the neuronal dynamics, the detection of spikes, and the fixed-point arithmetic on SpiNNaker.

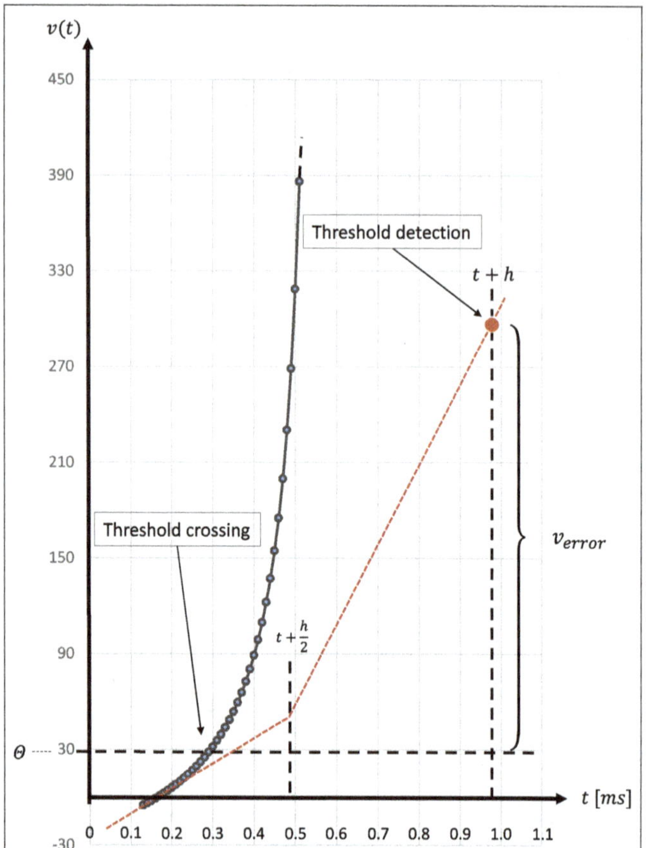

FIGURE 8 | Above threshold evolution of the state variable $v(t)$. The approximation in the evolution of $v(t)$ in the Equation (1) when using the semi-implicit symplectic Forward Euler method with a fixed-step size of $h/2 = 0.5$ ms (the red dotted line), where h refers to the 1 ms simulation time-step, causes $v(t)$ values to be well above the threshold and, thus, producing a propagating error over time. This is expressed in delayed spike times. The black solid line shows the evolution of $v(t)$ around threshold for a regular-spiking type Izhikevich neuron stimulated with a constant current of $I_{ext} = 5$ pA. For integration, the same Forward Euler method was used but with an integration step size of $h/100 = 0.01$ ms. The steep slope at threshold requires a precise threshold detection to prevent a numeric overflow.

3.4.2.1. Numeric integration scheme and precise threshold detection

When working with systems of ordinary differential equations (ODEs), it is important to make sensible decisions regarding the choice of a numeric integration scheme. To achieve accurate approximations of their solutions one must take into account not only the form of the equation but also the magnitude of the variables occurring in them (Dahmen and Reusken, 2005). Depending on these parameters, some ordinary differential equations can become *stiff*, i.e., requiring excessively small time steps for an *explicit* numerical iteration scheme (i.e., one that only uses the values of variables at preceding time-steps) to achieve acceptable accuracy and avoid numeric instabilities. Such equation systems require the use of an *implicit* scheme (i.e., one that finds a solution by solving an equation involving both the current values of variables and their later values). However, this method is computationally more expensive, entailing unnecessarily long run-times when applied to non-stiff systems (Strehmel and Weiner, 1995). The ODEs used to model neuronal behavior are often non-stiff, so that an explicit numerical iteration scheme is sufficient (Lambert, 1992).

The Izhikevich ODE system (Equations 1–3) is an example of such a non-stiff model, see Blundell et al. (2018b). Thus, in principle, the choice of an explicit method, namely the Forward Euler method, albeit in a semi-implicit symplectic variant, which is used in the C model, is correct. Nevertheless, the numerical integration scheme must be applied correctly, i.e., the step size must be chosen according to the desired maximum error. The (relatively large) selected step sizes of $h = 0.5$ ms for the integration of the membrane potential (Equation 1), and $h = 1.0$ ms for the recovery variable are not only questionable because no motivation is given for why two different step sizes are chosen for the same system of equations, but more importantly because no error estimate is implemented to guarantee that the integration scheme does in fact give a reasonable approximation of the solution of the ODE system. The algorithm of the original C model implementation is shown in Listing 1. Note the symplectic, or semi-implicit Forward Euler scheme, i.e., the update of u is based on an already updated value for v. In an unorthodox approach, the variable v is integrated in two 0.5 ms steps whilst u is integrated in one 1 ms step.

```
EVERY MILLISECOND:
{
  NEURON STATE UPDATE:
  {
    // for numerical stability
    // 2 integration steps within 1 ms
    v = v + 0.5 * (( 0.04 * v + 5.0 ) * v
        + 140.0 - u + I )
    v = v + 0.5 * (( 0.04 * v + 5.0 ) * v
        + 140.0 - u + I )
    u = u + a * ( b * v - u )
  }

  THRESHOLD DETECTION:
  {
    IF( v >= 30.0 )
    {
      v = c
      u = u + d
    }
  }
}
```

Listing 1 | C model: algorithm of updating the neuronal dynamics (given as pseudocode) as implemented in the original C model. The algorithm implements a fixed-step size semi-implicit symplectic Forward Euler method.

The spike onset of a regular-spiking Izhikevich neuron appears as a steep slope at threshold, and, due to the grid-constrained threshold detection in the C model, leads to values of $v(t)$ which can be two orders of magnitude higher than the threshold value $\theta = 30$ mV (Equation 3). In the C model, we observed values of $v(t) \leq 1700$. **Figure 8** graphically illustrates the error caused by this approximation. The value of $u(t)$ (Equation 2), which describes the threshold dynamics, evolves continuously, thus, v_{error} will induce an error to the threshold dynamic which propagates over time delaying all subsequent spike events.

Moreover, for efficiency, SpiNNaker uses fixed-point numerics. Numbers are held as 32-bit fixed-point values in a $s16.15$ representation, limited in range. Large values of $v(t)$ can lead to a fixed-point overflow, as discussed in greater detail below, which may then produce spike artifacts. The likelihood of this is even further increased by the fact that this value appears as a power of two in Equation (1). To demonstrate this, we adapted the algorithm shown in Listing 1 and added an additional integration step (see Listing 2). The neuronal activity, shown in **Figure 9**, exhibits spiking artifacts in the form of bursts of spikes with high spike rates.

```
EVERY MILLISECOND:
{
  NEURON STATE UPDATE:
  {
    REPEAT 3 TIMES:
    {
      v = v + 0.333 * (( 0.04 * v + 5.0 ) * v
          + 140.0 - u + I )
      u = u + 0.333 * a * ( b * v - u )
    }
  }

  THRESHOLD DETECTION:
  {
    IF( v >= 30.0 )
    {
      v = c
      u = u + d
      deliverSpikeEvent()
    }
  }
}
```

Listing 2 | SpiNNaker model: an algorithm of updating the neuronal dynamics (given as pseudo code). The algorithm is similar to the implementation shown in Listing 1 but uses three fixed size integration steps. The additional step increases the likelihood that large values of $v(t)$ are squared. This implementation may cause a numeric overflow.

The SpiNNaker software stack (Rowley et al., 2017b) provides an Izhikevich neuron model implementation optimized for efficiency for fixed-point processors, such as ARM. The implementation follows a new approach called Explicit Solver Reduction (ESR), described in Hopkins and Furber (2015): *"for merging an explicit ODE solver and autonomous ODE into one algebraic formula, with benefits for both accuracy and speed."* The SpiNNaker system is designed for simulations in biological real-time. The real-time capability is achieved at an integration step size of $h = 1$ ms which then corresponds to the simulation time-step, i.e., the same integration step size as the C model. At higher resolution, i.e., smaller integration time-steps, the simulation time increases accordingly. The SpiNNaker ESR implementation, at the same integration step size, does not exhibit such artifacts, but fails in in adequately reproducing the network states, as can be seen in the model substantiation assessment for Iteration I (top row of **Figure 7**).

In general, higher accuracy can be obtained by using smaller step sizes. However, for this model, using smaller steps to integrate whilst restricting spike detection and reset to a 1 ms grid results in a steep slope in the evolution of the membrane potential above threshold which rapidly reaches values that can not be represented with double precision (compare red dotted curve and black solid curve in **Figure 8**). We therefore propose a solution that combines a simple fixed-step size symplectic Forward Euler ODE solver and an exact off-grid threshold detection, while a spike event is still forced to a grid point. To be more specific, within each 1 ms simulation time-step h, the equations evolve in steps of $h/16$. The number of internal integration steps was chosen for two reasons. First, as a power of two, it can be represented in $s16.15$ without numerical error. Second, it represents a good compromise between the increased computational cost of smaller steps, and the increased overshoot in the membrane potential for larger steps. The algorithm is given as pseudo code in Listing 3. Please note the multiplication with 0.0625, avoiding a costly division. Spikes can be detected

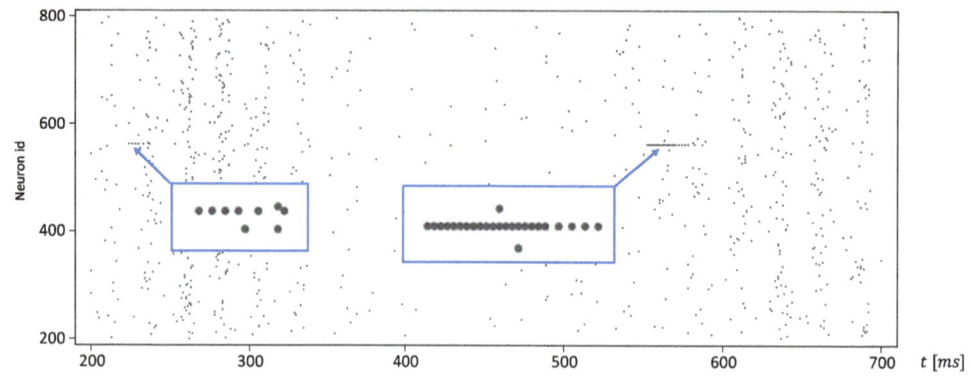

FIGURE 9 | Spike artifacts caused by fixed-point overflow. Large values of $v(t)$ can cause an overflow of the fixed-point data type, which may result in short spike-trains with higher rates (marked by blue boxes). Simulations on SpiNNaker using fixed-step size symplectic Forward Euler with an integration step size of $h/3 = 0.333$ ms and without precise threshold detection. (h refers to the simulation time-step of 1 ms).

(and the dynamics reset) after every internal step, however, as with the C model, spikes are emitted on the simulation grid with a resolution of 1 ms. Multiple spike events within one simulation time-step are thus potentially possible, but are merged into a single event. However, this seems to be a very rare event. Pauli et al. (2018) demonstrated that there was only a very slight change in average firing rate for this network model between a simulation locked to a 1 ms grid, as used here, and one carried out at a higher resolution of 0.1 ms. We thus consider this effect to be negligible in the following.

```
EVERY MILLISECOND:
{
  NEURON STATE UPDATE:
  {
    REPEAT 16 TIMES:
    {
      v = v + 0.0625 * (( 0.04 * v + 5.0 ) * v
          + 140.0 - u + I )
      u = u + 0.0625 * a * ( b * v - u )

      IF( v >= 30.0 )
      {
        v = c
        u = u + d
        SET spikeEventHasOccurred
      }
    }
  }

  THRESHOLD DETECTION:
  {
    IF( spikeEventHasOccurred )
    {
      deliverSpikeEvent()
    }
  }
}
```

Listing 3 | SpiNNaker model: an improved algorithm of updating the neuronal dynamics (given as pseudo code) that uses a fixed-step size symplectic Forward Euler method and precise threshold detection.

To assess the accuracy of our proposed solver and that of the implementation provided by the SpiNNaker framework, we performed single neuron simulations and compared the resultant membrane potentials to that produced by a Runge-Kutta-Fehlberg(4, 5) (rkf45) solver implementation from the GNU Scientific Library (GSL)[11]. The explicit Runge-Kutta-Fehlberg(4, 5) method is a good general-purpose integrator, and, compared to a simple Forward Euler, of a higher order. To serve as a reliable reference, the rkf45 algorithm was parametrized to integrate with an absolute error of 10^{-6}. The results are shown in **Figure 10**. Note that not only do the spike times for both the fixed-step size Euler and the ESR solvers lag behind the rkf45 solver, but due to the accumulation of v_{error}, the lag becomes larger during the course of the simulation, here reaching around 20 ms in a simulation of 500 ms duration containing five spikes. As the errors occur at spike times, higher spike rates lead to larger deviations. Thus, the course of the membrane potential of the fast-spiking type neuron is less accurate than for the regular-spiking type neuron. This applies also to an increasing injected current I, as this also leads to higher spike rates (data not shown). As the firing rate increases, the ESR lags more, such that fewer spikes are generated in the given time window. Our results show that even though the fixed-step size Euler scheme is simpler than ESR, it is a more accurate match to the single neuron dynamics.

3.4.2.2. Fixed-point numeric precision

Hardware floating point units are expensive in chip area, and thus lower the power efficiency of the system. Consequently, SpiNNaker stores numbers, i.e., membrane voltages and other neuron parameters, as 32-bit signed fixed-point values (Furber et al., 2013). Since the meaning of an n-bit binary word depends entirely on its interpretation, we can divide an n-bit word into an integer part i and a fractional part f by defining a *binary point* position. Calculations are then performed as if the numbers are simple two's complement integers. SpiNNaker uses a so called $s16.15$ representation, that is, a 32-bit signed fixed-point format with $i = 16, f = 15$ and a sign bit. The value range is small in comparison to a single or double precision data type. For the $si.f$ data types the value range is defined by:

$$-2^i \leq x \leq +2^i - 2^{-f}. \tag{5}$$

[11] https://www.gnu.org/software/gsl/

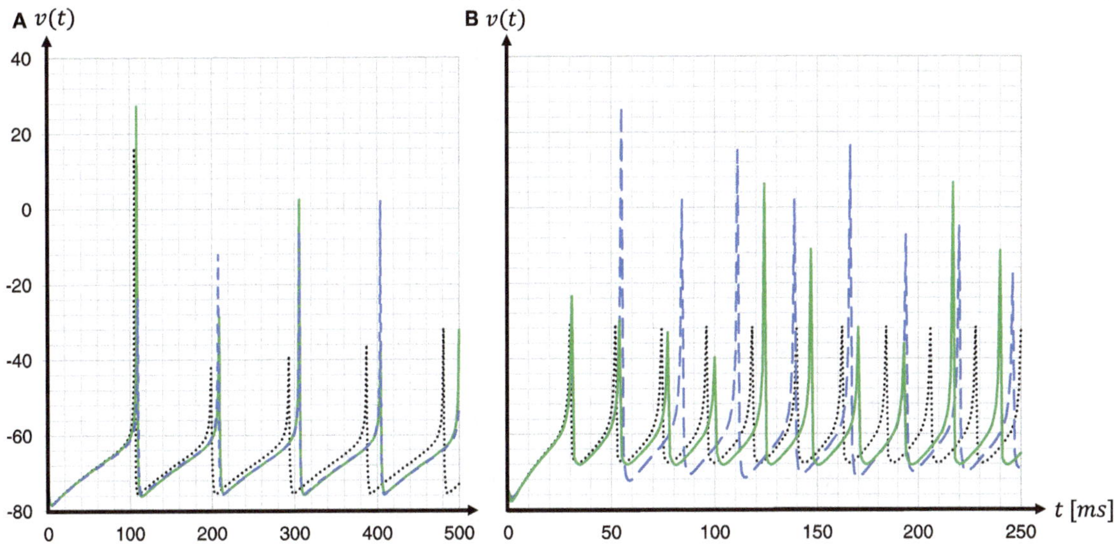

FIGURE 10 | Spike timing: comparison of different ODE solver implementations. Membrane potential $v(t)$ recorded for a regular-spiking **(A)** and fast-spiking **(B)** Izhikevich neuron, stimulated with a constant current of $I_{\text{ext}} = 5$ pA. The dynamics are solved by the original SpiNNaker ESR ODE solver implementation (blue dashed curves); a fixed-step size symplectic Forward Euler approach with precise threshold detection ($h/16 = 0.0625$ ms) (green solid curves); and, for comparison, a reference implementation of the GSL rkf45 ODE solver with an absolute integration error of 10^{-6} (black dotted curves). Both the SpiNNaker ESR and the fixed-step size Forward Euler implementations show considerable lags in the spike timing compared to the rkf45 reference implementation. While for the regular-spiking neuron **(A)** the SpiNNaker implementations have much the same accuracy, the fixed-step size Forward Euler approach with precise spike timing shows a substantial improvement over the ESR implementation for the fast-spiking neuron **(B)**.

The SpiNNaker $s16.15$ data type therefore ranges from $-2^{16} = -65536$ to $2^{16} - 2^{-15} = 65535.999969482$.

This data type does not saturate on SpiNNaker (Hopkins and Furber, 2015). This means that in case of a fixed-point overflow, the value wraps around producing a negative number. In neural network simulations this might be seen as spike artifacts, as demonstrated in **Figure 9**. Another aspect of fixed-point arithmetic and an additional source of numerical inaccuracy is that not every number can be accurately represented. For example: although small, the error in the $s16.15$ representation of the constant value 0.04 in Equation (1) induces a noticeable delay in the spike timing.
To represent a number in $si.f$, its value is shifted f bits to the left, i.e., multiplied by 2^f. For the constant value 0.04 in Equation (1) this yields:

$$0.04 \cdot 2^{15} = 1310.72_{(s16.15)}$$

The compiler stores the value as a 32-bit word while truncating the fraction:

$$0x0000051E$$

If the value is converted back, this leads to:

$$1310_{(s16.15)} \cdot 2^{-15} = 0.03997802$$

This loss in precision is significant. At the level of the dynamics of individual neurons, this difference is expressed in terms of delayed spike times. The following example may illustrate this: for the sake of simplicity we assume a membrane potential of $v(t_0) = -75$ mV while $u(t_0) = 0$ and $I(t_0) = 0$. The expected value for $v(t_1)$ in the Equation (1) is:

$$0.04 \cdot 75 \cdot 75 + 5 \cdot (-75) + 140 = -10.0000000$$

The same calculation in $s16.15$ leads to:

$$0.03997802 \cdot 75 \cdot 75 + 5 \cdot (-75) + 140 = -10.1236357$$

This slightly more negative value of $v(t)$ causes the threshold crossing to occur later and affects the dynamics on the network level.

The effect can be mitigated if critical calculations are performed with higher precision numbers, whereby the order of operations also plays a role. If, for example, the constant value 0.04 in Equation (1) is represented in $s8.23$, the numerical error can be reduced.

$$0.04 \cdot 2^{23} = 335544.32_{(s8.23)}$$

If the value which is truncated by the compiler is converted back, we then get:

$$335544_{(s8.23)} \cdot 2^{-23} = 0.039999962$$

If now the same calculation as in the beginning is performed, the result is significantly more precise.

$$0.039999962 \cdot 75 \cdot 75 + 5 \cdot (-75) + 140 = -10.00021375$$

The disadvantage, however, is the limited value range of the $s8.23$ representation which is:

$$-2^8 = -256 \quad \text{to} \quad 2^8 - 2^{-23} = 255.999999881$$

The simple fixed-step size symplectic Forward Euler method together with a precise threshold detection presented above ensures that values stay within limits. Furthermore, we point out that a $s8.23$ data type is not available on SpiNNaker, i.e., it is not supported by the ARM C compiler. To let the value $335544.32_{(s8.23)}$ appear as a $s16.15$ constant we can write:

$$335544.32_{(s16.15)} = 10.24 \cdot 2^{15}$$

In order to return to the original value, a right-shift operation of 8 bits is then required.

$$10.24 \cdot 2^{-8} = 0.04$$

In this context, the order in which the operations are carried out is also very important. For example, multiplying 10.24 with the power of two of the membrane potential may cause an overflow of the $s16.15$ data type. Combining all this leads to the following sequence of operations for the Equation (1).

$$\dot{v} = ((10.24 \cdot v) \cdot 0.00390625)) \cdot v + 5 \cdot v + 140 - u + I \quad (6)$$

In order to prevent the compiler from optimizing the code and perhaps arranging the operations in an inappropriate order, the critical calculations in the Equation (6) are placed in separate lines. This is shown as pseudo code in Listing 4. Note that suppressing optimization in this way works for the ARM C compiler, but can not be generalized. We verified this through an analysis of the generated assembler source code.

```
EVERY MILLISECOND:
{
  NEURON STATE UPDATE:
  {
    REPEAT 16 TIMES:
    {
      A = 10.24 * v
      A = A * 0.00390625
      A = A * v
      B = 5.0 * v + 140.0 - u + I

      v = v + 0.0625 * ( A + B )
      u = u + 0.0625 * a * ( b * v - u )

      IF( v >= 30.0 )
      {
        v = c
        u = u + d
        SET spikeEventHasOccurred
      }
    }
  }

  THRESHOLD DETECTION:
  {
    IF( spikeEventHasOccurred )
    {
      deliverSpikeEvent()
    }
  }
}
```

Listing 4 | SpiNNaker model: the same algorithm (given as pseudo code) as shown in Listing 3, but adds fixed-point conversion to the constant 0.04.

The above also applies to the Izhikevich neuron model parameters a and b which add an error to $u(t)$. Further, the example ignored that the state variables $v(t)$ and $u(t)$ are themselves fixed-point values that add numerical inaccuracy.

In the course of the implementation of the SpiNNaker Izhikevich neuron model, and the adaptations of the model during the verification and substantiation process, we added fixed-point data type conversion to all constant values involved in critical calculations, that is the constant value 0.04 in the Equation (1) and the neuron model parameters a and b.

To investigate the consequences of data type conversion for critical parameters on the accuracy of the solution of the dynamics, we simulated regular-spiking and fast-spiking Izhikevich neurons with and without fixed-point data type conversion, and compared the development of the membrane voltages to a Runge-Kutta-Fehlberg(4, 5) (rkf45) solver implementation of the GNU Scientific Library (GSL), thus, using the same verification method as before when choosing the integration scheme. The results are shown in **Figure 11**. For both neuron parameterizations, we achieved a substantial improvement in the spike timing. Compared to results for the regular-spiking neuron, in which the solver employing data type conversion is very close to the rkf45-reference, our implementation still lags behind the rkf45-reference for the fast-spiking neuron. This can be explained by the overshoot in $v(t)$ at threshold crossing, that, even if it is small, still exists, and propagates over time—and the more spikes emitted, the larger the error becomes.

3.4.2.3. *Substantiation*

As the C model was adapted during Iteration II, we can no longer speak of a *replication*. Therefore, before performing the model substantiation assessment, we needed to check whether the results of the modified model are compatible with the original, i.e., whether or not *result reproducibility* is preserved. We evaluated the development of polychronous groups in the modified C model using the analysis provided in Izhikevich (2006). We found that the number of polychronous groups was reduced by about 34%. Thus the network still shows the behavior reported in the original manuscript (Izhikevich, 2006), albeit in a weakened form. As it was demonstrated in Pauli et al. (2018) that the number of groups developed by the C model varies strongly with implementation details, including the solver algorithm of the neuron model, we consider this result to be within our acceptance criteria.

We then performed the model substantiation assessment as described in section 3.2 for the C and SpiNNaker models incorporating the refined neuron model implementations described above. Note that this included re-generating the reference data, due to the changes in the neuron model implementation.

The result of the network activity data analysis and its comparison is shown in the middle row of **Figure 7**. Our new ODE solver, implemented in both models, leads to a good match in the firing rates (FR) and the pairwise correlation coefficients (CC). We note, though, that the distributions are shifted from those expressed by the C implementation in Iteration I. The

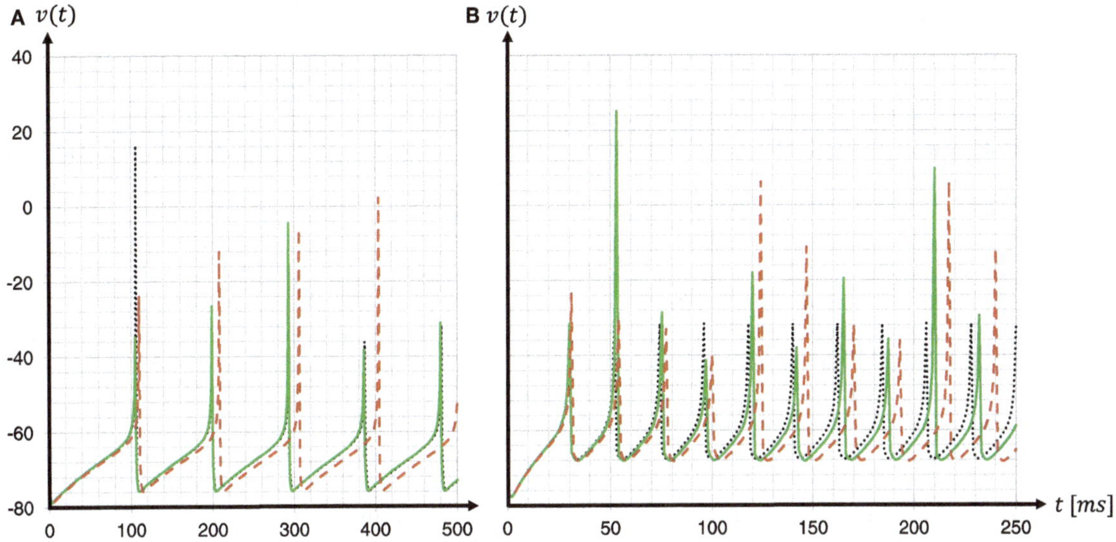

FIGURE 11 | Spike timing: with and without fixed-point data type conversion. The graphs show the development of the membrane voltages $v(t)$ with (green solid line) and without (red dashed line) fixed-point data type conversion for a regular-spiking type **(A)** and a fast-spiking type **(B)** Izhikevich neuron, that is stimulated with a constant current of $I_{ext} = 5pA$. For the ODE solver, the fixed-step size symplectic Forward Euler implementation with precise threshold detection was used ($h/16 = 0.0625$ ms). This is shown in comparison to a reference implementation of the GSL rkf45 ODE solver with an absolute integration error of 10^{-6} (black dotted line). For both neuron types, a substantial improvement in the spike timing can be seen.

shift of cross-correlation to lower values may well account for the smaller number of polychronous groups developed. Both the firing rates and the cross correlations also show small effect sizes after this iteration. In case of the CC distributions, the effect size has to be interpreted with care, as it assumes Gaussian-like distributions which is clearly violated by the bimodality of the CC distributions. Nevertheless, in combination with visual inspection and additional comparison measures, its application here provides a useful discrepancy quantification.

A discrepancy can still be seen between the distributions of the coefficients of variation (LV). The distribution for the SpiNNaker model is shifted toward lower values, indicating a higher degree of regularity than that of the C model. This is confirmed by the consistently high effect size obtained for the five reference network states. Therefore, we conclude that there is still a disagreement in the executable models, and that model substantiation assessment has not been achieved at the end of Iteration II.

3.4.3. Iteration III

The slight discrepancy in regularity observed in Iteration II allowed us to identify systematic differences in spike timing between the two models, hinting at an error in the numerical integration of the single neuron dynamics. Indeed, the visual comparison of the dynamics of individual neurons on SpiNNaker with a stand-alone C application that implements an identical fixed-step size symplectic Forward Euler ODE solver, revealed a small discrepancy in the sub-threshold dynamics, leading to a fixed delay in the spike timing. We identified an issue in the precise threshold detection algorithm as to be the cause.

3.4.3.1. Substantiation

The result that we achieved after resolving the issue and repeating the SpiNNaker simulations is shown in the bottom row of **Figure 7**. We observe a close match of all three distributions, consistently across the five reference network states. The comparison is not perfect, with the distribution of firing rates showing the largest discrepancy with only a subtle shift toward higher firing rates for the SpiNNaker simulation. The small discrepancies between the two implementations are quantified by the effect size, and demonstrate that we have achieved a considerable reduction of the mismatch as a result of the model verification and substantiation process. All effect sizes are classified in the range of small to medium according to Cohen (1988). While further iterations of the model implementation in the verification and substantiation process (see section 4 for suggestions) may further improve the effect size scores, for our purposes, we find the remaining mismatch in the range of acceptable agreement. We therefore conclude that the executable models are in close agreement at the end of Iteration III.

4. DISCUSSION

In this study, we introduced the concept of model verification and substantiation. In conjunction with the work presented in Gutzen et al. (2018), we demonstrated the application of a rigorous workflow assessing the level of agreement between the C implementation of the spiking network model proposed by Izhikevich (2006) and a reproduction of its underlying mathematical model on the SpiNNaker neuromorphic system. The choice of this network was motivated by its unorthodox implementation choices, examined in greater detail in Pauli et al.

(2018). These issues make it a particularly illustrative example for a reproduction on the SpiNNaker neuromorphic system and to demonstrate various aspects of source code and calculation verification.

After three iterations of the proposed workflow we concluded, on the basis of the substantiation assessment, that the executable models are in acceptable agreement. This conclusion is predicated on the domain of application and the expected level of agreement that we defined for three characteristic measures of the network activity. We emphasize that these definitions are set by the researcher: further iterations would be necessary, if, for example, we set a level of agreement requiring a spike-by-spike reproduction of the network activity data, as applied by Pauli et al. (2018).

We speculate that the remaining mismatch in the statistical measures at the end of Iteration III can be explained by the reduced precision in the representation of the synaptic weights on the SpiNNaker system. This source of error is introduced by the conversion of the double precision weight matrix exported from the C model and converted into a fixed-point representation when imported into the simulation on the SpiNNaker system. The absolute values of the synaptic weights after conversion are always smaller than its double origin, thus, negative weights increase, contributing to larger firing rates on SpiNNaker (see Iteration III in **Figure 7**). Another potential source of error, in terms of calculation verification, is related to the grid based simulation paradigm, i.e., the simulation time-step, with which spike events are delivered. Both the original C model implementation and the SpiNNaker system use a simulation time-step of 1 ms, which is larger than commonly used in spiking neural network simulations. Since both models are affected, the substantiation assessment can not give us further insight.

Although some of the verification tasks we applied, such as functional testing, are closely tied to model implementation details, the methodology presented in this work is transferable to similar modeling tasks, and could be further automated. The quantitative comparison of the statistical measures carried out in the substantiation was performed using the modular framework NetworkUnit[12] (NetworkUnit, RRID:SCR_016543), an open source Python module, presented in the companion study to this work (Gutzen et al., 2018). NetworkUnit facilitates the formalized application of standardized statistical test metrics that enable the quantitative validation of network models on the level of the population dynamics.

The model substantiation methodology we propose has a number of advantages. Firstly, from the point of view of computational neuroscience, simulation results should be independent of the hardware, at least on the level of statistical equivalence. In practice, implementations may be sensitive to issues such as 32/64-bit architecture or compiler versions. Thus, the underlying hardware used to simulate a model should be considered part of the model implementation. Applying our proposed model substantiation methodology allows a researcher an opportunity to discover and correct such weaknesses in the implementation. Secondly, in the case of new types of hardware, such as neuromorphic systems, the methodology used here can help to build confidence and uncover shortcomings. In the particular example investigated here, we were able to demonstrate that the numerical precision is a critical issue for the model's accuracy. Integrating the model dynamics at 1 ms resolution using 32-bit fixed-point arithmetic available on SpiNNaker (Furber et al., 2013) does not adequately reproduce the dynamics of the corresponding C model with floating point arithmetic. We propose an alternative integration strategy that does adequately reproduce the dynamics, but the more general point is that this study demonstrates how the use of a rigorous model substantiation methodology can contribute to fundamental open questions in neuromorphic computing, such as the required level of precision in the representation of variables. Finally, in neuroscience, models often function as discovery tools and hypothesis generators in cases where experimental data, against which a model could be validated, does not exist. Performing a substantiation assessment is an option to accumulate circumstantial evidence for a model's plausibility and self-consistency, although it cannot reveal whether a model reflects reality.

Beyond our introduction of the term *substantiation*, we have adopted the ACM (Association for Computing Machinery, 2016) terminology for reproducibility and replicability, as it seems most appropriate for our purposes. Alternative definitions exist, and terminology for research reproducibility is an ongoing theme of a controversial debate. The application of methodologies from model verification and validation (Thacker et al., 2004) to the field of neural network modeling and simulation can be of great value, but we have suggested some adaptations that, in our view, fit the domain better. In particular, the terms *mathematical model* and *executable model*, that we propose instead of using the terms *conceptual model* and *computerized model*, are intended to yield better separation of the entities they describe, so that, for example, implementation details are not falsely understood to belong to the mathematical model. This is important, as the classic "one model—one code" relationship does not typically apply to spiking neuron network models. Instead, they are implemented using general purpose neural simulation tools such as NEURON (Hines and Carnevale, 1997), Brian (Goodman and Brette, 2008), or NEST (Gewaltig and Diesmann, 2007), which can run many different models. In addition, model simulation codes may be partially generated by other tools (Blundell et al., 2018a). This scenario abstracts the implementation details away from the modeler, who can focus on analysis and modeling, and has the further advantage that individual components (such as neuron models) can be separately verified, and may subsequently serve as reliable references. We hope that our proposed terminology will help to pave the way to a more formalized approach for model verification and validation in the domain of neural network simulation.

In this study, we applied a number of standard methods from software engineering. This discipline is concerned with the application of a systematic, disciplined, quantifiable approach to the development, operation, and maintenance of software (Bourque and Fairley, 2014). Such methods include, for example, the application of clean code heuristics, test driven development,

[12]https://github.com/INM-6/NetworkUnit

continuous integration and agile development methodologies, with the common goal of building quality into software. The formalized model verification and substantiation workflow that we presented in this work should be seen in this context.

We note that software engineering methods, whilst critical for developing high quality software, are underutilized in computational science in general, and in computational neuroscience in particular. For the network model investigated here, it is important to emphasize that the awareness of software engineering methodology was even less widespread at the time of publication, and so the yardsticks for source code quality applicable by today's standards should be considered in their temporal distance. Credit must in any case be given for the unusual step of publishing the source code, allowing scientific transparency and making studies such as the current one, and that of Pauli et al. (2018), possible. Following formalized processes, such as the one described here, further aids transparency and comprehensibility, and reduces the risk of incorrect conclusions. Moreover, simulation tools as well as neuromorphic hardware platforms can benefit from formalized and automated verification and validation procedures, such that their reliability can be inherited by user-developed models that are simulated using those tools and frameworks. Most importantly, such standardized procedures are designed not to place an additional burden on researchers, but rather to open up simple avenues for computational neuroscientists to increase the rigor and reproducibility of their models.

In conclusion, we argue that the methods of software engineering, including the model verification and substantiation workflow presented here, as well as verification and validation methodologies in general, need to become a mainstream aspect of computational neuroscience. Simulation and analysis tools, frameworks and collaboration platforms are part of the research infrastructure on which scientists base their work, and thus should meet high software development standards. The consideration of the application of software engineering methodologies to scientific software development should start at the funding level, such that an assessment of the software engineering strategy is part of the evaluation of grant applications. Likewise, journals should become more selective with their acceptance of studies, and reject those for which no demonstration has been made of an attempt to verify the calculations. The use of standard tools goes a significant way to fulfilling this criterion, to the extent that the standard tools themselves are developed with a rigorous testing and verification methodology.

AUTHOR CONTRIBUTIONS

GT devised the project, the main conceptual ideas and workflows. GT performed the verification tasks, the implementation of the models and their refinement, and performed the numerical simulations. RG and MD designed the statistical analysis which was then carried out by RG. RG and MD have written the passage on analysis of spiking activity and contributed to the terminology section. IB contributed expertise on numeric integration. AM gave scientific and theoretical guidance. GT, RG, MD, and AM established the terminology. All authors provided critical feedback and helped shape the research, analysis, and manuscript.

FUNDING

This work was supported by the Helmholtz Association through the Helmholtz Portfolio Theme Supercomputing and Modeling for the Human Brain and the Initiative and Networking Fund, also by the European Union's Horizon 2020 Framework Program for Research and Innovation under Grant Agreement No. 720270 (Human Brain Project SGA1) and 785907 (Human Brain Project SGA2).

ACKNOWLEDGMENTS

We are greatful to Dimitri Plotnikov, Sandra Diaz, Alexander Peyser, Jochen Martin Eppler, Sonja Grün, Michael von Papen, Pietro Quaglio, Robin Pauli, and Philipp Weidel for the fruitful discussions throughout the project. We would especially like to thank Fahad Kahlid for his comments on an earlier version of the manuscript, and to our colleagues in the Simulation Lab Neuroscience for continuous collaboration.

REFERENCES

Association for Computing Machinery (2016). *Artifact Review and Badging*. Available online at: https://www.acm.org/publications/policies/artifact-review-badging(Accessed March 14, 2018).

Barba, L. A. (2018). Terminologies for reproducible research. *arXiv [Preprint]:1802.03311.*

Benureau, F. C. Y., and Rougier, N. P. (2017). Re-run, repeat, reproduce, reuse, replicate: transforming code into scientific contributions. *Front. Neuroinform.* 11:69. doi: 10.3389/fninf.2017.00069

Blundell, I., Brette, R., Cleland, T. A., Close, T. G., Coca, D., Davison, A. P., et al. (2018a). Code generation in computational neuroscience: a review of tools and techniques. *Front. Neuroinform.* 12:68. doi: 10.3389/fninf.2018.00068

Blundell, I., Plotnikov, D., Eppler, J., and Morrison, A. (2018b). Automatically selecting a suitable integration scheme for systems of differential equations in neuron models. *Front. Neuroinform.* 12:50. doi: 10.3389/fninf.2018.00050

Bourque, P., and Fairley, R. E., (eds.). (2014). *SWEBOK: Guide to the Software Engineering Body of Knowledge.* Los Alamitos, CA: IEEE Computer Society.

Cohen, J. (1988). *Statistical Power Analysis for the Behavioral Sciences.* New York, NY: Lawrence Erlbaum Associates.

Dahmen, W., and Reusken, A. (2005). *Numerik für Naturwissenschaftler.* Berlin; Heidelberg: Springer.

Davison, A., Brüderle, D., Eppler, J., Kremkow, J., Muller, E., Pecevski, D., et al. (2009). Pynn: a common interface for neuronal network simulators. *Front. Neuroinform.* 2:11. doi: 10.3389/neuro.11.011.2008

Furber, S. B., Lester, D. R., Plana, L. A., Garside, J. D., Painkras, E., Temple, S., et al. (2013). Overview of the spinnaker system architecture. *IEEE Trans. Comput.* 62, 2454–2467. doi: 10.1109/TC.2012.142

Gewaltig, M.-O., and Diesmann, M. (2007). NEST (NEural Simulation Tool). *Scholarpedia* 2:1430. doi: 10.4249/scholarpedia.1430

Goodman, D., and Brette, R. (2008). Brian: a simulator for spiking neural networks in python. *Front. Neuroinform.* 2:5. doi: 10.3389/neuro.11.005.2008

Goodman, S. N., Fanelli, D., and Ioannidis, J. P. A. (2016). What does research reproducibility mean? *Sci. Transl. Med.* 8:341ps12. doi: 10.1126/scitranslmed.aaf5027

Gutzen, R., von Papen, M., Trensch, G., Quaglio, P., Grün, S., and Denker, M. (2018). Reproducible neural network simulations: statistical methods for model validation on the level of network activity data. *Front. Neuroinform.* 12:90. doi: 10.3389/fninf.2018.00090

Hines, M. L., and Carnevale, N. T. (1997). The NEURON simulation environment. *Neural Comput.* 9, 1179–1209. doi: 10.1162/neco.1997.9.6.1179

Hopkins, M., and Furber, S. (2015). Accuracy and efficiency in fixed-point neural ode solvers. *Neural Comput.* 27, 2148–2182. doi: 10.1162/NECO_a_00772

Izhikevich, E. M. (2003). Simple model of spiking neurons. *IEEE Trans. Neural Netw.* 14, 1569–1572. doi: 10.1109/TNN.2003.820440

Izhikevich, E. M. (2006). Polychronization: computation with spikes. *Neural Comput.* 18, 245–282. doi: 10.1162/089976606775093882

Lambert, J. D. (1992). *Numerical Methods for Ordinary Differential Systems.* New York, NY: Wiley.

Martin, R. C., and Coplien, J. O. (2009). *Clean Code: A Handbook of Agile Software Craftsmanship.* Upper Saddle River, NJ: Prentice Hall.

Martis, M. S. (2006). Validation of simulation based models: a theoretical outlook. *Electron. J. Bus. Res. Methods* 4, 39–46.

Patil, P., Peng, R. D., and Leek, J. (2016). A statistical definition for reproducibility and replicability. *bioRxiv [Preprint].* doi: 10.1101/066803

Pauli, R., Weidel, P., Kunkel, S., and Morrison, A. (2018). Reproducing polychronization: a guide to maximizing the reproducibility of spiking network models. *Front. Neuroinform.* 12:46. doi: 10.3389/fninf.2018.00046

Plesser, H. E. (2018). Reproducibility vs. replicability: a brief history of a confused terminology. *Front. Neuroinform.* 11:76. doi: 10.3389/fninf.2017.00076

Rowley, A. G. D., Stokes, A. B., and Gait, A. D. (2017a). *Spinnaker New Model Template Lab Manual.* Manchester. Available online at: https://github.com/SpiNNakerManchester/SpiNNakerManchester.github.io/blob/master/spynnaker/4.0.0/NewNeuronModels-LabManual.pdf (Accessed March 14, 2018).

Rowley, A. G. D., Stokes, A. B., Knight, J., Lester, D. R., Hopkins, M., Davies, S., et al. (2017b). *PyNN on SpiNNaker Software 4.0.0.* doi: 10.5281/zenodo.1255864

Schlesinger, S., Crosbie, R. E., Gagn, R. E., Innes, G. S., Lalwani, C., Loch, J., et al. (1979). Terminology for model credibility. *Simulation* 32, 103–104.

Shinomoto, S., Shima, K., and Tanji, J. (2003). Differences in spiking patterns among cortical neurons. *Neural Comput.* 15, 2823–2842. doi: 10.1162/089976603322518759

Sommerville, I. (2015). *Software Engineering, 10th Edn.* Pearson Education.

Strehmel, K., and Weiner, R. (1995). *Numerik gewöhnlicher Differentialgleichungen.* Wiesbaden: B.G. Teubner.

Temple, S. (2011a). *AppNote 1 - SpiNN-3 Development Board.* Available online at: http://spinnakermanchester.github.io/docs/spinn-app-1.pdf (Accessed March 14, 2018).

Temple, S. (2011b). *AppNote 4 - SpiNNaker Datagram Protocol (SDP) Specification.* Available online at: http://spinnakermanchester.github.io/docs/spinn-app-4.pdf (Accessed March 14, 2018).

Thacker, B., Doebling, S., Hemez, F., Anderson, M., Pepin, J., and Rodriguez, E. (2004). *Concepts of Model Verification and Validation.* Los Alamos National Laboratory.

9

Re-run, Repeat, Reproduce, Reuse, Replicate: Transforming Code into Scientific Contributions

Fabien C. Y. Benureau[1,2,3*] *and Nicolas P. Rougier*[1,2,3]

[1] *INRIA Bordeaux Sud-Ouest, Talence, France,* [2] *Institut des Maladies Neurodégénératives, Université de Bordeaux, Centre National de la Recherche Scientifique UMR 5293, Bordeaux, France,* [3] *LaBRI, Université de Bordeaux, Bordeaux INP, Centre National de la Recherche Scientifique UMR 5800, Talence, France*

Correspondence:
Fabien C. Y. Benureau
fabien@benureau.com

Scientific code is different from production software. Scientific code, by producing results that are then analyzed and interpreted, participates in the elaboration of scientific conclusions. This imposes specific constraints on the code that are often overlooked in practice. We articulate, with a small example, five characteristics that a scientific code in computational science should possess: re-runnable, repeatable, reproducible, reusable, and replicable. The code should be executable (re-runnable) and produce the same result more than once (repeatable); it should allow an investigator to reobtain the published results (reproducible) while being easy to use, understand and modify (reusable), and it should act as an available reference for any ambiguity in the algorithmic descriptions of the article (replicable).

Keywords: replicability, reproducibility of results, reproducible science, reproducible research, computational science, software development, best practices

INTRODUCTION (R^0)

Replicability[1] is a cornerstone of science. If an experimental result cannot be re-obtained by an independent party, it merely becomes, at best, an observation that may inspire future research (Mesirov, 2010; Open Science Collaboration, 2015). Replication issues have received increased attention in recent years, with a particular focus on medicine and psychology (Iqbal et al., 2016). One could think that computational research would mostly be shielded from such issues, since a computer program describes precisely what it does and is easily disseminated to other researchers without alteration.

But precisely because it is easy to believe that if a program runs once and gives the expected results it will do so forever, crucial steps to transform working code into meaningful scientific contributions are rarely undertaken (Schwab et al., 2000; Sandve et al., 2013; Collberg and Proebsting, 2016). Computational research is plagued by replication problems, in part, because it seems impervious to them. Contrary to production software who provides a service geared toward a practical outcome, the motivation behind scientific code is to test a hypothesis. While in some instance production software and scientific code are indistinguishable, the reasons why they were created are different, and, therefore, so are the criteria to evaluate their success. A program

[1] *Reproducibility* and *replicability* are employed differently by different authors and in different domains (see for instance the report from the U.S. National Academies of Sciences, 2016). Here, we place ourselves in the context of computational works, where data is produced by a program. In this paper, we call a result *reproducible* if one can take the original source code, re-execute it and reobtain the original result. Conversely, a result is *replicable* if one can create a code that matches the algorithmic descriptions given in the published article and reobtain the original result.

can fail as a scientific contribution in many different ways for many different reasons. Borrowing the terms coined by Goble (2016), for a program to contribute to science, it should be re-runnable (R^1), repeatable (R^2), reproducible (R^3), reusable (R^4), and replicable (R^5). Let us illustrate this with a small example, a random walk (Hughes, 1995) written in Python:

LISTING 0: Random walk (R^0) raw code, archive

```
import random

x = 0
for i in xrange(10):
    step = random.choice([-1,+1])
    x += step
    print x,
```

In the code above, the `random.choice` function randomly returns either +1 or −1. The instruction "`for i in xrange(10):`" executes the next three indented lines ten times. Executed, this program would display:

Output

```
-1, 0, -1, 0, -1, 0, -1, 0, 1, 2
# with the steps being -1,+1,-1,+1,-1,+1,-1,+1,+1,+1
```

What could go wrong with such a simple program? Well...

RE-RUNNABLE (R^1)

Have you ever tried to re-run a program you wrote some years ago? It can often be frustratingly hard. Part of the problem is that technology is evolving at a fast pace and you cannot know in advance how the system, the software and the libraries your program depends on will evolve. Since you wrote the code, you may have reinstalled or upgraded your operating system. The compiler, interpreter or set of libraries installed may have been replaced with newer versions. You may find yourself battling with arcane issues of library compatibility—thoroughly orthogonal to your immediate research goals—to execute again a code *that worked perfectly before*. To be clear, it is impossible to write future-proof code, and the best efforts can be stymied by the smallest change in one of the dependencies. At the same time, modernizing an unmaintained ten-year-old code can reveal itself to be an arduous and expensive undertaking—and precarious, since each change risks affecting the semantics of the program. Rather than trying to predict the future or painstakingly dusting off old code, an often more straightforward solution is to recreate the old execution environment[2]. For this to happen however, the dependencies in terms of systems, software, and libraries must be made clear enough.

[2]To be clear, and although virtual machines are often a great help here, this is not always possible. It is, however, *always* more difficult when the original execution environment is unknown.

A *re-runnable* code is one that can be run again when needed, and in particular more than the one time that was needed to produce the results. It is important to notice that the re-runnability of a code is not an intrinsic property. Rather, it depends on the context, and becomes increasingly difficult as the code ages. Therefore, to be and remain re-runnable on the computers of other researchers, a re-runnable code should describe—with enough details to be recreated—an execution environment in which it is executable. As shown by Collberg and Proebsting (2016), this is far from being either obvious or easy.

LISTING 1: Re-runnable random walk (R^1) raw code, archive

```
# Tested with Python 3
import random

x = 0
walk = []
for i in range(10):
    step = random.choice([-1,+1])
    x += step
    walk.append(x)

print(walk)
```

In our case, the R^0 version of our tiny walker seems to imply that any version of Python would be fine. This not the case: it uses the print *instruction* and the `xrange` operator, both specific to Python 2. The print *instruction*, available in Python 2 (a version still widely used; support is scheduled to stop in 2020), has been deprecated in Python 3 (first released in 2008, almost a decade ago) in favor of a print *function*, while the `xrange` operator has been replaced by the `range` operator in Python 3. In order to try to future-proof the code a bit, we might as well target Python 3, as is done in the R^1 version. Incidentally, it remains compatible with Python 2. But whichever version is chosen, the crucial step here is to document it.

REPEATABLE (R^2)

The code is running and producing the expected results. The next step is to make sure that you can produce the same output over successive runs of your program. In other words, the next step is to make your program deterministic, producing *repeatable* output. Repeatability is valuable. If a run of the program produces a particularly puzzling result, repeatability allows you to scrutinize any step of the execution of the program by re-running it again with extraneous prints, or inside a debugger. Repeatability is also useful to prove that the program did indeed produce the published results. Repeatability is not always possible or easy (Diethelm, 2012; Courtès and Wurmus, 2015). But for sequential and deterministically parallel programs (Hines, and Carnevale, 2008; Collange et al., 2015) not depending on analog inputs, it often comes down to controlling the initialization of the pseudo-random number generators (RNG).

For our program, that means setting the seed of the `random` module. We may also want to save the output of the program to a file, so that we can easily verify that consecutive runs do produce the same output: eyeballing differences is unreliable and time-consuming, and therefore won't be done systematically.

LISTING 2: Re-runnable, repeatable random walk (R^2) raw code, archive

```
# Tested with Python 3
import random

random.seed(1) # RNG initialization

x = 0
walk = []
for i in range(10):
    step = random.choice([-1,+1])
    x += step
    walk.append(x)

print(walk)
# Saving output to disk
with open('results-R2.txt', 'w') as fd:
    fd.write(str(walk))
```

Setting seeds should be done carefully. Using 439 as a seed in the previous program would result in ten consecutive +1 steps[3], which—although a perfectly valid random walk—lend itself to a gross misinterpretation of the overall dynamics of the algorithm. Verifying that the qualitative aspects of the results and the conclusions that are made are not tied to a specific initialization of the pseudo-random generator is an integral part of any scientific undertaking in computational science; this is usually done by repeating the simulations multiple times with different seeds.

REPRODUCIBLE (R^3)

The R^2 code seems fine enough, but it hides several problems that come to light when trying to *reproduce* results. A result is said to be *reproducible* if another researcher can take the original code and input data, execute it, and re-obtain the same result (Peng et al., 2006). As explained by Donoho et al. (2009), scientific practice must expect that *errors are ubiquitous*, and therefore be robust to them. Ensuring reproducibility is a fundamental step toward this: it provides other researchers the means to verify that the code does indeed produce the published results, and to scrutinize the procedures it employed to produce them. As demonstrated by Mesnard and Barba (2017), reproducibility is hard.

For instance, the R^2 program will not produce the same results all the time. It will, because it is repeatable, produce the same results over repeated executions. But it will not necessarily do so over different execution environments. The cause is to be found in a change that occurred in the pseudo-random number generator between Python 3.2 and Python 3.3. Executed with Python 2.7–3.2, the code will produce the sequence −1, 0, 1, 0, −1, −2, −1, 0, −1, −2. But with Python 3.3–3.6, it will produce −1, −2, −1, −2, −1, 0, 1, 2, 1, 0. With future versions of the language, it may change still. For the R^3 version, we abandon the use of the `random.choice` function in favor of the `random.uniform` function, whose behavior is consistent across versions 2.7–3.6 of Python.

Because any dependency of a program—to the most basic one, the language itself—can change its behavior from one version to the other, executability (R^1) and determinism (R^2) are necessary but not sufficient for reproducibility. The exact execution environment used to produce the results must also be specified—rather than the broadest set of environments where the code can be effectively run. In other words, assertions such as "the results were obtained with CPython 3.6.1" are more valuable, in a scientific context, than "the program works with Python 3.x and above". With the increasing complexity of computational stacks, retrieving, and deciding what is pertinent (CPU architecture? operating system version? endianness?) might be non-trivial. A good rule of thumb is to include more information than necessary rather than not enough, and some rather than none.

Recording the execution environment is only the first step. The R^2 program uses a random seed but does not keep a trace of it except in the code. Should the code change after the production of the results, someone provided with the last version of the code will not be able to know which seed was used to produce the results, and would need to iterate through all possible random seeds, an impossible task in practice[4].

This is why result files should come alongside their context, i.e., an exhaustive list of the parameters used as well as a precise description of the execution environment, as the R^3 code does. The code itself is part of that context: the version of the code must be recorded. It is common for different results or different figures to have been generated by different versions of the code. Ideally, all results should originate from the same (and last) version of the code. But for long or expensive computations, this may not be feasible. In that case, the result files should contain the version of the code that was used to produce it. This information can be obtained from the version control software. This also allows, if some errors are found and corrected after some results have been obtained, to identify which ones should be recomputed. In R^3, the code records the git revision, and prevents execution if the repository holds uncommitted changes when the computation starts.

Published results should obviously come from versions of the code where every change and every file has been committed. This includes pre-processing, post-processing, and plotting code. Plotting code may seem mundane, but it is as vulnerable as any other piece of the code to bugs and errors. When it comes to checking that the reproduced data match the one published in the article, however, figures can reveal themselves to be imprecise and cumbersome, and sometimes plain unusable. To avoid having to manually overlay pixelated plots, published figures should be accompanied by their underlying data (coordinates of the plotted

[3]With CPython 3.3–3.6. See the next section for details.

[4]Here, with 2^{10} possibilities for a 10-step random walk, the seed used or another matching the generated sequence could certainly be found. For instance, 436 is the smallest positive integer seed to reproduce the results of R^0 with Python 2.7 (1,151, 3,800, 4,717 or 11,235,813 work as well). Such a search becomes intractable for a 100-step walk.

LISTING 3: Re-runnable, repeatable, reproducible random walk (R^3)
raw code, archive

```
# Copyright (c) 2017 N.P. Rougier and F.C.Y. Benureau
# Release under the BSD 2-clause license
# Tested with 64-bit CPython 3.6.2 / macOS 10.12.6
import sys, subprocess, datetime, random

def compute_walk():
    x = 0
    walk = []
    for i in range(10):
        if random.uniform(-1, +1) > 0:
            x += 1
        else:
            x -= 1
        walk.append(x)
    return walk

# If repository is dirty, don't run anything
if subprocess.call(("git", "diff-index",
                    "--quiet", "HEAD")):
    print("Repository is dirty, please commit first")
    sys.exit(1)

# Get git hash if any
hash_cmd = ("git", "rev-parse", "HEAD")
revision = subprocess.check_output(hash_cmd)

# Unit test
random.seed(42)
assert compute_walk() == [1,0,-1,-2,-1,0,1,0,-1,-2]

# Random walk for 10 steps
seed = 1
random.seed(seed)
walk = compute_walk()

# Display & save results
print(walk)
results = {
    "data"     : walk,
    "seed"     : seed,
    "timestamp": str(datetime.datetime.utcnow()),
    "revision" : revision,
    "system"   : sys.version}
with open("results-R3.txt", "w") as fd:
    fd.write(str(results))
```

points) in the supplementary data to allow straightforward numeric comparisons.

Another good practice is to make the code self-verifiable. In R^3, a short unit test is provided, that allows the code to verify its own reproducibility. Should this test fail, then there is little hope of reproducing the results. Of course, passing the test does not guarantee anything.

It is obvious that *reproducibility implies availability*. As shown in Collberg and Proebsting (2016), code is often unavailable, or only available upon request. While the latter may seem sufficient, changes in email address, changes in career, retirement, a busy inbox or poor archiving practices can make a code just as unreachable. Code *and* input data *and* result data should be available with the published article, as supplementary data, or through a DOI link to a scientific repository such as Figshare, Zenodo[5] or a domain specific database, such as ModelDB for computational neuroscience. The codes presented in this article are available in the GitHub repository github.com/rougier/random-walk and at doi.org/10.5281/zenodo.848217.

To recap, reproducibility implies re-runnability and repeatability and availability, yet imposes additional conditions. Dependencies and platforms must be described as precisely and as specifically as possible. Parameters values, the version of the code, and inputs should accompany the result files. The data and scripts behind the graphs must be published. Unit tests are a good way to embed self-diagnostics of reproducibility in the code. Reproducibility is hard, yet tremendously necessary.

REUSABLE (R^4)

Making your program reusable means it can be easily used, and modified, by you and other people, inside and outside your lab. Ensuring your program is reusable is advantageous for a number of reasons.

For you, first. Because the you now and the you in 2 years are two different persons. Details on how to use the code, its limitations, its quirks, may be present to your mind now, but will probably escape you in 6 months (Donoho et al., 2009). Here, comments and documentation can make a significant difference. Source code reflects the results of the decisions that were made during its creation, but not the reasons behind those decisions. In science, where the method and its justification matter as much as the results, those reasons are precious knowledge. In that context, a comment on how a given parameter was chosen (optimization, experimental data, educated guess), why a library was chosen over another (conceptual or technical reasons?) is valuable information.

Reusability of course directly benefits other researchers from your team and outside of it. The easier it is to use your code, the lower the threshold is for other to study, modify and extend it. Scientists constantly face the constraint of time: if a model is available, documented, and can be installed, run, and understood all in a few hours, it will be preferred over another that would require weeks to reach the same stage. A reproducible and reusable code offers a platform both *verifiable* and easy-to-use, fostering the development of derivative works by other researchers on solid foundations. Those derivative works contribute to the impact of your original contribution.

Having more people examining and using your code also means that potential errors have a higher chance to be caught. If people start using your program, they will most likely report bugs or malfunctions they encounter. If you're lucky enough, they might even propose either bug fixes or improvements, hence improving the overall quality of your software. This process contributes to the long-term reproducibility to the extent people continue to use and maintain the program.

[5]Online code repositories such as GitHub *are not* scientific repositories, and may disappear, change name, or change their access policy at any moment. Direct links to them are not perpetual, and, when used, they should always be supplemented by a DOI link to a scientific archive.

LISTING 4: Re-runnable, repeatable, reproducible, reusable random walk (R^4)
raw code, archive

```
# Copyright (c) 2017 N.P. Rougier and F.C.Y. Benureau
# Release under the BSD 2-clause license
# Tested with 64-bit CPython 3.6.2 / macOS 10.12.6
import sys, subprocess, datetime, random

def compute_walk(count, x0=0, step=1, seed=0):
    """Random walk
        count: number of steps
        x0   : initial position (default 0)
        step : step size (default 1)
        seed : seed for the initialization of the
            random generator (default 0)
    """
    random.seed(seed)
    x = x0
    walk = []
    for i in range(count):
        if random.uniform(-1, +1) > 0:
            x += 1
        else:
            x -= 1
        walk.append(x)
    return walk

def compute_results(count, x0=0, step=1, seed=0):
    """Compute a walk and return it with context"""
    # If repository is dirty, don't do anything
    if subprocess.call(("git", "diff-index",
                        "--quiet", "HEAD")):
        print("Repository is dirty, please commit")
        sys.exit(1)

    # Get git hash if any
    hash_cmd = ("git", "rev-parse", "HEAD")
    revision = subprocess.check_output(hash_cmd)

    # Compute results
    walk = compute_walk(count=count, x0=x0,
                        step=step, seed=seed)
    return {
        "data"       : walk,
        "parameters": {"count": count, "x0": x0,
                       "step": step, "seed": seed},
        "timestamp"  : str(datetime.datetime.utcnow()),
        "revision"   : revision,
        "system"     : sys.version}

if __name__ == "__main__":
    # Unit test checking reproducibility
    # (will fail with Python<=3.2)
    assert (compute_walk(10, 0, 1, 42) ==
            [1,0,-1,-2,-1,0,1,0,-1,-2])

    # Simulation parameters
    count, x0, seed = 10, 0, 1
    results = compute_results(count, x0=x0, seed=seed)

    # Save & display results
    with open("results-R4.txt", "w") as fd:
        fd.write(str(results))
    print(results["data"])
```

Despite all this, reusability is often overlooked, and it is not hard to see why. Scientists are rarely trained in software engineering, and reusability can represent an expensive endeavor if undertaken as an afterthought, for little tangible short-term benefits, for a codebase that might, after all, only see a single use. And, in fact, reusability is not as indispensable a requirement as re-runnability, repeatability, and reproducibility. Yet, some simple measures can tremendously increase reusability, and at the same time strengthen reproducibility and re-runnability over the long-term.

Avoid hardcoded or magic numbers. Magic numbers are numbers present directly in the source code, that do not have a name and therefore can be difficult to interpret semantically. Hardcoded values are variables that cannot be changed through a function argument or a parameter configuration file. To be modified, they involve editing the code, which is cumbersome and error-prone. In the R^3 code, the seed and the number of steps are respectively hardcoded and magic.

Similarly, code behavior should not be changed by commenting/uncommenting code (Wilson et al., 2017). Modification of the behavior of the code, required when different experiments examine slightly different conditions, should always be explicitly set through parameters accessible to the end-user. This improves reproducibility in two ways: it allows those conditions to be recorded as parameters in the result files, and it allows to define separate scripts to run or configuration files to load to produce each of the figures of the published paper. With documentation explaining which script or configuration file corresponds to which experiment, reproducing the different figures becomes straightforward.

Documentation is one of the most potent tools for reusability. A proper documentation on how to install and run the software often makes the difference whether other researchers manage to use it or not. A comment describing what each function does, however evident, can avoid hours of head-scratching. Great code may need few comments. Scientists, however, are not always brilliant developers. Of course, bad, complicated code should be rewritten until is simple enough to explain itself. But realistically, this is not always going to be done: there is simply not enough incentive for it. There, a comment that explains the intentions and reasons behind a block of code can be tremendously useful.

Reusability is not a strict requirement for scientific code. But it has many benefits, and a few simple measures can foster it considerably. To complement the R^4 version provided here, we provide an example repository of a re-runnable, repeatable, reproducible and reusable random walk code.

REPLICABLE (R^5)

Having made a software reusable offers an additional way to find errors, especially if your scientific contribution is popular. Unfortunately, this is not always effective, and some recent cases have shown that bugs can lurk in well-used open-source code, impacting the false positive rates of fMRI studies (Eklund et al., 2016), or the encryption of communications over the Internet (Durumeric et al., 2014). Let's be clear: the goal here is not to remove all bugs and mistakes from science. The goal is to have methods and practices in place that make possible for the inevitable errors that will be made to be caught and corrected by motivated investigators. This is why, as explained by Peng et al. (2006), *the replication of important findings by multiple independent investigators is fundamental to the accumulation of scientific evidence.*

Replicability is the implicit assumption that an article that does not provide the source code makes: that the description it provides of the algorithms is sufficiently precise and complete to re-obtain the results it presents. Here, replicating implies writing a new code matching the conceptual description of the article, in order to reobtain the same results. Replication affords robustness to the results because, should the original code contain an error, a different codebase creates the possibility that this error will not be repeated, in the same way that replicating a laboratory experiment in a different laboratory can ferret out subtle biases. While every published article should strive for replicability, it is seldom obtained. In fact, absent an explicit effort to make an algorithmic description replicable, there is little probability that it will be.

This is because most papers strive to communicate the main ideas behind their contribution in terms as simple and as clear as possible, so that the reader may be able to easily understand them. Trying to ensure replicability in the main text adds a myriad of esoteric details that are not conceptually significant and clutter the explanations. Therefore, unless the writer dedicates an addendum or a section of the supplementary information for technical details specifically aimed at replicability, the information will not be there because clarity and concision represent enticing incentives not to do so.

But even when those details are present, the best efforts may fall short because an oversight, a typo or a difference between what is evident for the writer and for the reader (Mesnard and Barba, 2017). Minute changes in the numerical estimation of a common first-order differential equation can have significant impact (Crook et al., 2013). Hence, a reproducible code plays an important role alongside its article: it is a objective catalog of all the implementation details.

A researcher seeking to replicate published results might first consider only the article. If she fails to replicate the results, she will consult the original code, and with it be able to pinpoint why her code and the code of the authors differ in behavior. Because a mistake on their part? Hers? Or a difference in a seemingly innocuous implementation detail? A fine analysis of why a particular algorithmic description is lacking or ambiguous or why a minor implementation decision is in fact crucial to obtain the published results is of great scientific value. Such an analysis can only be done with access to both the article and the code. With only the article, the researcher will often be unable to understand why she failed to replicate the results, and will naturally be inclined to only report replication successes.

Replicability, therefore, does not negate the necessity of reproducibility. In fact, it often relies on it. To illustrate this, let us consider what could be the description of the random walker, as it would be written in an article describing it:

> *The model uses the Mersene Twister generator initialized with the seed 1. At each iteration, a uniform number between −1 (included) and +1 (excluded) is drawn and the sign of the result is used for generating a positive or negative step.*

This description, while somewhat precise, forgoes—as it is common—the initialization of the variables (here the starting value of the walk: 0), and the technical details about which implementation of the RNG is used.

It may look innocuous. After all, the Python documentation, states that "Python uses the Mersenne Twister as the core generator. It produces 53-bit precision floats and has a period of 2**19937-1". Someone trying to replicate the work however might choose to use the RNG from the NumPy library. The NumPy library is extensively used in the science community, and it provides an implementation of the Mersene Twister generator too. Unfortunately, the way the seed is interpreted by the two implementations is different, yielding different random sequences.

LISTING 5: Replicated random walk (R^5) raw code, archive

```
# Copyright (c) 2017 N.P. Rougier and F.C.Y. Benureau
# Release under the BSD 2-clause license
# 64-bit CPython 3.6.2 / NumPy 1.12.0 / macOS 10.12.6
import random
import numpy as np

def _rng(seed):
    """Return a numpy random number generator
       initialized with seed as it would be with
       a python random generator.
    """
    rng = random.Random()
    rng.seed(seed)
    _, keys, _ = rng.getstate()
    rng = np.random.RandomState()
    state = rng.get_state()
    rng.set_state((state[0], keys[:-1], state[2],
                   state[3], state[4]))
    return rng

def walk(n, seed):
    """Random walk for n steps"""
    rng = _rng(seed)
    steps = 2 * (rng.uniform(-1, +1, n) > 0) - 1
    return steps.cumsum().tolist()

if __name__ == "__main__":
    # Unit test
    assert (walk(n=10, seed=42) ==
            [1,0,-1,-2,-1,0,1,0,-1,-2])

    # Random walk for 10 steps, with seed=1
    seed = 1
    path = walk(n=10, seed=seed)

    # Save & display results
    results = {"data": path, "seed": seed}
    with open("results-R5.txt", "w") as fd:
        fd.write(str(results))
    print(path)
```

Here we are able to replicate exactly[6] the behavior of the pure-Python random walker by setting the internal state of the NumPy RNG appropriately, but only because we have access to specific technical details of the original code (the use of the `random` module of the standard Python library of CPython 3.6.1), or to the code itself.

But there are still more subtle problems with the description given above. If we look more closely at it, we can realize that nothing is said about the specific case of `0` when generating a step. Do we have to consider `0` to be a positive or a negative step? Without further information and without the original code, it is up to the reader to decide. Likewise, the description is ambiguous regarding the first element of the walk. Is the initialization value included (it was not in our codes so far)? This slight difference might affect the statistics of short runs.

All these ambiguities in the description of an algorithm pile up; some are inconsequential (the `0` case has null probability), but some may affect the results in important ways. They are mostly inconspicuous to the reader and oftentimes, to the writer as well. In fact, the best way to ferret out the ambiguities, big and small, of an article is to replicate it. This is one of the reasons why the ReScience journal (Rougier et al., 2017) was created (the second author, Nicolas Rougier, is one of the editor-in-chief of ReScience). This open-access journal, run by volunteers, *targets computational research and encourages the explicit replication of already published research, promoting new and open-source implementations in order to ensure that the original research is reproducible.*

Code is a key part of a submission to the ReScience journal. During the review process, reviewers run the submitted code, may criticize its quality and its ease-of-use, and verify the reproduciblity of the replication. The Journal of Open Source Software (Smith et al., 2017) functions similarly: testing the code is a fundamental part of the review process.

CONCLUSION

Throughout the evolution of a small random walk example implemented in Python, we illustrated some of the issues that may plague scientific code. The code may be correct and of good quality, and still possess many problems that reduce its contribution to the scientific discourse. To make these problems explicit, we articulated five characteristics that a code should possess to be a useful part of a scientific publication: it should be re-runnable, repeatable, reproducible, reusable, and replicable.

Running old code on tomorrow's computer and software stacks may not be possible. But recreating the old code's execution environment may be: to ensure the long-term re-runnability of a code, its execution environment must be documented. For our example, a single comment went a long way to transform the R^0 code into the R^1 (re-runnable) one.

Science is built on verifying the results of others. This is harder to do if each execution of the code produce a different result. While for complex concurrent workflows this may not be possible, in all instances where it is feasible the code should be repeatable. This allows future researchers to examine exactly how a specific result was produced. Most of the time, what is needed is to set or record the initial state of the pseudo-random number generator, as what done in the R^2 (repeatable) version.

Even more care is needed to make a code reproducible. The exact execution environment, code and parameters used must be recorded and embedded in the results files, as the R^3 (reproducible) version does. Furthermore, the code must be made available as supplementary data with the whole computational workflow, from preprocessing steps to plotting scripts.

Making code reusable is a stretch goal that can yield tremendous benefits for you, your team, and other researchers. Taken into account during development rather than as an afterthought, simple measures can avoid hours of head-scratching for others, and for yourself—in a few years. Documentation is paramount here, even if it is a single comment per function, as it was done in the R^4 (reusable) version.

Finally, there is the belief that an article should suffice by itself: the descriptions of the algorithms present in the paper should suffice to reobtain (to replicate) the published results. For well-written papers that precisely dissociate conceptually significant aspects from irrelevant implementation details, that may be. But scientific practice should not assume the best of cases. Science assumes that errors can crop up everywhere. Every paper is a mistake or a forgotten parameter away from irreplicability. Replication efforts use the paper first, and then the reproducible code that comes along with it whenever the paper falls short of being precise enough.

In conclusion, the R^3 (reproducible) form should be accepted as the minimum scientific standard (Wilson et al., 2017). This means this should be actually checked by reviewers and publishers when code is part of a work worth being published. It's hardly the case today.

Compared to psychology or biology, the replication issues of computational works have reasonable and efficient solutions. But making sure that these solutions are adopted will not be solved by articles such as this one. Just like in other fields, we have to modify the incentives for the researchers to publish by adopting exigences, enforced domain-wide, on what constitutes an acceptable scientific computational work.

AUTHOR CONTRIBUTIONS

We both contributed equally to the ideas, the text and the code.

[6]Striving, as we do here, for a perfect quantitative match may seem unnecessary. Yet, in replication projects, in particular in computational research, quantitative comparisons are a simple and effective way to verify that the behavior has been reproduced. Moreover, they are particularly helpful to track exactly where the code of a tentative replication fails to reproduce the published results. For a discussion about statistical ways to assess replication see the report of the U.S. National Academies of Sciences (2016).

REFERENCES

Collange, S., Defour, D., Graillat, S., and Iakymchuk, R. (2015). Numerical reproducibility for the parallel reduction on multi- and many-core architectures. *Parallel Comput.* 49, 83–97. doi: 10.1016/j.parco.2015.09.001

Collberg, C., and Proebsting, T. A. (2016). Repeatability in computer systems research. *Commun. ACM* 59, 62–69. doi: 10.1145/2812803

Courtès, L., and Wurmus, R. (2015). "Reproducible and user-controlled software environments in HPC with Guix," in *2nd International Workshop on Reproducibility in Parallel Computing (RepPar)* (Vienne).

Crook, S. M., Davison, A. P., and Plesser, H. E. (2013). "Learning from the past: approaches for reproducibility in computational neuroscience," in *20 Years of Computational Neuroscience,* ed J. M. Bower (New York, NY: Springer), 73–102.

Diethelm, K. (2012). The limits of reproducibility in numerical simulation. *Comput. Sci. Eng.* 14, 64–72. doi: 10.1109/mcse.2011.21

Donoho, D. L., Maleki, A., Rahman, I. U., Shahram, M., and Stodden, V. (2009, January). Reproducible research in computational harmonic analysis. *Comput. Sci. Eng.* 11, 8–18. doi: 10.1109/mcse.2009.15

Durumeric, Z., Payer, M., Paxson, V., Kasten, J., Adrian, D., Halderman, J. A., et al. (2014). "The matter of heartbleed," in *Proceedings of the 2014 Conference on Internet Measurement Conference - IMC'14* (Vancouver, BC: ACM Press).

Eklund, A., Nichols, T. E., and Knutsson, H. (2016). Cluster failure: why fMRI inferences for spatial extent have inflated false-positive rates. *Proc. Natl. Acad. Sci. U.S.A.* 113, 7900–7905. doi: 10.1073/pnas.1602413113

Goble, C. (2016). "What is reproducibility? The R*brouhaha," in *First International Workshop on Reproducible Open Science (Hannover).* Available online at: http://repscience2016.research-infrastructures.eu/img/CaroleGoble-ReproScience2016v2.pdf (September 9, 2016).

Hines, M. L., and Carnevale, N. T. (2008). Translating network models to parallel hardware in NEURON. *J. Neurosci. Methods* 169, 425–455. doi: 10.1016/j.jneumeth.2007.09.010

Hughes, B. D. (1995). *Random Walks and Random Environments.* Oxford; New York, NY: Clarendon Press; Oxford University Press.

Iqbal, S. A., Wallach, J. D., Khoury, M. J., Schully, S. D., and Ioannidis, J. P. A. (2016). Reproducible research practices and transparency across the biomedical literature. *PLoS Biol.* 14:e1002333. doi: 10.1371/journal.pbio.1002333

Mesirov, J. P. (2010). Accessible reproducible research. *Science* 327, 415–416. doi: 10.1126/science.1179653

Mesnard, O., and Barba, L. A. (2017). Reproducible and replicable computational fluid dynamics: it's harder than you think. *Comput. Sci. Eng.* 19, 44–55. doi: 10.1109/mcse.2017.3151254

Open Science Collaboration (2015). Estimating the reproducibility of psychological science. *Science* 349:aac4716. doi: 10.1126/science.aac4716

Peng, R. D., Dominici, F., and Zeger, S. L. (2006). Reproducible epidemiologic research. *Am. J. Epidemiol.* 163:783. doi: 10.1093/aje/kwj093

Rougier, N., Hinsen, K., Alexandre, F., Arildsen, T., Barba, L., Benureau, F., et al. (2017, July). Sustainable computational science: the ReScience initiative. *ArXiv e-prints. arXiv:1707. 04393.*

Sandve, G. K., Nekrutenko, A., Taylor, J., and Hovig, E. (2013). Ten simple rules for reproducible computational research. *PLoS Comput. Biol.* 9:e1003285. doi: 10.1371/journal.pcbi.1003285

Schwab, M., Karrenbach, N., and Claerbout, J. (2000). Making scientific computations reproducible. *Comput. Sci. Eng.* 2, 61–67. doi: 10.1109/5992.881708

Smith, A., Niemeyer, K. E., Katz, D., Barba, L., Githinji, G., Gymrek, M., et al. (2017, July). Journal of Open Source Software (JOSS): design and first-year review. *ArXiv e-prints. arXiv:170 7.02264.*

U.S. National Academies of Sciences, Engineering, and Medicine (2016). *Statistical Challenges in Assessing and Fostering the Reproducibility of Scientific Results: Summary of a Workshop,* ed M. Schwalbe. Washington, DC: The National Academies Press.

Wilson, G., Bryan, J., Cranston, K., Kitzes, J., Nederbragt, L., and Teal, T. K. (2017, June). Good enough practices in scientific computing. *PLOS Comput. Biol.* 13:e1005510. doi: 10.1371/journal.pcbi.100551

10

BindsNET: A Machine Learning-Oriented Spiking Neural Networks Library in Python

Hananel Hazan, Daniel J. Saunders*, Hassaan Khan, Devdhar Patel, Darpan T. Sanghavi, Hava T. Siegelmann and Robert Kozma*

Biologically Inspired Neural and Dynamical Systems Laboratory, College of Computer and Information Sciences, University of Massachusetts Amherst, Amherst, MA, United States

***Correspondence:**
Hananel Hazan
hananel@hazan.org.il
Daniel J. Saunders
djsaunde@cs.umass.edu

The development of spiking neural network simulation software is a critical component enabling the modeling of neural systems and the development of biologically inspired algorithms. Existing software frameworks support a wide range of neural functionality, software abstraction levels, and hardware devices, yet are typically not suitable for rapid prototyping or application to problems in the domain of machine learning. In this paper, we describe a new Python package for the simulation of spiking neural networks, specifically geared toward machine learning and reinforcement learning. Our software, called `BindsNET`[1], enables rapid building and simulation of spiking networks and features user-friendly, concise syntax. `BindsNET` is built on the `PyTorch` deep neural networks library, facilitating the implementation of spiking neural networks on fast CPU and GPU computational platforms. Moreover, the `BindsNET` framework can be adjusted to utilize other existing computing and hardware backends; e.g., `TensorFlow` and `SpiNNaker`. We provide an interface with the OpenAI `gym` library, allowing for training and evaluation of spiking networks on reinforcement learning environments. We argue that this package facilitates the use of spiking networks for large-scale machine learning problems and show some simple examples by using `BindsNET` in practice.

Keywords: GPU-computing, spiking Network, PyTorch, machine learning, python (programming language), reinforcement learning (RL)

1. INTRODUCTION

The recent success of deep learning models in computer vision, natural language processing, and other domains (LeCun et al., 2015) have led to a proliferation of machine learning software packages (Jia et al., 2014; Abadi et al., 2015; Chen et al., 2015; Tokui et al., 2015; Al-Rfou et al., 2016; Paszke et al., 2017). GPU acceleration of deep learning primitives has been a major proponent of this success (Chetlur et al., 2014), as their massively parallel operation enables rapid processing of layers of independent nodes. Since the biological plausibility of deep neural networks is often disputed (Stork, 1989), interest in integrating the algorithms of deep learning with long-studied ideas in neuroscience has been mounting (Marblestone et al., 2016), both as a means to increase machine learning performance and to better model learning and decision-making in biological brains (Wang et al., 2018).

[1]`BindsNET` code is available at https://github.com/Hananel-Hazan/bindsnet. To install the version of the code used for this paper, use `pip install bindsnet=0.2.2`. Benchmarking code for this paper can be found in the `examples/benchmark` directory.

Spiking neural networks (SNNs) (Maass, 1996, 1997; Kistler and Gerstner, 2002) are sometimes referred to as the "third generation" of neural networks because of their potential to supersede deep learning methods in the fields of computational neuroscience (Wall and Glackin, 2013) and biologically plausible machine learning (ML) (Bengio et al., 2015). SNNs are also thought to be more practical for data-processing tasks in which the data has a temporal component since the neurons which comprise SNNs naturally integrate their inputs over time. Moreover, their binary (spiking or no spiking) operation lends itself well to fast and energy efficient simulation on hardware devices.

Although spiking neural networks are not widely used as machine learning systems, recent work shows that they have the potential to be. SNNs are often trained with unsupervised learning rules to learn a useful representation of a dataset, which may then be used as features for supervised learning methods (Diehl and Cook, 2015; Kheradpisheh et al., 2016; Ferr et al., 2018; Hazan et al., 2018; Saunders et al., 2018). Trained deep neural networks may be converted to SNNs (Rueckauer et al., 2017; Rueckauer and Liu, 2018) and implemented in hardware while maintaining good image recognition performance (Diehl et al., 2015), demonstrating that SNNs can in principle compete with deep learning methods. In similar lines of work (Hunsberger and Eliasmith, 2015; Lee et al., 2016; O'Connor and Welling, 2016; Huh and Sejnowski, 2017; Mostafa, 2018; Wu et al., 2018), the popular back-propagation algorithm (or variants thereof) has been applied to differentiable versions of SNNs to achieve competitive performance on standard image classification datasets, providing additional evidence in support of the potential of spiking networks for ML problem solving. Finally, ideas from reinforcement learning can be used to efficiently train spiking neural networks for object classification or other tasks (Florian, 2007; Mozafari et al., 2018).

The membrane potential (or voltage) of a spiking neuron is often described by ordinary differential equations. The membrane potential of the neuron is increased or decreased by *presynaptic* inputs, depending on their sign and strength. In the case of the leaky integrate-and-fire (LIF) model (Kistler and Gerstner, 2002) and several other models, the neuron is constantly decaying to a *rest potential* v_{rest}. If a neuron integrates enough input and reaches its *threshold voltage* v_{thr}, it emits a spike which travels to downstream neurons via synapses, its *post-synaptic* effect modulated by synaptic strengths, and its voltage is reset to some value v_{reset}. Synapses between neurons can also have their own dynamics, which are modified by prescribed learning rules or external reward signals.

Several software packages for the discrete-time simulation of SNNs exist, with varying levels of biological realism and support for hardware platforms. Many such solutions, however, were not developed to target ML applications, and often feature abstruse syntax resulting in steep learning curves for new users. Moreover, packages with a large degree of biological realism may not be appropriate for problems in ML, since they are computationally expensive to simulate and may require a large degree of hyper-parameter tuning. Real-time hardware implementations of SNNs exist as well, but cannot support the rapid prototyping that some software solutions can.

Motivated by the foregoing shortcomings, we present the `BindsNET` spiking neural networks library, which is developed on top of the popular `PyTorch` deep learning library (Paszke et al., 2017). At its core, the software allows users to build, train, and evaluate SNNs composed of groups of neurons and their connections. The learning of connection weights is supported by various algorithms from the biological learning literature (Hebb, 1949; Markram et al., 1997). A separate module provides an interface to the OpenAI `gym` (Brockman et al., 2016) reinforcement learning (RL) environments library from `BindsNET`. A `Pipeline` object is used to streamline the interaction between spiking networks and RL environments, removing many of the messy details from the purview of the experimenter. Still other modules provide functions such as loading of ML datasets, encoding of raw data into spike train network inputs, plotting of network state variables and outputs, and evaluation of SNN as ML models.

The paper is structured as follows: we begin in section 2 with an assessment of the existing SNN simulation software and hardware implementations. In section 3, the `BindsNET` library is described in details, emphasizing the motivation of creating each software module, describing their functionalities, and they way the inter-operate when solving a specific task. Code snippets and simple case studies are introduced in section 4 to demonstrate the breadth of possible `BindsNET` applications. Desirable directions and features of future developments are listed in 5, while potential research impacts are assessed in section 6.

2. REVIEW OF SNN SOFTWARE PACKAGES

2.1. Objectives of SNN Simulations

In the last two decades, neural networks have become increasingly prominent in machine learning and artificial intelligence research, leading to a proliferation of efficient software packages for their training, evaluation, and deployment. On the other hand, the simulation of the "third generation" of neural networks (SNNs) has not been able to reach its full potential, due in part to their inherent complexity and computational requirements. However, spiking neurons excel at remembering a short-term history of their activation and feature efficient binary communication with other neurons, a useful feature in reducing energy requirements on neuromorphic hardware. Spiking neurons exhibit more properties from their biological counterpart than the computing units utilized by deep neural networks, which may constitute an important advantage in terms of practical computational power or ML performance.

Researchers that want to conduct experiments with networks of spiking neurons for ML purposes have a number of options for SNN simulation software. Many frameworks exist, but each is tailored toward specific application domains. In this section, we describe the existing relevant software libraries and the challenges associated with each, and contrast these with the strengths of our package.

We believe that the chosen simulation framework must be easy to develop in, debug, and run, and, most importantly, support the level of biological complexity desired by its users. We express a preference to maintain consistency in development by using a single programming language, and for it to be affordable or an open source project. We describe whether and how these aspects are realized in each competing solution.

2.2. Comparison of State-of-Art Simulation Packages

Many spiking neural network frameworks exist, each with a unique set of use cases. Some focus on the biologically realistic simulation of neurons, while others on high-level spiking network functionality. To build a network to run even the simplest machine learning experiment, one will face multiple difficult design choices: Which biological properties should the neurons and the network have? e.g., how many GABAergic neurons or NMDA/AMPA receptors should be used, or what form of synaptic dynamics? Many such options exist, some of which may or may not have a significant impact on the performance of an ML system.

Several prominent SNN simulation packages are compared in **Table 1**. For example, `NEST` (Gewaltig and Diesmann, 2007), `BRIAN` (Stimberg et al., 2014), and `ANNarchy` (Vitay et al., 2015) focus on accurate biological simulation from sub-cellular components and biochemical reactions, to complex models of single neurons, all up to the network level. Other popular biologically realistic platforms are `NEURON` (Carnevale and Hines, 2006), `Genesis` (Cornelis et al., 2012). These simulation platforms target the neuro-biophysics community and neuroscientists that wish to simulate multicompartment neuron models, in which each compartment is a different part of the neuron with different functionalities, morphological details, and shape. These packages are able to simulate large SNNs on various types of systems, from laptops all the way up to HPC systems. However, each simulated component must be *homogeneous*, meaning that it must be built with a single type of neuron and a single type of synapse. If a researcher wants to simulate multiple types of neurons utilizing various synapse types, it may be difficult in these frameworks. For a more detailed comparison of development time, model performance, and varieties of models of neurons available in these libraries see (Tikidji-Hamburyan et al., 2017).

A major benefit of the `BRIAN`, `ANNarchy`, `NEST`, and `NEURON` packages is that, besides the built-in modules for neuron and connection objects, the programmer is able to specify the dynamics of neurons and connections using differential equations. This eliminates the need to manually specify the dynamic properties of each new neuron or connection object in code. The equations are compiled into fast `C++` code in the case of `ANNarchy`, vectorised and linear algebraic operations using `NumPy` and Basic Linear Algebra Subprograms (BLAS) in the case of `BRIAN2`, and to a mix of Python and native C-like language (hoc) (Hines et al., 2009) which are responsible for SNN simulation in the case of `NEURON`. In addition, in the `NEST` package, the programmer can combine pre-configured objects (which accepts arguments) to create SNNs. In all of these libraries, significant changes to the operation of the network components requires modification of the underlying code, a difficult task which gets in the way of fast network prototyping and breaks the continuity of the programming. At this time, `BindsNET` does not support the solution of arbitrary differential equations describing neural dynamics, rather, for simplicity, several popular neuron types are provided for the user to chose from.

Frameworks such as `NeuCube` (Kasabov, 2014) and `Nengo` (Bekolay et al., 2014) focus on high-level behaviors of spiking neural networks and may be used for machine learning experimentation. `NeuCube` supports rate coding-based spiking networks, and `Nengo` supports simulation at the level of spikes, firing rates, or high-level, abstract neural behavior. `NeuCube` attempts to map spatiotemporal input data into three-dimensional SNN architectures; however, it is not an open source project, and therefore is somewhat restricted in scope and usability. `Nengo` is often used to simulate high-level functionality of brains or brain regions, as a cognitive modeling toolbox implementing the Neural Engineering Framework (Stewart, 2012) rather than a machine learning framework. `Nengo` is an open source project, written in Python, and supports a `Tensorflow` (Abadi et al., 2015) backend to improve simulation speed and exploit some limited ML functionality. It also has options for deploying neural models on dedicated hardware platforms; e.g., SpiNNaker (Plana et al., 2011). `CARLsim` (Beyeler et al., 2015) and `NeMo` (Fidjeland et al., 2009) also focus on the high-level aspects of SNNs and are thus good candidates for applications in machine learning. Both allow the simulation of large spiking networks built with Izhikevich neurons (Izhikevich, 2003) with realistic synaptic dynamics as their fundamental computational unit, and support accelerated computation with GPU hardware. Like the frameworks before, low-level simulation code is written in `C++` for efficiency, but programmers can interact with them with a simulator-independent `PyNN` Python library (Davison et al., 2008), or in `MATLAB` or `Java`.

The `GeNN` (GPU-enhanced neuronal networks) library Yavuz et al. (2016) is an environment that enables simulation of SNNs on CPUs or NVIDIA GPUs via code generation technology. Networks are defined in a `C`-style API, and the code for simulating them (on CPU or GPU) are automatically generated by `GeNN`. The recent `BRIAN2genn` package Stimberg et al. (2018) (in beta release) can be used to convert network models written in `BRIAN2` to run on NVIDIA GPUs using the `GeNN` library, by invoking `BRIAN2`'s `set_device()` function to execute code in an external framework. Although this platform targets both CPUs and GPUs (a central feature of the `BindsNET` library), it requires an (often costly) intermediate code generation step between network prototyping and deployment (see **Figure 11** for an illustration of this issue). It is also difficult to intervene on the generated code when running;

TABLE 1 | Comparison between spiking neural network simulation libraries.

Simulator	Affiliation	Open source	Simulation	OpenMP	GPU	Programming languages
ANNarchy	Chemnitz University Germany	Yes	Clock-driven	Yes	Yes	C++ with Python interface
(Py)NEST	University of Freiburg Germany	Yes	Hybrid	Yes	No	C++ with Python interface
CARLsim	University of California Irvine, CA, US	Yes	Clock-driven	Yes	Yes	C++ with PyNN support
NeMo	Imperial College London, UK	Yes	Clock-driven	Yes	Yes	C++ with Python & PyNN support
PyNN	Open Community	Yes	Various	Yes	Yes	Python Interface only
Nengo AI	University of Waterloo Canada	Yes	Clock-driven	Partially	Yes	C++ with Python wrapper
SpiNNaker	Manchester University UK	Yes	Event-driven	No	No	C++ with PyNN & sPyNNaker support
Brian 2	Ecole Normale Superieure Paris, France	Yes	Clock-driven	Yes	No	C++ with Python wrapper
Brain2GeNN (GeNN)	University of Sussex UK	Yes	Clock-driven	Yes	Yes	C++ with Python wrapper
NeuCube	Auckland University New Zealand	No	?	?	?	MATLAB
BindsNET	University Massachusetts Amherst, US	Yes	Clock-driven	Yes	Yes	C++ with Python wrapper

e.g., clamping synapses if certain criteria are met, or changing learning rates as the simulation progresses.

Many of the above packages are written in more than one programming language: the core functionality is implemented in a lower-level language (e.g., C++) to achieve good performance with low overhead, and the code exposed to the user of the package is written in a higher-level language (e.g., Python or MATLAB) to enable fast prototyping. If such frameworks are not tailored to the needs of a user, have steep learning curves, or aren't flexible enough to create a desired model, the user may have to program in both high- and low-level languages to make changes to the required internal components. The authors have encountered this difficulty with the `BRIAN2` library in particular, since certain segments of simulation functionality is regulated to generated code, which is difficult or impossible to modify while, for example, training a SNN for a machine learning task. This issue is likely to appear in similar software frameworks; e.g., `GeNN` and `ANNarchy`.

`BindsNET` relies on PyTorch for its matrix computations in order to perform efficient simulation of spiking neural networks. Without changing the details of the mathematical operations, `BindsNET` can in principle be connected to various hardwares, e.g., FPGA, ASIC, DSP, or ARM, to execute the simulations. One may design an API to compile spiking networks created in `BindsNET` to run on designated hardware instead of using PyTorch as the simulation workhorse. In this way, `BindsNET` can be seen as a bridge between the software and hardware domains, enabling researchers to rapidly test software prototypes on CPUs or GPUs, and eventually deploy the simulation to fast, energy efficient dedicated hardware. At the moment, no such API exists, but may be added in a future release of the library.

3. PACKAGE STRUCTURE

A summary of all the software modules of the `BindsNET` package is included in **Figure 1**.

Many `BindsNET` objects use the `torch.Tensor` data structure for computation; e.g., all objects supporting the `Nodes` interface use `Tensors` to store and update state variables such as spike occurrences or voltages. The `Tensor` object is a multi-dimensional matrix containing elements of a single data type; e.g., integers or floating points numbers with 8, 16, 32, or 64 bits of precision. They can be easily moved between devices with calls to `Tensor.cpu()` or `Tensor.cuda()`, and can target GPU devices by default with the statement `torch.set_default_tensor_type('torch.cuda.FloatTensor')`.

3.1. SNN Simulation

`BindsNET` provides a `Network` object (in the `network` module) which is responsible for the coordination of one or many `Nodes` and `Connections` objects, and supports the use of `Monitors` for recording the state variables of these components. A time step parameter `dt` is the sole (optional) argument to the `Network` constructor, which controls the temporal resolution of simulation. The `run(inpts, time)`

BindsNET	
network	contains the Network object and submodules for network components
network / Network	spiking neural network; responsible for coordination of neurons and connections
network / nodes	groups of neurons of arbitrary size and dimensionality
nodes / Input	neurons with user-specified spiking activity
nodes / McCullochPittsNodes	implements the McCulloch-Pitts neuron model
nodes / IFNodes	implements the integrate-and-fire (IF) neuron model
nodes / LIFNodes	implements the leaky integrate-and-fire (LIF) neuron model
nodes / IzhikevichNodes	implements the Izhikevich neuron model
network / topology	connectivity between groups of neurons
topology / Connection	all-to-all connectivity between neurons (dense weight matrix)
topology / SparseConnection	sparse connectivity between neurons (sparse weight matrix)
topology / Conv2dConnection	two-dimensional convolution of presynaptic neurons (convolutional weight kernels)
network / monitors	record time-varying state variables of arbitrary objects.
monitors / Monitor	record state variable(s) from a single BindsNET object
monitors / NetworkMonitor	record state variable(s) from all components of a Network
environment	reinforcement learning environments
environment / GymEnvironment	thin wrapper of the gym RL environments library
environment / DatasetEnvironment	thin wrapper around arbitrary dataset for use in pipeline
datasets	downloading, pre-processing, and iteration over popular ML datasets
datasets / MNIST	handwritten digits dataset (28x28, 60K train, 10K test)
datasets / CIFAR-10	10-class natural image dataset (32x32x3, 50K train, 10K test)
datasets / CIFAR-100	100-class natural image dataset (32x32x3, 50K train, 10K test)
encoding	conversion of numerical data into binary spikes
encoding / bernoulli	conversion of non-negative data into Bernoulli-distributed spikes
encoding / poisson	conversion of non-negative data into spikes with exponentially-distributed inter-arrival times
encoding / rank_order_coding	conversion of non-negative data into one spike per neuron with times inversely proportional to intensity
learning	methods for updating connection parameters of topology objects
learning / hebbian	hebbian modification method for connections update
learning / post_pre	simple STDP rule based on pre- and post-synaptic neural activity
learning / m_stdp	reward-modulated STDP rule
learning / m_stdp_et	reward-modulated STDP rule with eligibility trace
pipeline	contains Pipeline object and feedback functions
pipeline / Pipeline	smoothly integrates a network, environment, and encoding and feedback functions
pipeline / action	functions for mapping network activity to actions in an environment
action / select_random	selects random action in action space
action / select_multinomial	samples an action from a probability distribution parametrized by a vector of spikes
evaluation	quantification of SNNs as machine learning models
evaluation / assign_labels	assign data labels to neurons based on their spiking activity on trainin data
evaluation / all_activity	classify data using spikes and labels from all neurons
evaluation / proportion_weighting	weigh spikes from neurons by the proportion of spiking activity per data label
analysis	tools for assessing state and evolution of network components
analysis / plotting	online (during simulation) plotting functions
analysis / visualization	offline (after simulation) plotting functions
models	network architectures from the spiking neural networks literature
models / DiehlAndCook2015	SNN trained to classify data using STDP and a competitive mechanism

FIGURE 1 | Depiction of the `BindsNET` directory structure and description of major software modules.

function implements synchronous updates (for a number of time steps $\frac{\texttt{time}}{\texttt{dt}}$) of all network components. This function calls `get_inputs()` to calculate pre-synaptic inputs to all `Nodes` instances (alongside user-defined inputs in `inpts`) as a subroutine. A `reset_()` method invokes resetting functionality of all network components, namely for resetting state variables back to default values. Saving and loading of networks to and from disk is implemented, permitting re-use of trained connection weights or other parameters.

The `Nodes` abstract base class in the `nodes` module specifies the abstract functions `step(inpts, dt)` and `reset_()`. The first is called by the `run()` function of a `Network` instance to carry out a single time step's update, and the second resets spikes, voltages, and any other recorded state variables to default values. Implementations of the `Nodes` class include `Input` (neurons with user-specified or fixed spikes) `McCullochPittsNodes` (McCulloch-Pitts neurons), `IFNodes` (integrate-and-fire neurons), `LIFNodes` (leaky integrate-and-fire neurons), and `IzhikevichNodes` (Izhikevich neurons). Other neurons or neuron-like computing elements may be implemented by extending the `Nodes` abstract class. Many `Nodes` object support optional arguments for customizing neural attributes such as threshold, reset, and resting potential, refractory period, membrane time constant, and more. It should be noted that some `Nodes` objects' behavior does not depend on the `dt` parameters; for example, the `McCullochPittsNodes` object has no memory of previous time steps (stateless), and yet it may still be embedded in a SNN simulation.

The `topology` module is used to specify interactions between `Nodes` instances, the most generic of which is implemented in the `Connection` object. The `Connection` is aware of *source* (pre-synaptic) and *target* (post-synaptic) `Nodes`, as well as a matrix of weights `w` of connections strengths. By default, connections do not implement any learning of connection weights, but do so through the inclusion of an `update_rule` argument. Several canonical learning rules from the biological learning literature are implemented in the `learning` module, including Hebbian learning (`Hebbian`), a variant of spike-timing-dependent plasticity (STDP) (`PostPre`), and less well-known methods such as reward-modulated STDP (`MSTDP`). The optional argument `norm` to the `Connection` specifies a desired sum of weights per target neuron, which is enforced by the parent `Network` during each call of `run()`. A `SparseConnection` object is available for specifying connections where certain weights are fixed to zero; however, this does not yet available for learning functionality due to a lack of adequate support for sparse `Tensor` in the PyTorch library. The `Conv2dConnection` object implements a two-dimensional convolution operation (using PyTorch's `torch.nn.conv2d` function) and supports all update rules from the `learning` module. The `LocallyConnectedConnection` implements a two-dimensional convolutional layer without shared weights; i.e., each input region is associated with a different set of filter weights (Bruna et al., 2013; Saunders et al., 2018).

3.2. Machine and Reinforcement Learning

`BindsNET` is being developed with machine and reinforcement learning applications in mind. At the core of these efforts is the `learning` module, which contains functions which can be attached to `Connection` objects to modify them during SNN simulation. By default, connections are instantiated with no learning rule. The `Hebbian` rule ("fire together, wire together") symmetrically strengthens weights when pre- and post-synpatic spikes occur temporally close together, and the `PostPre` rule implements a simple form of STDP in which weights are increased or decreased according to the relative timing of pre- and post-synaptic spikes, with user-specified (possibly asymmetric) learning rates. The reward-modulated STDP (`MSTDP`) and reward-modulated STDP with eligibility trace (`MSTDPET`) rules of Florian (2007) are also implemented for use in basic reinforcement learning experiments. In general, any learning rule can be used with any connection types and other network components, but it is up to the researcher to choose the right method for their experiment.

The `datasets` module provides a means to download, pre-process, and iterate over machine learning datasets. For example, the `MNIST` object provides this functionality for the MNIST handwritten digits dataset. Several other datasets are supported besides, including CIFAR-10, CIFAR-100, (Krizhevsky and Hinton, 2009) and Spoken MNIST. The samples from a dataset can be encoded into spike trains using the `encoding` module, currently supporting several functions for creating spike trains from non-negative data based on different statistical distributions and biologically inspired transformations of stimuli. Encoding functions include `poisson()`, which converts data representing firing rates into Poisson spike trains with said firing rates, and `rank_order()`, which converts data into single spikes per neuron temporally ordered by the intensity of the input data (Thorpe and Gautrais, 1998). Spikes may be used as input to SNNs, or even to other ML systems. A submodule `preprocess` of `datasets` allows the user to apply various pre-processing techiques to raw data; e.g., cropping, subsampling, binarizing, and more.

The `environment` module provides an interface into which a SNN, considered as a reinforcement learning agent, can take input from and enact actions in a reinforcement learning environment. The `GymEnvironments` object comprises of a generic wrapper for `gym` (Brockman et al., 2016) RL environments and calls its `reset()`, `step(action)`, `close()`, and `render()` functionality, while providing a default pre-processing function `preprocess()` for observations from each environment. The `step(action)` function takes an `action` in the `gym` environment, which returns an observation, reward value, an indication of whether the episode has finished, and a dictionary of (name, value) pairs containing additional information. Another object, `DatasetEnvironment`, provides a generic wrapper around objects from the `datasets` module, allowing these to be used as a component in a `Pipeline` instance (see section 3.3). The `environment.action` module provides methods for mapping one or more network layers' spikes to actions in the environment; e.g., `select_multinomial()` treats a (normalized) vector of spikes as a probability distribution from which to sample an action for the environment's similarly-sized action space.

Simple methods for the evaluation of SNNs as machine learning models are implemented in the `evaluation` module. In the context of unsupervised learning, the `assign_labels()` function assigns data labels to neurons corresponding to the class of data on which they spike most during network training (Diehl and Cook, 2015). These labels are to classify new data using methods like `all_activity()` and `proportion_weighting()` (Hazan et al., 2018). We have recently added `logreg_fit` and `logreg_predict` methods for fitting and predicting on categorical data with the logistic regression implementation borrowed from the `scikit-learn` library (Pedregosa et al., 2011). We plan to add additional "read-out" methods in the near future, such as *k*-nearest neighbor (KNN) and support vector machines (SVMs).

A collection of network architectures is defined in the `models` module. For example, the network structure of Diehl and Cook (2015) is implemented by the `DiehlAndCook2015` object, which supports arguments such as `n_neurons`, `excite`, `inhib`, etc. with reasonable default values.

3.3. The Pipeline Object

As an additional effort to ease prototyping of machine learning systems comprising spiking neural networks, we have provided the `Pipeline` object to compose an environment, network, an encoding of environment observations, and a mapping from network activity to the environment's action space. The `Pipeline` also provides optional arguments for visualization of the environment and network state variables during network operation, skipping or recording observations on a regular basis, the length of the simulation per observation (defaults to 1 time step), and more. The main action of the pipeline can be explained as a four-step, recurring process, implemented in the pipeline `step()` function:

1. An action is selected based on the activity of one or more of the network's layers during the last one or more time steps
2. This action is used as input to the environment's `step()` function, which returns a new observation, a scalar reward, whether the simulation has finished, and any additional information particular to the environment
3. The observation returned from the environment is converted into spike trains according to the user-specified encoding function (either custom or from the `encoding` module) and request simulation time
4. The spike train-encoded observation is used as input to the network.

Alongside the required arguments for the `Pipeline` object (`network`, `environment`, `encoding`, and `action`), there are a few keyword arguments that are supported, such as `history` and `delta`. The `history_length` argument indicates that a number of sequential observations are to maintained in order to calculate differences between current observations and those stored in the `history` data structure. This implies that only new information in the environment's observation space is delivered as input to the network on each time step. The `delta` argument (default 1) specifies an interval at which observations are stored in `history`. This may be useful if observations don't change much between consecutive steps; then, we should wait some `delta` time steps between taking observations to expect significant differences. As an example, combining `history_length = 4` and `delta = 3` will store observations {0, 3, 6, 9}, {3, 6, 9, 12}, {6, 9, 12, 15}, etc. A few other keyword arguments for handling console output, plotting, and more exist and are detailed in the `Pipeline` object documentation.

A functional diagram of the `Pipeline` object is depicted in **Figure 2**.

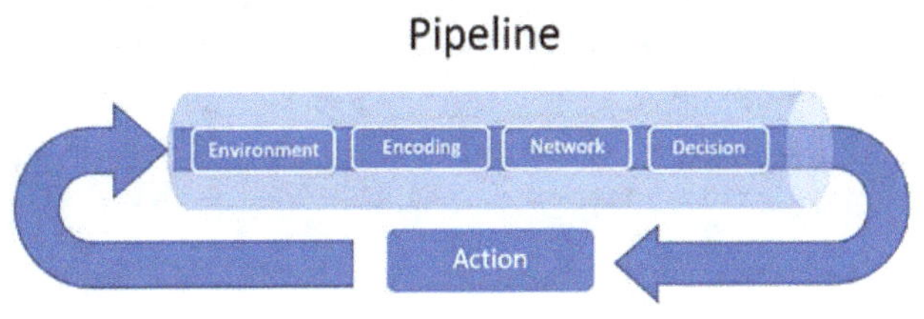

FIGURE 2 | A functional diagram of the `Pipeline` object. The four-step process involves an encoding function, network computation, converting network outputs into actions in an environment's action space, and a simulation step of the environment. An encoding function converts non-spiking observations from the environment into spike inputs to the network, and a `action` function maps network spiking activity into a non-spiking quantity: an action, fed back into the environment, where the procedure begins anew. Other modules come into play in various supporting roles: the network may use a `learning` method to update connection weights, or the environment may simply be a thin wrapper around a dataset (in which case there is no feedback), and it may be desirable to plot network state variables during the reinforcement learning loop.

3.4. Visualization

`BindsNET` contains useful visualization tools that provide information during or after network or environment simulation. Several generic plotting functions are implemented in the `analysis.plotting` module; e.g., `plot_spikes()` and `plot_voltages()` create and update plots dynamically instead of recreating figures at every time step. These functions are able to display spikes and voltages with a single call. Other functions include `plot_weights()` (displays connection weights), `plot_input()` (displays raw input data), and `plot_performance()` (displays time series of performance metric). Other visualization libraries in the Python ecosystem such as `matplotlib` can be used to plot network state variables or other data as users of BindsNET may require for more complicated use cases not covered by the `plotting` module.

The `analysis.visualization` module contains additional plotting functionality for network state variables after simulation has finished. These tools allow experimenters to analyze learned weights or spike outputs, or to summarize long-term behaviors of their SNN models. For example, the `weights_movie()` function creates an animation of a `Connection`'s weight matrix from a sequence of its values, enabling the visualization of the trajectory of connection weight updates.

3.5. Adding New BindsNET Features

To extend BindsNET, one can extend certain abstract objects found in the package with the desired functionality. In the following, we discuss how new neuron models, connection types, and learning rules can be custom-defined by users and developers of BindsNET. Other BindsNET objects (e.g., `Monitors`, `Datasets`, etc.) can be defined in a similar fashion.

3.5.1. Neuron Models

The abstract class `Nodes` implements functionality that is common to all neuron types. It defines the abstract functions `step()` and `reset_()`, which one can choose to override in child classes, or to One can define a new `Nodes` object by writing a class of the form:

```
class NewNodes(Nodes):
    def __init__(self, n, shape, traces, ...):
        ...
    def step(self, inpt, dt):
        ...
    def reset_(self):
        ...
```

All three functions typically call the similarly-named `Nodes` abstract class functions, but it is possible to completely re-define the functions as needed. The abstract base class `AbstractInput` is also available for defining node types with user-defined inputs (e.g., for simulating constant current injection with the `RealInput` object).

At present, BindsNET does not automatically solve state variable dynamics equations (as does, for example, the `BRIAN` simulator Goodman and Brette, 2009); instead, the user must define the neuron difference equation themselves in the body of the `step()` function. We implement Euler integration as part of our emphasis on efficient computation. Automatic solution of dynamics equations may be added in a future release of BindsNET.

3.5.2. Connection Types

The class `AbstractConnection` implements functionality common to all connection objects. It defines the abstract methods `compute(s)`, `update(dt)`, `normalize()`, and `reset_()`. Users of BindsNET can define their own connection types by creating a class that inherits from `AbstractConnection`. To define a new connection object, one must write a class of the form:

```
class NewConnection(AbstractConnection):
    def __init__(self, source, target, **kwargs):
        ...
    def compute(self, s):
        ...
    def update(self, dt, **kwargs):
        ...
    def normalize(self):
        ...
    def reset_(self):
        ...
```

3.5.3. Learning Rules

The abstract class `LearningRule` defines functions common to all learning rules. It defines the abstract method `update(dt)`, used to update a connection's synapse strengths in some fashion. Typically, this method makes use of pre- and post-synaptic neuron spikes and / or spike traces in order to calculate some local learning rule; e.g., `PostPre` STDP. However, users of BindsNET may want to construct learning rules than depend on non-local information; e.g., the `MSTDP` and `MSTDPET` rules require a `reward` keyword argument to modulate the sign and strength of synapse weight updates. To define a new learning rule, one can write a class as follows:

```
class NewLearningRule(LearningRule):
    def __init__(self, connection, nu, weight_decay):
        ...
    def update(self, dt, **kwargs):
        ...
```

4. EXAMPLES OF USING `BINDSNET` TO SOLVE MACHINE LEARNING TASKS

We present some simple example scripts to give an impression of how `BindsNET` can be used to build spiking neural networks implementing machine learning functionality. `BindsNET` is built with the concept of encapsulation of functionality to make it faster and easier for generalization and prototyping. Note in the examples below the compactness of the scripts: fewer lines of code are needed to create a model, load a dataset, specify their interaction in terms of a pipeline, and run a training loop. Of course, these commands rely on many lines of underlying code, but the user no longer has to implement them for each experimental script. If changes in the available parameters are not enough, the experimenter can intervene by making changes in the underlying code in the model without changing language or environment, thus preserving the continuity of the coding environment.

4.1. Unsupervised Learning

The `DiehlAndCook2015` object in the `models` module implements a slightly simplified version of the network architecture discussed in Diehl and Cook (2015). A minimal working example of training a spiking neural network to learn, without labels, a representation of the MNIST digit dataset is given in **Figure 3**, and state variable-monitoring plots are depicted in **Figure 4**. The `Pipeline` object is used to hide the messy details of the coordination between the dataset, encoding function, and network instance. Code for additional plots or console output may be added to the training loop for monitoring purposes as needed.

The main goal of the present paper is to introduce the `BindsNET` software framework, while a systematic evaluation of the implementation and comparison with other SNN platforms is the objective of ongoing or future studies. Nevertheless, it is important to show that `BindsNET` measures up to its peers. To illustrate the performance of `BindsNET`, here we introduce some preliminary results; further details are given in Saunders et al. (2018) and Hazan et al. (2018). In the case of MNIST dataset, `BindsNET`'s classification performance reaches 95%, which is on a par with the `BRIAN`-based implementations reported in Diehl and Cook (2015). Moreover, `BindsNET`'s flexible platform allowed extensive exploration of learning rules and hyper-parameters, and we have shown that our approach can reach or exceed `BRIAN`'s accuracy with smaller SNNs. Moreover, as training progresses, the accuracy of our approach using `BindsNET` increases rapidly at the early stage of learning, using much less examples than alternative methods (Hazan et al., 2018). Again, in the present work we do not aim at a systematic evaluation of the solutions based on `BindsNET`, but the initial results are promising, and extensive work is in progress.

```
from bindsnet.datasets import MNIST
from bindsnet.encoding import poisson
from bindsnet.pipeline import Pipeline
from bindsnet.models import DiehlAndCook2015
from bindsnet.environment import DatasetEnvironment

# Build Diehl & Cook 2015 network.
network = DiehlAndCook2015(n_inpt=784, n_neurons=400, exc=22.5,
                           inh=17.5, dt=1.0, norm=78.4)

# Specify dataset wrapper environment.
environment = DatasetEnvironment(dataset=MNIST(path='../../data/MNIST'),
                                 train=True, download=True, intensity=0.25)

# Build pipeline from components.
pipeline = Pipeline(network=network, environment=environment,
                    encoding=poisson, time=350, plot_interval=1)

# Train the network.
for i in range(60000):
    pipeline.step()
    network.reset_()
```

FIGURE 3 | Accompanying plots to the unsupervised training of the `DiehlAndCook2015` spiking neural network architecture. The network is able to learn prototypical examples of images from the training set, and on a test images, the excitatory neuron with the most similar filter should fire the most. This network structure is able to achieve 95% accuracy on the MNIST digits (Diehl and Cook, 2015; Hazan et al., 2018). **(A)** Raw input and "reconstructed" input, computed by summing Poisson-distributed spike trains over the time dimension. **(B)** Spikes from the excitatory and inhibitory layers of the `DiehlAndCook2015` model. **(C)** Voltages from the excitatory and inhibitory layers of the `DiehlAndCook2015` model. **(D)** Reshaped 2D label assignments of excitatory neurons, assigned based on activity on examples from the training data. **(E)** Reshaped 2D connection weights from input to excitatory layers. The network is able to learn distinct prototypical examples from the dataset, corresponding to the categories in the data.

4.2. Supervised Learning

We used a simple two-layer spiking neural network to implement supervised learning of the Fashion-MNIST image dataset (Xiao et al., 2017). An minimal example of training a spiking network to classify the data is given in **Figure 5**, with plotting outputs depicted in **Figure 6**. A layer of 100 excitatory neurons is split into 10 groups of size 10, one for each category. On each input example, we observe the label of the data and clamp a randomly selected excitatory neuron from its group to spike on every time step. This forces the neuron to adjust its filter weights toward the shape of current input example.

4.3. Reinforcement Learning

A three layer SNN is built to compute on spikes encoded from Breakout observations. The input layer takes the spike encoding of a 80x80 image which has been downsampled and binarized from the observations from the `GymEnvironment`. The output layer consists of 4 neurons which correspond to the 4 possible actions for the Breakout game. The result of this computation is spiking activity in the output layer, which are converted into actions in the game's action space by using a softmax function on the sum of the spikes in the output layer. The simulation of both the network and the environment are interleaved and appear to operate in parallel. The SNN combined with the softmax function gives a stochastic policy for the RL environment and the user may apply any reinforcement learning algorithm to modify the parameters of the SNN to change the policy. For a more complete view of the details involved in constructing an SNN and deploying a `GymEnvironment` instance, see the script depicted in **Figure 7** and accompanying displays in **Figure 8**.

4.4. Reservoir Computing

Reservoir computers are typically built from three parts: (1) an encoder that translates input from the environment that is fed to it, (2) a dynamical system based on randomly connected neurons (the *reservoir*), and (3) a readout mechanism. The readout is often trained via gradient descent to perform classification or regression on some target function. `BindsNET` can be used to build reservoir computers using spiking neurons with little effort, and machine learning functionality from `PyTorch` can be co-opted to learn a function from states of the high-dimensional reservoir to desired outputs. Code in for defining and simulating a simple reservoir computer is given in **Figure 9**, and plots to monitor simulation progress are shown in **Figure 10**. The outputs of the reservoir computer on the CIFAR-10 natural image dataset are used as transformed inputs to a logistic regression model. The logistic regression model is then trained to recognize the categories based on the features produced by the reservoir.

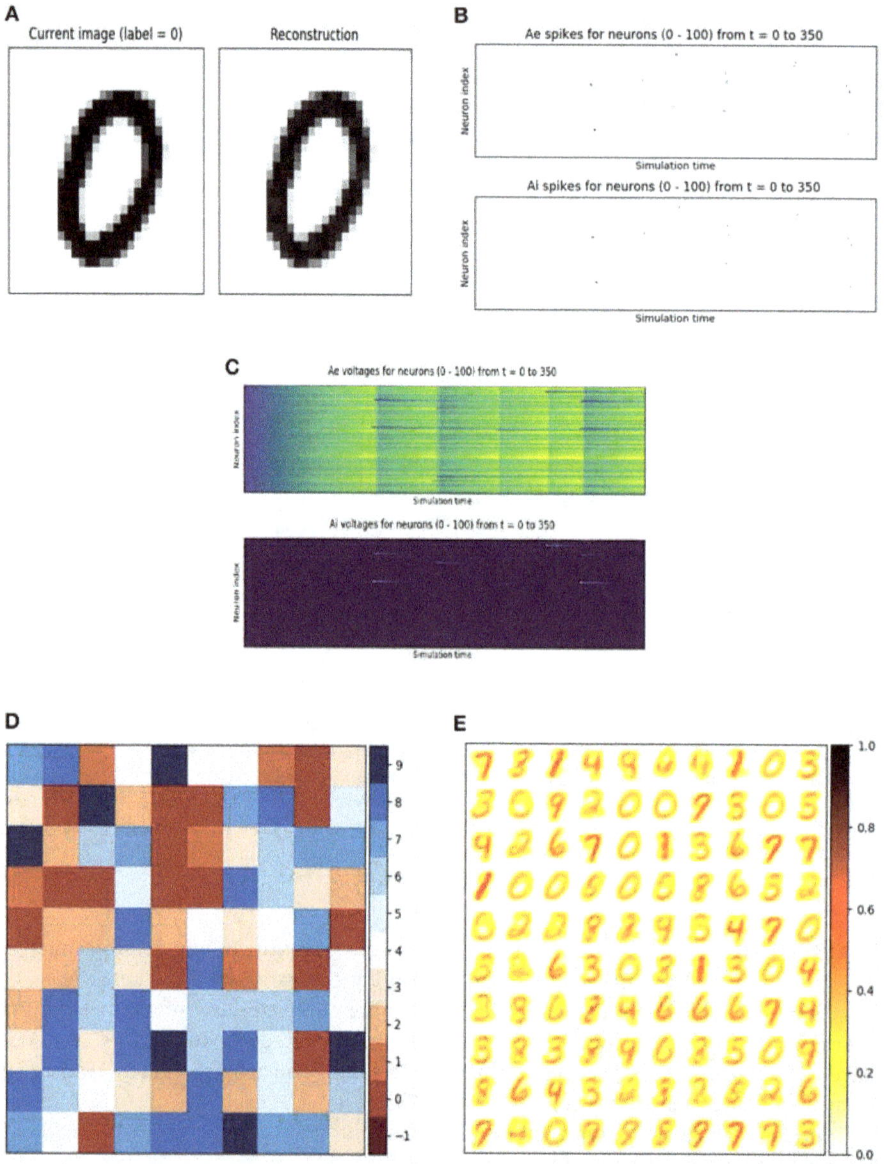

FIGURE 4 | Unsupervised learning of the MNIST handwritten digits in `BindsNET`. The `DiehlAndCook2015` model implements a simple spike timing-dependent plasticity rule between input and excitatory neuron populations as well as a competitive inhibition mechanism to learn prototypical digit filters from raw data. The `DatasetEnvironment` wraps the `MNIST` dataset object so it may be used as a component in the `Pipeline`. The network is trained on one pass through the 60K-example training data for 350ms each, with state variables (voltages and spikes) reset after each example.

4.5. Benchmarking

In order to compare several competing SNN simulators, we devised a simple simulation and benchmarked our software on it against other, similar frameworks. We simulated a network with a population of n Poisson input neurons with firing rates (in Hertz) drawn randomly from $U(0, 100)$, connected all-to-all with a equally-sized population of leaky integrate-and-fire (LIF) neurons, with connection weights sampled from $\mathcal{N}(0, 1)$. We varied n systematically from 250 to 10,000 in steps of 250, and ran each simulation with every library for 1,000ms with a time resolution $dt = 1.0$. We tested `BindsNET` (with CPU and GPU computation), `BRIAN2`, `PyNEST` (the Python interface to the NEST SLI interface that runs the `C++ NEST` core simulator), `ANNarchy` (with CPU and GPU computation), and `BRIAN2genn` (the `BRIAN2` front-end to the `GeNN` simulator). The `Nengo` and `NEURON` simulators were considered, but in both cases, we were unable to implement the benchmarked network structure. This speaks to the expressiveness or relative difficulty of using these competing simulation libraries as compared to `BindsNET`. Several packages, including `BRIAN` and `PyNEST`, allow the setting of certain global preferences; e.g., the number of CPU threads, the number of OpenMP

```
import torch
from bindsnet.network import Network
from bindsnet.datasets import FashionMNIST
from bindsnet.network.monitors import Monitor
from bindsnet.network.topology import Connection
from bindsnet.network.nodes import RealInput, IFNodes

# Network building.
network = Network()

input_layer = RealInput(n=784, sum_input=True)
output_layer = IFNodes(n=10, sum_input=True)
network.add_layer(input_layer, name='X')
network.add_layer(output_layer, name='Y')

input_connection = Connection(input_layer, output_layer, norm=150, wmin=-1, wmax=1)
network.add_connection(input_connection, source='X', target='Y')

# State variable monitoring.
time = 25  # No. of simulation time steps per example.
for l in network.layers:
    m = Monitor(network.layers[l], state_vars=['s'], time=time)
    network.add_monitor(m, name=l)

# Load Fashion-MNIST data.
images, labels = FashionMNIST(path='../../data/FashionMNIST', download=True).get_train()

# Run training.
grads = {}
lr, lr_decay = 1e-2, 0.95
criterion = torch.nn.CrossEntropyLoss()
spike_ims, spike_axes, weights_im = None, None, None
for i, (image, label) in enumerate(zip(images.view(-1, 784) / 255, labels)):
    # Run simulation for single datum.
    inpts = {'X': image.repeat(time, 1), 'Y_b': torch.ones(time, 1)}
    network.run(inpts=inpts, time=time)

    # Retrieve spikes and summed inputs from both layers.
    label = torch.tensor(label).long()
    spikes = {l: network.monitors[l].get('s') for l in network.layers}
    summed_inputs = {l: network.layers[l].summed for l in network.layers}

    # Compute softmax of output activity, get predicted label.
    output = spikes['Y'].sum(-1).softmax(0).view(1, -1)
    predicted = output.argmax(1).item()

    # Compute gradient of loss and do SGD update.
    grads['dl/df'] = summed_inputs['Y'].softmax(0)
    grads['dl/df'][label] -= 1
    grads['dl/dw'] = torch.ger(summed_inputs['X'], grads['dl/df'])
    network.connections['X', 'Y'].w -= lr * grads['dl/dw']

    # Decay learning rate.
    if i > 0 and i % 500 == 0:
        lr *= lr_decay

    network.reset_()
```

FIGURE 5 | A two-layer spiking neural network (a `RealNodes` object connected all-to-all with a `IFNodes` object) is trained with an approximated stochastic gradient descent algorithm using the Fashion-MNIST image dataset. The back-propagation algorithm operates on the `summed_inputs` to the groups of `Nodes`, while predictions are made based on the output layer's spiking activity.

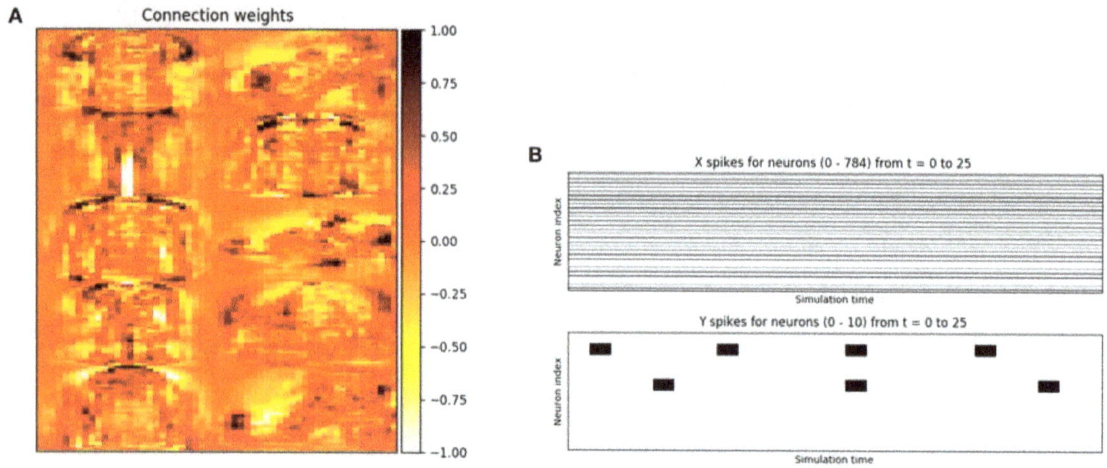

FIGURE 6 | Accompanying plots for the supervised training of a simple two-layer spiking neural network on the Fashion-MNIST dataset. The set of 10 28 × 28 tiled weights shown in (a) each correspond to a different class of Fashion-MNIST data. The plot of the input neurons' activity in (b) is simply the scaled input data, constant over the simulation length. This network architecture trained with stochastic gradient descent (SGD) achieves 85% test accuracy on this dataset. **(A)** Weights from the supervised spiking neural network trained on the Fashion-MNIST dataset. Each 28 × 28 region corresponds to the filter responsible for detecting a unique category of data. One can make out the profile of objects depicted in the filters; e.g., shirts, sneakers, and trousers. **(B)** Real-valued input activity and spikes from the input and output layers of the two-layer network, respectively.

processes, etc. We chose these settings for our benchmark study in an attempt to maximize each library's speed, but note that `BindsNET` requires no setting of such options. Our approach, inheriting the computational model of `PyTorch`, appears to make the best use of the available hardware, and therefore makes it simple for practicioners to get the best performance from their system with the least effort.

All simulations run on Ubuntu 16.04 LTS with Intel(R) Xeon(R) CPU E5-2687W v3 @ 3.10GHz, 128Gb RAM @ 2133MHz, and two GeForce GTX TITAN X (GM200) GPUs. Python 3.6 is used in all cases except for simulation with `ANNarchy`, which requires Python 2.7. Clock time was recorded for each simulation run. The results are depicted in **Figure 11**.

As can be noticed in the **Figure 11**, `PyNEST` simulation runs are cut off for $n > 2.5$K, and `ANNarchy` (on CPUs) for $n >$ 5K, due to the fact that, after this point, their simulation time far outstrips those of the other libraries. With small networks ($n <$ 2.5K), the CPU-only version of the `BindsNET` simulation is faster than the `BRIAN2` simulation; yet, this relationship reverses as the number of simulated neurons grows. However, in larger networks ($n > 1.5$K), the GPU-only `BindsNET` simulator is faster than `BRIAN2`, and is competitive in simulation time in the case of smaller networks. The `BRIAN2genn` simulator is very fast, with near-constant simulation time of approximately 0.2s; however, it requires a roughly 25s compilation period, no matter the network size, before simulation can begin. Somewhat similarly, simulation with `ANNarchy` using GPU computation is rather fast, but requires an super-linear increase in compilation time as the size of the network grows.

Therefore, `BindsNET` constitutes a speed-competitive alternative to several popular existing SNN simulation libraries. Although our benchmark study is far from comprehensive, it demonstrates a particular use case for which `BindsNET` is perhaps preferable to other methods; i.e., in the case of feedforward networks with all-to-all connectivity. Similar studies can be done to assess its performance relative to the competition in other SNN architectural regimes. We expect that, in different applications, other libraries will perform better in terms of speed or memory usage, and it is up to the experimenter to choose the best software for the simulation task. As stated previously, our approach is best for rapid prototyping and testing of SNNs on CPUs and GPUs alike, which is demonstrated in part by the foregoing benchmark analysis. In particular, a major advantage of using the `BindsNET` library for GPU computation is that it requires no compilation step intermediate between network definition and simulation, as opposed to the `BRIAN2genn` and `ANNarchy` libraries. This is well-suited to machine learning experimentation, which often requires many iterations of model building and hyper-parameter tuning that may be hindered by re-compilation before each attempt.

5. ONGOING DEVELOPMENTS

`BindsNET` is still at an early stage of development, and thus there is much room for future work and improvement. Since it is an open source project and because there is considerable interest in the research community in using SNNs for machine learning purposes, we are optimistic that there will be numerous community contributions to the library. Indeed, we believe that public interest in the project, along with the strong support of the libraries on which it depends, will be an important driving factor in its maturation and proliferation of features. We mention some specific implementation goals:

- Additional neuron types, learning rules, datasets, encoding functions, etc. Added features should take

```
import torch

from bindsnet.network import Network
from bindsnet.pipeline import Pipeline
from bindsnet.encoding import bernoulli
from bindsnet.network.topology import Connection
from bindsnet.environment import GymEnvironment
from bindsnet.network.nodes import Input, LIFNodes
from bindsnet.pipeline.action import select_softmax

# Build network.
network = Network(dt=1.0)

# Layers of neurons.
inpt = Input(n=80 * 80, shape=[80, 80], traces=True)
middle = LIFNodes(n=100, traces=True)
out = LIFNodes(n=4, refrac=0, traces=True)

# Connections between layers.
inpt_middle = Connection(source=inpt, target=middle, wmin=0, wmax=1e-1)
middle_out = Connection(source=middle, target=out, wmin=0, wmax=1)

# Add all layers and connections to the network.
network.add_layer(inpt, name='Input Layer')
network.add_layer(middle, name='Hidden Layer')
network.add_layer(out, name='Output Layer')
network.add_connection(inpt_middle, source='Input Layer', target='Hidden Layer')
network.add_connection(middle_out, source='Hidden Layer', target='Output Layer')

# Load SpaceInvaders environment.
environment = GymEnvironment('BreakoutDeterministic-v4')
environment.reset()

# Build pipeline from specified components.
pipeline = Pipeline(network, environment, encoding=bernoulli,
                    action_function=select_softmax, output='Output Layer',
                    time=100, history_length=1, delta=1,
                    plot_interval=1, render_interval=1)

# Run environment simulation for 100 episodes.
for i in range(100):
    # initialize episode reward
    reward = 0
    pipeline.reset_()
    while True:
        pipeline.step()
        reward += pipeline.reward
        if pipeline.done:
            break
    print("Episode " + str(i) + " reward:", reward)
```

FIGURE 7 | A spiking neural network that accepts input from the `BreakoutDeterministic-v4` `gym` Atari environment. The observations from the environment are downsampled and binarized. The `history` and `delta` keyword arguments are used to create difference images before they are converted into Bernoulli-distributed vectors of spikes, one per time step. The output layer of the network has 4 neurons in it, each representing a different action in the Breakout game. An action is selected at each time step using the `select_softmax` feedback function, which treats the summed spikes over each output layer neuron as a probability distribution over actions.

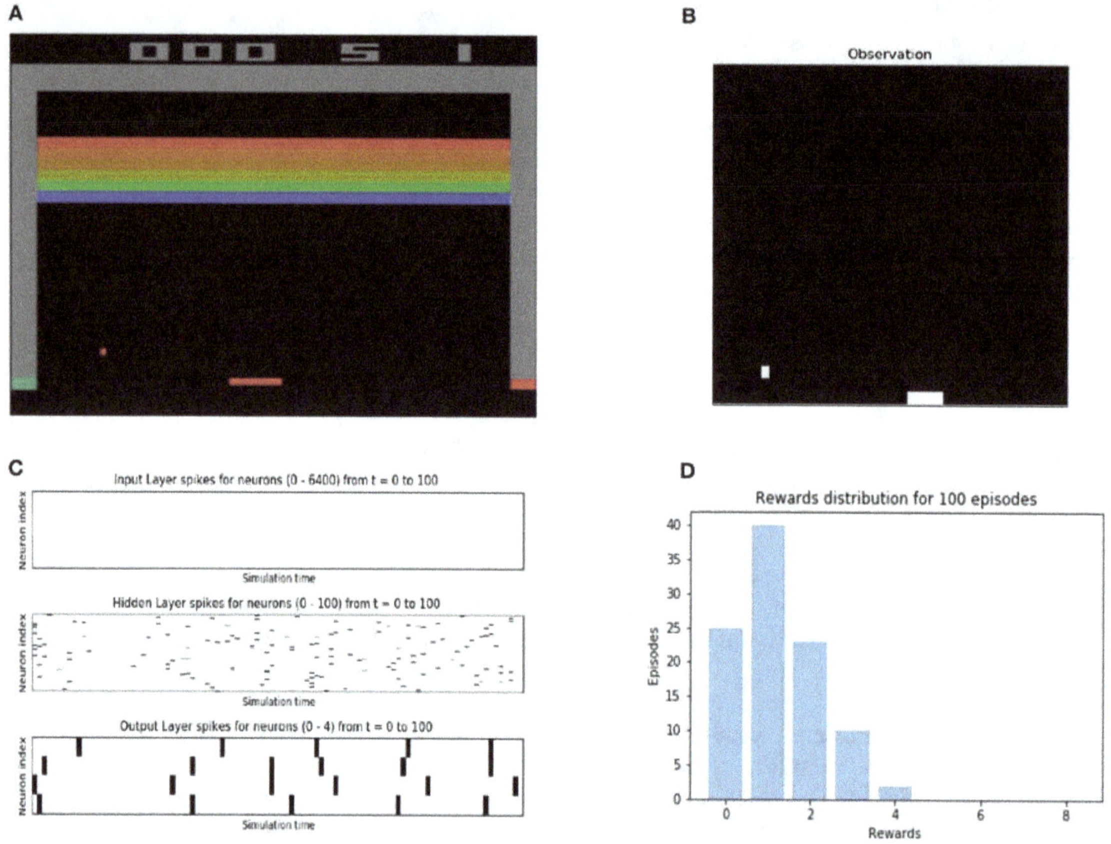

FIGURE 8 | Accompanying plots for a custom spiking neural network's which interacts with the `BreakoutDeterministic-v4` reinforcement learning environment. Spikes of all neuron populations are plotted, and the Breakout game is rendered, as well as the downsampled, `history`- and `delta`-altered observation, which is presented to the network. The performance of the network on 100 episodes of Breakout is also plotted. (note: The absence of spikes in the Input layer is due to the the large size of the layer and the way `matplotlib` library handles it. It is not a bug in our code). **(A)** Raw output from the Breakout game, provided by the OpenAI `gym render()` method. **(B)** Pre-processed output from breakout game environment used as input to the SNN. **(C)** Spikes from the Input, Hidden, and Output layers of the spiking neural network. **(D)** The reward distribution of the initialized network on 100 episodes of Breakout.

priority based on the needs of the users of the library.

- Specialization of machine learning and reinforcement learning algorithms for spiking neural networks. These may take the form of additional learning rules, or more complicated training methods that operate at the network level rather than on individual synapses.
- Tighter integration with `PyTorch`. Much of `PyTorch`'s neural network functions are useful in the spiking neural network context (e.g., `Conv2dConnection`), and will benefit from inheriting from them.
- Automatic conversion of deep neural network models implemented in `PyTorch` or specified in the `ONNX` format to near-equivalent spiking neural networks (as in Diehl et al., 2015).
- Performance optimization: improving the performance of library primitives will save time on all experiments with spiking neural networks. A high-priority feature is the use of sparse spike vectors and connection weights for efficient linear algebra operations.
- Automatic smoothing of SNNs: approximating spiking neurons as differentiable operations (Hunsberger and Eliasmith, 2015) will enable the use of backpropagation to train networks easily transferable to SNNs. The `torch.autograd` automatic differentiation library (Paszke et al., 2017) can then be applied to optimize the parameters of spiking networks for ML problems.

6. DISCUSSION

We have presented the `BindsNET` open source package for rapid biologically inspired prototyping of spiking neural networks with a machine learning-oriented approach. `BindsNET` is developed entirely in Python and is built on top of other mature Python libraries that lend their power to utilize multi-CPU or multi-GPU hardware configurations. Specifically, the ML tools and powerful data structures of `PyTorch` are a central part of `BindsNET`'s operation. `BindsNET` may also interface with the `gym` library to connect spiking neural networks to reinforcement learning

```
import torch
import torch.nn as nn
from bindsnet.datasets import MNIST
from bindsnet.network import Network
from bindsnet.encoding import poisson_loader
from bindsnet.network.monitors import Monitor
from bindsnet.network.topology import Connection
from bindsnet.network.nodes import LIFNodes, Input

# Define logistic regression model using PyTorch.
class LogisticRegression(nn.Module):
    def __init__(self, input_size, num_classes):
        super(LogisticRegression, self).__init__()
        self.linear = nn.Linear(input_size, num_classes)

    def forward(self, x):
        return self.linear(x)

# Build a simple, two layer, "input-output" network.
network = Network(dt=1.0)
inpt = Input(784, shape=(28, 28)); network.add_layer(inpt, name='I')
output = LIFNodes(625, thresh=-52 + torch.randn(625)); network.add_layer(output, name='O')
network.add_connection(Connection(inpt, output, w=torch.randn(inpt.n, output.n)), 'I', 'O')
network.add_connection(Connection(output, output, w=0.5 * torch.randn(output.n, output.n)), 'O', 'O')
network.add_monitor(Monitor(output, ['s'], time=250), name='output_spikes')

# Get MNIST training images and labels and create data loader.
images, labels = MNIST(path='../../data/MNIST').get_train()
loader = zip(poisson_loader(images * 0.25, time=250), iter(labels))

# Run training data on reservoir and store (spikes per neuron, label) pairs.
training_pairs = []
for i, (datum, label) in enumerate(loader):
    network.run(inpts={'I': datum}, time=250)
    training_pairs.append([network.monitors['output_spikes'].get('s').sum(-1), label])
    network.reset_()

    if (i + 1) % 50 == 0: print('Train progress: (%d / 500)' % (i + 1))
    if (i + 1) == 500: print(); break  # stop after 500 training examples

# Create and train logistic regression model on reservoir outputs.
model = LogisticRegression(625, 10); criterion = nn.CrossEntropyLoss()
optimizer = torch.optim.SGD(model.parameters(), lr=0.1)

# Train the logistic regression model on (spikes, label) pairs.
for epoch in range(10):
    for i, (s, label) in enumerate(training_pairs):
        optimizer.zero_grad(); output = model(s)
        loss = criterion(output.unsqueeze(0), label.unsqueeze(0).long())
        loss.backward(); optimizer.step()

# Get MNIST test images and labels and create data loader.
images, labels = MNIST(path='../../data/MNIST').get_test();
loader = zip(poisson_loader(images * 0.25, time=250), iter(labels))

# Run test data on reservoir and store (spikes per neuron, label) pairs.
test_pairs = []
for i, (datum, label) in enumerate(loader):
    network.run(inpts={'I': datum}, time=250)
    test_pairs.append([network.monitors['output_spikes'].get('s').sum(-1), label])
    network.reset_()

    if (i + 1) % 50 == 0: print('Test progress: (%d / 500)' % (i + 1))
    if (i + 1) == 500: print(); break  # stop after 500 test examples

# Test the logistic regresion model on (spikes, label) pairs.
correct, total = 0, 0
for s, label in test_pairs:
    output = model(s); _, predicted = torch.max(output.data.unsqueeze(0), 1)
    total += 1; correct += int(predicted == label.long())

print('Accuracy of logistic regression on 500 test examples: %.2f %%\n' % (100 * correct / total))
```

FIGURE 9 | A recurrent neural network built from 625 spiking neurons accepts inputs from the CIFAR-10 natural images dataset. An *input* population is connected all-to-all to an *output* population of LIF neurons with weights draw from the standard normal distribution, which has voltage thresholds drawn from $\mathcal{N}(-52, 1)$ and is recurrently connected to itself with weights drawn from $\mathcal{N}(0, \frac{1}{2})$. The reservoir is used to create a high-dimensional, temporal representation of the image data, which is used to train and test a logistic regression model created with `PyTorch`.

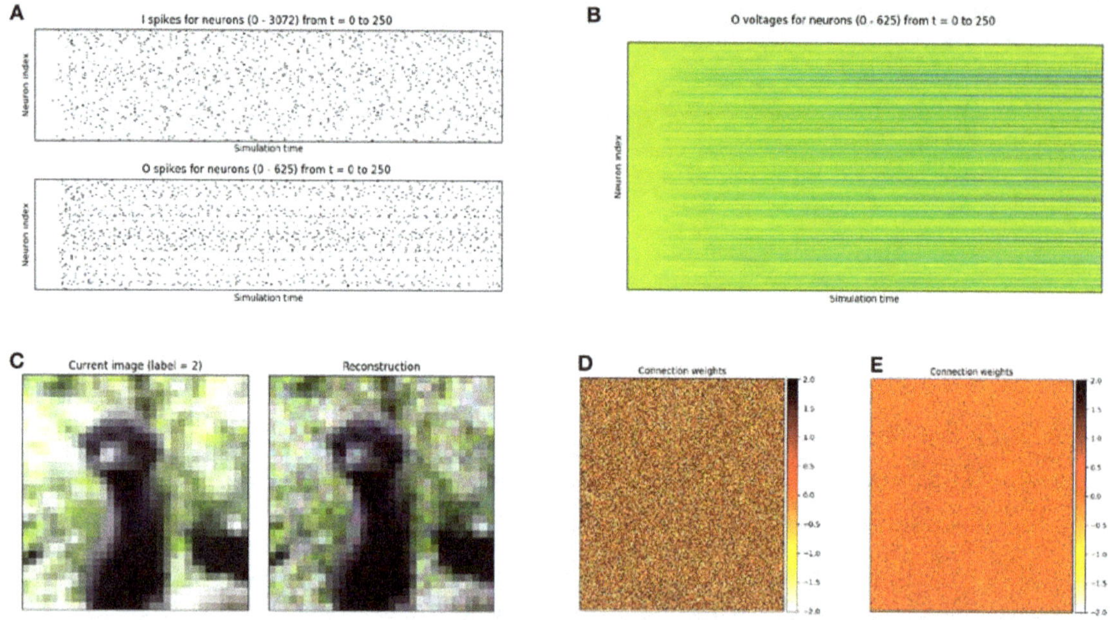

FIGURE 10 | Plots accompanying another reservoir computing example, in which an input population of size equal to the CIFAR-10 data dimensionality is connected to a population of 625 LIF neurons, which is recurrently connected to itself. **(A)** Spikes recorded from the input and output layers of the two layer reservoir network. **(B)** Voltages recorded from the output of the two layer reservoir network. **(C)** Raw input and its reconstruction, computed by summing Poisson-distributed spike trains over the time dimension. **(D)** Weights from input to output neuron populations, initialized initialized from the distribution $\mathcal{N}(0, 1)$. **(E)** Recurrent weights of the output population, initialized from the distribution $\mathcal{N}(0, \frac{1}{2})$.

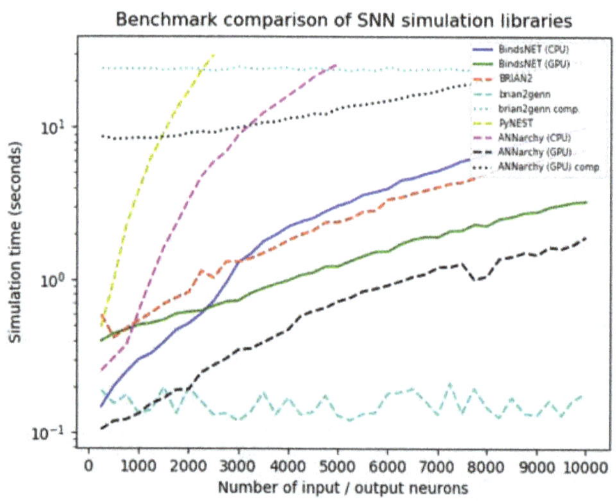

FIGURE 11 | Benchmark comparison results from a number of SNN simulation frameworks. Variability in benchmarked times is likely due to randomness in the simulation and fluctuations in CPU load.

environments. In sum, `BindsNET` represents an additional and attractive alternative for the research community for the purpose of developing faster and more flexible tools for SNN experimentation.

`BindsNET` comprises a spiking neural network simulation framework that is easy to use, flexible, and efficient. Our library is set apart from other solutions by its ML and RL focus; complex details of the biological neuron are eschewed in favor of high-level functionality. Computationally inclined researchers may be familiar with the underlying `PyTorch` functions and syntax, and excited by the potential of the third generation of neural networks for ML problems, driving adoption in both ML and computational neuroscience communities. This combination of ML programming tools and neuroscientific ideas may facilitate the further integration of biological neural networks and machine learning. To date, spiking neural networks have not been widely applied in ML and RL problems; having a library aimed at such is a promising step toward exciting new lines of research.

Researchers interested in developing spiking neural networks for use in ML or RL applications will find that `BindsNET` is a powerful and easy tool to develop their ideas. To that end, the biological complexity of neural components has been kept to a minimum, and high-level, qualitative functionality has been emphasized. However, the experimenter still has access to and control over groups of neurons at the level of membrane potentials and spikes, and connections at the level of synapse strengths, constituting a relatively low level of abstraction. Even with such details included, it is straightforward to build large and flexible network structures and apply them to real data. We believe that the ease with which our framework allows researchers to reason about spiking neural networks as ML models, or as RL agents, will enable advancements in biologically plausible machine learning, or further fusion of ML with neuroscientific concepts.

Although `BindsNET` is similar in spirit to the `Nengo` (Bekolay et al., 2014) neural and brain modeling software in that both packages can utilize a deep learning library as a "backend" for computation, `Nengo` optionally uses `Tensorflow` in a limited fashion while `BindsNET` uses `PyTorch` by default, for all network simulation functionality (with the `torch.Tensor` object). Additionally, for users that prefer the flexibility and the imperative execution of `PyTorch`, `BindsNET` inherits these features and is developed with many of the same design principles in mind. `BindsNET` has advantages with respect to other simulation libraries using GPU computation, which require costly compilation steps between network building and deployment. `BindsNET` does not need these expensive intermediate steps as it uses "eager" execution of `PyTorch` regardless of the actual simulation hardware.

Hardware platforms for spiking neural network computations have advantages over software simulations in terms of performance and power consumption. For example, SpiNNaker (Plana et al., 2011) combines cheap, generic, yet dedicated CPU boards together to create a powerful SNN simulation framework in hardware. Other platforms (e.g., TrueNorth Akopyan et al., 2015, HRL, and Braindrop) involve the design of a new chip. A novel development is Intel's Loihi platform for spike-based computation, outperforming all known conventional solutions (Davies et al., 2018). Other solutions are based on programmable hardware, like FPGAs which transform neural equations to configurations of electronic gates in order to speed up computation. More specialized hardware such as ASIC and DSP can be used to parallelize and therefore accelerate the calculations. In order to conduct experiments in the hardware domain, one must usually learn a specific programming language targeted to the hardware platform, or carefully adapt an existing experiment to the unique hardware environment under the constraints as enforced by chip designers. In either case, this is not an ideal situation for researchers who want rapid prototyping and testing. `BindsNET` platform introduces a flexibility, which can be exploited in future hardware developments, in particuliar in machine learning problems.

`BindsNET` is a simple yet attractive option for those looking to quickly build flexible SNN prototypes backed by an easy-to-use yet powerful deep learning library. It encourages the conception of spiking networks as machine learning models or reinforcement learning agents, and is one of the first of its kind to provide a seamless interface with machine learning and reinforcement learning environments. The library is supported by several mature and feature-full open source software projects, and benefits from their growth and continuous improvements. Considered as an extension of the `PyTorch` library, `BindsNET` represents a natural progression from second generation neural networks to third generation SNNs.

AUTHOR CONTRIBUTIONS

HS and RK initiated the research, produced the conceptual framework, and coordinated the ongoing development efforts. RK and HH conceived and design principles of the BindsNET package. HH and DJS wrote the BindsNET code and the initial version of the manuscript. DJS lead the efforts to create a standardized BindsNET code according to Python specification. HK and DTS helped with improving and testing the BindsNET code. All authors contributed to the revisions and producing the final manuscript.

ACKNOWLEDGMENTS

This work has been supported in part by Defense Advanced Research Project Agency Grant, DARPA/MTO HR0011-16-l-0006 and by National Science Foundation Grant NSF-CRCNS-DMS-13-11165.

REFERENCES

Abadi, M., Agarwal, A., Barham, P., Brevdo, E., Chen, Z., Citro, C., et al. (2015). *TensorFlow: Large-Scale Machine Learning on Heterogeneous Systems.* Available online at: tensorflow.org

Akopyan, F., Sawada, J., Cassidy, A. S., Alvarez-Icaza, R., Arthur, J. V., Merolla, P., et al. (2015). Truenorth: Design and tool flow of a 65 mw 1 million neuron programmable neurosynaptic chip. *IEEE Trans. Comput. Aid. Design Integr. Circ. Syst.* 34, 1537–1557. doi: 10.1109/TCAD.2015.2474396

Al-Rfou, R., Alain, G., Almahairi, A., Angermueller, C., Bahdanau, D., Ballas, N., et al. (2016). Theano: a Python framework for fast computation of mathematical expressions. *arXiv e-prints:abs/1605.02688.*

Bekolay, T., Bergstra, J., Hunsberger, E., DeWolf, T., Stewart, T. C., Rasmussen, D., et al. (2014). Nengo: a python tool for building large-scale functional brain models. *Front. Neuroinformat.* 7:48. doi: 10.3389/fninf.2013.00048

Bengio, Y., Lee, D., Bornschein, J., and Lin, Z. (2015). Towards biologically plausible deep learning. *CoRR:abs/1502.04156.*

Beyeler, M., Carlson, K. D., Chou, T.-S., Dutt, N. D., and Krichmar, J. L. (2015). "Carlsim 3: a user-friendly and highly optimized library for the creation of neurobiologically detailed spiking neural networks," in *2015 International Joint Conference on Neural Networks (IJCNN)* (Killarney), 1–8.

Brockman, G., Cheung, V., Pettersson, L., Schneider, J., Schulman, J., Tang, J., et al. (2016). Openai gym. *CoRR*, abs/1606.01540.

Bruna, J., Zaremba, W., Szlam, A., and LeCun, Y. (2013). Spectral networks and locally connected networks on graphs. *CoRR:abs/1312.6203.*

Carnevale, N. T., and Hines, M. L. (2006). *The NEURON Book.* Cambridge: University Press.

Chen, T., Li, M., Li, Y., Lin, M., Wang, N., Wang, M., et al. (2015). Mxnet: A flexible and efficient machine learning library for heterogeneous distributed systems. *CoRR:abs/1512.01274.*

Chetlur, S., Woolley, C., Vandermersch, P., Cohen, J., Tran, J., Catanzaro, B., et al. (2014). cudnn: Efficient primitives for deep learning. *CoRR:abs/1410.0759.*

Cornelis, H., Rodriguez, A. L., Coop, A. D., and Bower, J. M. (2012). Python as a federation tool for genesis 3.0. *PLoS ONE* 7:e29018. doi: 10.1371/journal.pone.0029018

Davies, M., Srinivasa, N., Lin, T.-H., Chinya, G., Cao, Y., Choday, S. H., et al. (2018). Loihi: a neuromorphic manycore processor with on-chip learning. *IEEE Micro* 38, 82–99. doi: 10.1109/MM.2018.112130359

Davison, A. P., Brüderle, D., Eppler, J. M., Kremkow, J., Müller, E., Pecevski, D., et al. (2008). Pynn: a common interface for neuronal network simulators. *Front. Neuroinformat.* 2:11. doi: 10.3389/neuro.11.011.2008

Diehl, P. U., and Cook, M. (2015). Unsupervised learning of digit recognition using spike-timing-dependent plasticity. *Front. Comput. Neurosci.* 9:99. doi: 10.3389/fncom.2015.00099

Diehl, P. U., Neil, D., Binas, J., Cook, M., Liu, S. C., and Pfeiffer, M. (2015). "Fast-classifying, high-accuracy spiking deep networks through weight and threshold balancing. in *2015 International Joint Conference on Neural Networks (IJCNN)*, 1–8.

Ferr, P., Mamalet, F., and Thorpe, S. J. (2018). Unsupervised feature learning with winner-takes-all based stdp. *Front. Comput. Neurosci.* 12:24. doi: 10.3389/fncom.2018.00024

Fidjeland, A., Roesch, E. B., Shanahan, M., and Luk, W. (2009). "Nemo: a platform for neural modelling of spiking neurons using gpus," *2009 20th IEEE International Conference on Application-specific Systems, Architectures and Processors*, 137–144.

Florian, R. V. (2007). Reinforcement learning through modulation of spike-timing-dependent synaptic plasticity. *Neural Comput.* 19, 1468–1502. doi: 10.1162/neco.2007.19.6.1468

Gewaltig, M.-O., and Diesmann, M. (2007). Nest (neural simulation tool). *Scholarpedia* 2:1430. doi: 10.4249/scholarpedia.1430

Goodman, D. F. M., and Brette, R. (2009). The Brian simulator. *Front. Neurosci.* 3:192-7. doi: 10.3389/neuro.01.026.2009

Hazan, H., Saunders, D. J., Sanghavi, D. T., Siegelmann, H. T., and Kozma, R. (2018). "Unsupervised learning with self-organizing spiking neural networks," *IEEE/INNS International Joint Conference on Neural Networks (IJCNN2018)* (Rio de Janeiro), 493–498.

Hebb, D. O. (1949). *The Organization of Behavior: A Neuropsychological Theory.* New York, NY: Wiley.

Hines, M., Davison, A., and Muller, E. (2009). Neuron and python. *Front. Neuroinformat.* 3:1. doi: 10.3389/neuro.11.001.2009

Huh, D., and Sejnowski, T. J. (2017). Gradient Descent for Spiking Neural Networks. *ArXiv e-prints.*

Hunsberger, E., and Eliasmith, C. (2015). Spiking deep networks with lif neurons. *CoRR:abs/1510.08829.*

Izhikevich, E. M. (2003). Simple model of spiking neurons. *IEEE Trans. Neural Netw.* 14, 1569–1572. doi: 10.1109/TNN.2003.820440

Jia, Y., Shelhamer, E., Donahue, J., Karayev, S., Long, J., Girshick, R., et al. (2014). Caffe: Convolutional architecture for fast feature embedding. *arXiv [Preprint] arXiv:1408.5093.*

Kasabov, N. K. (2014). Neucube: a spiking neural network architecture for mapping, learning and understanding of spatio-temporal brain data. *Neural Netw.* 52, 62–76. doi: 10.1016/j.neunet.2014.01.006

Kheradpisheh, S. R., Ganjtabesh, M., Thorpe, S. J., and Masquelier, T. (2016). Stdp-based spiking deep neural networks for object recognition. *CoRR:abs/1611.01421.*

Kistler, W. M., and Gerstner, W. (2002). *Spiking Neuron Models. Single Neurons, Populations, Plasticity.* Cambridge, UK: Cambridge University Press.

Krizhevsky, A., and Hinton, G. (2009). *Learning Multiple Layers of Features from Tiny Images.* Master's thesis, Department of Computer Science, University of Toronto.

LeCun, Y., Bengio, Y., and Hinton, Y. (2015). Deep learning. *Nature* 521, 436–444. doi: 10.1038/nature14539

Lee, J. H., Delbruck, T., and Pfeiffer, M. (2016). Training deep spiking neural networks using backpropagation. *Front. Neurosci.* 10:508. doi: 10.3389/fnins.2016.00508

Maass, W. (1996). Lower bounds for the computational power of networks of spiking neurons. *Neural Comput.* 8, 1–40. doi: 10.1162/neco.1996.8.1.1

Maass, W. (1997). Networks of spiking neurons: the third generation of neural network models. *Neural Netw.* 10, 1659–1671. doi: 10.1016/S0893-6080(97)00011-7

Marblestone, A. H., Wayne, G., and Kording, K. P. (2016). Toward an integration of deep learning and neuroscience. *Front. Comput. Neurosci.* 10:94. doi: 10.3389/fncom.2016.00094

Markram, H., Luebke, J., Frotscher, M., and Sakmann, B. (1997). Regulation of synaptic efficacy by coincidence of postsynaptic aps and epsps. *Science* 275, 213–215. doi: 10.1126/science.275.5297.213

Mostafa, H. (2018). Supervised learning based on temporal coding in spiking neural networks. *IEEE Trans. Neural Netw. Learn. Syst.* 29, 3227–3235. doi: 10.1109/TNNLS.2017.2726060

Mozafari, M., Kheradpisheh, S. R., Masquelier, T., Nowzari-Dalini, A., and Ganjtabesh, M. (2018). First-spike based visual categorization using reward-modulated stdp. *IEEE Trans. Neural Netw. Learn. Syst.* 29, 6178–6190. doi: 10.1109/TNNLS.2018.2826721

O'Connor, P., and Welling, M. (2016). Deep spiking networks. *CoRR:abs/1602.08323.*

Paszke, A., Gross, S., Chintala, S., Chanan, G., Yang, E., DeVito, Z., et al. (2017). "Automatic differentiation in pytorch," in *NIPS-W*, (Long Beach, CA).

Pedregosa, F., Varoquaux, G., Gramfort, A., Michel, V., Thirion, B., Grisel, O., et al. (2011). Scikit-learn: machine learning in Python. *J. Mach. Learn. Res.* 12, 2825–2830.

Plana, L. A., Clark, D. M., Davidson, S., Furber, S. B., Garside, J. D., Painkras, E., et al. (2011). SpiNNaker: design and implementation of a gals multicore system-on-chip. *J. Emerg. Technol. Comput. Syst.* 7, 17:1–17:18. doi: 10.1145/2043643.2043647

Rueckauer, B., and Liu, S. (2018). "Conversion of analog to spiking neural networks using sparse temporal coding," in *2018 IEEE International Symposium on Circuits and Systems (ISCAS)* (Florence), 1–5.

Rueckauer, B., Lungu, I.-A., Hu, Y., Pfeiffer, M., and Liu, S.-C. (2017). Conversion of continuous-valued deep networks to efficient event-driven networks for image classification. *Front. Neurosci.* 11:682. doi: 10.3389/fnins.2017.00682

Saunders, D. J., Siegelmann, H. T., Kozma, R., and Ruszinkó, M. (2018). "Stdp learning of image features with spiking neural networks," in *IEEE/INNS International Joint Conference on Neural Networks (IJCNN2018)* (Rio de Janeiro), 4906–4912.

Stewart, T. C. (2012). *A Technical Overview of the Neural Engineering Framework.* Technical report, Centre for Theoretical Neuroscience.

Stimberg, M., Goodman, D., Benichoux, V., and Brette, R. (2014). Equation-oriented specification of neural models for simulations. *Front. Neuroinformat.* 8:6. doi: 10.3389/fninf.2014.00006

Stimberg, M., Goodman, D. F. M., and Nowotny, T. (2018). Brian2genn: a system for accelerating a large variety of spiking neural networks with graphics hardware. *bioRxiv.*

Stork, D. G. (1989). "Is backpropagation biologically plausible?," in *International 1989 Joint Conference on Neural Networks*, vol.2 (Washington, DC), 241–246.

Thorpe, S., and Gautrais, J. (1998). "Rank order coding," in *Proceedings of the Sixth Annual Conference on Computational Neuroscience : Trends in Research, 1998: Trends in Research, 1998*, CNS '97 (New York, NY: Plenum Press), 113–118.

Tikidji-Hamburyan, R. A., Narayana, V., Bozkus, Z., and El-Ghazawi, T. A. (2017). Software for brain network simulations: a comparative study. *Front. Neuroinformat.* 11:46. doi: 10.3389/fninf.2017.00046

Tokui, S., Oono, K., Hido, S., and Clayton, J. (2015). "Chainer: a next-generation open source framework for deep learning," in *Proceedings of Workshop on Machine Learning Systems (LearningSys) in The Twenty-ninth Annual Conference on Neural Information Processing Systems (NIPS).* Available online at: http://learningsys.org/papers/LearningSys_2015_paper_33.pdf

Vitay, J., Dinkelbach, H., and Hamker, F. (2015). Annarchy: a code generation approach to neural simulations on parallel hardware. *Front. Neuroinformat.* 9:19. doi: 10.3389/fninf.2015.00019

Wall, J., and Glackin, C. (2013). Spiking neural network connectivity and its potential for temporal sensory processing and variable binding. *Front. Comput. Neurosci.* 7:182. doi: 10.3389/fncom.2013.00182

Wang, J. X., Kurth-Nelson, Z., Kumaran, D., Tirumala, D., Soyer, H., Leibo, J. Z., et al. (2018). Prefrontal cortex as a meta-reinforcement learning system. *Nat. Neurosci.* 22, 860–868. doi: 10.1038/s41593-018-0147-8

Wu, Y., Deng, L., Li, G., Zhu, J., and Shi, L. (2018). Spatio-temporal backpropagation for training high-performance spiking neural networks. *Front. Neurosci.* 12:331. doi: 10.3389/fnins.2018.00331

Xiao, H., Rasul, K., and Vollgraf, R. (2017). Fashion-mnist: a novel image dataset for benchmarking machine learning algorithms. *CoRR:abs/1708.07747.*

Yavuz, E., Turner, J. P., and Nowotny, T. (2016). Genn: a code generation framework for accelerated brain simulations. *Sci. Reports* 6:18854. doi: 10.1038/srep18854

11

Reproducing Polychronization: A Guide to Maximizing the Reproducibility of Spiking Network Models

Robin Pauli [1*†], *Philipp Weidel* [1†], *Susanne Kunkel* [2,3] *and Abigail Morrison* [1,4]

[1] *Institute of Neuroscience and Medicine (INM-6) and Institute for Advanced Simulation (IAS-6) and JARA BRAIN Institute I, Jülich Research Centre, Jülich, Germany,* [2] *Faculty of Science and Technology, Norwegian University of Life Sciences, Ås, Norway,* [3] *Department of Computational Science and Technology, School of Computer Science and Communication, KTH Royal Institute of Technology, Stockholm, Sweden,* [4] *Institute of Cognitive Neuroscience, Faculty of Psychology, Ruhr-University Bochum, Bochum, Germany*

Correspondence:
Robin Pauli
r.pauli@fz-juelich.de

† These authors have contributed equally to this work.

Any modeler who has attempted to reproduce a spiking neural network model from its description in a paper has discovered what a painful endeavor this is. Even when all parameters appear to have been specified, which is rare, typically the initial attempt to reproduce the network does not yield results that are recognizably akin to those in the original publication. Causes include inaccurately reported or hidden parameters (e.g., wrong unit or the existence of an initialization distribution), differences in implementation of model dynamics, and ambiguities in the text description of the network experiment. The very fact that adequate reproduction often cannot be achieved until a series of such causes have been tracked down and resolved is in itself disconcerting, as it reveals unreported model dependencies on specific implementation choices that either were not clear to the original authors, or that they chose not to disclose. In either case, such dependencies diminish the credibility of the model's claims about the behavior of the target system. To demonstrate these issues, we provide a worked example of reproducing a seminal study for which, unusually, source code was provided at time of publication. Despite this seemingly optimal starting position, reproducing the results was time consuming and frustrating. Further examination of the correctly reproduced model reveals that it is highly sensitive to implementation choices such as the realization of background noise, the integration timestep, and the thresholding parameter of the analysis algorithm. From this process, we derive a guideline of best practices that would substantially reduce the investment in reproducing neural network studies, whilst simultaneously increasing their scientific quality. We propose that this guideline can be used by authors and reviewers to assess and improve the reproducibility of future network models.

Keywords: reproducibility, polychronization, spiking network models, spike-timing dependent plasticity, synchrony

1. INTRODUCTION

Reproducing computational models of networks of spiking point neurons seems like it should be easy. Neuron and synapse models are described as systems of ordinary differential equations with a few additional conditions and constraints. By specifying the parameters, the initial conditions, and any stimulus to the network, the dynamics of any reproduced network should be at least statistically equivalent, or even identical if external sources of random numbers are handled appropriately.

However, this optimistic attitude rarely survives the experience of trying to reproduce a model from a paper. As contributors to the NEST simulator (Gewaltig and Diesmann, 2007), the authors have reproduced a variety of models to create examples. A major source of frustration is inadequate specification of numbers. Parameters are sometimes missing from the description in the paper. This can be in an overt manner, e.g., τ_{m} occurs in the neuron model equations but its value is not stated anywhere, or occur covertly, such that the parameter is not even mentioned in the text. Another common issue with parameters is that the value used in the paper is not the value used for the simulation. Sometimes the number is rounded to a smaller number of decimal places, sometimes it is plain wrong, sometimes the unit is wrong, and sometimes the author fails to mention, for example, a multiplicative factor. Similarly, initial conditions can be incompletely or incorrectly specified, for example the authors state that the initial values for a given parameter are drawn from a certain random distribution, but fail to mention it is truncated.

A further area of divergence is inadequate specification of implementation. One example of this would be for the truncated distribution mentioned above, the authors do not state the behavior when a number is drawn outside of the bounds: clip to bounds or re-draw? Other examples include the choice of the numeric solver of model dynamics and issues to do with event ordering in plastic synapse models – if a pre- and post-synaptic spike arrive simultaneously at a synapse implementing spike-timing dependent plasticity, which happens first, depression or facilitation?

It is worth noting that the two types of insufficient specification are of quite different natures and cannot necessarily be addressed by the same approach. For the majority of current spiking point neuron models, the number of parameters to be specified is large but not ridiculously so. Thus it is reasonable to expect that they all be mentioned explicitly in the main text of a manuscript or in its **Supplementary Material**. This issue was partially addressed by Nordlie et al. (2009), who developed a break-down of network models into components (e.g., neuron model, connectivity, stimulus etc.) which can then be expressed in tables with a standardized layout. The experience of the authors is that the exercise of filling out these tables brings parameters to light that might otherwise have been overlooked, however it does not provide any protection against wrong values or secret multiplicative factors as discussed above.

In contrast, a complete specification of the implementation cannot be sensibly captured in tables, as it is "how" rather than "what" information. Whereas some aspects can be explained in the text of a manuscript, comprehensive coverage cannot be expected, firstly because it would make manuscripts technically dense to the point of unreadability, and secondly because human readable language is rife with ambiguities that would hamper an accurate reproduction of the described model. Because of these specification issues it is often not possible to reproduce a model from a paper without contacting the authors and extracting more information.

Clearly, then, sharing model code should be seen as part of a modeler's obligation to enable reproducibility of his or her study. This is easily achieved on a variety of platforms. However, downloading a model code from such a platform and running it on your own machine does not constitute reproducing a study in the strong sense. Using the definitions proposed by the Association for Computing Machinery (2016), we will refer to this as *replication*, i.e., different team, same experimental set-up (see Plesser, 2018 for a summary and analysis of different technical definitions for reproduction and replication). At best, it simply shows that the model code is portable and generates the reported results. At worst, it does nothing, since availability of code does not entail that this code can be run on your machine, as tragically documented by Topalidou et al. (2015) and on a more industrial scale (but outside the neuroscience context) by Collberg and Proebsting (2016).

The ReScience Initiative (Rougier et al., 2017) seeks to address this issue by providing a home for *reproductions* of model studies (i.e., different team, different experimental set-up). The reproductions published there are open-source implementations of published research that are tested, commented, and reviewed. However, it would be preferable if the original publications were intrinsically reproducible, rather than requiring intense post-publication efforts by others. To achieve this, it is important not only for researchers to put greater effort into making their code available and comprehensible, but also for reviewers to be able to quickly evaluate any factors that might undermine its reproducibility.

In this article, we develop a guideline for spiking neuronal network modelers to present their work in such a way as to minimize the effort of other scientists to reproduce it. As we believe that concrete illustrations are necessary to convincingly motivate recommendations, we provide these by reproducing a seminal study in computational neuroscience, a minimal network generating polychronous groups (Izhikevich, 2006). We analyze which features of the model and analysis code (and description in the manuscript) support, and which hinder, the reproduction of the study. From each of these features, we derive a corresponding recommendation that, if followed by future studies, would increase their reproducibility.

The choice of this source material is motivated by the following considerations. Firstly, the author took the (then) highly unusual step of making the model code available, both in the manuscript itself (MATLAB) and in downloadable form (MATLAB and C++). Secondly, despite the availability of the code, the model is rather challenging to reproduce, due to a number of non-standard models and numerics choices, thus making it a fruitful source of recommendations.

We would like to emphasize that the choice is purely demonstrative, and almost any study with published code could have been used for our purposes; indeed the authors' own work has not come up to the standards we propose. Furthermore, we point out that many of the technical solutions we propose were not available at the time the source material was published.

In the first phase (section 2.2), we establish a baseline by downloading the author's C++ code and carrying out some minimal modifications to enable it to run locally. In the second phase we demonstrate that our best-effort initial attempt to reproduce the study's results using a NEST implementation of the network fail (section 3.2), and focus our efforts on creating an implementation capable of reproducing results identical on the level of individual spikes and synaptic weights. For this implementation, various artifacts (e.g., connectivity matrix) need to be exported from the original implementation into NEST. Therefore, in the the third phase we develop a stand-alone NEST implementation and investigate how well it reproduces the original results (section 3.3). We demonstrate that the original network has a second activity mode unreported in the original study.

In section 3.4, we manipulate the stand-alone NEST implementation to investigate various issues with respect to numerics and model features that we discovered in the preceding phases, and in section 3.5 we perform an analogous investigation of the main analysis algorithm provided as part of the original code. In this way, we uncover unreported major dependencies on coding errors and implementation (rather than conceptual) choices such as the background noise, the resolution of the neuron update and the thresholding parameter of the analysis algorithm. The series of recommendations that we derive from reproducing the original model and investigating its sensitivity to parameters and implementation details are gathered and discussed in section 3.6.

Our results demonstrate that putting effort into code presentation and study design to boost its reproducibility does not just make it easier for future researchers to independently confirm the results and/or extend the model. It also increases the scientific quality of the study, by reducing the risk that results have been distorted by avoidable coding errors, inappropriate choices of numerics, or highly specific parameter settings.

2. METHODS

Our implementation of the model and all materials used for this study are publicly available on GitHub[1] under MIT license.

2.1. Polychronization Network Model

The polychronization network model as described in Izhikevich (2006) is inspired by a patch of cortical tissue. The network model contains 1,000 neurons, of which 800 are modeled as excitatory and 200 modeled as inhibitory, as described in Izhikevich (2004). Throughout the simulation the neurons are stimulated by the unusual method of randomly selecting one neuron in each millisecond step, and applying a direct current of 20 pA to it for the duration of that step, reliably evoking a spike.

The neurons in the original network model are connected as follows: for each inhibitory neuron, 100 targets are selected from the excitatory population, not permitting multapses or autapses. Inhibitory synaptic connections are static with a weight of -5 mV and argued to be local, and thus have a delay of 1 ms. For the excitatory neurons, the 100 targets are selected at random from the whole network, also not permitting multapses or autapses. Excitatory synaptic connections are plastic, the detailed dynamics of which are described in section 3.4.2. The delays for these connections are highly structured: they are evenly spread between 1 and 20 ms, i.e., exactly five outgoing connections of each neuron have the delay 1 ms, exactly five connections have the delay 2 ms, and so on. The model parameters are summarized in tables in the **Supplementary Materials**.

2.2. Preparing the Polychronization Network Model for Replication

We downloaded the C++ source code `poly_spnet.cpp` from the author's website[2] and installed it locally. The original code could not be compiled with the standard g++ compiler under Ubuntu 16.04 LTS. Some minor adjustments were necessary to make the code compile and run, which are given in the **Supplementary Material**. We note that there are differences between the MATLAB code published in Izhikevich (2006) and that available for download, and between both MATLAB versions and the C++ code. Unless stated otherwise, all remarks on features of "the original code" refer to the C++ version used as the basis of this study.

The source code is a single standalone script that comprises both simulation and the analysis, including identification of polychronous groups. In order to later compare the statistics of groups found by the original simulation code and by the NEST re-implementations, we re-structured the code to separate the analysis from the simulation, writing the neural activity (spike times and membrane potentials) in NEST-formatted text files, and the network connectivity in JSON format.

We checked that using the separated versions of the simulation script and analysis script serially yields identical results to running the downloaded code with integrated simulation and analysis. This enabled us to run the same analysis on data produced by the original code and by implementations in NEST, rather than having to chase down disparities in simulation and analysis code simultaneously. In the following, we refer to this slightly modified version of the downloaded code as the "original network model".

The recommendations that we compile in section 3.6.1 are mostly inspired by this initial process of assessing and adapting the original source code.

2.2.1. NEST

Network simulations are either carried out using Izhikevich's homebrewed network simulator written in C++ or using NEST 2.14. (Peyser et al., 2017). The source code for the Izhikevich

[1] https://github.com/INM-6/reproducing-polychronization

[2] https://www.izhikevich.org/publications/spnet.htm

synapse model is publicly available on GitHub in a branch of a fork of the NEST repository. Due to the model's multiple idiosyncrasies and numerical issues reported on in this article (see section 3.2.2 and section 3.4), it does not fulfill the quality standards for NEST and so will not be merged to the master branch of the main repository and included with future releases of NEST.

2.3. Experiments

2.3.1. YAML

In order to investigate the dynamics of the model under study, we defined several experiments described in section 3.4. In the experiments we varied parameters such as stimuli, delay distributions and numeric resolution. For each experiment we wrote a distinct parameter file in YAML ("Yet Another Markup Language" or "YAML Ain't Markup Language") which makes the workflow very clear and modular. All YAML files are available in the repository and in the **Supplemental Material** in tabular form.

2.3.2. Polychronous Group Finding Algorithm

For our data analysis we used two different versions of the algorithm which finds polychronous groups. For the first version, we extracted the original algorithm from Izhikevich's C++ code and adapted it such that it uses our JSON data format. We confirmed that our adaptation does not change the original results by comparing the found groups on a given dataset.

This C++ version of the algorithm finds groups by running a full network simulation, in which a specific group of neurons is stimulated and the network response recorded. As the delay distribution is hardcoded in the structure of the algorithm and the integration timestep is fixed to 1 ms, it is not possible to apply this algorithm to experiments in which we changed these parameters. We therefore wrote a second algorithm in Python that runs a NEST simulation, in which we can easily alter the integration timestep or delay distribution.

For the Python version of the algorithm we tried to be as close as possible to the original C++ version, but generalized to be applicable to all parameter sets. Starting from a pivot neuron, we iterate over all triplets of neurons ("anchor neurons") forming synapses with at least 95% of the maximal weight to this pivot neuron. We then determine all other neurons which are targeted by this triplet, start a NEST simulation, and stimulate the targeted neurons in the order of their delay relative to the pivot neuron, with the corresponding weight from the triplet. We record the network response and consider the triplet and all neurons emitting a spike during the simulation as part of a polychronous group. After the NEST simulation finishes we scan the connectivity for connections between the neurons participating in this group and define the "layer of a neuron" as the length of the chain of pre-synaptic neurons within the group. Finally, following the original algorithm, the group is only considered to be relevant if the longest path is larger than seven layers and all three anchor neurons participate in the activation of the group. We point out that setting the minimum layer threshold lower than seven leads to a rapid increase of the number of groups. The Python version deviates from the original C++ code, as we found errors in the original code that we fixed in our version. For example, for large groups, the original code exhibits an array index overflow, leading to erroneous spike delivery during group detection. Moreover, the original code often misses one last spike in the network response; this reduces the group size and longest path by one, leading to a reduced number of relevant groups.

Compared to the original algorithm, our Python version typically finds twice as many polychronous groups. However, conceptually the two algorithms seem to be approximately equivalent as nearly all (>99%) groups found by the original version are also found by the Python version. Thus, we consider the Python version to be a "generous" evaluation of the number of groups with respect to the original version. A detailed discussion of the group finding algorithm and the definition of polychrony can be found in section 3.5.

2.3.3. Activity Metrics

To estimate firing rates, we binned the spikes of all excitatory (inhibitory) neurons in bins of 5 ms. We then divided by the number of excitatory (inhibitory) neurons to calculate the average rate of one neuron in the population f_{pop} in spks/s. The single neuron variability is expressed by the coefficient of variation (CV) of the inter-spike interval distribution, $CV = \sigma(ISI)/\mu(ISI)$. The synchrony of the network dynamics is calculated as the Fano factor (FF) of the population averaged spike counts $N(t)$ with $\text{FF} = \sigma(N(t))^2/\mu(N(t))$. To estimate the spectral characteristic of the network, we applied a Fourier transformation on the population rate f_{pop} of the excitatory neurons, following Izhikevich (2006). We calculated the peak frequency in the range between $20 - 500$ Hz and categorized the network activity as having a low gamma peak if its maximum amplitude fell in the range $35 - 50$ Hz, and a high gamma peak if the maximum amplitude fell in the range $50 - 100$ Hz.

2.3.4. Snakemake

Snakemake is a script based workflow management system which allows reproducible and scalable data analysis (Köster and Rahmann, 2012). The complexity of our simulations, involving several different versions of neuron, synapse and network models as well as analysis scripts was massively eased by using snakemake. It allows its users to run their analysis on laptops and clusters, visualize the workflow (see **Figure 1**) and manage the data in a consistent and efficient way. Using a workflow manager enables us to keep track of the files generated by the original code, the slightly modified version of the original code and the various experiments conducted in sections 3.4 and 3.5. Snakemake links the version of the program to the data it created, such that it can re-run specific sections of a workflow depending on what parts were changed.

2.4. Workflow

In order to investigate the dynamics and performance of the model under study on different sets of parameters (see our recommendations in section 3.6.3), we simulated the model many times under different conditions which led to a rather complex workflow. This is illustrated in **Figure 1** for the example of comparing the bitwise reproduction to the

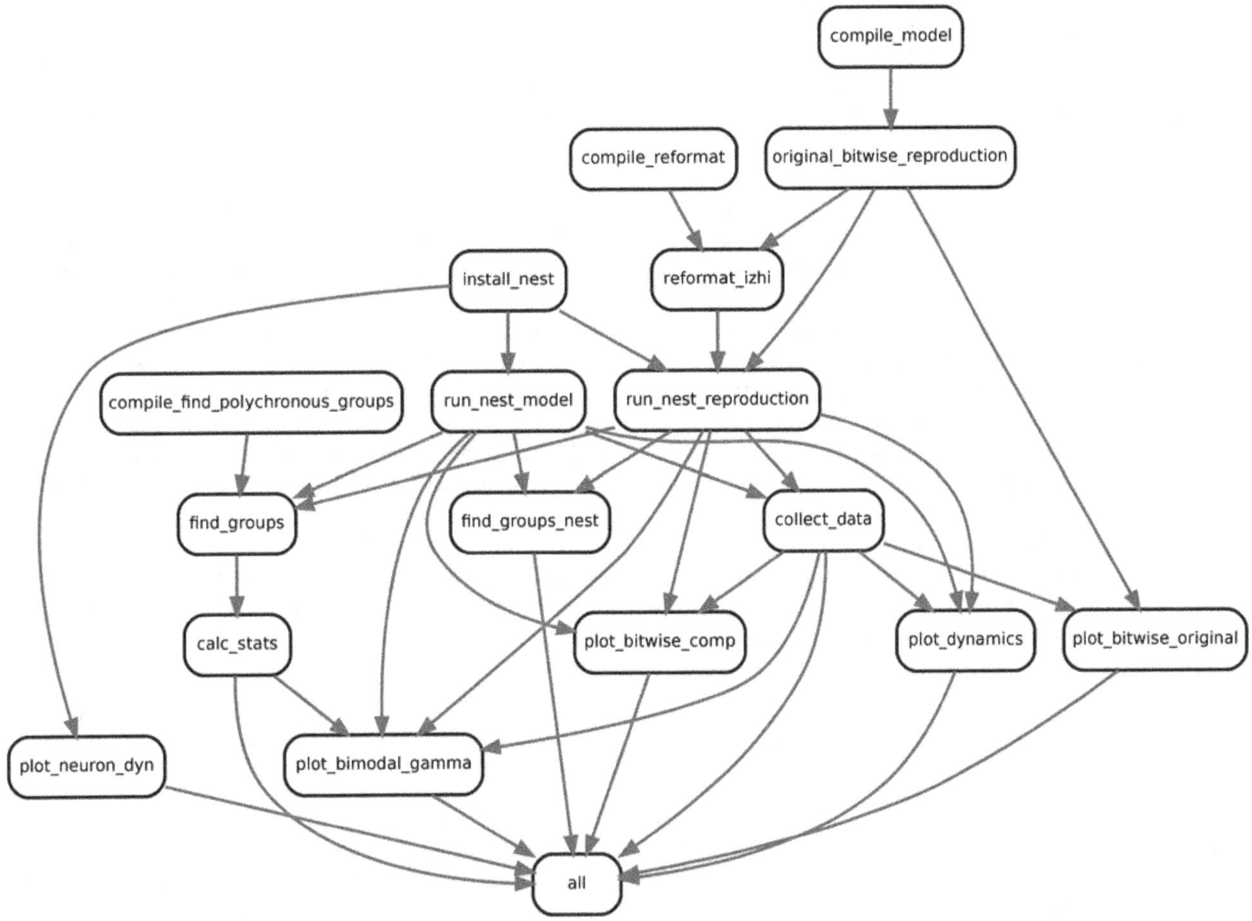

FIGURE 1 | Example visualization of the snakemake workflow for comparing the bitwise reproduction and the qualitative model. Shown are the rulenames defined and their input output relationships.

qualitative reproduction. Shown are the rulenames (labels in the boxes) defined and their input-output (arrow between boxes) relationships, for example *collect_data* where the arrows indicate that the defined rule uses input, i.e., a data file from *run_nest_model* and its output is used by *plot_dynamics*.

First, to prepare the simulations we have to compile and install all dependencies including the original model in C++ (*compile_model*), the tools for reformatting the original data to JSON (*compile_reformat*), the original algorithm to find polychronous groups (*compile_find_polychronous_groups*) and NEST (*install_nest*). Next, we run the original model (*original_bitwise_reproduction*) and reformat the produced data to use the JSON dataformat (*reformat_izhi*). The output of the original model is used to initialize the neurons, connectivity and stimuli in the NEST bitwise reproduction. We run the bitwise reproduction (*run_nest_reproduction*) and the qualitative reproduction (*run_nest_model*), which is independent of the output of the original model. Afterwards we collect all data (*collect_data*) and run the algorithm for finding polychronous groups (*find_groups* and *find_groups_nest*). Finally we calculate group statistics (*calc_stats*) and activity statistics and plot the relevant data (*plot_dynamics*). The box with label *all* is a dummy target used to define all files that should be produced by the workflow. This is used by Snakemake to generate the dependency tree in **Figure 1**. This workflow is repeated automatically 10 times for all experiments and 100 times for bitwise reproduction and qualitative reproduction using Snakemake. After generation of the necessary files, the plots for the single neuron dynamics (**Figure 9**), group analysis (**Figure 8**) and the bi-modal dynamic states (**Figures 5, 7**) are produced.

3. RESULTS

3.1. Replicating the Polychronization Network Model

The polychronization network model was proposed by Izhikevich (2006) as a minimal spiking neural network model capable of exhibiting polychronization, consisting of randomly coupled point neurons expressing STDP (see section 2.1 for a detailed network description). In addition to the network model, an algorithm for detecting polychronous groups was provided in this study. A polychronous group is a group of neurons connected in such a way that neural activity propagates in a reliable and stereotypical fashion due to the interplay between synaptic delays and the activation times of neurons. Izhikevich (2006) illustrates the concept of polychrony in a comprehensible way and links to higher neural processes such as cognition, computation, attention and consciousness.

Our execution of the original network model, prepared for execution on our system as described in section 2.2, successfully replicates the main results reported in that study. Executing the original network model on our system results in 18,000 s of network activity, exhibiting slow oscillations and gamma rhythms (interpreted by the original study as "sleep-like" and "implicated in cognitive tasks"). After simulation, the original polychronous group finding algorithm (see section 2.3.2) identifies 4,305 polychronous groups in the connectivity of the network model. The final weight distribution and power spectrum can be seen in **Figure 2**.

3.2. Identical Reproduction

In order to reproduce a network model in machine precision it is not enough to parameterize the network model identically. The issue of reproducibility goes deeper than the model specification itself. For example the choice of compiler, the order in which numerical operations are executed or the underlying hardware the model is run on can lead to rounding errors; these accumulate over a long simulation time and therefore lead to different results. Without providing the original code with provenance tracking and raw data, a model can therefore not be reproduced identically as there is no possibility to compare the exact results, i.e., every spike and every weight (Ghosh et al., 2017).

The original raw data was not provided, but given that the original code is written in C++, as is NEST, we determined that it should be possible to replicate the results yielded by the original C++ version on our machines with a NEST version on the same machine. This is not what is normally understood as "reproduction of a neural network model," which would typically only aim for statistical equivalence of aggregate findings, e.g., firing rates, mean number of groups, etc. For such measures, environmental features such as the operating system or compiler version should not play a role; if they do, this suggests the model is inherently excessively sensitive. However, we take this step here to ensure we have captured all details of the neuron and synapse model used in the original network model.

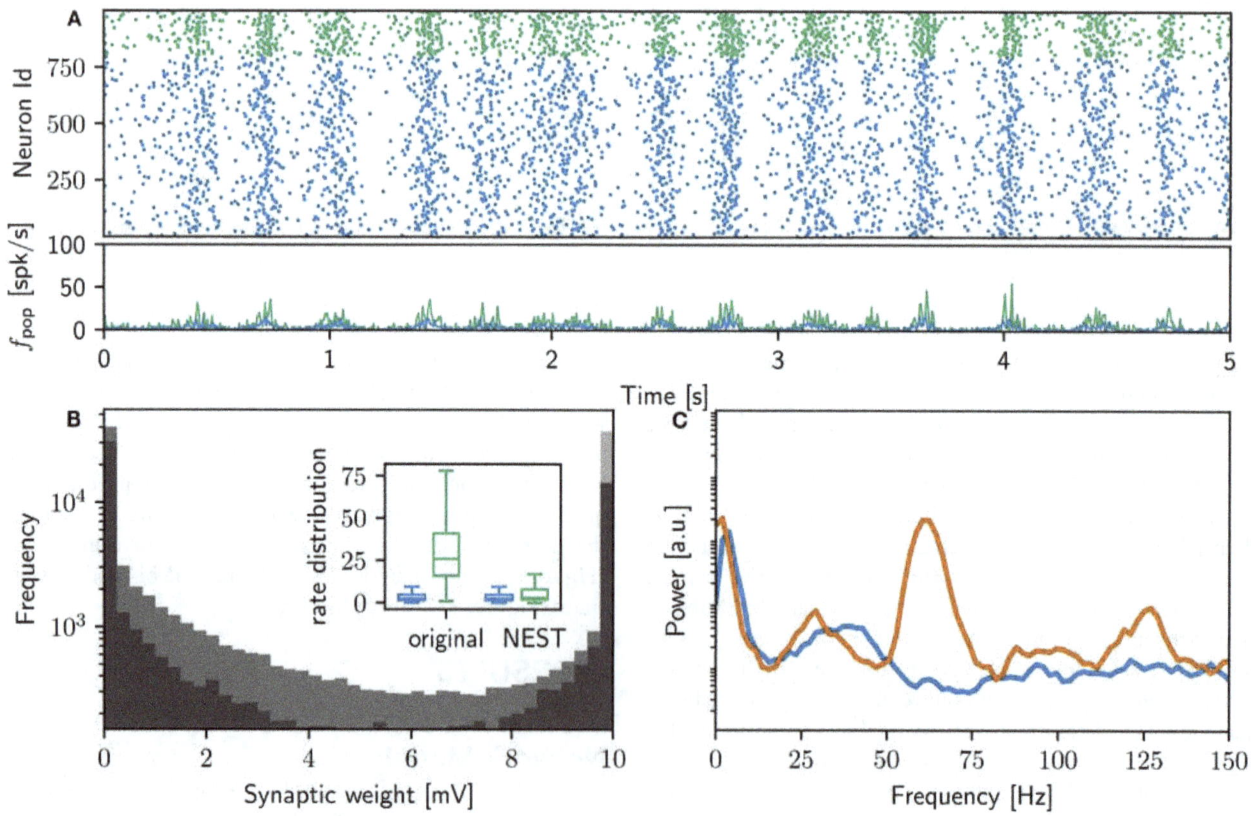

FIGURE 2 | Comparison of initial NEST network model with original. **(A)** Spike raster plot and rate envelope generated by the NEST simulation in the final 10 s (17,990 – 18,000) for inhibitory (green) and excitatory (blue) neurons. **(B)** Final weight distribution (frequency plotted on a logarithmic scale) for the original (dark gray) and NEST (light gray) simulations. Inset: rate distributions over the final 10 s displayed as box plots for the excitatory and inhibitory populations in the original and NEST simulations, colors as above. **(C)** Power spectrum of the rate envelope over the final 10 s for the excitatory population in the original (orange curve) and NEST (blue curve) simulations.

3.2.1. Initial Iteration

The Izhikevich neuron model (Izhikevich, 2004) used in the original code already existed in the NEST code base, but we needed to implement the synapse model based on the text description in Izhikevich (2006) and the modified version of source code as described in section 2.2.

The original network model has three sources of randomness: the selection of which neurons to connect, the initial values of the membrane potentials, and the noise stimulation, implemented as a direct current delivered to one randomly selected neuron in each millisecond. We therefore modified the original version to save the connectivity matrix, the initial values of the membrane potentials and the order of neuron stimulation to file; these are then read in and applied by the NEST simulation. Additionally, we modified the original to allow the seed for the random number generator to be set as a parameter, thus enabling multiple runs of the model to be carried out in our snakemake workflow (see section 2.4).

Figure 2A shows a raster plot of the spiking activity in the final 10 s of simulation in our initial iteration of trying to replicate the original model identically; the rate distributions are strikingly different, in particular the inhibitory rate of the NEST model is low compared with the original version (see **Figure 2B**, inset). The power spectra (**Figure 2C**) reveal that the strong gamma peak exhibited by the original model is not present in the NEST simulation. The weight distribution is also different; whilst still maintaining a bimodal character, the NEST simulation has a larger number of maximum weights (**Figure 2B**). Using the original algorithm to find polychronous groups we were able to find five groups in ten iterations with different random seeds.

These results show that despite the best, good-faith attempt of a group of researchers with considerable experience in developing neuron, synapse and network models, it was not possible to reproduce the neuron and synapse dynamics described in Izhikevich (2006) in one pass, even though the source code was available for inspection. Our first iteration fails to reproduce the key findings of the original study, either in terms of network dynamics or in terms of the generation of polychronous groups. Not only does this demonstrate that reproduction of computational models can be challenging even for experienced modelers with access to the original model code, it also raises the possibility that the aforementioned key findings are dependent on implementation details of the synapse and neuron models.

3.2.2. Final Iteration

It took a great investment of time to iteratively adapt the NEST simulation described above such that it yielded identical results to the original version. There were a number of disparities in the respective neuron and synapse models, including priority assigned to simultaneous events in the synapse model, ordering of neuron update, implementation of exponential functions, and ordering of mathematical operations.

These algorithmic and numeric aspects are (understandably) not discussed in the text description of the manuscript, underlining once again the importance of sharing the code. However, neither can they be readily found by examining the C++ code, as it is rather hard to comprehend in detail for the following reasons:

- It is uncommented (or commented only with the corresponding lines from the MATLAB version of the code)
- It exhibits low encapsulation; neuronal and synaptic updates are mixed throughout the simulation code, and synaptic interactions rely on long nested sequences of indexing rather than meaningfully named functions
- Numerics are not always standard, e.g., multiplication by 0.95 in each time step rather than using an exponential function
- Parameters are not always given meaningful names and defined in one place, such as the beginning of the script or in a separate parameter file; moreover, some appear as "magic numbers" in the middle of the code

We note that the MATLAB code is somewhat better commented, but the discrepancies between the sources mean that comments in one do not necessarily help to understand the other. However, even with a perfectly structured and commented source code it would be difficult to find all disparities, as there are many special cases in the particular synaptic plasticity algorithm used in the original network model. It would be very challenging to think of all possible special cases and check by mental simulation of the two codes whether each one would be handled identically.

Consequently, it was necessary to write several specific tests for the neuron and synapse model in both the original version and the NEST implementation in order to progressively eliminate discrepancies until they all came to light (see section 3.6.2 in the recommendations). By comparing their responses to identical input, especially border cases, it was possible to track down the algorithmic differences between the models. In the case of NEST, writing scripts to test a synapse or neuron with a particular input is easy, because it is a modular simulation tool written in a general purpose fashion, i.e., not optimized for a specific network model. In contrast, as the homebrewed original version is neither modular nor general, testing the behavior of individual elements required some creative modifications (see our recommendations in section 3.6.2).

The main discrepancies between the original version and our initial attempt, which we resolved in the bitwise reproduction, were as follows:

- The STDP spike pairing in the original model is of type nearest-neighbor, whereas the default pairing in NEST is all-to-all (see Morrison et al., 2008 for a review)
- The original neuron model processes incoming spikes at the beginning of a timestep, rather than the end, as in NEST, leading to a shift in delivery times of 1 ms and thus overall weaker synapses (see STDP windows of the initial and bitwise reproduction in **Figure 4**)
- For border cases, e.g., synchronous spiking of pre- and post-synaptic neurons, the original synapse model applies the LTP and LTD in a different order from our initial reproduction
- The original C++ model applies a decaying term to the eligibility trace before adding it to the synaptic weights, whereas our initial attempt (and the MATLAB version)

applied it afterwards:

```
wdev ← wdev * 0.9;
weight ← weight + 0.01 + wdev;
```

Note that the C++ and MATLAB versions of the code diverge in their handling of the eligibility trace, and the variables `wdev` and `weight` (the buffered weight changes and the current synaptic weight), are known as `sd` and `s` in the original code.

These four disparities in the synapse model lead to the largest differences in the two models. However, even after aligning these, we observed that the spike trains of the original and our re-implementation could be identical for several hours of simulation before some small differences in spike timings ultimately led to complete divergence. This was due to some extremely small (i.e., around machine precision) deviations, which were inflated by the instable numerical integration. We therefore had to additionally adjust all numerical operations to be in the same order as in the original code, and reverse any conversions to standard numerics.

- In the eligibility trace, replace $\exp(-\Delta t/20)$ by $0.95^{\Delta t}$
- In the neuron update, replace
  `0.04 * v * v + 5 * v + 140. - u + I`
  by
  `(0.04 * v + 5) * v + 140. - u + I`
- In the synapse update, replace
  `wdev*= 0.9; weight += 0.01 + wdev;`
  by
  `weight += 0.01 + wdev * 0.9;`

Finally, after detailed investigation and adjustments to the NEST implementation of the neuron and synapse model, the NEST simulation yielded identical results to the original version over the entire 18,000 s simulation period. **Figure 3** shows a raster plot of the spiking activity in the final 10 s of simulation for a NEST network model that replicates the original model identically. It is unquestionable that if the original study had complied with the recommendations in section 3.6.2, the process of identically reproducing the results would have been far less complicated.

The rate of the inhibitory population is high compared to the NEST network activity shown in **Figure 2**, and the oscillations in the gamma band are more strongly represented, as can be seen in the power spectrum in the bottom right panel. The bottom left panel demonstrates, for an example inhibitory neuron (top) and an example excitatory neuron (bottom), that the spike times of the NEST simulation coincide with those of the original. The membrane potential in the NEST simulation is recorded after the numeric update step, but before spikes are detected and the membrane potential set back to resting potential. This leads to the

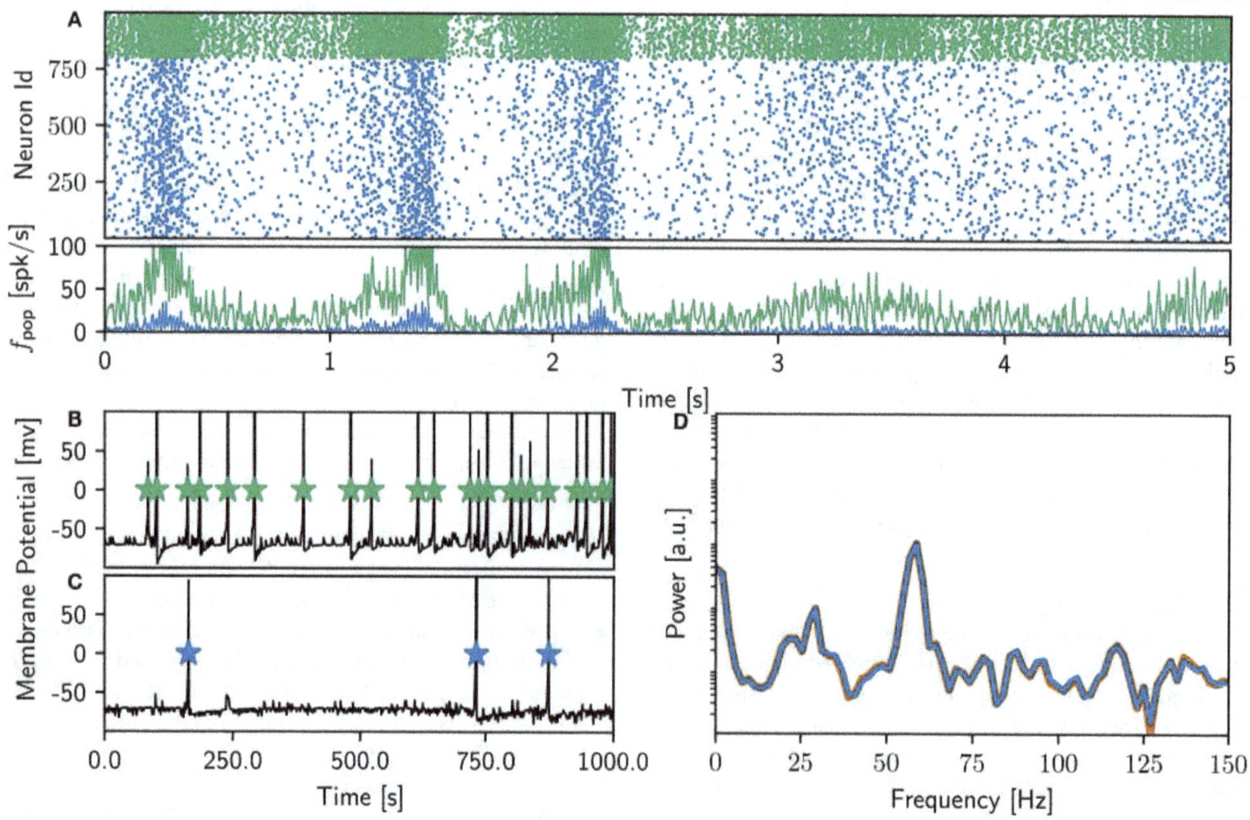

FIGURE 3 | Comparison of bitwise identical NEST network model to original. **(A)** Spike raster plot and rate envelope generated by the NEST simulation in the final 10 s (17,990 – 18,000) for inhibitory (green) and excitatory (blue) neurons. **(B)** membrane potential for a selected inhibitory neuron from the NEST simulation and spike times of corresponding neuron from original code. **(C)** As in **(B)** for a selected excitatory neuron. **(D)** Power spectrum of the rate envelope over the final 10 s for the excitatory population from the NEST (blue curve) and original (orange curve) simulation.

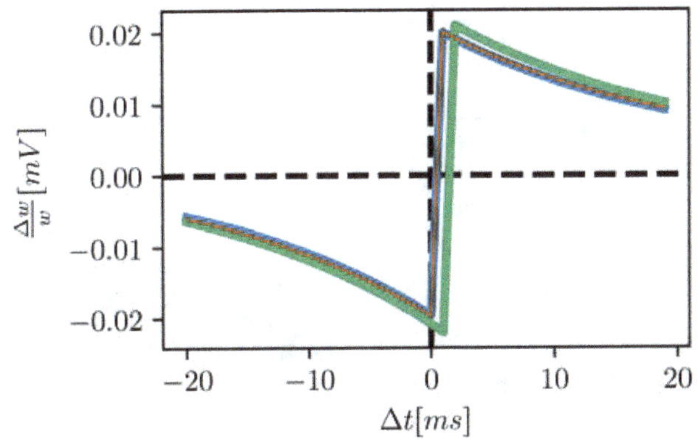

FIGURE 4 | STDP windows of alternative STDP implementations: initial implementation (green), bitwise identical implementation (blue) qualitatively equivalent implementation (orange). Our initial attempt is similar to the bitwise identical reproduction, but shifted by 1 ms to positive delays. The windows of the bitwise identical and qualitatively equivalent implementations coincide.

membrane potential reaching values of above 100 mV, frequently reaching values of around 1,000 mV (**Figure 9**). This indicates numerical instabilities when simulating the neuron model with a resolution of 1 ms, which we investigate further in section 3.4.4.

The original study showed an analysis of the polychronous groups for exactly one run. To investigate the properties of the distribution of groups, we performed 100 runs of the bitwise identical NEST simulation using different random seeds. Surprisingly, we discovered that the network model does not converge to a single dynamic and structural state, as demonstrated in **Figure 5**. In the majority of cases (87%), the network activity results in a power spectrum with a high gamma peak around 60 Hz, as previously shown in **Figures 2C, 3D**. However, the rest of the simulation runs result in a lower peak at 40 Hz, an eventuality not reported in the original study. The full collection of power spectra is shown in **Figure 5A**. The two dynamical states correspond to two alternate structural states. For the high gamma state, the maximum weight of 10 mV occurs for delays between 12 and 14 ms and for the low gamma state, this maximum occurs for a delay of 20 ms (**Figure 5B**).

Analyzing the polychronous groups (**Figure 5C**) reveals that the two dynamical/structural states described above develop significantly different numbers of groups. The distribution of numbers of groups detected is shown in **Figure 5C**. For the high gamma state, the mean number of groups detected was 2,500 with a inter quartile range (IQR) of 1,300, with a minimum of 1,200 and a maximum of 23,000 over the 87 trials resulting in that state. For the 13 low gamma runs, a mean of 1,600 groups with an IQR of 1,400 were detected (minimum: 700; maximum: 29,000). Notably, both distributions are lower than the figure of 5,000 − 6,000 reported in the original study.

3.3. Qualitative Reproduction

The network model developed in section 3.2 replicates the original results precisely, but this does not coincide with the common understanding of reproducing a model. Firstly, requiring equality of floating-point numbers at machine resolution is too strict, and generally not practicable - here we had the advantage that the original code and the code of the target simulator NEST are both in C++, and so identical sequences of mathematical operations will be compiled into identical machine code. Secondly, all pseudorandom elements need to be extracted from the original code in order to initialize the code used for reproducing the model.

We therefore developed a network model that reproduces the original in the commonly understood sense, i.e., all concepts of the original are faithfully translated into the new framework. Specifically, the sources of randomness (connectivity, membrane potential initialization and neuron stimulation) are replaced with analogous routines within the NEST simulation script, and hence there is no dependence on output from the original model. Moreover, the numerics of the synapse model comply with standard forms, and the simulation is parallelized for multithreaded execution.

It could be argued that such a qualitative reproduction should also integrate the neuron dynamics at a finer resolution than the 1 ms used in the original version, as the resolution of a simulation or the algorithm chosen to numerically solve the dynamics should not be considered a conceptual element of a model. However, it turns out that the numerical integration of the dynamics is critical for the model behavior, which we examine in greater detail in section 3.4. We therefore remained with the original numerical choices to create the qualitative reproduction of the model.

Figures 6, 7 demonstrates that the qualitative reproduction captures the key features of the original model. The raster plots are visually similar to those shown in **Figure 3A**, an impression supported by the similarity of the rate distributions (**Figure 6B**, inset) and the power spectra (**Figure 6C**) to those of the original model. Likewise, the final weight distributions (**Figure 6B**) overlap almost completely. In line with the bitwise reproduction, simulations exhibiting a high gamma peak yield more groups than the simulations exhibiting a low gamma peak (median 2,700, IQR 1,300 vs. median 1,500 IQR: 800; **Figure 7C**).

However, despite the apparent good match between the qualitative reproduction and the original, analyzing the activity from 100 simulation runs with different random seeds reveals that the proportion of high gamma and low gamma states have reversed (14 high gamma simulations, 86 low gamma simulations) with respect to the bitwise identical reproduction (compare **Figure 5A** and **Figure 7A**).

A full investigation of the mechanism by which the network converges to one dynamic state or the other, and the implementational differences between the bitwise identical and qualitatively equivalent NEST simulations that cause a differentiation in the respective likelihoods of these states, lies outside the scope of the current manuscript. However, this result does highlight the importance of the recommendation made in section 3.6.3: performing multiple runs so that one can discover, and report, alternate dynamical states for a network model. A researcher may have implemented everything correctly, and yet still fail to reproduce key results, if he or she was unlucky enough

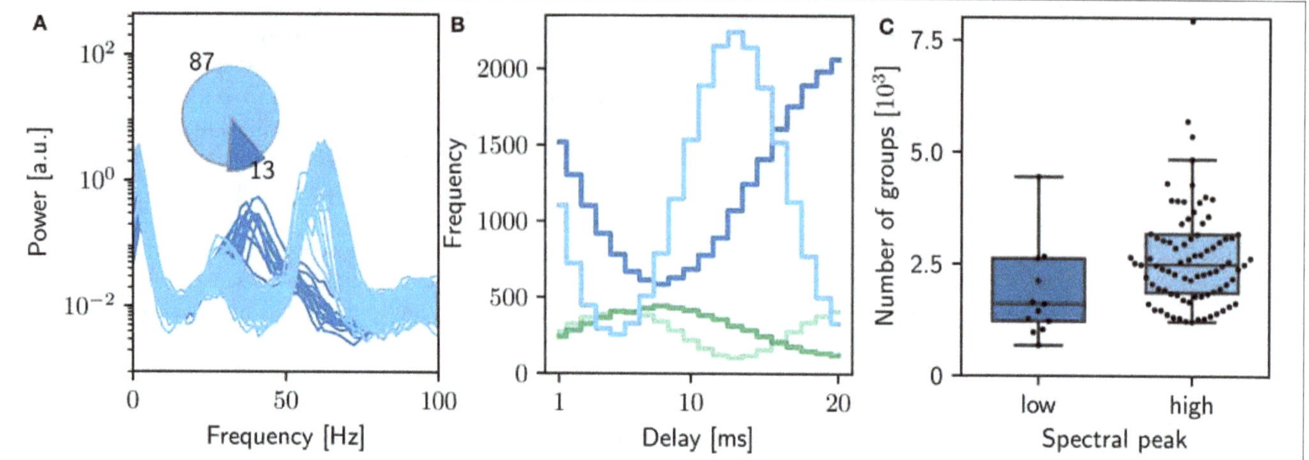

FIGURE 5 | Sensitivity of network dynamics of the bitwise identical NEST implementation to choice of random seed. **(A)** Power spectrum of the rate envelope over the final 10 s for the excitatory population for 100 different seeds. Light blue curves indicate runs resulting in a high gamma peak (60 Hz), dark blue curves those with a low gamma peak (40 Hz). Inset shows the proportion in which these two activity profiles occur. **(B)** The equilibrium distribution of weights (Maximum 10 mV, blue curves; minimum 0 mV, green curves) as functions of the delay in the high (light) and low (dark) gamma dynamical states. **(C)** Relationship between dynamical state and number of polychronous groups found. Boxes show median and interquartile range (IQR); whiskers show additional 1.5 × IQR or limits of distribution.

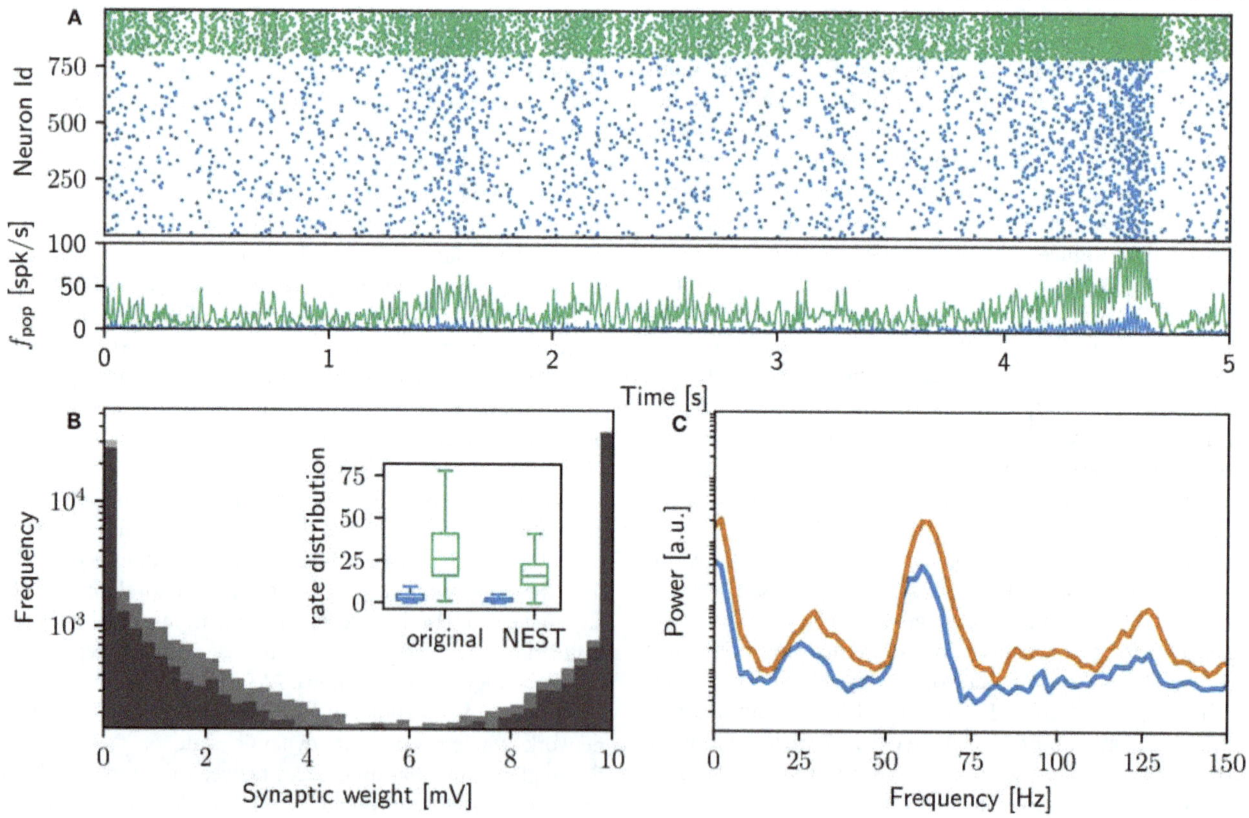

FIGURE 6 | Comparison of qualitatively equivalent NEST network model to original. **(A)** Spike raster plot and rate envelope generated by the NEST simulation in the final 10 s (17, 990 – 18, 000) for inhibitory (green) and excitatory (blue) neurons. **(B)** Final weight distribution (frequency plotted on a logarithmic scale) for the original (light gray) and NEST (dark gray) simulations. Inset: rate distributions over the final 10 s displayed as box plots for the excitatory and inhibitory populations in the original and NEST simulations, colors as above. **(C)** Power spectrum of the rate envelope over the final 10 s for the excitatory population in the original (orange curve) and NEST (blue curve) simulations, colors as above.

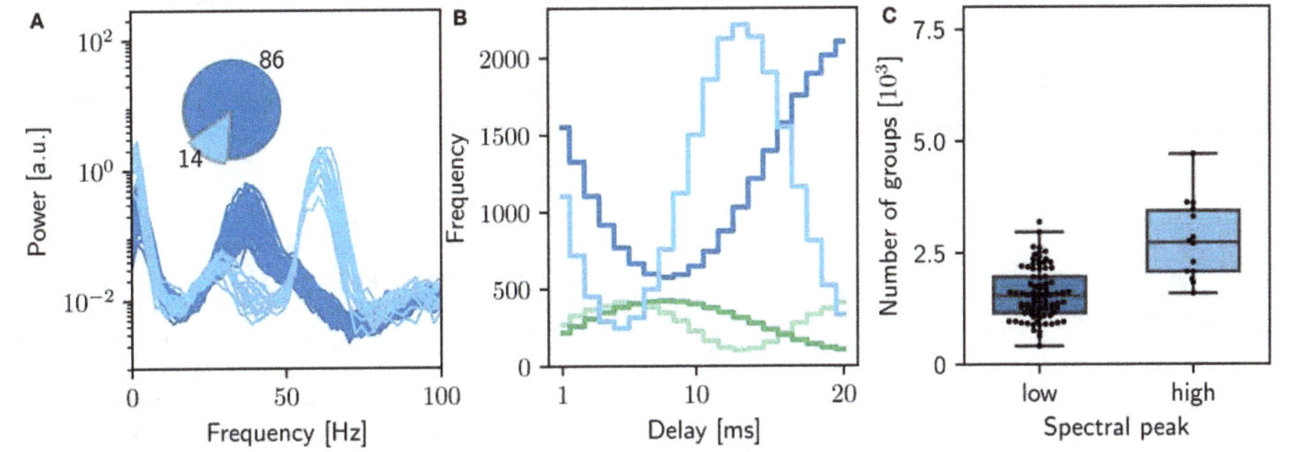

FIGURE 7 | Sensitivity of network dynamics of the qualitatively equivalent NEST implementation to choice of random seed. **(A)** Power spectrum of the rate envelope over the final 10 s for the excitatory population for 100 different seeds. Light blue curves indicate runs resulting in a high gamma peak (60 Hz), dark blue curves those with a low gamma peak (40 Hz). Inset shows the proportion in which these two activity profiles occur. **(B)** The equilibrium distribution of weights (Maximum 10 mV, blue curves; minimum 0 mV, green curves) as functions of the delay in the high (light) and low (dark) gamma dynamical states. **(C)** Relationship between dynamical state and number of polychronous groups found. Boxes show median and interquartile range (IQR); whiskers show additional 1.5 × IQR or limits of distribution.

to select a random seed that caused the network to converge to an unreported, but completely valid, dynamical regime.

3.4. Generalizing Reproduction

Creating a scientific model by necessity requires making simplifying assumptions. In order to draw credible conclusions on how the brain works from the results of simulating a simplified model, it is therefore important to be vigilant that it is not precisely those simplifying assumptions that cause the reported phenomena. Moreover, when a mathematical model is implemented in code for simulation, this introduces the risk that the numerical approach chosen is not suitable to evaluate the model dynamics with adequate accuracy. If the numerics are not suitable, the reported phenomena may be contaminated with misleading numerical artifacts. Even if the simplifying assumptions are valid, and the numerics well-chosen, the selection of parameters may give results that are a special case, and not representative either of the model or of the targeted physical system.

Obviously, it is generally not practicable to test the generality of the results with respect to every aspect of the model. However, it is certainly possible to analyze a network model to identify conceptual, parameter and numeric choices that have a high risk of being critical, and examine those with greater rigor (see our recommendations in section 3.6.3). To demonstrate this, we pinpointed a number of such choices during the process outlined in the previous sections, and modified the qualitative reproduction developed in section 3.3 accordingly to test them. Each modification is quite simple, and either relaxes an assumption (hidden or otherwise), shifts a parameter or alters the numerics of the dynamic components of the network model. On the basis of these generalizing reproductions of the original model, we can then determine to what extent the originally reported results are dependent on these. For all modifications, we made sure that the network dynamics are similar to the original model. The average network firing rate in the final 10 s is in the range between 2 and 8 Hz (compared with 2–5 Hz of the original). Raster plots, weight distributions, power spectra and parameters can be found in the **Supplementary Materials**. The results are summarized in **Figure 8**.

3.4.1. Stimulus

In the original network model, the neurons are stimulated throughout the simulation by the unusual method of randomly selecting one neuron in each millisecond step, and applying a direct current of 20 pA to it for the duration of that step. We replace this stimulation model with a more widely-used and biologically plausible scenario, in which each neuron receives an independent Poissonian spike train with synaptic weight of 10 mV and rate of 40 Hz, tuned such that the excitatory and inhibitory rates in the final second of simulation are closely matched to the original values ($\sim$ 3 spks/s).

In comparison to the original results, this scenario yields significantly different results in respect to the group statistics. Although the statistics for the longest path remain similar to the original results (data not shown), the number of found groups are reduced by around 90% to a median of 291 with an IQR of 24 (see **Figure 8A** *Poisson Stimulus*).

3.4.2. Plasticity Model

Izhikevich describes the plasticity in the original model as STDP with a time constant of $\tau_+ = \tau_- = 20$ ms, $A_+ = 0.1$ mV and $A_- = -0.12$ mV without dependence on the current strength of the synapse, i.e., of the form described by Song et al. (2000), amongst others. This form of additive STDP is known to yield bimodally distributed synaptic strengths which does not fit well to experimental observations. Clearly, an STDP rule resulting in a unimodal distribution of weights would generate qualitatively

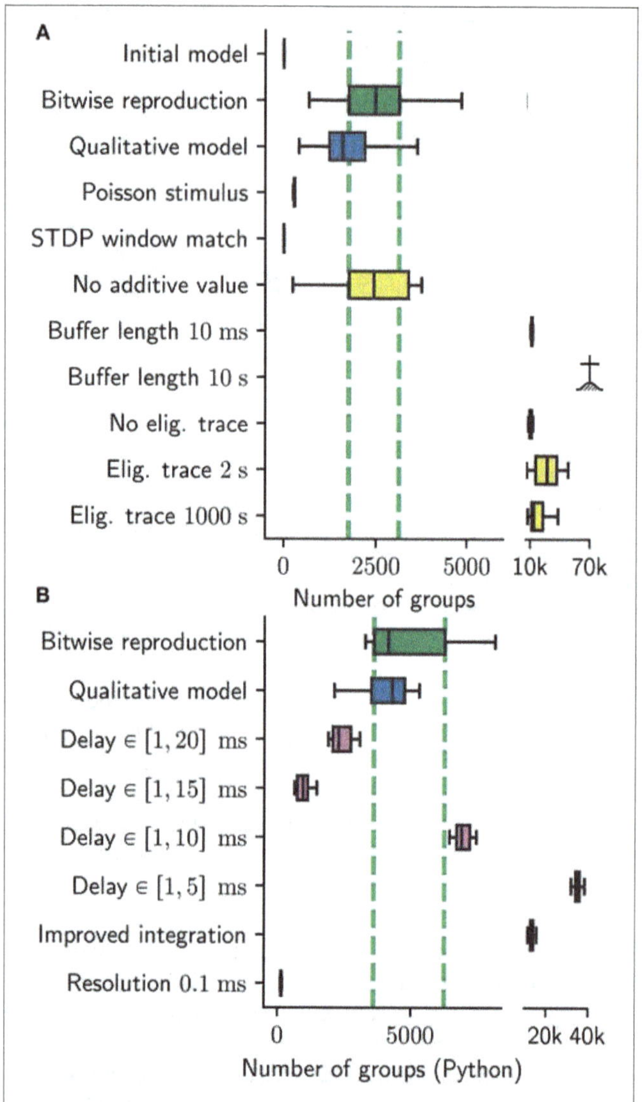

FIGURE 8 | Sensitivity of number of groups found to various parameters. Number of groups found for **(A)** the original group finding algorithm, **(B)** the Python group finding algorithm. Note the different scales; the Python algorithm find about twice as many groups (see section 2.3.2). Boxes show median and interquartile range (IQR); whiskers show additional 1.5 × IQR or limits of distribution. Group statistics are measured over 100 realizations in the case for bitwise reproduction and qualitative model in **(A)** and over ten realizations otherwise. Colors indicate type of experiment: Bitwise reproduction (green), qualitative reproduction (blue), altered connectivity (violet), altered plasticity mechanism (yellow). The IQR of the number of found groups for the bitwise reproduction are indicated by vertical dashed green lines; ⊥ indicates algorithm failure due to too many groups (memory consumption exploded).

different results, but this is well known and does not need to be examined in this context. Instead, we turn our attention to several assumptions and parameters, for which biological motivation is not always easily identifiable:

1. In order to calculate the weight change the pre- and post-synaptic activity is filtered with an exponential kernel using the time constants stated above. In the default STDP synapses in NEST, the LTP/LTD traces are increased by A_+/A_- leading to an "all to all" matching between pre- and post-synaptic spike pairs. The synapse model presented by Izhikevich (2006) caps the traces to a maximum value of A_+/A_-, leading to a "nearest neighbor" matching.
2. Synaptic weights are not updated directly after the occurrence of pre- and post-synaptic spikes. Instead, weight changes are accumulated in a separate buffer for one biological second. At the end of each simulated second, weight changes are applied to all plastic synapses simultaneously.
3. Before applying the buffered weight changes to the synaptic strengths, the buffered values are multiplied with 0.9. This reduced value is applied as an increment to the corresponding synapse and also kept as a start value for the next second. Although this mechanism lacks any biological counterpart, we refer to it as the "eligibility trace" as it introduces a very long time constant of 10 s to the model. The stated intention is to have smoother development of the synaptic weights instead of the rapid and volatile development in additive STDP (Gütig et al., 2003).
4. Additionally to the weight update due to STDP, each synapse is strengthened every second by a constant value of 0.01 mV. The stated motivation is to reactivate and strengthen silent neurons.

We relax these assumptions in the following ways:

1. We change the "nearest neighbor" matching to "all to all" matching. Notably, the STDP windows for a single pre/post pair look exactly the same in both cases. Interestingly, the version with "all to all" matching finds maximally 11 groups which underlines the sensitivity of the model to the exact implementation of STDP (**Figure 8A** *STDP window match*).
2. We vary the duration of buffering the synaptic changes in both directions. For a duration of 10 ms the simulation yields considerably more groups (median: 11, 200, IQR: 910 see **Figure 8A** *Buffer length* 10 ms). The model also seems to be sensitive to larger buffering times, as the number of groups exploded for an increased buffer duration (10 s) such that a quantitative analysis was not possible: all runs crashed due to memory limitations of our cluster (**Figure 8A** *Buffer length* 10 s).
3. We replace the multiplication with 0.9 with an exponential decay and run the simulation for two extreme choices for the time constant: 2 s and 1,000 s, translating to a multiplicative factors of roughly 0.6 and 1.0. For the 2 s version we find 27, 000 groups in median with a high variance expressed in an IQR of 21, 600 groups (**Figure 8A** *Eligibility trace 2 s*).
The 1, 000 s time constants yields 13, 500 groups with an IQR of 11, 200 (**Figure 8A** *Eligibility trace 1,000 s*). In both cases the network is exclusively in the high gamma state. In a further experiment we disabled this eligibility trace completely. To this end, we updated the weights with the full value of the buffer after 1 s, and reset the buffered values to zero. This experiment also yields significantly more groups (10, 000) than the original model with an IQR of 2, 000 (**Figure 8A** *No eligibility trace*).

We conclude that the model results are rather sensitive to this parameter, for which we can ascertain neither a plausible biological motivation nor a reason why 0.9 would be a good choice. Presumably this factor is needed to make the groups more stable over time, which is one of the main findings of the original manuscript.

4. We investigate the role of the constant additive value by setting it to zero. This seems to be completely irrelevant as the group statistics (median 2,400 and IQR 1,600) hardly changes with respect to the original model (**Figure 8A** *No additive value*). We criticize this parameter as unnecessary, introducing additional complexity to the plasticity model adding, to our understanding, no benefit.

3.4.3. Connectivity

The delays in the connections are highly structured: they are evenly spread between 1 and 20 ms, i.e., exactly five outgoing connections of each neuron have the delay 1 ms, exactly five connections have the delay 2 ms, and so on. Izhikevich (2006) argues that this very wide distribution is biologically motivated, because connections between remote neurons, that have to pass through white matter, can easily be so long. However, this is incompatible with the connection probability of 0.1, which suggests a population of neurons within the same cortical microcircuit, and thus a distribution of delays up to, at most, 2 ms.

We relax the assumptions on the connectivity in two ways. First, we simulate with a uniform distribution of delays, i.e., each delay is randomly selected between 1 and 20 ms. Second, we additionally restrict the upper limit to 15, 10, and 5 ms.

Unfortunately, the original group finding algorithm is not able to analyze this data as this particular delay distribution is hard wired in the C++ code, as is the integration timestep investigated in the next section. It was therefore necessary to create a more general version of this algorithm in Python, instantiating a NEST simulation, thus allowing us to perform equivalent analysis on all of our data. Due to errors in the original code which we did not re-implement in Python, our version of the algorithm finds around twice as many groups, including almost all (>99%) of the groups found by the original algorithm. A description of the Python implementation can be found in section 2.3.2, and we provide an in-depth discussion of the errors and definition of polychrony in section 3.5. If the original code had been designed in a flexible way allowing for potential changes to the model and its implementation, as suggested in our recommendations in section 3.6.2, the time-consuming re-implementation of the group finding algorithm would not have been necessary.

In the experiments mentioned above, we find only a weak dependence of the group statistics on the delay distribution in the range between 10 − 20 ms. In the cases of 20, 15, and 10 ms, the simulations yield 2,200, 900, and 7,000 groups in median with IQRs of 700, 400, and 500 respectively (**Figure 8B** *delay 20 / 15 / 10 ms*). In the case of 5 ms, the group statistics exhibit an extremely high median number of 35,000 with IQR of 1,800 (**Figure 8B** *delay 5 ms*). In all cases the gamma oscillations are lost, meaning (in Izhikevich's interpretation) that the network model stays "sleeping" and never "wakes up." For the simulation with 5 ms maximal delays, the network exhibits strong synchronization around 27 Hz. We thus conclude that the choice of delay range beyond that found within a local cortical area is critical for the model behavior, and as such should be clearly reported.

3.4.4. Neuron Integration and Resolution

The neuron model in the original version is integrated in 1 ms steps using a form of forward Euler integration scheme:

```
v[i]+=0.5*((0.04*v[i]+5)*v[i]+140-u[i]+I[i]);
v[i]+=0.5*((0.04*v[i]+5)*v[i]+140-u[i]+I[i]);
u[i]+=a[i]*(0.2*v[i]-u[i]);
```

where v represents the membrane potential and u a membrane recovery variable. This is a symplectic, or semi-implicit scheme, i.e., the update of u is based on an already updated value for v. We note several unusual features of this scheme that may result in numeric artifacts. Firstly, the forward Euler integration is a first order method, which, whilst computationally inexpensive, is less accurate than higher order methods. Secondly, the choice of 1 ms as the integration time step is ten times longer than usual in computational neuroscience models, and may give inaccurate results on the single neuron level, especially in combination with the first order integration scheme. Finally, the variable v is integrated in two 0.5 ms steps whilst u is integrated in one 1 ms step. On the network level, forcing spikes onto a 1 ms time grid may result in artefactual synchrony (Hansel et al., 1998; Morrison et al., 2007), which would in turn affect the STDP dynamics.

To consider the results of a simulation to be representative of the dynamics of the underlying model, we would expect them to show no qualitative changes if the model is re-run at a higher resolution. However, the numerical integration used in the original code is not sufficiently stable, as evidenced by the membrane voltage frequently reaching values around 1,000 mV (see **Figure 9A**). Consequently, simply reducing the timestep to 0.1 ms may well change the single neuron dynamics, and, in turn, the network dynamics. Therefore, to investigate whether the 1 ms timestep induces artefactual synchrony, we have to carefully control for all the model features that are affected by the choice of timestep.

We first adapt the neuron model to separate the numerical instability issue from the locking of spikes to a 1 ms grid, by introducing integration substeps, see also Trensch et al. (in press) for an in-depth analysis of increasing the accuracy of integration of the Izhikevich model by this method. Thus the original configuration is simulated with 1 ms resolution and one integration substep: (1.0, 1). We also examine a configuration in which the numerics are integrated at a higher resolution using ten 0.1 ms substeps: (1.0, 10). For this configuration, if the membrane potential crosses threshold in any substep, no further substeps are carried out in that 1 ms timestep. The spike is emitted at the end of the timestep, along with the corresponding update/reset of the dynamic variables u and v. We call this the "locked" configuration, as the dynamics is integrated with high resolution but the spikes and associated neuron reset is locked to the lower

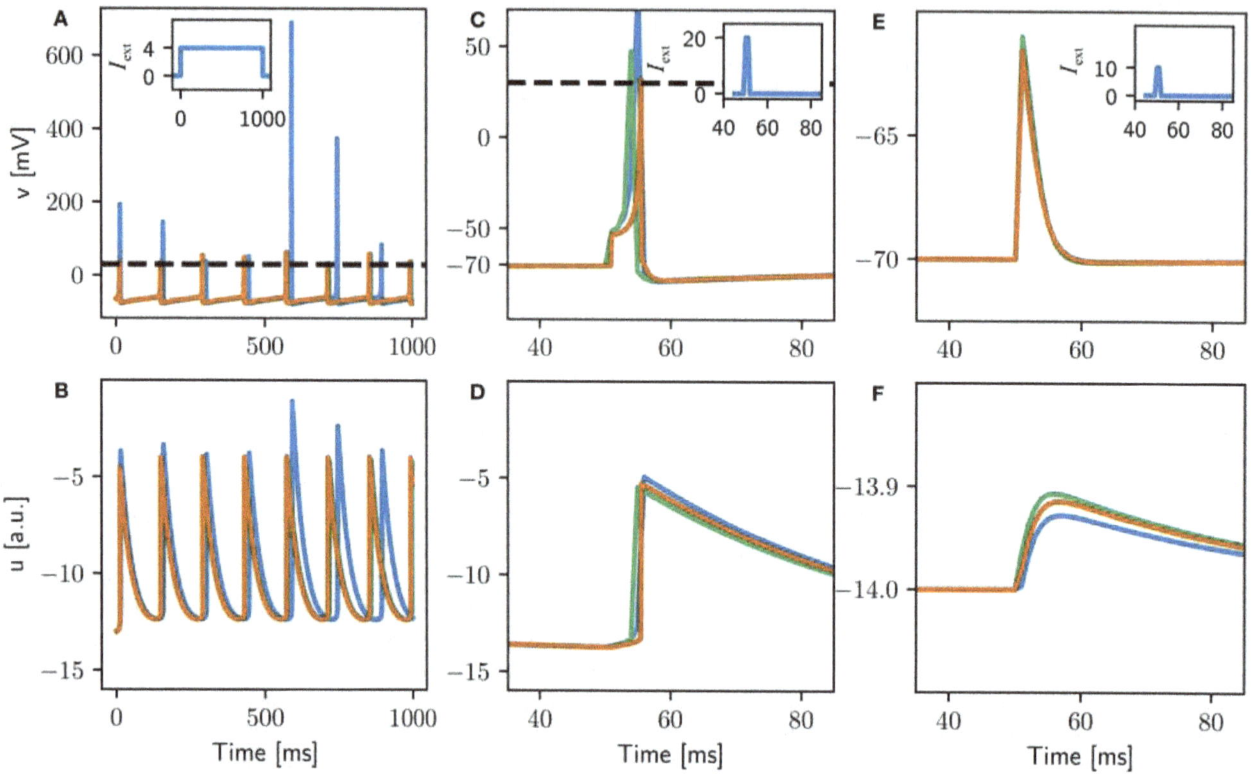

FIGURE 9 | Comparison of the evolution of the membrane potential v (top) and the membrane recovery variable u (bottom) for three different configurations of the adapted Izhikevich neuron. The *original* configuration is simulated with a 1 ms timestep (blue curves). The *locked* configuration performs the integration of the dynamics with a 0.1 ms timestep, but spikes can only be emitted on the 1 ms grid (green curves). The *high resolution* configuration is simulated with a 0.1 ms timestep (orange curves). Insets depict applied currents. Dashed black line depicts action potential threshold. **(A,B)** Constant input of 4 pA. **(C,D)** Two synchronous spikes of maximal weight arriving at 50 ms and evoking an action potential. **(E,F)** One spike of maximal weight arriving at 50 ms which does not evoke an action potential.

resolution grid. As a comparison, we also investigate a "high resolution" configuration, in which the dynamics integration and the spike generation and reset occur on a 0.1 ms grid: $(0.1, 1)$.

As the synaptic interaction in the original is modeled as a direct current for the duration of the 1 ms timestep in which it arrives, simply decreasing the timestep for the high resolution configuration would decrease the effect a spike has on the postsynaptic neuron. To adjust the synaptic weights and plasticity accordingly, we apply three criteria:

- Two synchronous incoming spikes of maximal weights elicit a post synaptic spike (as defined in Izhikevich, 2006)
- The post synaptic potential (PSP) evoked by a spike with maximal weight is conserved
- The STDP windows match

The adjusted parameters are summarized in **Table 1**, and the single neuron dynamics for the three configurations is illustrated in **Figure 9**. Unlike the original configuration, the high resolution and locked configurations exhibit a stable integration with no excessive peaks in the variables u and v when stimulated by a constant input current (**Figures 9A,B**). The firing rates of all three configurations are very close (see **Table 1**), but the locked and high resolution configurations exhibit a coefficient of variation two orders of magnitude lower than the original. The high coefficient of variation can therefore be ascribed to the numerical instability in the integration. All three configurations fit to the firing scheme of regular spiking as described in Izhikevich (2004).

The responses of the three configurations to spiking input (**Figures 9C–F**) indicate that the first two criteria stated above have been fulfilled (data not shown for third criterion), indicating that the three configurations can be meaningfully compared in a full network simulation. Note that the curves for the locked and high resolution configurations are still distinguishable, because the high resolution configuration can emit spikes on a 0.1 ms grid whereas the locked configuration can only emit them on a 1 ms grid.

To remove synchronization artifacts in the full network simulation of the high resolution configuration due to the distribution of delays in multiples of 1 ms, we draw the delays for the excitatory-excitatory connections from a uniform distribution between 1.0 and 20.0 ms with a resolution of 0.1 ms. To allow the fairest comparison, for all configurations we use the original input stimulus (one neuron made to fire randomly selected to fire each millisecond by current injection of an input

TABLE 1 | Comparison between the parameters, dynamics, and number of groups found for the original, locked, and high resolution neuron configurations.

	Original	Locked	High resolution
PARAMETERS			
Resolution	1.0	1.0	0.1
Integration steps	1	10	1
Delay distribution	$\in [1, 20]$ 1 ms steps	$\in [1, 20]$ 1 ms steps	$\in [1, 20]$ 0.1 ms steps
Initial synaptic weight	6 mV	6 mV	50 mV
Max synaptic weight	10 mV	10 mV	85 mV
LTP	0.1	0.1	0.85
LTD	−0.12	−0.12	−1.02
Const add value	0.1 mV	0.1 mV	0.85 mV
SINGLE NEURON DYNAMICS (4pA CURRENT INPUT)			
Firing rate	6.83 spks/s	7.10 spks/s	7.13 spks/s
CV	0.124	0.004	0.003
NETWORK DYNAMICS (LOW GAMMA)			
Firing rate	3.28 ± 0.36 spks/s	2.73 ± 0.04 spks/s	2.84 ± 0.04 spks/s
CV	0.39 ± 0.04	0.43 ± 0.02	0.43 ± 0.01
Fano factor (1.0 ms bin)	2.21	2.29	1.89
Fano factor (0.5 ms bin)	12.20	12.34	2.91
Spectral peak	≈ 40 Hz	≈ 27 Hz	≈ 25 Hz
GROUPS FOUND			
	$4,300 \pm 2,900$	$13,000 \pm 1,100$	151 ± 25

current of twice maximal synaptic weight), as we previously showed in section 3.4.1 that a Poissonian stimulus reduces the number of groups found by around 90%. The network activity for the full network simulations of the locked and high resolution exhibits average firing rates that are very close to each other and slightly lower than the original; the coefficients of variation are comparable across all three configurations (around 3 spks/s and 0.4, respectively, see **Table 1**). The spectral peak is found at around 40 Hz for the original, but around 25 Hz for the locked and high resolution configurations. We thus conclude that the gamma band oscillation is an artifact of the low resolution of the integration step. In terms of synchrony, the Fano factor measured with a binsize of 1.0 ms yields slightly higher values for the original and locked configurations (2.21, 2.29) than for the high resolution configuration (1.89). However, with a bin size of 0.5 ms the synchrony induced by the 1.0 ms spike locking is clearly visible. The original and locked configurations have a much increased Fano factor of around 12, whereas the high resolution network simulation increases only slightly to around 3.

Applying our Python reproduction of the polychronous group finding algorithm to the network results of all three configurations yields 4,300 (IQR 2,900) groups for the original, 13,000 (IQR 1,100) groups for the locked, and 151 (IQR 25) groups for the high resolution configuration. These results are indicated by the labels *Improved integration* and *Resolution* 0.1 ms in **Figure 8B**.

Thus, in summary, the key difference between the original and the locked configuration is that the latter integrates the dynamics without the numerical instabilities of the former. Resolving this issue causes an increase in the number of groups by a factor of three. The difference between the locked and the high resolution simulation is that spikes and delays occur on a 0.1 ms grid rather than a 1 ms grid. This decreases the number of groups found by a factor of 90 (and by a factor of 30 from the original).

We therefore conclude that the number of groups found is strongly influenced by the choice of a 1 ms timestep and delay resolution, although the network dynamics, in terms of firing rate and coefficient of variation, is not. In particular, the original study significantly overstates the number of groups to be found in such networks, due to the artificial synchrony induced by these implementational (rather than conceptional) choices. Using standard numerics or testing the robustness of the results for a higher simulation precision as recommended in section 3.6.3 could have prevented this misinterpretation in the original study.

3.5. Definition of Polychrony

In section 3.4, we examined the sensitivity of polychronous group generation to parameter settings and model assumptions, given comparable network dynamics. We now turn our attention to the group finding algorithm itself. As stated in the previous section, it was necessary to re-implement the original analysis script in order to investigate the effects of alternative choices of delay distribution and integration timestep.

In this process we found several aspects of the original algorithm, briefly outlined in section 2.3.2, that warrant further discussion and investigation. First, we note that the identification of a polychronous group is based on an analysis of the connectivity, rather than the activity. The original manuscript reports that $\sim$ 90% of the groups which are found to be stable over 24 h of simulation time can also be found to be active in the

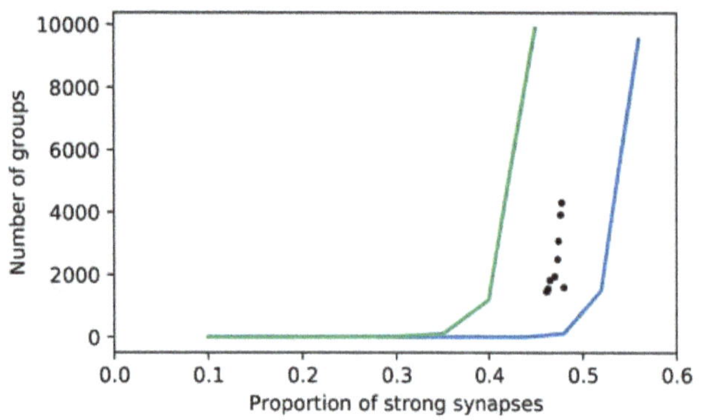

FIGURE 10 | Number of groups identified by the original algorithm as a function of the proportion of excitatory synapses that are strong. Realizations of the bitwise identical reproduction; black dots. Surrogate data with connections randomly selected to be strong (excitatory-excitatory synapses only—all excitatory-inhibitory synapses are strong); blue curve. Surrogate data with connections randomly selected to be strong (all excitatory); green curve.

spiking activity. However, this part of the analysis is not part of the available online materials, and so we were not able to confirm this relationship.

Second, we found three major errors in the C++ implementation of the algorithm:

- During the simulation phase, the spike delivery buffer often overflows, leading to a spike being delivered at the wrong time. Although this mainly happens in large groups, we consider this to be a critical error as exact spike timings are necessary to reliably activate groups.
- A group is only valid if the maximum layer, the longest chain of neurons within the group, is greater than, or equal to seven. However, the calculation of layers depends on an arbitrary sorting of neuron ids and also on the time of activation of those neurons. This leads to errors in which neurons are assigned to the wrong layer. If this results in a sub-threshold number of layers, the group will be considered invalid and not counted.
- The maximal duration of the simulation is set to 1 ms after the last spike delivery, however two simultaneous spike arrivals lead to a postsynaptic spike generation of up to 4 ms later. This last spike is thus overlooked in the original algorithm. This is a crucial error, as missing the last spike can result in a reduced number of layers identified for a group, and therefore to the group being considered invalid (i.e., less than seven layers).

In our re-implementation of the algorithm we fixed these errors; as a result, our algorithm finds around twice as many groups, but including more than 99% of those found by the original algorithm.

Thirdly, we note that the motivation for many of the conditions underlying the definition of a polychronous group is unclear; for example, the exclusion of weak synapses from the analysis, or the classification of groups that are activated by only one or two neurons as invalid. In particular, the analysis algorithm sets the seemingly arbitrary conditions that a polychronous group has to consist of at least six neurons and seven layers. The choice of the number of layers has a profound effect on the number of groups found. Reducing it to five increases the number of groups found in the original model from 4, 305 to 27, 116, whereas increasing it to ten decreases the number to 608. As no scientific justification is given for the choice of seven, we speculate that it was chosen for aesthetic reasons. In any case, the strong dependence of the results on the choice of thresholding parameter indicate that it should be explicitly stated as a model critical parameter, even though it is not a parameter of the network model.

To get an understanding of how many groups are found with respect to those expected from a network with random connectivity, we performed a surrogate analysis. The original C++ code provides a similar functionality, by shuffling the excitatory-excitatory connections. However, it is not clear why the number of groups found with this shuffling defines the null hypothesis, given that the excitatory-inhibitory connections also adapt during the course of the simulation (and almost all become strong). Regarding the strength of these as a given introduces a bias. Moreover, the functionality does not allow the proportion of strong synapses to be considered as an independent variable. We therefore developed a surrogate analysis in which excitatory connections (either just excitatory-excitatory, or all excitatory) are randomly drawn with a given probability of being strong. The results are shown in **Figure 10**.

In line with the original findings, networks with randomly selected strong excitatory-excitatory synapses exhibit fewer groups (using the original group finding algorithm) than those where the strong synapses develop due to network activity. The proportion of random strong synapses must be increased to around ∼ 50% in order to find as many groups as in the "grown" networks, where the proportion of strong synapses is around ∼ 45%. Note that in this setting, 20% of synapses are automatically strong, being the excitatory-inhibitory connections. However, if the strong synapses are randomly selected from all excitatory synapses, the opposite tendency is found: only around ∼ 40% strong synapses are required for the group finding algorithm to identify as many groups as in the grown network. Hence, the algorithm finds either more or fewer groups in grown networks than random networks, depending on what assumption is used to generate the latter.

We therefore conclude that the provided analysis script is an additional factor undermining the reproducibility of the original study. It contains coding errors that distort the results, making it likely that a researcher trying to re-implement the analysis would generate substantially different numbers of groups, even if the network model had been reproduced identically. These errors could have been avoided, or at least made more visible, by clean code features such as encapsulation and commenting, as discussed in section 3.2.2 and summarized in section 3.6.2. Moreover, there is an unstated strong dependence on an apparently arbitrary threshold parameter, and the null hypothesis from which positive results are to be distinguished is not well motivated. For future research into polychronous groups, we would therefore suggest following a different analytic approach. Some alternative methods (none of which were available at the time of publication of the original study) are discussed in section 4.3.

3.6. Recommendations

In carrying out the steps outlined in sections 2.2–3.5, we identified which features of the code and the methodology of the original study support reproducing the results, and which hinder it. From these we derive a series of recommendations that, if followed, would not only increase the reproducibility of a given study, but also its scientific credibility, by reducing the risk that results are dependent on implementational details.

These can be roughly divided into three categories, although of course there is overlap. On the most basic level, it is important to make the code available and executable. This includes topics such as sharing and providing an installation guide, as well as information about the versions used of model code and any dependencies. On the next level, we provide recommendations on how to make it comprehensible and testable. This covers topics from low-level artifacts like commenting and naming of parameters and functions, to more abstract issues such as appropriate organization of the code and unit tests for components. Finally, our work revealed that computational models may easily contain undesirable implementation dependencies. Whereas it is not feasible to comprehensively test for all of them, we emphasize the importance of using existing standards as much as possible, both for accuracy and comprehensibility. In addition, we uncovered an alternative dynamical mode of the original network, with a lower peak in the power spectrum, which occurs in a minority of simulation runs. This illustrates the importance of carrying out multiple runs of models to uncover any dependency on the random seed used.

3.6.1. Make Code Available and Executable

Recommendation: share the code

We would certainly not have been able to reproduce the simulation results either identically or qualitatively if the author had not provided the complete source. This applies not only to the network model but also to the analysis of the results. As there are many options for sharing the code in a sustainable fashion, as listed below, "available from the author on request" should not be considered an adequate fulfillment of this recommendation. Moreover, the code should be accessible for the reviewers when an article is submitted to a journal, and not deferred until publication, so that the reviewers can form an opinion of its reproducibility.

ModelDB. ModelDB[3] is a database for computational and conceptual models in neuroscience. One can choose to share the code on ModelDB itself or as a weblink to the code. ModelDB provides a direct link between publication and source code of the model. Additionally, the database can be searched by keywords, for example for specific neuron models, types of plasticity or brain regions. Since a model can even be entered into ModelDB as a link to another hosting platform, there is really no reason not to make an entry.

Zenodo. Zenodo[4] makes it possible to assign a DOI to a certain version of the code. The code version will also be archived on the CERN cloud infrastructure. The model code can be stored in a github repository and then linked and archived via Zenodo.

GitHub, GitLab, Bitbucket. Web-based hosting services such as GitHub, GitLab, and Bitbucket[5,6,7] are mainly based on git, a standard and widely used tool in collaborative software development. The advantage of sharing model code through git is that it facilitates opening up the code to the community.

Open Source Brain. The Open Source Brain platform is a web resource for publishing and sharing models in the field of computational neuroscience with a strong focus on open source technologies. The submitted models can be visualized and their parameter spaces and dynamics can be explored in browser-based simulations (Gleeson et al., 2018).

Collaboratory. The collaboratory is a web portal designed within the Human Brain Project intended to improve the quality of collaboration between many possibly international parties (Senk et al., 2017). It allows scientists to share data, collaborate on code and re-use models and methods, and enables tracking and crediting researchers for their contributions.

Recommendation: provide an installation guide

The single stand-alone C++ program downloaded for this study was easy to install. However, more complicated set-ups with dependencies on other applications (e.g., simulation or analysis tools) require more work. An installation guide takes (most of) the guesswork out of it. An installation guide should not only include the exact steps and commands to install the software, but should also name the platform and operating system on which the authors tested the installation steps. Additionally, it should mention a complete list of software dependencies.

Recommendation: use a version control system

In the current investigation, the downloaded script did not match the paper, and the C++ and MATLAB versions did not match each other. Therefore it was not clear which version of the code had been used to generate the reported results. More generally, models are often developed further after being published, which leads to increasing divergence between the description in the manuscript and the current version of the model. A version control system such as git, SVN or Mercurial helps to keep different versions accessible, and enables users and scientists to understand the changes to the implementation of a model.

Recommendation: provide provenance tracking

To reproduce the study, we used specific versions of NEST and various Python packages. However, sometimes different versions

[3]https://senselab.med.yale.edu/modeldb/

[4]https://zenodo.org/

[5]https://github.com/

[6]https://gitlab.com/

[7]https://bitbucket.org

of software applications vary significantly in their performance (Gronenschild et al., 2012) or just have non-compatible APIs. The manuscript and the installation guide should be specific about which versions of software were used to generate the results.

3.6.2. Make Code Comprehensible and Testable

Recommendation: modularize the code

Separating simulation and data analysis makes it possible to use the two independently. In this study, it allowed us to apply a new analysis to the original simulation results and, vice versa, the original analysis code to our implementation of the model. Without the possibility to apply exactly the same analysis to different implementations, we would not have been able to discover the causes of the disparities between the original network model and our initial attempts to reproduce it.

Recommendation: encapsulate the code

Encapsulation gathers data and the methods that operate on it into cohesive units. This is a similar principle to modularization. Using methods with meaningful names rather than operating directly on data makes the code easier to comprehend; compare:

```
I[i]+=s[firings[k][1]][delays[firings[k][1]][t-firings[k][0][j]];
```

and

```
deliver_spike(post_neuron,weight(pre_neuron, post_neuron))
```

Further, it makes the code less error prone, as complex access/operation routines are defined in one place and parameterized, rather than repeated throughout the code. Finally, it facilitates testing, see below.

Recommendation: write flexible code

Code flexibility is a precondition for efficient testing of model robustness toward changes on both the implementation level (e.g., smaller integration time step) and the modeling level (e.g., different parameter values). Testing the generalized reproducibility of the model (see section 3.4) was a tedious and time-consuming process due to several model features being hardwired into the simulation and analysis code. Routines should be written as general as possible to avoid these problems; using standard tools (see next section) will tend to mitigate this issue automatically.

Recommendation: provide tests

Reproducing the synapse model was challenging, because there were discrepancies between our initial model and the original and handling specific combinations of pre- and post-synaptic spikes that were not defined in the original publication. To avoid this situation, novel network elements such as neuron, synapse or stimulus models should be accompanied by tests that define the output of the model for representative or critical inputs. This documents the behavior of the model, especially for border cases, in much greater detail than it would be reasonable to include in a text description.

Recommendation: comment the code

Using comments substantially increases the comprehensibility of the code, and thus the ability of a researcher to re-implement it in a different framework. Comments should explain *what* complex code sections are doing, but often straightforward code sections are greatly enhanced by a comment explaining *why* they are performing their operations.

Recommendation: parameterize meaningfully and consistently

Parameters should be given meaningful names such that they can be understood when they occur in an expression. Parameter definitions should be gathered in parameter files, or at the beginning of a stand-alone script, rather than spread throughout. Raw numbers (other than 0 and 1) should not appear in expressions, as this reduces the comprehensibility of the code, and they are easy to overlook as parameters that influence the behavior of the model.

Recommendation: use parameter files

Models often rely on a set of parameters which should be either declared in the beginning of the source code, or, if there are more than a few parameters, in a separate file. To aid comprehensibility, if there is more than one experiment conducted with one model there should be a dedicated parameter file for each experiment, with a corresponding human-readable table as proposed by Nordlie et al. (2009).

Recommendation: use tables to communicate parameters

It is easy to overlook a parameter when writing a text description of a network model. Use of structured tables, such as those proposed by Nordlie et al. (2009) acts as a reminder to record all the model parameters and their values, and present them in a comprehensible and easily referable fashion for the reader.

3.6.3. Reduce Risk of Implementation Dependencies

Recommendation: use standard tools

Tools that are created and maintained by a group of developers over a period of time and have a substantial user base will generally have more consistently applied coding standards, documentation and tests than a homebrewed single-purpose application. All these aspects increase the comprehensibility of the code and reduce the risk that it contains numeric or algorithmic errors. Given the current excellent availability of open source tools for simulation and data analysis, using standard tools should be preferred over homebrew as far as possible. Novel network elements (e.g., neuron model) or analyses should ideally be handled by contributing features to open source tools, or at least formating them as compatible patches. The use of homebrewed simulation or analysis tools should be clearly motivated, and such code should comply with the recommendations set out here.

Recommendation: use standard numerics

Using standard numerics lowers the risk of introducing rounding or other numeric errors and also makes it easier to understand the code.

Recommendation: perform multiple realizations

A robust model will generate statistically equivalent results for different choices of the random seed. Variable behavior should be reported; this is not only relevant for a reader's ability to evaluate the explanatory power of the model, it is also important for reproducibility to be aware that the model can yield substantially different results.

Recommendation: test model robustness

Proofs of model robustness with regard to implementation details, parameter values, and higher-level modeling choices boost the quality and credibility of the presented scientific results. A basic requirement of model robustness is that an outcome of a simulation that is reported as model behavior should not change qualitatively if the simulation is repeated with higher precision. In case of the model that we investigate here, increasing the simulation resolution significantly affects the number of polychronous groups found (see section 3.4.4), and hence, renders the main result of the study questionable. Such checks should always be carried out if there is a risk that the results might be distorted by artificial synchrony or numeric instabilities.

4. DISCUSSION

In this article, we have demonstrated that even if model code is available and can be executed on a local machine with only minimal modifications (section 3.1), this is only a first step toward enabling reproduction of a study. By taking the publicly available model code of a well-known study (Izhikevich, 2006) and attempting to reproduce it in NEST, we uncovered a variety of barriers to reproducibility (sections 3.2, 3.3). From each of these barriers, we derive a recommendation that would lower or remove it.

These recommendations are explained in detail in the previous section, and for convenience we have gathered them into a checklist, which is available in the **Supplementary Material**. This checklist can be used by researchers to evaluate and improve the reproducibility of their neuronal network model before submitting an article. Similarly, a reviewer can use it to rapidly assess the likely reproducibility of a submitted model, without having to expend considerable time trying to actually reproduce it.

Beyond the practical steps that can be taken to improve the quality of model code and related artifacts, in the course of our study we have identified several unusual assumptions and numerics choices in the original simulation and analysis code, and investigated to what extent the reported model behavior depends on them (sections 3.4, 3.5).

With regards to the model code, in the case of the implementation of background noise (random selection in each millisecond of a neuron to fire), the non-standard features of the plasticity model, and the extremely long range of delays, making a choice that was better biologically founded (or at least removed complexity that did not have a clear biological foundation) resulted in a reduction or increase in the number of groups found by an order of magnitude. In the case of the simulation resolution, despite careful matching of network and single neuron dynamics, in a network running at a higher resolution of 0.1 ms, we found a massive reduction of groups compared to either the original network, or one with 0.1 ms integration but spikes locked to a 1.0 ms grid. This last finding is of particular concern, as it demonstrates that the majority of the polychronous groups reported in the original study can be attributed to artificial synchrony brought about by an unsuitable choice of numerics (low resolution).

Similarly, with regards to the analysis code, we discovered a series of coding errors that distorted the findings, and strong dependencies on both a thresholding parameter (lacking a biological motivation) and the assumptions defining the null hypothesis.

Thus we conclude that the main reported results of the original study generalize very poorly. The number of groups found varies substantially with each aspect we investigated, with the exception of the additive factor in the plasticity model, which seems to have no effect. We argue that had the dependence of the findings on a very specific configuration of modeling and implementation choices been apparent, the original study would not have been as influential as it has been.

Clearly, it is not possible to check for all parameter and implementation choices, and it is reasonable to assume that the authors of the current study have more computational resources at their disposal for such analyses than were available to the author of the original. This notwithstanding, we note that it is the obligation of authors to evaluate their choices and assumptions critically, and to be transparent about which ones are necessary for the reported results. Analogously, it is the obligation of reviewers to use their expertise to identify potential dependencies and request additional simulations to uncover them.

As discussed in the next section, following the set of recommendations laid out in section 3.6 would not only increase the ability of researchers to independently verify the findings of neuronal network studies, but would decrease the likelihood that such findings are subject to highly specific parameter and implementation choices.

4.1. Relationship of the Reproducibility Guideline to Scientific Quality

The reproducibility guideline is divided into three categories. The first category contains recommendations that allow researchers to reproduce identical results, which includes also the case where a researcher wants to rerun a simulation at a later point in time. The second category of recommendations facilitate qualitative reproduction by others, primarily through effective communication of the model code and parameters. The recommendations of the third category principally address model robustness. All three categories are important for the quality and credibility of the presented scientific results, but on different levels. By following the recommendations of the first category, a researcher can be transparent about exactly what experiments were carried out using which software. Following the second category provides evidence to other researchers that the study was conducted in a structured way. Moreover, a study that follows these recommendations invites other researchers to investigate the model independently. A study that follows the third category of recommendations demonstrates the researchers' ability to critically assess their own work, their willingness to disclose limitations, and their openness to potential refutation of the results by other researchers in future studies.

4.2. Limitations of the Reproducibility Guideline

The reproducibility guideline developed in the course of this study is not intended as a definitive document, and the authors welcome suggestions for further recommendations to increase the currently poor record of reproducibility in neuronal network modeling studies. In particular, our guideline is aimed at the reproducibility of networks of point (or few-compartment) neuron models. Where as much of it is likely applicable to networks of biophysical neuron models with thousands of compartments (commenting code is never a bad idea), some recommendations are likely to be inappropriate (e.g., using tables to communicate parameters) and some important aspects that boost reproducibility may well have been overlooked entirely. The adaptation of the guideline to such models lies outside the expertise of the authors. We suspect that domain specific languages such as NEUROML (Gleeson et al., 2018) have an important role to play here, as they provide unambiguous, standardized, and machine-readable representations of complex neurons and their connectivity.

4.3. Alternative Methods for Detecting Polychronous Groups

Izhikevich (2006) introduces a method to find polychonous groups in the connectivity data of the presented spiking neural network model. Although the concept is fruitful in this very specific case, it does not generalize to other means. More general methods (e.g., Torre et al., 2013; Quaglio et al., 2017; Russo and Durstewitz, 2017) have recently been developed for the detection of repeated precise spike sequences in electrophysiological recordings. Such methods do not use any assumption of the underlying connectivity and could be applied to the simulated spiking activity in order to find active patterns without the prior detection of potential polychronous groups in the connection profile. With these methods the same kind of analysis could be performed as in Izhikevich (2006) with the advantageous possibility of comparing the results to experimental data in order to confirm the validity of the model.

5. CONCLUSION AND OUTLOOK

Based on our work to reproduce the network presented by Izhikevich (2006), we conclude that the more points in the guideline are adhered to, the easier it will be to reproduce a study of a network of spiking neurons, and the higher quality the study will be. Whereas journals are beginning to take issues such as availability of model code more seriously than before, the current study clearly demonstrates that this is a necessary but not sufficient condition for reproducibility. We propose that the editorial boards of journals in computational neuroscience go considerably further, and provide their reviewers with clearly defined reproducibility criteria, for which we provide a draft. Only in this way can we achieve a substantial change in attitude and approach in our field.

AUTHOR CONTRIBUTIONS

SK and AM created a prototype of the project. RP created all figures. RP, PW, and AM investigated and eliminated the discrepancies between the original code and the NEST model. RP and PW performed the analysis and simulations. SK, PW, and RP created the NEST group finding algorithm. All authors jointly wrote the manuscript.

ACKNOWLEDGMENTS

We acknowledge the Initiative and Networking Fund of the Helmholtz Association, the Helmholtz Association through the Helmholtz Portfolio Theme Supercomputing and Modeling for the Human Brain, the German Research Foundation (DFG; KFO 219, TP9) and the European Union's Horizon 2020 research and innovation programme under grant agreement no. 720270 (HBP SGA 1) and no. 754304 (DEEP-EST). We thank P. Quaglio, G. Trensch, and R. Gutzen for fruitful discussions.

REFERENCES

Association for Computing Machinery (2016). *Artifact Review and Badging.* Available online at: https://www.acm.org/publications/policies/artifact-review-badging (Accessed March 14, 2018).

Collberg, C., and Proebsting, T. A. (2016). Repeatability in computer systems research. *Commun. ACM* 59, 62–69. doi: 10.1145/2812803

Gewaltig, M.-O., and Diesmann, M. (2007). NEST (NEural Simulation Tool). *Scholarpedia* 2:1430. doi: 10.4249/scholarpedia.1430

Ghosh, S. S., Poline, J.-B., Keator, D. B., Halchenko, Y. O., Thomas, A. G., Kessler, D. A., et al. (2017). A very simple, re-executable neuroimaging publication. *F1000Research* 6:124. doi: 10.12688/f1000research.10783.2

Gleeson, P., Cantarelli, M., Marin, B., Quintana, A., Earnshaw, M., Piasini, E., et al. (2018). Open Source Brain: a collaborative resource for visualizing, analyzing, simulating and developing standardized models of neurons and circuits. *bioRxiv.* [Preprint]. Available online at: https://www.biorxiv.org/content/early/2018/01/11/229484

Gronenschild, E. H. B. M., Habets, P., Jacobs, H. I. L., Mengelers, R., Rozendaal, N., van Os, J., et al. (2012). The effects of FreeSurfer version, workstation type, and Macintosh operating system version on anatomical volume and cortical thickness measurements. *PLoS ONE* 7:e38234. doi: 10.1371/journal.pone.0038234

Gütig, R., Aharonov, R., Rotter, S., and Sompolinsky, H. (2003). Learning input correlations through nonlinear temporally asymmetric hebbian plasticity. *J. Neurosci.* 23, 3697–3714. doi: 10.1523/JNEUROSCI.23-09-03697.2003

Hansel, D., Mato, G., Meunier, C., and Neltner, L. (1998). On numerical simulations of integrate-and-fire neural networks. *Neural Comput.* 10, 467–483.

Izhikevich, E. M. (2004). Which model to use for cortical spiking neurons? *IEEE Trans. Neural Netw.* 15, 1063–1070. doi: 10.1109/TNN.2004.832719

Izhikevich, E. M. (2006). Polychronization: computation with spikes. *Neural Comput.* 18, 245–282. doi: 10.1162/089976606775093882

Köster, J., and Rahmann, S. (2012). Snakemake–a scalable bioinformatics workflow engine. *Bioinformatics* 28, 2520–2522. doi: 10.1093/bioinformatics/bts480

Morrison, A., Diesmann, M., and Gerstner, W. (2008). Phenomenological models of synaptic plasticity based on spike timing. *Biol. Cybernet.* 98, 459–478. doi: 10.1007/s00422-008-0233-1

Morrison, A., Straube, S., Plesser, H. E., and Diesmann, M. (2007). Exact subthreshold integration with continuous spike times in discrete-time neural network simulations. *Neural Comput.* 19, 47–79. doi: 10.1162/neco.2007.19.1.47

Nordlie, E., Gewaltig, M.-O., and Plesser, H. E. (2009). Towards reproducible descriptions of neuronal network models. *PLoS Comput. Biol.* 5:e1000456. doi: 10.1371/journal.pcbi.1000456

Peyser, A., Sinha, A., Vennemo, S. B., Ippen, T., Jordan, J., Graber, S., et al. (2017). NEST 2.14.0. doi: 10.5281/zenodo.882971

Plesser, H. E. (2018). Reproducibility vs. replicability: a brief history of a confused terminology. *Front. Neuroinformatics* 11:76. doi: 10.3389/fninf.2017.00076

Quaglio, P., Yegenoglu, A., Torre, E., Endres, D. M., and Grün, S. (2017). Detection and evaluation of spatio-temporal spike patterns in massively parallel spike train data with spade. *Front. Comput. Neurosci.* 11:41. doi: 10.3389/fncom.2017.00041

Rougier, N. P., Hinsen, K., Alexandre, F., Arildsen, T., Barba, L. A., Benureau, F. C., et al. (2017). Sustainable computational science: the ReScience initiative. *PeerJ Comp. Sci.* 3:e142. doi: 10.7717/peerj-cs.142

Russo, E., and Durstewitz, D. (2017). Cell assemblies at multiple time scales with arbitrary lag constellations. *Elife* 6:e19428. doi: 10.7554/eLife.19428

Senk, J., Yegenoglu, A., Amblet, O., Brukau, Y., Davison, A., Lester, D. R., et al. (2017). "A collaborative simulation-analysis workflow for computational neuroscience using HPC," in *High-Performance Scientific Computing*, eds E. Di Napoli, M. A. Hermanns, H. Iliev, A. Lintermann, and A. Peyser (Cham: Springer International Publishing), 243–256.

Song, S., Miller, K. D., and Abbott, L. F. (2000). Competitive Hebbian learning through spike-timing-dependent synaptic plasticity. *Nat. Neurosci.* 3:919. doi: 10.1038/78829

Topalidou, M., Leblois, A., Boraud, T., and Rougier, N. P. (2015). A long journey into reproducible computational neuroscience. *Front. Comput. Neurosci.* 9:30. doi: 10.3389/fncom.2015.00030

Torre, E., Picado-Muiño, D., Denker, M., Borgelt, C., and Grün, S. (2013). Statistical evaluation of synchronous spike patterns extracted by frequent item set mining. *Front. Comput. Neurosci.* 7:132. doi: 10.3389/fncom.2013.00132

Trensch, G., Gutzen, R., Blundell, I., Denker, M., and Morrison, A. (in press). Rigorous neural network simulations: model cross-validation for boosting the correctness of simulation results. *Front. Neuroinformatics.*

12

Using NEURON for Reaction-Diffusion Modeling of Extracellular Dynamics

Adam J. H. Newton [1,2], Robert A. McDougal [1,3], Michael L. Hines [1] and William W. Lytton [2,4]*

[1] Department of Neuroscience, Yale University, New Haven, CT, United States, [2] SUNY Downstate Medical Center, The State University of New York, New York, NY, United States, [3] Center for Medical Informatics, Yale University, New Haven, CT, United States, [4] Neurology, Kings County Hospital Center, Brooklyn, NY, United States

***Correspondence:**
Adam J. H. Newton
adam.newton@downstate.edu

Development of credible clinically-relevant brain simulations has been slowed due to a focus on electrophysiology in computational neuroscience, neglecting the multiscale whole-tissue modeling approach used for simulation in most other organ systems. We have now begun to extend the NEURON simulation platform in this direction by adding extracellular modeling. The extracellular medium of neural tissue is an active medium of neuromodulators, ions, inflammatory cells, oxygen, NO and other gases, with additional physiological, pharmacological and pathological agents. These extracellular agents influence, and are influenced by, cellular electrophysiology, and cellular chemophysiology—the complex internal cellular milieu of second-messenger signaling and cascades. NEURON's extracellular reaction-diffusion is supported by an intuitive Python-based *where/who/what* command sequence, derived from that used for intracellular reaction diffusion, to support coarse-grained macroscopic extracellular models. This simulation specification separates the expression of the conceptual model and parameters from the underlying numerical methods. In the volume-averaging approach used, the macroscopic model of tissue is characterized by *free volume fraction*—the proportion of space in which species are able to diffuse, and *tortuosity*—the average increase in path length due to obstacles. These tissue characteristics can be defined within particular spatial regions, enabling the modeler to account for regional differences, due either to intrinsic organization, particularly gray vs. white matter, or to pathology such as edema. We illustrate simulation development using spreading depression, a pathological phenomenon thought to play roles in migraine, epilepsy and stroke. Simulation results were verified against analytic results and against the extracellular portion of the simulation run under FiPy. The creation of this NEURON interface provides a pathway for interoperability that can be used to automatically export this class of models into complex intracellular/extracellular simulations and future cross-simulator standardization.

Keywords: reusability, computer simulation, multiscale modeling, spreading depression, stroke

1. INTRODUCTION

Computational neuroscience has had an historical focus on electrophysiology, with consequent neglect not only of the accompanying chemophysiology that directly underlies neural function, but also of the brain as a complex organ within which neuronal networks are embedded (De Schutter, 2008). This neglect is of particular importance as we try to adapt our models for understanding of brain disease, many of which are associated with changes in extracellular concentrations of ions, metabolites, transmitters, or toxins in various parts of the brain (Mulugeta et al., 2018). These extracellular concentration changes then cause alterations in reactions and reaction rates involving cellular elements including specific and nonspecific receptors, ion channels, and intracellular signaling pathways. In order to begin to fill out modeling of the brain as a whole organ, we have developed an extracellular modeling extension for the NEURON modeling platform (Carnevale and Hines, 2006), a widely used simulation tool that has been used in over 1900 neuroscience publications, with around 600 models freely available on ModelDB (McDougal et al., 2017).

NEURON has always allowed modelers to describe arbitrarily complex phenomena with their own "mod" files, optionally including verbatim C-code, thereby permitting arbitrary programming to be done to augment the package. This left the user with complex code which intermingled model specifics with the numerics, making reuse difficult. One of the guiding principles of simulator development, both for NEURON and for other simulators, has been to promote reproducibility, reusability, and credibility by providing a consistent numerics-independent way to specify models. In the reaction-diffusion domain, the NEURON *rxd* module simplified and standardized the description of accumulation, reaction and diffusion (McDougal et al., 2013). This module has been used to study calcium dynamics in both physiological and pathological conditions (Neymotin et al., 2014, 2016). We have now expanded the *rxd* module to include macroscopic volume averaged description of extracellular space (ECS). This is appropriate for spatial discretization on the order of 10 μm to produce simulations up to centimeters (Nicholson and Phillips, 1981; Nicholson, 1995). The *rxd* macroscopic model of tissue is parameterized by free volume fraction—the proportion of space unoccupied by cells, blood vessels, etc.; and tortuosity—the increase in a diffusing particle's path-length due to obstacles.

In the following sections we give details of the development of the extracellular *rxd* module, with examples to demonstrate the utility of the Python interface. We then show some details of the numerical methods underling the module's interface and techniques used to improve performance for large simulations, providing several tests to verify *rxd* simulation results. We give a basic example of clinically-relevant simulation by demonstrating the phenomenon of *spreading depression*, a pathological condition thought to play a role in a variety of conditions including mirgraine, epilepsy, and stroke (Wei et al., 2014).

2. OBJECTIVES

As with cells of other solid organs, neurons exist in a highly active medium, influenced by bioactive chemicals whose concentrations change rapidly through: (1) passive diffusion, (2) active deposit and clearance from other cells, and (3) binding or other reactions with extracellular species (Syková and Nicholson, 2008). These important tissue-level *chemophysiological* influences have been neglected by computational neuroscience for a variety of reasons, including the aforementioned focus on electrophysiology. Primarily, however, simulators have been unable to support this level of interaction due to the difficulty of reconciling the small spatial scale of single cell and local network simulation with the large millimeter (mouse) or centimeter (primate) scale of the brain as an organ. This type of broad multiscale modeling naturally requires compromises at both ends, and across the temporal scales as well. We set out to extend NEURON to handle this domain by providing a coarsely-discretized extracellular domain within which cells and networks can be embedded, creating *mosaic models* where different parts are provided at different levels of detail. The coarse scale permits relatively rapid simulation runs, but is sufficiently detailed to set parameters based on currently available experimental measures. Other spatial scales will be added to this mosaic in the future.

A major focus for both the original *rxd* module and this extension is ease-of-use. This goal is partly achieved by separating the user from the details of the numerics enhancing reproducibility by making it easy to identify the conceptual model. Additionally, the *rxd* Python interface subserves this goal by providing relatively simple, biologically-intuitive representations that allow the user to focus on the translation of the conceptual model by specifying (1) regions: *where?* — in this case the ECS; (2) species in each region: *who?* — an ionic species, a peptide, a transmitter, etc.; and (3) transformations *what?* — reactions between species, signaling across a membrane, or transits involving the same species across a membrane.

Providing consistent modeling of both intracellular and extracellular space also ensures conservation of mass. The total amount of a substance of interest will be conserved within the simulation, despite moving in and out of subcellular compartments, or in and out of cells, via currents, active transport, or vesicular release.

3. EXAMPLES

We present two related examples to demonstrate the use of the *rxd* module to model extracellular concentrations: (1) simple potassium diffusion, and (2) spreading depression. In each case we begin by specifying the region for the dynamics, here the ECS. We then identify the species involved. Finally, their interactions with each other or with fixed agents are identified. The code for these examples are available at ModelDB (http://modeldb.yale.edu/238892) (McDougal et al., 2017).

3.1. Potassium Diffusion in ECS

This example shows potassium diffusion through a box of ECS, with spatial uptake represented phenomenologically as a reaction. We demonstrate each of the stages required to specifying a model. First, to use extracellular *rxd*, we import it from NEURON and enable it:

```
from neuron import crxd as rxd
rxd.options.enable.extracellular = True
```

3.1.1. Region

We then specify the specific extracellular region;

```
ecs = rxd.Extracellular(xlo=-500, ylo=-500,
    zlo=-500, xhi=500, yhi=500,
    zhi=500, dx=10,
    volume_fraction=0.2,
    tortuosity=1.6)
```

(xlo,ylo,zlo) and (xhi,yhi,zhi) define the lower left back and upper right front corners of a 3D box in micrometers. dx is the size of a side of a cubic voxel; alternatively dx can be a 3-element tuple to specify voxel length, height and depth. The optional argument volume_fraction is the free volume fraction or porosity, the accessible portion of extracellular volume. The tortuosity is the average multiplicative increase in path length a particle must travel due to obstacles. The effective diffusion coefficient is the free diffusion coefficient divided by the square of the tortuosity. Here, the free volume fraction (0.2) and tortuosity (1.6) were set to typical values for brain (Syková and Nicholson, 2008). Both the volume fraction and the tortuosity can be scalar values as shown here. Alternatively, arrays the size of the extracellular space, or functions that take the *x*, *y*, *z* coordinates as arguments can be used (section 3.2.1). Extracellular concentrations are given relative to free volume, i.e., the total amount in a voxel divided by free volume of the voxel.

3.1.2. Species

To create extracellular potassium, we use the same rxd.Species call as would be used for intracellular diffusion; the difference is in the first argument that gives the extracellular region.

```
k = rxd.Species(ecs, name='k',
    d=2.62, charge=1,
    initial=lambda nd: 40
      if nd.x3d**2 + nd.y3d**2 + nd.z3d**2
      < 100**2 else 3.5,
    ecs_boundary_conditions=3.5)
```

Where d (the free diffusion coefficient) is set to $2.62\mu m^2/ms$ for K^+(Samson et al., 2003), where *d* has been increased to reflect a higher temperature of 37°C by using the Stokes-Einstein equation, assuming viscosity of the extracellular fluid to be the same as water. Anisotropic diffusion is supported by passing a 3-tuple for diffusion coefficients in 3 dimensions. Initial conditions can be a scalar value for the whole region, an array matching the region $\left(\text{i.e., } \left\lceil \frac{\texttt{xhi} - \texttt{xlo}}{\texttt{dx}} \right\rceil, \left\lceil \frac{\texttt{yhi} - \texttt{ylo}}{\texttt{dy}} \right\rceil, \left\lceil \frac{\texttt{zhi} - \texttt{zlo}}{\texttt{dz}} \right\rceil\right)$ or an anonymous (lambda) function, as shown here. The lambda function is given a NodeExtracellular as argument, allowing the model to specify initial concentration depending on the location (x3d, y3d, z3d). If the species exists in both intracellular rxd.Region and the ECS then the initial function will receive both NodeExtracellular and either Node1D or Node3D from the class rxd.node. This multiplicity of regions, where the same location is represented in both the intracellular space and the ECS is due to using an interposition of intracellular and extracellular space handled by ECS free volume fraction, instead of by using excluded volume. The initial function can assign values by first checking region is equal to the defined ecs. The default boundary conditions for the ECS are Neumann (zero flux). Dirichlet boundary conditions can be specified with the keyword argument ecs_boundary_conditions set to the desired concentration. Concentrations are in mM.

3.1.3. Reactions

Extracellular reactions are specified using rxd.Rate, rxd.Reaction and rxd.MultiCompartmentReaction as described in the *rxd* tutorial (McDougal, 2018). We consider the case of excess potassium in the ECS, which is primarily taken up by astrocytes (MacAulay and Zeuthen, 2012). A wide variety of modeling options are available for explicitly modeling these cells at various levels of complexity (Wei et al., 2014; Conte et al., 2018). Here we demonstrate the phenomenological model of astrocytic buffering from (Bazhenov et al., 2004; Krishnan and Bazhenov, 2011). This model treats astrocytes as a chemical buffer that could take up excess K^+ but would then release K^+ when ECS levels dropped.

$$[K][A] \underset{k_b}{\overset{k_f}{\rightleftharpoons}} [AK] \tag{1}$$

where *A* is the concentration of free astrocyte "buffering" capacity and *AK* is the concentration of bound potassium. By default mass-action kinetics are assumed, so the stoichiometry is implicit. The rate of change in unbound astrocyte capacity A used in the following example is then given by; kf*[K]*[A] - kb[AK] mM/ms. Alternative kinetics can be specified with the keyword argument mass_action=False. The rates would then be assumed to be the full forward and reverse rates, and change in unbound buffer would be kf-kb mM/ms. The initial condition Amax represents the total capacity of glial to buffer K^+ (in mM), in this phenological model it represents the density of astrocyte uptake/binding sites. These sites are immobile: d=0.

The specification of kf uses the exponential of an rxd.Species. This is achieved in Python by importing the rxd.rxdmath module, which provides the same library of functions as the Python math module. However while Python math functions require numeric arguments the rxd.rxdmath allows rxd.Species to be used, as in the following example;

```
from neuron.rxd import rxdmath
kb = 0.0008     #backward rate mM/ms
kth = 15.0      #k threshold
kf = kb/(1.0 + rxdmath.exp(-(k - kth)/1.15))
```

```
Amax = 10 #uptake/release site density

A = rxd.Species(ecs,name='astrocyte',
    d=0, initial=Amax)
AK = rxd.Species(ecs,name='bound',
    d=0, initial=0)

astrocytes = rxd.Reaction(k + A, AK, kf,
            kb)
```

3.2. Cortical Spreading Depression

The preceding simulation framework can be used to develop a model of spreading depression (SD). SD is a wave of near complete depolarizations of neurons that propagates in gray matter at 2-7 mm/min and lasts for ~1 min. This phenomena is highly reproducible and is associated with several pathological conditions, including; migraines, ischemic stroke, traumatic brain injury and epilepsy (Somjen, 2004). An early mechanistic model attributed the depolarization to an increase in extracellular K^+ (Grafstein, 1956). A positive feedback loop underlies SD: high extracellular K^+ activates cells whose depolarization opens K^+ channels which release more K^+ into extracellular space.

To produce this positive feedback between ECS and cellular physiology, we simulate a realistic density of 90,000 cells/mm^3 embedded in 1mm^3 of ECS with diffusion of both K^+ and Na^+. Each neuron has a soma and dendrite with the Hodgkin-Huxley complement of channels (naf, kdr, gleak) as well as kleak and nap (persistent Na^+ channel) with parameters based on Conte et al. (2018). This initial simplified model omits several mechanisms likely to contribute to spreading depolarization, including slow Ca^{2+}-dependent K^+ currents. More importantly, we omit neurons Na-K-ATPase, a major mechanism for restoring ion gradients. As noted above, glial Na-K-ATPase is partially modeled by the field of K^+ sink.

An initial spherical bolus of 40 mM K^+ of radius 100 μm was placed in the center of the ECS to trigger SD. In the absence of astrocytic uptake, the SD wave front propagated at 1.69 mm/min. High astrocyte capacity of 500 mM (Bazhenov et al., 2004) immediately removed the free K^+, preventing SD. At a far lower astrocyte density of 10 mM, SD did occur (**Figure 1**). SD speed was reduced by 70% compared to the no-astrocyte case (**Figure 2**).

3.2.1. Cerebral Edema

The volume-averaged macroscopic description of tissue can be characterized by free volume fraction and tortuosity. Both vary across brain regions (Nicholson and Syková, 1998), as well as during the sleep-wake cycle (Xie et al., 2013) and under pathological conditions (Hrabětová and Nicholson, 2000). A major pathological condition that decreases free volume fraction and increases tortuosity is cytotoxic edema, which is caused by cell swelling resulting in reduced ECS. In the case of ischemia (stroke), edema will be greatest at the ischemia core, the central location where metabolites have been cut-off through lack of blood flow. At the core we reduced free volume fraction to 0.07 and increased tortuosity to 1.8 (Zoremba et al., 2008). Outside of the core, there is a penumbra where cell function and ECS characteristic are less abnormal. The penumbra in turn is surrounded by normal tissue. The notion of 3 concentric volumes is a gross approximation since there is fall-off of damage as one passes from central core to normal tissue at the outside. We therefore simulated SD with cerebral edema using a linear change in the free volume fraction and tortuosity parameters from central core outward.

The characteristics of the ECS were specified with functions:

```
Lx, Ly, Lz = 1000, 1000, 1000
alpha0, alpha1 = 0.07, 0.2
tort0, tort1 = 1.8, 1.6
r0 = 100

def alpha(x, y, z) :
  return (alpha0 if x**2 + y**2 + z**2
  < r0**2
  else min(alpha1, alpha0 +(alpha1
  -alpha0) *((x**2+y**2+z**2)**0.5-r0)/
  (Lx/2)))

def tort(x, y, z) :
  return (tort0 if x**2 + y**2 + z**2
  < r0**2
  else max(tort1, tort0 - (tort0
  -tort1) *((x**2+y**2+z**2)**0.5-r0)/
  (Lx/2)))

ecs = rxd.Extracellular(-Lx/2.0, -Ly/2.0,
  -Lz/2.0, Lx/2.0, Ly/2.0, Lz/2.0, dx=10,
  volume_fraction=alpha, tortuosity=tort)
```

We repeated the SD simulation in the ischemic context. Although diffusion was slowed by the increased tortuosity, the effect was less than the speed-up obtained due to reduced volume fraction. With the reduced volume fraction, less K^+ was required to propagate the wave (**Figure 2**).

This simple model demonstrates the utility and simplicity of the expanded *rxd* module. However, it only included diffusion of K^+ and Na^+. Other relevant species could be added to make the simulation more closely comparable to the clinical situation. Adding glutamate would produce further depolarization through synaptic receptors and could contribute to both excitotoxicity (cell damage due to excessive depolarization and calcium) and to the propagation of SD (Kager et al., 2000; Hübel et al., 2017). Demonstrating excitotoxicity would also suggest adding diffusion of calcium, which is also involved in the induction and propagation of SD. Chloride contributes to K^+ homoeostasis via Cl-K cotransport and also regulates cell osmolarity (Hübel and Ullah, 2016).

In order to explicitly simulate uptake by astrocytes `rxd.MultiCompartmentReaction` would be used to define stoichiometrically-defined flux between intracellular and extracellular regions. A more sophisticated model of astrocytes would include gap junctions, allowing astrocytes to maintain a lower membrane potential facilitating K^+ uptake. Such a model could also include spatial buffering, where K^+ is transported via astrocytes rather than diffusion in the ECS (Gardner-Medwin, 1983). While the buffering in this simple model is neuroprotective, astrocytes also play an adverse role in

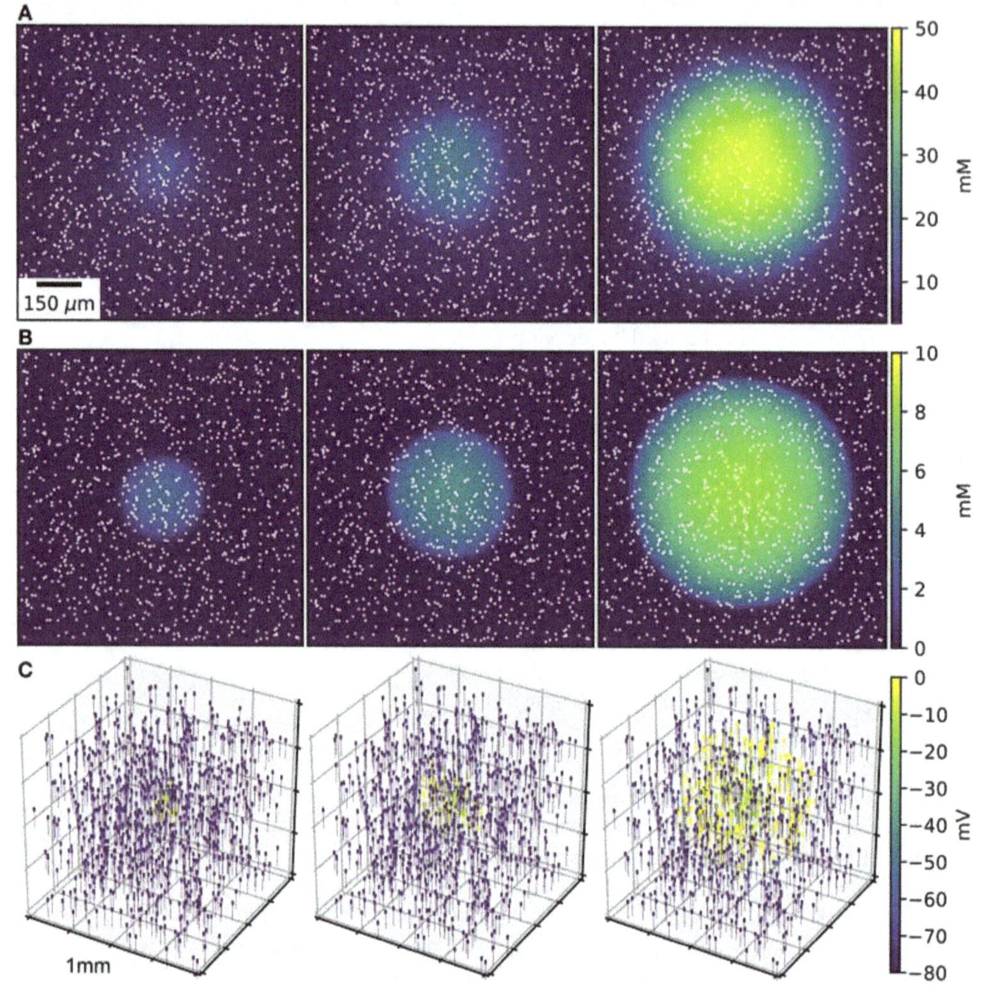

FIGURE 1 | SD wave Time points at 10, 20, 30 s, with concentrations averaged over the depth of 1 mm^3 of ECS. **(A)** Extracellular K^+ with glial uptake and Dirichlet boundary conditions. **(B)** Glial uptake occupancy. **(C)** Membrane potential for 1,000 of the 90,000 cells [their locations are shown in **(A,B)** by white points]. Video available in Supplementary Data.

SD, as gap-junction mediated calcium waves may be related to the initiation and amplification of SD, facilitating propagation over longer distances (Nedergaard et al., 1995).

These simulations focused on the wave of cell depolarization and omitted the silencing of electrical activity that follows—looking at the spreading depolarization rather than at the specifics of the spreading depression itself (Dreier, 2011). This second phase of neuronal inactivity may be related to depolarization blockade, as well as to synaptic plasticity and the accumulation of extracellular adenosine (Frenguelli and Wall, 2016; Cozzolino et al., 2018).

4. IMPLEMENTATION DETAILS

We provide a Python interface for specifying the model for ease of use and reproducibility; for performance reasons the numerical details are implemented in C and connected to Python using `ctypes`. This separation between interface and numerics allows the user to see a standard approach to modeling the ECS, where species and reactions are immediately apparent when examining a model. Parameters can be read directly from the Python code or obtained by querying the model through the Python console. In the future, parameters will also be accessible via a graphical user interface (GUI).

4.1. Model Specification Aids Reproducibility

The concise, declaratory syntax for model specification has been slightly augmented since introduction of the original *rxd* module introduced with NEURON 7.3. However, all models implemented using a previous version of the *rxd* module will continue to work with the expanded version. Because of the vast difference in spatial scale between the intracellular and extracellular volumes, distinct modeling techniques are used to support diffusion in region `rxd.Extracellular`.

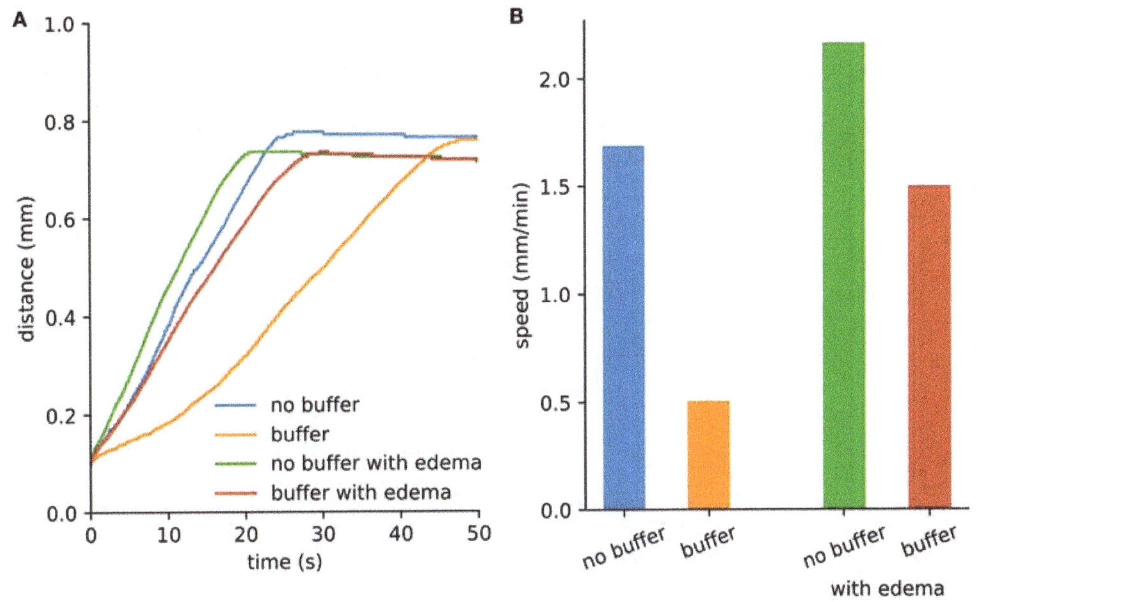

FIGURE 2 | Spreading depression spread faster with edema. **(A)** Maximum distance from the center where extracellular K^+ exceeds 15 mM. The extent was limited by the loss of K^+ at the Dirichlet boundary. **(B)** Wave speed from the first 10 s of SD.

4.2. Finite-Volume Alternating Direction Implicit Method

We used the Douglas-Gunn Alternating Direction Implicit method (DG-ADI) for diffusion in the ECS (Douglas and Gunn, 1964). DG-ADI divides each time step into three sub-steps (Equations A1–A3). The first deals with the diffusion operator in the x-direction, the second in the y-direction and the third in the z-direction. DG-ADI is computationally efficient with worst case runtime $\mathcal{O}(N)$ for N voxels. DG-ADI also provides an embarrassingly parallel workload. If the size of the extracellular space is $N_x \times N_y \times N_z$, then there are $N_y \times N_z$ independent operations for (Equation A1), $N_x \times N_z$ for (Equation A2) and $N_x \times N_y$ for (Equation A3). The finite volume method discretization (Equation A15) can be modified to account for heterogeneous diffusion coefficients and free volume fractions (Equation A16), while ensuring conservation of mass (**Figure 5A**). The details of the numerical scheme are given in Appendix A.

4.3. Just-in-Time Compiled Reactions

Reaction-diffusion performance is further improved by using compiled reactions. Reactions are now parsed into C code which is compiled Just-In-Time (JIT). For example, the reaction given in section 3.1.3 produces the following C code;

```
#include <math.h>
#include <rxdmath.h>
void reaction(double* species_ecs,
    double* rhs)
{
    double rate;
    rate = -((species_ecs[2])*(0.0008))
      +(((0.0008)/(1.0+exp((
          -(species_ecs[0]-(15.0)))/(1.15))))
        *(species_ecs[1]))*(species_ecs[0]);
    rhs[1] = (-1)*rate;
    rhs[0] = (-1)*rate;
    rhs[2] = (1)*rate;
}
```

The 0 index of the `species_ecs` and `rhs` arrays corresponds to `k`, `1` to `A` and `2` to `AK`. The C code for the reactions are compiled into a dynamic library using the C compiler distributed with the operating system or distributed with NEURON. The compiled library is loaded and provides a function pointer that is used to numerically approximate the Jacobian. This allows function overloading, so the same method is used to process all extracellular reactions. The Jacobian for the reaction is solved using the Meschach library (Stewart and Leyk, 1994) included with the NEURON distribution. `rxd.rxdmath` supports all the mathematical functions in the math module. Most of these are defined in the GNU C Library `math.h`. Additional functions have been added in `rxdmath.h`.

4.4. Parallel Implementation

Extracellular reaction-diffusion benefits from two forms of parallelization; multithreading and multiprocessor (**Figure 3**). Multithreading, implemented with POSIX threads, uses shared memory. The number of *rxd* threads `n` can be set by calling `rxd.nthread(n)`.

A thread pool is created at the start of the simulation; the calculations required for both diffusion (DG-ADI) and reactions are distributed across the available threads in the pool. The *rxd* threads are independent of NEURON threads used for electrophysiology, which are accessed via

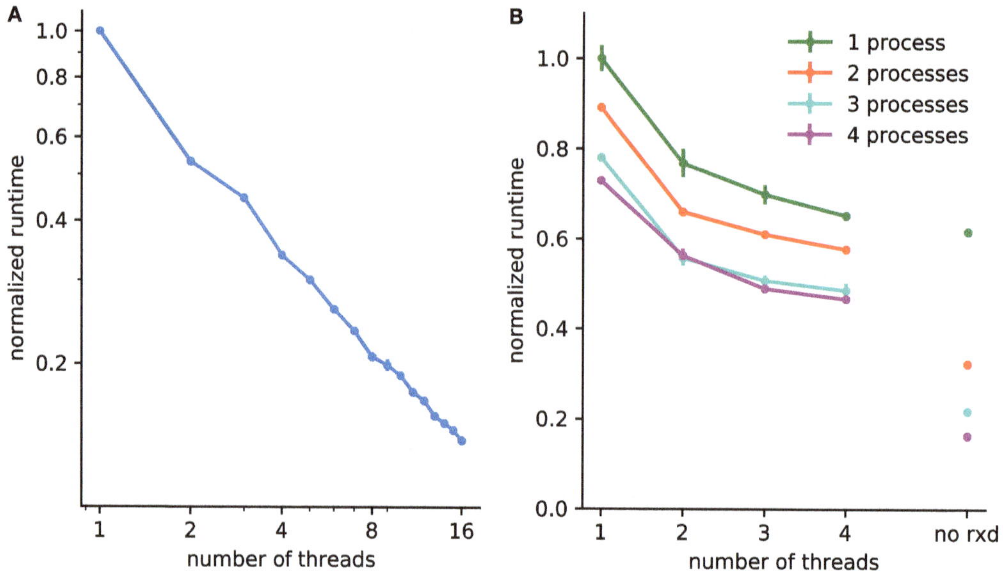

FIGURE 3 | Reduction in runtime with parallelization. **(A)** 5x speedup with 8 threads with 250^3 (15,625,000) extracellular voxels for example in section 3.1. **(B)** A spreading depression example with 1mm^3 tissue, with 250,000 two compartment neurons and 150^3 (3,375,000) voxels. Electrophysiology accounts for 62% of the runtime with one process (with 38% due to extracellular *rxd*), this is reduced to 22% when four processes are used, increasing the relative burden of extracellular *rxd* to 78%. Walltime minimum and standard error are shown for 5 runs of each simulation performed on a 24 core system (4 Intel Xeon L5640 processors).

`ParallelContext.nthreads`. Independent pools are used because these are independent problems: (1) electrophysiology: ParallelContext threads split computations either by cell, or by cell section (multi-split method; Hines et al., 2008) (2) diffusion and reaction: DG-ADI. Although DG-ADI is trivially parallelizable, we do not achieve optimal scaling (**Figure 3A**). Performance is limited by the overhead of the relatively large non-contiguous memory access required, and the need to coordinate with the NEURON time step.

The multiprocessor approach, implemented with the Message Passing Interface (MPI) is primarily intended for large neuronal network models. The network that is embedded within the ECS may in this case be purely electrophysiological or may also include intracellular *rxd*. In either case, the speed-up from using MPI is entirely due to network speed-up; each processor solves the entire ECS reaction-diffusion space independently. All cellular influx and efflux are made available to all processors. This simple approach was adopted after demonstrating that communication overhead dominated over calculation when the ECS was split across processors. Multiprocessor and multithreading can be used together, with MPI reducing the runtime for the intracellular *rxd* for electrophysiology and for networks, multiple threads reducing runtime for ECS reaction-diffusion (**Figure 3B**).

5. VERIFICATION AND VALIDATION

We verified the numerical implementation by (1) comparing a simple model with its analytic solution; and (2) confirming conservation of mass, (3) comparing results with FiPy, a finite volume PDE solver (Guyer et al., 2009).

5.1. Comparison With Analytic Results

A simple model with an analytic solution is an initial cube of elevated concentration diffusing in a closed boxed. It is solved by integrating the Green's function over the initial conditions and matching the Neumann boundary conditions with the method of images (Appendix B). A direct comparison to the numerical method is obtained by integrating over the central voxel and dividing by volume to obtain the average concentration at the center (Equation A20). There is close agreement between the numerical solution provided by the *rxd* module and this analytic solution (**Figure 4**).

5.2. Conservation of Mass

When using Neumann (zero flux) boundary conditions the finite volume method will conserve mass. This provides a basic numerical and algorithmic verification that can be applied even to complex models. The example of section 3.2.1 can be modified so *rxd* manages both intracellular and extracellular concentrations. Multiplying the extracellular concentration by the volume fraction and the voxel volume and the intracellular concentration by the segment volume gives the total amount of K^+. The change in total amount of K^+ (**Figure 5A**) was on the order of floating point accuracy ($\sim 10^{-12}$).

5.3. FiPy Comparison

We modeled a morphologically detailed reconstruction of a rat hippocampal CA1 pyramidal neuron obtained from NeuroMorpho.Org `NMO_00227` (Ishizuka et al., 1995; Ascoli et al., 2007), with constant outgoing ion flux corresponding to a current density of 1mA/cm^2 of K^+ (**Figure 5B**).

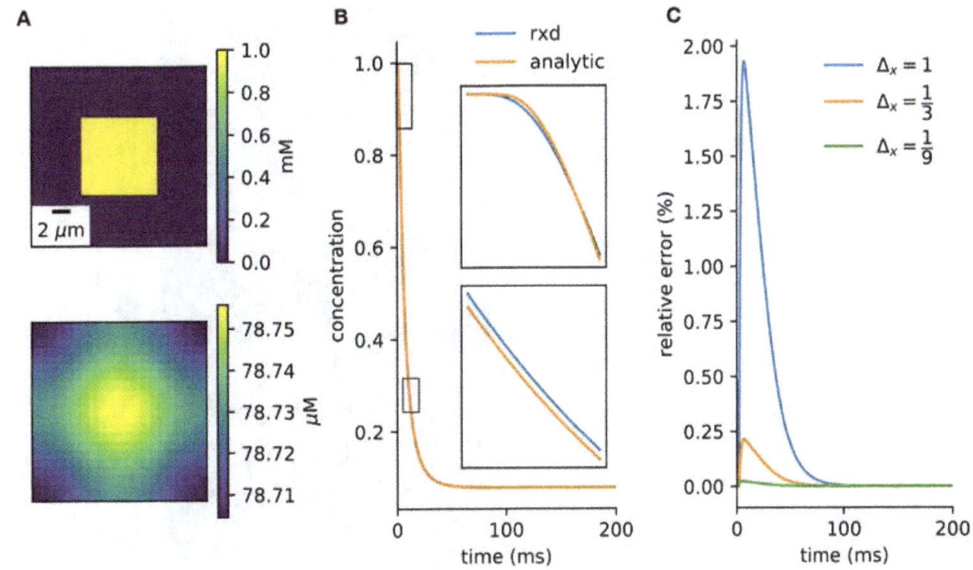

FIGURE 4 | Verification against analytic solution. **(A)** Cross-section of initial conditions (top) and after 100ms (bottom). 9 μm^3 cube diffuses in a 21 μm^3 cube. **(B)** Concentration of center voxel compared to analytic solution (Equation A20), with insets at two 2.5 ms periods ($\Delta x = 1$ μm, $\Delta t = 0.1$ ms). **(C)** Relative error tends toward zero with finer spatial discretization.

In *rxd* objects provide point sources, and occupied space is represented by the free volume fraction and tortuosity. We exported the point sources from the NEURON simulation and used them with the FiPy solver (**Figure 5C**). Differences were $\leq$5 nM, with largest differences at the sites of efflux (**Figure 5D**). The sum of absolute differences was 0.03% of the total concentration at $t = 1$s.

6. DISCUSSION

The original *rxd* package expanded multiscale modeling in NEURON from the electrophysiological scales of neurites, cells and networks into chemophysiological scales of spines, subcellular organelles, interactomics, metabolomics, proteomics. This further development of the module into the domain of extracellular space considerably extends the scope of chemophysiology into the vast distances of interneuronal space. Computational performance for this large-scale problem is improved by the use of multi-threading parallelization of DG-ADI algorithm for diffusion, multiprocessor parallelization for electrophysiology, and JIT compilation of reactions. The ECS module implementation was verified against an analytic solution, a test of conservation, and by comparison to an established simulator.

The extension to whole-organ simulation in the brain is particularly important for the development of multiscale modeling for clinical applications (Hunt et al., 2018; Mulugeta et al., 2018). In the past, large neural simulations have typically been neuronal networks which focus exclusively on the electrical activity of neurons and their mutual influence via chemical and electrical synapses. Such neuronal network simulations have effectively operated in a vacuum, omitting the effects of nonsynaptic neuromodulators, neuromodulatory gases, ions, glia, metabolites, etc. These physiological agents also play pathophysiological roles, for example the excessive ion concentrations seen in spreading depression, and the lack of metabolites that causes tissue damage from ischemia and stroke. Pharmacological agents used in treatments are also broadcast diffusively, as are agents and effects associated with microglia. Mechanical factors from brain trauma and current in electrical stimulation follow their respective tissue impedance boundaries. Many pathological disorders, particularly stroke and traumatic brain injury, involve large volumes of tissue. For this reason, the initial development of our new extension has focused on coarse spatial discretization in order to accommodate large distances, permitting representative neuronal networks to be seeded in a mosaic of locations within the volume.

6.1. Large Volume Averaged Approach

Electrophysiological models in NEURON can specify currents either in absolute terms or as current densities. In the latter case, membrane surface area must be used to calculate the current. The ECS *rxd* module identifies ion flux from currents, which are then placed in the corresponding voxel of the ECS simulation. Macroscopic measure of ion diffusion in bulk tissue observed experimentally with ion selective sensors, biosensors, and fast-scan cyclic voltammetry can be used to constrain parameters (Budygin et al., 2000; Dale et al., 2005; Nicholson and Hrabětová, 2017).

Currently, we support two boundary conditions: Neumann boundary conditions (constant boundary flux) and Dirichlet conditions (constant boundary concentration). Neumann boundary conditions are appropriate for *in-vivo* models where we are simulating a piece of brain in continuity with other similar pieces of brain. In this case, any substance that

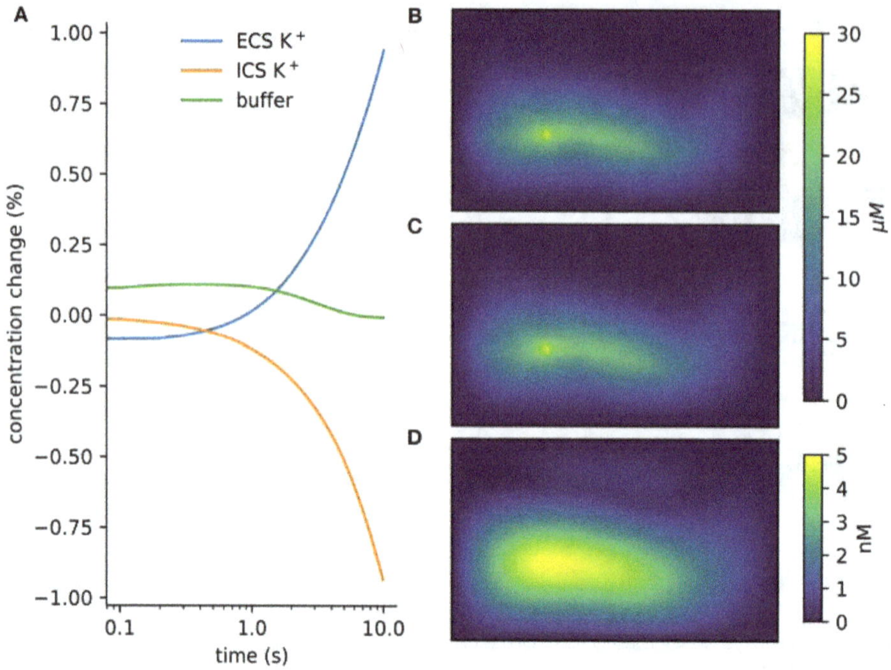

FIGURE 5 | Verification and validation. **(A)** Conservation of mass for verification: $< 10^{-12}$ change with currents from 1,000 neurons in tissue with heterogeneous diffusion. **(B)** *rxd* simulation of 1mA/cm^2 constant K^+ flux from a traced rat hippocampal CA1 pyramidal neuron and Dirichlet boundary conditions, concentrations at 1 s (averaged over depth). **(C)** Comparable solution using FiPy with identical current fluxes. **(D)** Difference between *rxd* and FiPy concentrations results (note scale in nM).

leaves the simulated space would be replaced by substance from neighboring regions. Conversely Dirichlet conditions (constant boundary) are appropriate if the region modeled is not representative, as occurs under pathological conditions such as the core area of a stroke. In this case perturbations in extracellular concentrations are expected to be restored sufficiently far from their source. In both cases, clearance can still be modeled using NEURON models or extracellular reactions to represent transport through the blood-brain-barrier. If the ECS is made large enough relative to simulation duration, the choice of boundary conditions will not have a significant effect on results.

6.2. Multiple Uses of Extracellular Reaction-Diffusion Simulation

There are many forms of extracellular extra-synaptic signaling between cells. Here we have illustrated the utility of the module with a simple model for spreading depression, where the "signal" is a change in ion concentration. The extracellular *rxd* module has a wide range of potential applications tracking the variety of substances of both physiological and pathological relevance. For example, neurotoxic substances such as free radicals diffuse away from areas of damaged tissue; amyloid-β oligomers may diffuse away from specific cells creating misfolding of protein in remote cells (Waters, 2010). Both synaptic spillover and nonsynaptic release provide diffusing of neurotransmitters (e.g., glutamate and excitotoxicity), and of neuromodulators: dopamine, acetylcholine, norepinephrine, adenosine, etc. For example, dopamine (DA) in striatum is released by axonal projections from midbrain, and diffuses in a local region before reuptake by DA transporter (Sulzer et al., 2016). Models of striatal activity in physiological (Humphries et al., 2010) or pathological conditions (Migliore et al., 2008; Blackwell et al., 2018) would benefit by including this extracellular dopamine spread. Simulating extracellular dopamine would follow the same procedure described in section 3.1; specifying the region with tortuosity and porosity, the species with its diffusion coefficient and boundary conditions and the reactions that remove it from the ECS including the kinetics of DA transporters.

6.3. Future Development

The ECS simulation developed here will provide the broadest spatial scale for future multiscale models that will add additional methods at smaller scales. These multiple methods will interconnect so as to be used together in single multiscale simulations that coordinate a broad range of spatial and temporal scales, that could not be assessed using a uniform fine discretization, or uniform algorithms throughout. At the finest scales, stochastic methods will be used to better understand the variability seen at small scale, for example in synaptic clefts. Additional simulation method currently being addressed include techniques for understanding bulk tissue current flow to simulate deep and transcranial current stimulation. Whether induced externally or produced by local field potentials (Lindén et al., 2014), bulk electric field effects will not only depolarize or hyperpolarize cells, but will also affect diffusion of ions and other charged species i.e., the phenomenon of electrodiffusion. Not only are ions affected by the field, ions also produce a field that will affect other ions, potentially producing fields of order hundreds of microvolts over 1mm of tissue (Halnes et al., 2016; Solbrå et al., 2018). Such gradients are likely to have an even greater influence in SD, where there is a large redistribution of ions.

There are a number of other important organ-level processes that are particularly important for brain pathology. These include blood flow which is of importance for understanding stroke, and mechanical properties of importance for understanding traumatic brain injury. Additional processes that are unique to the brain would include CSF production, flow and reuptake; and status of the blood-brain barrier. More controversial is the role of advection—fluid flow. The brain lacks a lymphatic system for waste clearance, and the small spaces between cells, ~40 nm, are too small to support advection (Jin et al., 2016; Holter et al., 2017). It has been hypothesized to instead use a *glymphatic system* that establishes fluid flow via glial astrocytic aquaporin-4 channels, driven by pulsations from respiration and heartbeat. Fluid would flow via astrocytes oriented to provide the pathways that cannot be supported by the interstitium (Iliff et al., 2012).

All of these processes are currently the subject of multiscale modeling at varying degrees of sophistication (Anderson and Vadigepalli, 2016; Linninger et al., 2016; Calvetti et al., 2018; Durka et al., 2018; Zhao et al., 2018). Although it would not be practical to incorporate these many types of simulation within NEURON, there will be possibilities for cross-simulator communication providing complex multiphysics simulations in the future (Djurfeldt et al., 2010). In the meantime, some aspects of this complexity can be readily incorporated without considering the details: for example, brain vascularization can be modeled as a "metabolite field" that would take account of the greater availability of oxygen and glucose at locations within, and reduced availability in the *watershed areas* that lie between, the major artery distribution trees.

The term *mosaic modeling* may be used to describe these complex multiscale, multiphysics, multialgorithmic, multidimensional simulations—the mosaic involves pieces of a cell or of a brain simulated with different dimensionality, different algorithms, and different discretizations. An example at the cellular level are spines, which are best handled stochastically and in three dimensions, while the rest of the cell is handled deterministically and as a one dimensional branched tree structure (Lin et al., 2017a,b). Similarly, in the ECS, small spaces such as synapses require a microscopic approach that is not practical for bulk tissue modeling. In the future, these pieces of the mosaic will be adapted from approaches currently used by other simulators. For example, one approach at small scales is to track individual particles, done by Smoldyn (Andrews, 2012) and MCell (Stiles and Bartol, 2001; Franks et al., 2002). Another small-volume technique uses averaged volumetrics as done by the ENOS platform, which has also been used for high resolution models of glutamatergic synapses and their interaction with glia (Bouteiller et al., 2008). Other platforms that support intracellular diffusion will also be mined for additional techniques, including STEPS (Wils and De Schutter, 2009), NeuroRD (Brandi et al., 2011), MOOSE (Ray and Bhalla, 2008).

AUTHOR CONTRIBUTIONS

WL, MH, RM, and AN expanded the rxd module. WL, RM, and AN created the examples and wrote the paper.

FUNDING

Supported by NIH grant R01 MH086638.

ACKNOWLEDGMENTS

We thank Prof. Charles Nicholson, Prof. Sabina Hrabětová and Dr. Jan Hrabe for their advice on modeling the extracellular space. We thank Prof. David Terman who provided the inspiration and channel kinetics for the spreading depression simulations.

REFERENCES

Anderson, W. D., and Vadigepalli, R. (2016). Modeling cytokine regulatory network dynamics driving neuroinflammation in central nervous system disorders. *Drug Discov. Today Dis. Models* 19, 59–67. doi: 10.1016/j.ddmod.2017.01.003

Andrews, S. S. (2012). "Spatial and stochastic cellular modeling with the smoldyn simulator," in *Bacterial Molecular Networks. Methods in Molecular Biology (Methods and Protocols)*, Vol. 804, eds J. van Helden, A. Toussaint, and D. Thieffry (New York, NY: Springer).

Ascoli, G. A., Donohue, D. E., and Halavi, M. (2007). Neuromorpho. org: a central resource for neuronal morphologies. *J. Neurosci.* 27, 9247–9251. doi: 10.1523/JNEUROSCI.2055-07.2007

Bazhenov, M., Timofeev, I., Steriade, M., and Sejnowski, T. J. (2004). Potassium model for slow (2-3 hz) *in vivo* neocortical paroxysmal oscillations. *J. Neurophysiol.* 92, 1116–1132. doi: 10.1152/jn.00529.2003

Blackwell, K. T., Salinas, A. G., Tewatia, P., English, B., Hellgren Kotaleski, J., and Lovinger, D. M. (2018). Molecular mechanisms underlying striatal synaptic plasticity: Relevance to chronic alcohol consumption and seeking. *Eur. J. Neurosci.* doi: 10.1111/ejn.13919. [Epub ahead of print].

Bouteiller, J. M., Baudry, M., Allam, S. L., Greget, R. J., Bischoff, S., and Berger, T. W. (2008). Modeling glutamatergic synapses: insights into mechanisms regulating synaptic efficacy. *J. Integr. Neurosci.* 7, 185–197. doi: 10.1142/S0219635208001770

Brandi, M., Brocke, E., Talukdar, H. A., Hanke, M., Bhalla, U. S., Kotaleski, J. H., et al. (2011). Connecting moose and neurord through music: towards a communication framework for multi-scale modeling. *BMC Neurosci.* 12:P77. doi: 10.1186/1471-2202-12-S1-P77

Budygin, E. A., Kilpatrick, M. R., Gainetdinov, R. R., and Wightman, R. M. (2000). Correlation between behavior and extracellular dopamine levels in rat striatum:

comparison of microdialysis and fast-scan cyclic voltammetry. *Neurosci. Lett.* 281, 9–12. doi: 10.1016/S0304-3940(00)00813-2

Calvetti, D., Capo Rangel, G., Gerardo Giorda, L., and Somersalo E(2018). A computational model integrating brain electrophysiology and metabolism highlights the key role of extracellular potassium and oxygen. *J. Theor. Biol.* 446, 238–258. doi: 10.1016/j.jtbi.2018.02.029

Carnevale, N. T., and Hines, M. L. (2006). *The NEURON Book*. Cambridge, UK: Cambridge University Press.

Conte, C., Lee, R., Sarkar, M., and Terman, D. (2018). A mathematical model of recurrent spreading depolarizations. *J. Comput. Neurosci.* 44, 203–217. doi: 10.1007/s10827-017-0675-3

Cozzolino, O., Marchese, M., Trovato, F., Pracucci, E., Ratto, G. M., Buzzi, M. G., et al. (2018). Understanding spreading depression from headache to sudden unexpected death. *Front. Neurol.* 9:19. doi: 10.3389/fneur.2018.00019

Dale, N., Hatz, S., Tian, F., and Llaudet, E. (2005). Listening to the brain: microelectrode biosensors for neurochemicals. *Trends Biotechnol.* 23, 20–428. doi: 10.1016/j.tibtech.2005.05.010

De Schutter, E. (2008). Why are computational neuroscience and systems biology so separate? *PLoS Comput. Biol.* 4:e1000078. doi: 10.1371/journal.pcbi.1000078

Djurfeldt, M., Hjorth, J., Eppler, J. M., Dudani, N., Helias, M., Potjans, T. C., et al. (2010). Run-time interoperability between neuronal network simulators based on the MUSIC framework. *Neuroinformatics* 8:43–60. doi: 10.1007/s12021-010-9064-z

Douglas, J., and Gunn, J. E. (1964). A general formulation of alternating direction methods. *Numer. Math.* 6, 428–453. doi: 10.1007/BF01386093

Dreier, J. P. (2011). The role of spreading depression, spreading depolarization and spreading ischemia in neurological disease. *Nat. Med.* 17:439. doi: 10.1038/nm.2333

Durka, M. J., Wong, I. H., Kallmes, D. F., Pasalic, D., Mut, F., Jagani, M., et al. (2018). A data-driven approach for addressing the lack of flow waveform data in studies of cerebral arterial flow in older adults. *Physiol. Meas.* 39:015006. doi: 10.1088/1361-6579/aa9f46

Franks, K. M., Bartol, T. M., and Sejnowski, T. J. (2002). A monte carlo model reveals independent signaling at central glutamatergic synapses. *Biophys. J.* 83, 2333–2348. doi: 10.1016/S0006-3495(02)75248-X

Frenguelli, B. G., and Wall, M. J. (2016). Combined electrophysiological and biosensor approaches to study purinergic regulation of epileptiform activity in cortical tissue. *J. Neurosci. Methods* 260, 202–214. doi: 10.1016/j.jneumeth.2015.09.011

Gardner-Medwin, A. (1983). Analysis of potassium dynamics in mammalian brain tissue. *J. Physiol.* 335, 393–426. doi: 10.1113/jphysiol.1983.sp014541

Grafstein, B. (1956). Mechanism of spreading cortical depression. *J. Neurophysiol.* 19, 154–171. doi: 10.1152/jn.1956.19.2.154

Guyer, J. E., Wheeler, D., and Warren, J. A. (2009). FiPy: partial differential equations with Python. *Comput. Sci. Eng.* 11, 6–15. doi: 10.1109/MCSE.2009.52

Halnes, G., Mäki-Marttunen, T., Keller, D., Pettersen, K. H., Andreassen, O. A., and Einevoll, G. T. (2016). Effect of ionic diffusion on extracellular potentials in neural tissue. *PLoS Comput. Biol.* 12:e1005193. doi: 10.1371/journal.pcbi.1005193

Hines, M. L., Markram, H., and Schürmann, F. (2008). Fully implicit parallel simulation of single neurons. *J. Comput. Neurosci.* 25, 439–448. doi: 10.1007/s10827-008-0087-5

Holter, K. E., Kehlet, B., Devor, A., Sejnowski, T. J., Dale, A. M., Omholt, S. W., et al. (2017). Interstitial solute transport in 3d reconstructed neuropil occurs by diffusion rather than bulk flow. *Proc. Natl. Acad. Sci. U.S.A.* 114, 9894–9899. doi: 10.1073/pnas.1706942114

Hrabetová, S., and Nicholson, C. (2000). Dextran decreases extracellular tortuosity in thick-slice ischemia model. *J. Cereb. Blood Flow Metab.* 20, 1306–1310. doi: 10.1097/00004647-200009000-00005

Hübel, N., Hosseini-Zare, M. S., Žiburkus, J., and Ullah, G. (2017). The role of glutamate in neuronal ion homeostasis: a case study of spreading depolarization. *PLoS Comput. Biol.* 13:e1005804. doi: 10.1371/journal.pcbi.1005804

Hübel, N., and Ullah, G. (2016). Anions govern cell volume: a case study of relative astrocytic and neuronal swelling in spreading depolarization. *PLoS ONE* 11:e0147060. doi: 10.1371/journal.pone.0147060

Humphries, M. D., Wood, R., and Gurney, K. (2010). Reconstructing the three-dimensional gabaergic microcircuit of the striatum. *PLoS Comput. Biol.* 6:e1001011. doi: 10.1371/journal.pcbi.1001011

Hunt, C. A., Erdemir, A., Lytton, W. W., MacGabhann, F., Sander, E. A., Transtrum, M. K., et al. (2018). The spectrum of Mechanism-Oriented models and methods for explanations of biological phenomena. *Processes* 6:56. doi: 10.3390/pr6050056

Iliff, J. J., Wang, M., Liao, Y., Plogg, B. A., Peng, W., Gundersen, G. A., et al. (2012). A paravascular pathway facilitates csf flow through the brain parenchyma and the clearance of interstitial solutes, including amyloid β. *Sci. Transl. Med.* 4, 147ra111–147ra111. doi: 10.1126/scitranslmed.3003748

Ishizuka, N., Cowan, W. M., and Amaral, D. G. (1995). A quantitative analysis of the dendritic organization of pyramidal cells in the rat hippocampus. *J. Comp. Neurol.* 362, 17–45. doi: 10.1002/cne.903620103

Jin, B.-J., Smith, A. J., and Verkman, A. S. (2016). Spatial model of convective solute transport in brain extracellular space does not support a glymphatic mechanism. *J. Gen. Physiol.* 148, 489–501. doi: 10.1085/jgp.201611684

Kager, H., Wadman, W. J., and Somjen, G. G. (2000). Simulated seizures and spreading depression in a neuron model incorporating interstitial space and ion concentrations. *J. Neurophysiol.* 84, 495–512. doi: 10.1152/jn.2000.84.1.495

Krishnan, G. P., and Bazhenov, M. (2011). Ionic dynamics mediate spontaneous termination of seizures and postictal depression state. *J. Neurosci.* 31, 8870–8882. doi: 10.1523/JNEUROSCI.6200-10.2011

Lin, Z., Tropper, C., McDougal, R. A., Patoary, M. N. I., Lytton, W. W., Yao, Y., et al. (2017a). Multithreaded stochastic pdes for reactions and diffusions in neurons. *ACM Trans. Model. Comput. Simul.* 27:7. doi: 10.1145/2987373

Lin, Z., Tropper, C., Yao, Y., Mcdougal, R. A.,Ishlam Patoary, M. N., Lytton, W. w., et al. (2017b). Load balancing for multi-threaded pdes of stochastic reaction-diffusion in neurons. *J. Simul.* 11:267. doi: 10.1057/s41273-016-0033-x

Lindén, H., Hagen, E., Leski, S., Norheim, E. S., Pettersen, K. H., and Einevoll, G. T. (2014). Lfpy: a tool for biophysical simulation of extracellular potentials generated by detailed model neurons. *Front. Neuroinform.* 7:41. doi: 10.3389/fninf.2013.00041

Linninger, A. A., Tangen, K., Hsu, C.-Y., and Frim, D. (2016). Cerebrospinal fluid mechanics and its coupling to cerebrovascular dynamics. *Annu. Rev. Fluid Mech.* 48, 219–257. doi: 10.1146/annurev-fluid-122414-034321

MacAulay, N., and Zeuthen, T. (2012). Glial K^+ clearance and cell swelling: key roles for cotransporters and pumps. *Neurochem. Res.* 37, 2299–2309. doi: 10.1007/s11064-012-0731-3

McDougal, R. A. (2018). *Reaction-Diffusion Tutorials*. Available online at: https://neuron.yale.edu/neuron/static/docs/rxd/index.html

McDougal, R. A., Hines, M. L., and Lytton, W. W. (2013). Reaction-diffusion in the neuron simulator. *Front. Neuroinform.* 7:28. doi: 10.3389/fninf.2013.00028

McDougal, R. A., Morse, T. M., Carnevale, T., Marenco, L., Wang, R., Migliore, M., et al. (2017). Twenty years of modeldb and beyond: building essential modeling tools for the future of neuroscience. *J. Comput. Neurosci.* 42, 1–10. doi: 10.1007/s10827-016-0623-7

Migliore, M., Cannia, C., and Canavier, C. C. (2008). A modeling study suggesting a possible pharmacological target to mitigate the effects of ethanol on reward-related dopaminergic signaling. *J. Neurophysiol.* 99, 2703–2707. doi: 10.1152/jn.00024.2008

Mulugeta, L., Drach, A., Erdemir, A., Hunt, C. A., Horner, M., Ku, J. P., et al. (2018). Credibility, replicability, and reproducibility in simulation for biomedicine and clinical applications in neuroscience. *Front. Neuroinform.* 12:18. doi: 10.3389/fninf.2018.00018

Nedergaard, M., Cooper, A. J., and Goldman, S. A. (1995). Gap junctions are required for the propagation of spreading depression. *Dev. Neurobiol.* 28, 433–444. doi: 10.1002/neu.480280404

Neymotin, S. A., Dura-Bernal, S., Lakatos, P., Sanger, T. D., and Lytton, W. W. (2016). Multitarget multiscale simulation for pharmacological treatment of dystonia in motor cortex. *Front. Pharmacol.* 7:157. doi: 10.3389/fphar.2016.00157

Neymotin, S. A., McDougal, R. A., Hines, M., and Lytton, W. W. (2014). Calcium regulation of hcn supports persistent activity associated with working memory: a multiscale model of prefrontal cortex. *BMC Neurosci.* 15:P108. doi: 10.1186/1471-2202-15-S1-P108

Nicholson, C. (1995). Interaction between diffusion and michaelis-menten uptake of dopamine after iontophoresis in striatum. *Biophys. J.* 68, 1699–1715. doi: 10.1016/S0006-3495(95)80348-6

Nicholson, C., and Hrabetová, S. (2017). Brain extracellular space: the final frontier of neuroscience. *Biophys. J.* 113, 2133–2142. doi: 10.1016/j.bpj.2017.06.052

Nicholson, C., and Phillips, J. (1981). Ion diffusion modified by tortuosity and volume fraction in the extracellular microenvironment of the rat cerebellum. *J. Physiol.* 321, 225–257. doi: 10.1113/jphysiol.1981.sp013981

Nicholson, C., and Syková, E. (1998). Extracellular space structure revealed by diffusion analysis. *Trends Neurosci.* 21, 207–215. doi: 10.1016/S0166-2236(98)01261-2

Ray, S., and Bhalla, U. (2008). PyMOOSE: interoperable scripting in Python for MOOSE. *Front. Neuroinform.* 2:6. doi: 10.3389/neuro.11.006.2008

Samson, E., Marchand, J., and Snyder, K. A. (2003). Calculation of ionic diffusion coefficients on the basis of migration test results. *Mater. Struct.* 36, 156–165. doi: 10.1007/BF02479554

Solbrå, A., Bergersen, A. W., van den Brink, J., Malthe-Sørenssen, A., Einevoll, G. T., and Halnes, G. (2018). A Kirchhoff-Nernst-Planck framework for modeling large scale extracellular electrodiffusion surrounding morphologically detailed neurons. *bioRxiv* [Preprint]. 261107. doi: 10.1101/261107

Somjen, G. G. (2004). *Ions in the Brain: Normal Function, Seizures, and Stroke.* New York, NY: Oxford University Press.

Stewart, D. E., and Leyk, Z. (1994). *Meschach: Matrix Computations in C,* Vol. 32. Canberra ACT: Centre for Mathematics and its Applications, Australian National University.

Stiles, J. R., and Bartol, T. M. (2001). "Monte carlo methods for simulating realistic synapticmicrophysiology usingmcell," in *Computational Neuroscience: Realistic Modeling for Experimentalists,* ed E. De Schutter, (Boca Raton, FL: CRC Press), 87–127.

Sulzer, D., Cragg, S. J., and Rice, M. E. (2016). Striatal dopamine neurotransmission: regulation of release and uptake. *Basal Ganglia,* 6, 123–148. doi: 10.1016/j.baga.2016.02.001

Syková, E., and Nicholson, C. (2008). Diffusion in brain extracellular space. *Physiol. Rev.* 88, 1277–1340. doi: 10.1152/physrev.00027.2007

Waters, J. (2010). The concentration of soluble extracellular amyloid-β protein in acute brain slices from crnd8 mice. *PLoS ONE* 5:e15709. doi: 10.1371/journal.pone.0015709

Wei, Y., Ullah, G., and Schiff, S. J. (2014). Unification of neuronal spikes, seizures, and spreading depression. *J. Neurosci.* 34, 11733–11743. doi: 10.1523/JNEUROSCI.0516-14.2014

Wils, S., and De Schutter, E. (2009). Steps: modeling and simulating complex reaction-diffusion systems with python. *Front. Neuroinfor.* 3:15. doi: 10.3389/neuro.11.015.2009

Xie, L., Kang, H., Xu, Q., Chen, M. J., Liao, Y., Thiyagarajan, M., et al. (2013). Sleep drives metabolite clearance from the adult brain. *Science* 342, 373–377. doi: 10.1126/science.1241224

Zhao, W., Choate, B., and Ji, S. (2018). Material properties of the brain in injury-relevant conditions–experiments and computational modeling. *J. Mech. Behav. Biomed. Mater.* 80, 222–234. doi: 10.1016/j.jmbbm.2018.02.005

Zoremba, N., Homola, A., Slais, K., Vorísek, I., Rossaint, R., Lehmenkühler, A. et al. (2008). Extracellular diffusion parameters in the rat somatosensory cortex during recovery from transient global ischemia/hypoxia. *J. Cereb. Blood Flow Metab.* 28, 1665–1673. doi: 10.1038/jcbfm.2008.58

13

Uncertainpy: A Python Toolbox for Uncertainty Quantification and Sensitivity Analysis in Computational Neuroscience

Simen Tennøe [1,2], Geir Halnes [1,3] and Gaute T. Einevoll [1,3,4]*

[1] Centre for Integrative Neuroplasticity, University of Oslo, Oslo, Norway, [2] Department of Informatics, University of Oslo, Oslo, Norway, [3] Faculty of Science and Technology, Norwegian University of Life Sciences, Ås, Norway, [4] Department of Physics, University of Oslo, Oslo, Norway

***Correspondence:**
Gaute T. Einevoll
gaute.einevoll@nmbu.no*

Computational models in neuroscience typically contain many parameters that are poorly constrained by experimental data. Uncertainty quantification and sensitivity analysis provide rigorous procedures to quantify how the model output depends on this parameter uncertainty. Unfortunately, the application of such methods is not yet standard within the field of neuroscience. Here we present Uncertainpy, an open-source Python toolbox, tailored to perform uncertainty quantification and sensitivity analysis of neuroscience models. Uncertainpy aims to make it quick and easy to get started with uncertainty analysis, without any need for detailed prior knowledge. The toolbox allows uncertainty quantification and sensitivity analysis to be performed on already existing models without needing to modify the model equations or model implementation. Uncertainpy bases its analysis on polynomial chaos expansions, which are more efficient than the more standard Monte-Carlo based approaches. Uncertainpy is tailored for neuroscience applications by its built-in capability for calculating characteristic features in the model output. The toolbox does not merely perform a point-to-point comparison of the "raw" model output (e.g., membrane voltage traces), but can also calculate the uncertainty and sensitivity of salient model response features such as spike timing, action potential width, average interspike interval, and other features relevant for various neural and neural network models. Uncertainpy comes with several common models and features built in, and including custom models and new features is easy. The aim of the current paper is to present Uncertainpy to the neuroscience community in a user-oriented manner. To demonstrate its broad applicability, we perform an uncertainty quantification and sensitivity analysis of three case studies relevant for neuroscience: the original Hodgkin-Huxley point-neuron model for action potential generation, a multi-compartmental model of a thalamic interneuron implemented in the NEURON simulator, and a sparsely connected recurrent network model implemented in the NEST simulator.

Keywords: uncertainty quantification, sensitivity analysis, features, polynomial chaos expansions, quasi-Monte Carlo method, software, computational modeling, Python

SIGNIFICANCE STATEMENT

A major challenge in computational neuroscience is to specify the often large number of parameters that define neuron and neural network models. Many of these parameters have an inherent variability, and some are even actively regulated and change with time. It is important to know how the uncertainty in the model parameters affects the model predictions. To address this need we here present Uncertainpy, an open-source Python toolbox tailored to perform uncertainty quantification and sensitivity analysis of neuroscience models.

1. INTRODUCTION

Computational modeling has become a useful tool for examining various phenomena in biology in general (Brodland, 2015) and neuroscience in particular (Koch and Segev, 1998; Dayan and Abbott, 2001; Sterratt et al., 2011). The field of neuroscience has seen the development of ever more complex models, and models now exist for large networks of biophysically detailed neurons (Izhikevich and Edelman, 2008; Merolla et al., 2014; Markram et al., 2015).

Computational models typically contain a number of parameters that for various reasons are uncertain. A typical example of an uncertain parameter in a neural model can be the conductance g_x of a fully open ion channel of a specific type x. Despite the parameter uncertainty, it is common practice to construct models that are deterministic in the sense that single numerical values are assigned to each parameter.

Uncertainty quantification is a means to quantify the uncertainty in the model output that arises from uncertainty in the model parameters. Instead of assuming fixed model parameters as in a deterministic model (as illustrated in **Figure 1A**), one assigns a distribution of possible values to each model parameter. The uncertainty in the model parameters is then propagated through the model and gives rise to a distribution in the model output (as illustrated in **Figure 1B**).

Sensitivity analysis is tightly linked to uncertainty quantification and is the process of quantifying how much of the output uncertainty each parameter is responsible for Saltelli (2002b). A small change in a parameter the model is highly sensitive to, leads to a comparatively large change in the model output. Similarly, variations in a parameter the model has a low sensitivity to, result in comparatively small variations in the model output.

Given that most neuroscience models contain a variety of uncertain parameters, the need for systematic approaches to quantify what confidence we can have in the model output is pressing. The importance of uncertainty quantification and sensitivity analysis of computational models is well known in a wide variety of fields (Leamer, 1985; Beck, 1987; Turanyi and Turányi, 1990; Oberkampf et al., 2002; Sharp and Wood-Schultz, 2003; Marino et al., 2008; Najm, 2009; Rossa et al., 2011; Wang and Sheen, 2015; Yildirim and Karniadakis, 2015). Due to the prevalence of inherent variability in the parameters of biological systems, uncertainty quantification and sensitivity analysis are at least as important in neuroscience. Toward this end we have created Uncertainpy[1], a Python toolbox for uncertainty quantification and sensitivity analysis, tailored toward neuroscience models.

The uncertainty in a model parameter may have many origins. It may be due to (i) measurement uncertainty or (ii) lack of experimental techniques that enable the parameter to be measured. The uncertainty can also be due to an inherent biological variability, meaning the value of a parameter can vary (iii) between neurons of the same species (Edelman and Gally, 2001; Hay et al., 2013), or (iv) dynamically within a single neuron due to plasticity or homeostatic mechanisms (Marder and Goaillard, 2006). Additionally, some models include parameters that are (v) phenomenological abstractions, and therefore do not represent directly measurable physical entities. They might, for example, represent the combined effect of several physical processes. The above uncertainties can generally be divided into two main classes: aleatory uncertainties and epistemic uncertainties. Epistemic uncertainty reflects a lack of knowledge, and can in principle be reduced to zero by acquiring additional information. Aleatory uncertainty, on the other hand, is uncertainty due to inherent variability of the parameters. The importance of distinguishing between aleatory and epistemic uncertainties has evoked some debate (Ferson and Ginzburg, 1996; Hora, 1996; Oberkampf et al., 2002; Ferson et al., 2004; Kiureghian and Ditlevsen, 2009; Mullins et al., 2016), but the distinction is important for how to interpret the results of an uncertainty quantification. Parameters with epistemic uncertainties produce an uncertainty as to whether or not we have acquired the "correct" result, while parameters with aleatory uncertainties reflect the true variability of the system.

A common way to avoid addressing the uncertainty in measured parameters is to use the means of several experimental measurements. This can be problematic since the underlying distribution of a set of parameters can be poorly characterized by the mean and variance of each parameter (Golowasch et al., 2002). Additionally, during model construction, a subset of the uncertain parameters are commonly treated as *free parameters*. This means the parameters are tuned by the modeler to values that make the model output match a set of experimental constraints. An example is fitting an ion-channel conductance g_x so the membrane potential of a neuron model reproduces an experimentally measured voltage trace. Whatever method used, the tuning procedure does not guarantee a unique solution for the correct parameter set, since it is often the case that a wide range of different parameter combinations give rise to similar model behavior (Bhalla and Bower, 1993; Beer et al., 1999; Goldman et al., 2001; Golowasch et al., 2002; Prinz et al., 2004; Tobin, 2006; Halnes et al., 2007; Schulz et al., 2007; Taylor et al., 2009; Marder and Taylor, 2011).

When we have uncertain parameters, but nevertheless choose to use a single set of fixed parameter values, it is a priori difficult to assess to what degree we can trust the model result. Performing an uncertainty quantification enables us to properly take the effects of the uncertain parameters into account, and it quantifies what confidence we can have in the model output.

[1]https://github.com/simetenn/uncertainpy

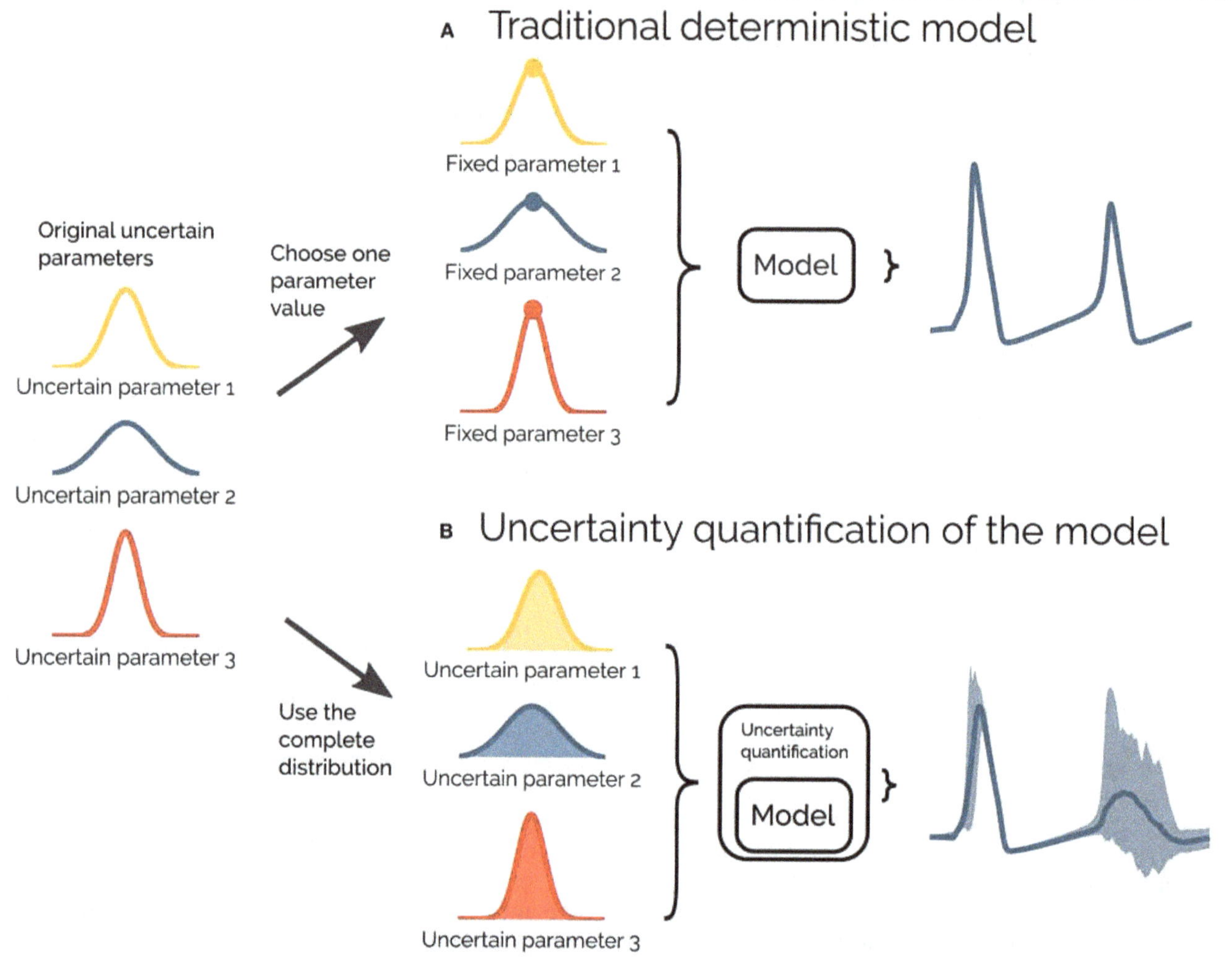

FIGURE 1 | Illustration of uncertainty quantification of a deterministic model. **(A)** A traditional deterministic model where each input parameter has a chosen fixed value, and we get a single output of the model (gray). **(B)** An uncertainty quantification of the model takes the distributions of the input parameters into account, and the output of the model becomes a range of possible values (light gray).

An uncertainty quantification enables us to model the naturally occurring variation in the parameters of biological systems. It also increases our understanding of the model by quantifying how the uncertain parameters influence the model output. Additionally, performing an uncertainty quantification makes comparing two model outputs, as well as a model output and an experimental result, more informative. By knowing the distribution of the model output we can better quantify how similar (or different) the two model outputs, or model output and experimental result, are.

Performing a sensitivity analysis provides insight into how each parameter affects different aspects of the model, and it gives us a better understanding of the relationship between the parameters (and by extent the biological mechanisms) and the output of the model (Marino et al., 2008). A model-based sensitivity analysis can thus help to guide the experimental focus (Zi, 2011). Knowing how sensitive the model is to changes in each parameter, enables us to take special care to obtain accurate measures of parameters with a high sensitivity, while more crude measures are acceptable for parameters with a low sensitivity.

Sensitivity analysis is also useful in model reduction contexts and when performing parameter estimations (Degenring et al., 2004; Zi, 2011; Snowden et al., 2017). A parameter that the model has a low sensitivity to, can essentially be set to any fixed value (within the explored distribution), without greatly affecting the variance of the model output. In some cases, such an analysis can even justify leaving out entire mechanisms from a model. For example, if a single neuron model is insensitive to the conductance of a given ion channel g_x, this ion channel could possibly (but not necessarily) be removed from the model with only small changes to the model behavior.

Unfortunately, a generally accepted practice of uncertainty quantification and sensitivity analysis does not currently exist within the field of neuroscience, and models are commonly presented without including any form of uncertainty quantification or sensitivity analysis. When an effort is made in that direction, it is still common to use rather simple, so-called One-At-A-Time methods, where one examines how much the model output changes when varying one parameter at a time (see e.g., De Schutter and Bower, 1994; Blot and Barbour, 2014; Kuchibhotla et al., 2017). Such approaches do not account for potential dependencies between the parameters, and thereby miss correlations within the often multi-dimensional parameter space (Borgonovo and Plischke, 2016). Other methods that have been applied are local methods, which are multi-dimensional, but confined to exploring small perturbations surrounding a single point in the parameter space (see e.g., Gutenkunst et al., 2007; Blomquist et al., 2009; O'Donnell et al., 2017). Such methods can thus not explore the effects of arbitrarily broad uncertainty distributions for the parameters.

Methods for uncertainty quantification and sensitivity analysis that take the entire parameter space into account are often called global methods (Borgonovo and Plischke, 2016; Babtie and Stumpf, 2017). Global methods are only occasionally used within the field of neuroscience (see e.g., Halnes et al., 2009; Torres Valderrama et al., 2015). The most well-known of the global methods is the (quasi-)Monte Carlo method, which relies on randomly sampling the parameter distributions, followed by calculating statistics from the resulting model outputs. The problem with the (quasi-)Monte Carlo method is that it is computationally very demanding, particularly for computationally expensive models. A means to obtain similar results in a much more efficient way, is provided by the recent mathematical framework of polynomial chaos expansions (Xiu and Hesthaven, 2005). Polynomial chaos expansions are used to approximate the model with a polynomial (as a surrogate model), on which the uncertainty and sensitivity analysis can be performed much more efficiently.

To lower the threshold for neuroscientists to perform uncertainty quantification and sensitivity analysis, we have created Uncertainpy, an open-source Python toolbox for efficient uncertainty quantification and sensitivity analysis. Uncertainpy aims to make it quick and easy to get started with uncertainty quantification and sensitivity analysis. Just a few lines of Python code are needed, without any need for detailed prior knowledge of uncertainty or sensitivity analysis. Uncertainpy implements both the quasi-Monte Carlo method and polynomial chaos expansions. The toolbox is model-independent and treats the model as a "black box," meaning that uncertainty quantification can be performed on already existing models without needing to modify the model equations or model implementation.

Whereas its statistical methods are generally applicable, Uncertainpy is tailored for neuroscience applications by having a built-in capability for recognizing characteristic features in the model output. This means Uncertainpy does not merely perform a point-to-point comparison of the "raw" model output (e.g., a voltage trace). When applicable, Uncertainpy also recognizes and calculates the uncertainty in model response features, for example the spike timing and action-potential shape for neural models and firing rates and interspike intervals for neural networks.

To present Uncertainpy, we start this paper with an overview of the theory behind uncertainty quantification and sensitivity analysis in section 2, with a focus on the (quasi-)Monte Carlo method and polynomial chaos expansions. In section 3 we explain how to use Uncertainpy, and give details on how the uncertainty quantification and sensitivity analysis are implemented. In section 4 we illustrate the use of Uncertainpy by showing four different case studies where we perform uncertainty analysis of: (i) a cooling coffee-cup model (Newton's law of cooling) to illustrate the uncertainty analysis on a conceptually simple model, (ii) the original Hodgkin-Huxley point-neuron model for action potential generation, (iii) a comprehensive multi-compartmental model of a thalamic interneuron, and (iv) a sparsely connected recurrent network model (Brunel network). The final section of section 4 gives a comparison of the performance, that is, numerical efficacy, of the quasi-Monte Carlo method and polynomial chaos expansions using the original Hodgkin-Huxley model as an example. We end with a discussion and some future prospects in section 5.

2. THEORY ON UNCERTAINTY QUANTIFICATION AND SENSITIVITY ANALYSIS

Uncertainty quantification and sensitivity analysis provide rigorous procedures to analyze and characterize the effects of parameter uncertainty on the output of a model. The methods for uncertainty quantification and sensitivity analysis can be divided into global and local methods. Local methods examine how the model output changes with small perturbations around a fixed point in the parameter space. Global methods, on the other hand, take the whole range of parameters into consideration.

The global methods can be divided into intrusive and non-intrusive methods. Intrusive methods require changes to the underlying model equations and are often challenging to implement. Models in neuroscience are often created with the use of advanced simulators such as NEST (Peyser et al., 2017) and NEURON (Hines and Carnevale, 1997). Modifying the underlying equations of models using such simulators is a complicated task best avoided. Non-intrusive methods, on the other hand, consider the model as a black box and can be applied to any model without needing to modify the model equations or model implementation. Global, non-intrusive methods are therefore the methods of choice in Uncertainpy. The uncertainty calculations in Uncertainpy are mainly based on the Python package *Chaospy* (Feinberg and Langtangen, 2015), which provides global, non-intrusive methods for uncertainty quantification and sensitivity analysis. Additionally, Uncertainpy uses the package *SALib* (Herman and Usher, 2017) to perform sensitivity analysis with the quasi-Monte Carlo method.

In this section, we go through the theory behind the methods for uncertainty quantification and sensitivity analysis used in Uncertainpy. We start by introducing the notation used in this paper (section 2.1). Next, we introduce the statistical measurements for uncertainty quantification (section 2.2) and sensitivity analysis (section 2.3). Further, we give an introduction to the (quasi-)Monte Carlo method (section 2.4) and polynomial chaos expansions (section 2.5), the two methods used to perform the uncertainty analysis in Uncertainpy. We next explain how Uncertainpy handles cases with statistically dependent model parameters (section 2.6). Finally, we explain the concept and benefits of performing a feature-based analysis (section 2.7). We note that detailed insight into the theory of uncertainty quantification and sensitivity analysis is not a prerequisite for *using* Uncertainpy, so the more practically oriented reader may choose to skip this section, and go directly to the user guide in section 3.

2.1. Problem Definition

Consider a model U that depends on space $\boldsymbol{x}$ and time t, has d uncertain input parameters $\mathbf{Q} = [Q_1, Q_2, \ldots, Q_d]$, and gives the output Y:

$$Y = U(\boldsymbol{x}, t, \mathbf{Q}). \tag{1}$$

The output Y can have any value within the output space Ω_Y and has an unknown probability density function ρ_Y. The goal of an uncertainty quantification is to describe the unknown ρ_Y through statistical metrics. We are only interested in the input and output of the model, and we ignore all details on the inner workings of the model. The model U is thus considered a black box and may represent any model, for example a spiking neuron model that returns a voltage trace, or a neural network model that returns a spike train.

We assume the model includes uncertain parameters that can be described by a multivariate probability density function $\rho_{\mathbf{Q}}$. Examples of parameters that can be uncertain in neuroscience are the conductance of a single ion channel or the synaptic weight between two types of neurons in a neural network. If the uncertain parameters are statistically independent, the multivariate probability density function $\rho_{\mathbf{Q}}$ can be given as separate univariate probability density functions ρ_{Q_i}, one for each uncertain parameter Q_i. The joint multivariate probability density function for the independent uncertain parameters is then:

$$\rho_{\mathbf{Q}} = \prod_{i=1}^{d} \rho_{Q_i}. \tag{2}$$

In cases where the uncertain input parameters are statistically dependent variables, the multivariate probability density function $\rho_{\mathbf{Q}}$ must be defined directly. It should be noted that with statistically dependent parameters we here mean that there is a dependence between the input parameters. When drawing parameters from the joint probability function, by drawing one parameter we influence the probability of drawing specific values for the other parameters. Thus, we do not refer to dependencies between how the input parameters affect the model *output*. We assume the probability density functions are known and are not here concerned with how they are determined. They may be the product of a series of measurements, a parameter estimation, or educated guesses.

2.2. Uncertainty Quantification

As mentioned, the goal of an uncertainty quantification is to describe the unknown distribution of the model output ρ_Y through statistical metrics. The two most common statistical metrics used in this context are the mean $\mathbb{E}$ (also called the expectation value) and the variance $\mathbb{V}$. The mean is defined as:

$$\mathbb{E}[Y] = \int_{\Omega_Y} y\rho_Y(y)dy, \tag{3}$$

and tells us the expected value of the model output Y. The variance is defined as:

$$\mathbb{V}[Y] = \int_{\Omega_Y} \left(y - \mathbb{E}[Y]\right)^2 \rho_Y(y)dy, \tag{4}$$

and tells us how much the output varies around the mean.

Another useful metric is the $(100 \cdot x)$-th percentile P_x of Y, which defines a value below which $100 \cdot x$ percent of the model outputs are located. For example, 5% of the evaluations of a model will give an output lower than the 5th percentile. The $(100 \cdot x)$-th percentile is defined as:

$$x = \int_{-\infty}^{P_x} \rho_Y(y)dy. \tag{5}$$

We can combine two percentiles to create a prediction interval I_x, which is a range of values within which a $100 \cdot x$ percentage of the outputs Y occur:

$$I_x = \left[P_{(x/2)}, P_{(1-x/2)}\right]. \tag{6}$$

The 90% prediction interval gives us the interval within which 90% of the Y outcomes occur, which also means that 5% of the outcomes are above and 5% are below this interval.

2.3. Sensitivity Analysis

A sensitivity analysis quantifies how much of the uncertainty in the model output each uncertain parameter is responsible for. Several different sensitivity measures exist, for a review of methods for sensitivity analysis see Saltelli et al. (2007), Hamby (1994), and Zi (2011). Uncertainpy uses variance-based sensitivity analysis and computes the commonly considered Sobol sensitivity indices (Sobol, 1990). This sensitivity analysis is global, non-intrusive and allows the effects of interactions between parameters within the model to be studied (Zi, 2011). (Two parameters are said to interact if they have a non-additive effect on the output (Saltelli et al., 2007).)

The Sobol sensitivity indices quantify how much of the variance in the model output each uncertain parameter is responsible for. If a parameter has a low sensitivity index, variations in this parameter result in comparatively small variations in the final model output. Similarly, if a parameter has a high sensitivity index, a change in this parameter leads to a large change in the model output.

There are several types of Sobol indices. The first-order Sobol sensitivity index S_i measures the direct effect each parameter has on the variance of the model:

$$S_i = \frac{\mathbb{V}[\mathbb{E}[Y|Q_i]]}{\mathbb{V}[Y]}. \tag{7}$$

Here, $\mathbb{E}[Y|Q_i]$ denotes the expected value of the output Y when the parameter Q_i is fixed. The first-order Sobol sensitivity index tells us the expected reduction in the variance of the model when we fix parameter Q_i. The sum of the first-order Sobol sensitivity indices cannot exceed one, and is only equal to one if no interactions are present (Glen and Isaacs, 2012).

Higher order Sobol indices exist and give the sensitivity due to interactions between a parameter Q_i and various other parameters. It is customary to only calculate the first and total-order indices (Saltelli et al., 2010). The total Sobol sensitivity index S_{Ti} includes the sensitivity of both the first-order effects, as well as the sensitivity due to interactions between a given parameter Q_i and all combinations of the other parameters (Homma and Saltelli, 1996). It is defined as:

$$S_{Ti} = 1 - \frac{\mathbb{V}[\mathbb{E}[Y|Q_{-i}]]}{\mathbb{V}[Y]}, \tag{8}$$

where Q_{-i} denotes all uncertain parameters except Q_i. The sum of the total Sobol sensitivity indices is equal to or greater than one, and is only equal to one if there are no interactions between the parameters (Glen and Isaacs, 2012). When the goal is to use sensitivity analysis to fix parameters with low sensitivity, it is recommended to use the total-order Sobol indices.

We might want to compare Sobol indices across different features (introduced in section 2.7). This can be problematic when we have features with a different number of output dimensions. In the case of a zero-dimensional output, the Sobol indices are a single number and for a one-dimensional output we get Sobol indices for each point in time. To better be able to compare the Sobol indices across such features, we also calculate the average of the first-order Sobol indices $\overline{S}_i$, and total-order Sobol indices $\overline{S}_{Ti}$.

2.4. (Quasi-)Monte Carlo Method

A typical way to obtain the statistical metrics mentioned above is to use the (quasi-)Monte Carlo method. We give a brief overview of the Monte Carlo and quasi-Monte Carlo method here, for a more comprehensive review see Lemieux (2009).

The general idea behind the standard Monte Carlo method is quite simple. A set of parameters is randomly drawn from the joint multivariate probability density function ρ_Q of the parameters. The model is then evaluated for the sampled parameter set. This process is repeated thousands of times, and statistical metrics such as the mean and variance are computed from the resulting series of model outputs. The accuracy of the Monte Carlo method, and by extent the number of samples required, is independent of the number of uncertain parameters. Additionally, the Monte Carlo method makes no assumptions about the model. However, a limitation of the Monte Carlo method is that a very high number of model evaluations are required to get reliable statistics. If the model is computationally expensive, the Monte Carlo method may thus require insurmountable computer power.

The quasi-Monte Carlo method improves upon the standard Monte Carlo method by using variance-reduction techniques to reduce the number of model evaluations needed. This method is based on increasing the coverage of the sampled parameter space by distributing the samples more evenly. Fewer samples are then required to obtain a given accuracy. Instead of randomly selecting parameters from ρ_Q, the samples are selected using a low-discrepancy sequence such as the Sobol sequence or Hammersley sequence (Hammersley, 1960; Sobol, 1967). The quasi-Monte Carlo method is faster than the Monte Carlo method, as long as the number of uncertain parameters is sufficiently small, and the model is sufficiently smooth (Lemieux, 2009).

Uncertainpy allows the quasi-Monte Carlo method to be used to compute the statistical metrics. When this option is chosen, the metrics are computed as follows. With N_s model evaluations, which gives the results $\boldsymbol{Y} = [Y_1, Y_2, \ldots, Y_{N_s}]$, the mean is given by

$$\mathbb{E}[Y] \approx \frac{1}{N_s}\sum_{i=1}^{N_s} Y_i, \tag{9}$$

and the variance by

$$\mathbb{V}[Y] \approx \frac{1}{N_s - 1}\sum_{i=1}^{N_s}(Y_i - \mathbb{E}[Y])^2. \tag{10}$$

Prediction intervals are found by sorting the model evaluations $\boldsymbol{Y}$ in an ascending order, and then finding the $(100 \cdot x/2)$-th and $(100 \cdot (1 - x/2))$-th percentiles. The Sobol indices can be calculated using Saltelli's method (Saltelli, 2002a; Saltelli et al., 2010). The number of samples required by this method is:

$$N_s = N(d + 2), \tag{11}$$

where N is the number of samples required to get a given accuracy with the quasi-Monte Carlo method. This means that the number of samples required by both the Monte Carlo method and the quasi-Monte Carlo method for sensitivity analysis depends on the number of uncertain parameters. Due to how the samples are selected in Saltelli's method, when selecting N samples for the uncertainty quantification (which give $N_s = N$), we get $N_s = N(d + 2)/2$ samples for the sensitivity analysis. The chosen number of samples N is effectively halved.

It should be noted that there is no guarantee that each set of sampled parameters will produce a valid model evaluation. For example, the spike width will not be defined for a model that produces no spikes. The (quasi-)Monte Carlo method is robust for such missing model results when performing an uncertainty quantification, as long as the number of valid model evaluations is relatively high. However, for the sensitivity analysis the (quasi-) Monte Carlo method using Saltelli's approach requires that there are no missing model results. A suggested workaround (Herman and Usher, 2017) is to replace invalid model evaluations with the mean of the evaluations[2]. This workaround introduces an error depending on the number of missing evaluations but enables us to still calculate the Sobol indices. This workaround is used in Uncertainpy.

[2]https://github.com/SALib/SALib/issues/134

2.5. Polynomial Chaos Expansions

A recent mathematical framework for efficient uncertainty quantification and sensitivity analysis is that of polynomial chaos expansions (Xiu and Hesthaven, 2005). This method calculates the same statistical metrics as the (quasi-)Monte Carlo method but is typically much faster (Xiu and Hesthaven, 2005; Crestaux et al., 2009; Eck et al., 2016). For the Hodgkin-Huxley model, we find that polynomial chaos expansions require one to three orders of magnitude fewer model evaluations than the quasi-Monte Carlo method (see section 4.5). We here give a short review of polynomial chaos expansions, for a comprehensive review see Xiu (2010).

Polynomial chaos expansions are typically much faster than the (quasi-)Monte Carlo method as long as the number of uncertain parameters is relatively low, typically smaller than about 20 (Xiu and Hesthaven, 2005; Crestaux et al., 2009; Eck et al., 2016). This means polynomial chaos expansions require far fewer model evaluations than the (quasi-)Monte Carlo method to obtain the same accuracy. It is often the case that neuroscience models have fewer than about 20 parameters, and even for models with a higher number of uncertain parameters, polynomial chaos expansions can be used for selected subsets of the parameters.

The main limitation of polynomial chaos expansions is that the required number of model evaluations scales worse with an increasing number of uncertain parameters than the (quasi-)Monte Carlo method does. This is the reason why the (quasi-)Monte Carlo method becomes better at around 20 uncertain parameters. Another limitation of the polynomial chaos expansions is that the performance is reduced if the output has a non-smooth behavior with respect to the input parameters (Eck et al., 2016).

The exact gain in efficiency when using polynomial chaos expansions instead of the quasi-Monte Carlo method is problem dependent. However, Crestaux et al. (2009) examined three different benchmark problems with three, twelve, and five uncertain parameters. They found that the error in the polynomial chaos expansions converged as N_s^{-6}, N_s^{-2}, and between N_s^{-1} and $N_s^{-3/4}$, respectively. In comparison, the error of the quasi-Monte Carlo method converged as $\sim N_s^{-3/4}$ for each of the problems. Polynomial chaos expansions thus have a much faster convergence for the first two benchmark problems, while the convergences were essentially the same for the last problem. The last benchmark problem was non-smooth, which led to the slower convergence of the polynomial chaos expansions. Still, even in the worst-case example considered in Crestaux et al. (2009), the convergence of the polynomial chaos expansions was essentially as good as for the quasi-Monte Carlo method.

The general idea behind polynomial chaos expansions is to approximate the model U with a polynomial expansion $\hat{U}$:

$$U \approx \hat{U}(\boldsymbol{x}, t, \mathbf{Q}) = \sum_{n=0}^{N_p-1} c_n(\boldsymbol{x}, t)\boldsymbol{\phi}_n(\mathbf{Q}), \tag{12}$$

where $\boldsymbol{\phi}_n$ are polynomials, and c_n are expansion coefficients. The number of expansion factors N_p is given by

$$N_p = \binom{d+p}{p}, \tag{13}$$

where p is the polynomial order. The polynomials $\phi_n(\mathbf{Q})$ are chosen so they are orthogonal with respect to the probability density function $\rho_{\mathbf{Q}}$, which ensures useful statistical properties.

When creating the polynomial chaos expansion, the first step is to find the orthogonal polynomials $\boldsymbol{\phi}_n$. In Uncertainpy this is done using the so-called three-term recurrence relation (Xiu, 2010) if available, otherwise the discretized Stieltjes method (Stieltjes, 1884) is used. The next step is to estimate the expansion coefficients c_n. The non-intrusive methods for doing this can be divided into two classes, point-collocation methods and pseudo-spectral projection methods, both of which are implemented in Uncertainpy.

Point collocation is the default method used in Uncertainpy. This method is based on demanding that the polynomial approximation is equal to the model output evaluated at a set of collocation nodes drawn from the joint probability density function $\rho_{\mathbf{Q}}$. This demand results in a set of linear equations for the polynomial coefficients c_n, which can be solved by the use of regression methods. The regression method used in Uncertainpy is Tikhonov regularization (Rifkin and Lippert, 2007). Hosder et al. (2007) recommends using $N_s = 2(N_p + 1)$ collocation nodes.

Pseudo-spectral projection methods are based on least squares minimization in the orthogonal polynomial space and calculate the expansion coefficients c_n through numerical integration. The integration uses a quadrature scheme with weights and nodes, and the model is evaluated at these nodes. The number of samples is determined by the quadrature rule. The quadrature method used in Uncertainpy is Leja quadrature, with Smolyak sparse grids to reduce the number of required nodes (Smolyak, 1963; Narayan and Jakeman, 2014). Pseudo-spectral projection is only used in Uncertainpy when requested by the user.

Of these two methods, point collocation is robust toward invalid model evaluations as long as the number of remaining evaluations is high enough, while spectral projection is not (Eck et al., 2016).

Several of the statistical metrics of interest can be obtained directly from the polynomial chaos expansion $\hat{U}$. The mean is simply

$$\mathbb{E}[Y] \approx c_0, \tag{14}$$

and the variance is

$$\mathbb{V}[Y] \approx \sum_{n=1}^{N_p-1} \gamma_n c_n^2, \tag{15}$$

where γ_n is a normalization factor defined as

$$\gamma_n = \mathbb{E}\left[\boldsymbol{\phi}_n^2(\mathbf{Q})\right]. \tag{16}$$

The first and total-order Sobol indices can also be calculated directly from the polynomial chaos expansion (Sudret, 2008; Crestaux et al., 2009). On the other hand, the percentiles (Equation 5), and thereby the prediction interval (Equation 6), must be estimated by using $\hat{U}$ as a surrogate model and then performing the same procedure as for the (quasi-)Monte Carlo method.

2.6. Dependency Between Uncertain Parameters

One of the underlying assumptions when creating the polynomial chaos expansions is that the model parameters are independent. However, dependent parameters in neuroscience models are quite common (Achard and De Schutter, 2006). Fortunately, models containing dependent parameters can be analyzed with Uncertainpy by the aid of the Rosenblatt transformation from Chaospy (Rosenblatt, 1952; Feinberg and Langtangen, 2015). Briefly explained, the idea is to create a reformulated model $\widetilde{U}(\boldsymbol{x}, t, \boldsymbol{R})$ based on an independent parameter set $\boldsymbol{R}$, and then perform polynomial chaos expansions on the reformulated model. The Rosenblatt transformation is used to construct the reformulated model so it gives the same output (and statistics) as the original model, i.e.,:

$$\widetilde{U}(\boldsymbol{x}, t, \boldsymbol{R}) = U(\boldsymbol{x}, t, \boldsymbol{Q}). \tag{17}$$

For more information on the use of the Rosenblatt transformation, see the Uncertainpy documentation[3] or Feinberg and Langtangen (2015).

2.7. Feature-Based Analysis

When measuring the membrane potential of a neuron, the precise timing of action potentials often varies between recordings, even if the experimental conditions are the same. This behavior is typical for biological systems. Since the experimental data displays such variation, it is often meaningless and misleading to base the success of a computational model on a direct point-to-point comparison between a particular experimental recording and model output (Druckmann et al., 2007; Van Geit et al., 2008). A common modeling practice is therefore to have the model reproduce essential features of the experimentally observed dynamics, such as the action-potential shape or action-potential firing rate (Druckmann et al., 2007). Such features are typically more robust across different experimental measurements, or across different model simulations, than the raw data or raw model output itself, at least if sensible features have been chosen.

Uncertainpy takes this aspect of neural modeling into account and is constructed so that it can extract a set of features relevant for various common model types in neuroscience from the raw model output. Examples include the action potential shape in single neuron models and the average interspike interval in neural network models. Thus Uncertainpy performs an uncertainty quantification and sensitivity analysis not only on the raw model output but also on a set of relevant features selected by the user. Lists of the implemented features are given in section 3.4, and the value of a feature-based analysis is illustrated in two of the case studies (sections 5.3 and 5.4).

3. USER GUIDE FOR UNCERTAINPY

Uncertainpy is a Python toolbox, tailored to make uncertainty quantification and sensitivity analysis easily accessible to the computational neuroscience community. The toolbox is based on Python, since Python is a high level, open-source language in extensive and increasing use within the scientific community (Oliphant, 2007; Einevoll, 2009; Muller et al., 2015). Uncertainpy works with both Python 2 and 3, and utilizes the Python packages Chaospy (Feinberg and Langtangen, 2015) and SALib (Herman and Usher, 2017) to perform the uncertainty calculations. In this section, we present a guide on to how to use Uncertainpy. We do not present an exhaustive overview, and only show the most commonly used classes, methods and method arguments. We refer to the online documentation[4] for the most recent, complete documentation. A complete case study with code is shown in section 4.1.

Uncertainpy is easily installed by following the instructions in section 3.8. After installation, we get access to Uncertainpy by simply importing it:

```
import uncertainpy as un
```

Performing an uncertainty quantification and sensitivity analysis with Uncertainpy includes three main components:

1. The **model** we want to examine.
2. The **parameters** of the model.
3. Specifications of **features** in the model output.

The model and parameters are required components, while the feature specifications are optional. The three (or two) components are brought together in the `UncertaintyQuantification` class. This class performs the uncertainty calculations and is the main class the user interacts with. In this section, we explain how to use `UncertaintyQuantification` with the above components, and introduce a few additional utility classes.

3.1. The Uncertainty Quantification Class

The `UncertaintyQuantification` class is used to define the problem, perform the uncertainty quantification and sensitivity analysis, and save and visualize the results. Among others, `UncertaintyQuantification` takes the arguments:

```
UQ = un.UncertaintyQuantification(
    # Required
    model=...,
    parameters=...,
    # Optional
    features=...
)
```

[3]http://uncertainpy.readthedocs.io/

[4]http://uncertainpy.readthedocs.io/

The `model` argument is either a `Model` instance (section 3.2) or a model function (section 3.2.2). The `parameters` argument is either a `Parameters` instance or a parameter dictionary (section 3.3). Lastly, the `features` argument is either a `Features` instance (section 3.4) or a list of feature functions (section 3.4.1). In general, using the class instances as arguments give more options, while using the corresponding functions are slightly easier. We go through how to use each of these classes and corresponding functions in the next three sections.

After the problem is set up, an uncertainty quantification and sensitivity analysis can be performed by using the `UncertaintyQuantification.quantify` method. Among others, `quantify` takes the optional arguments:

```
data = UQ.quantify(
     method="pc"|"mc",
     pc_method="collocation"|"spectral",
     single=False
)
```

The `method` argument allows the user to choose whether Uncertainpy should use polynomial chaos expansions (`"pc"`) or the quasi-Monte Carlo method (`"mc"`) to calculate the relevant statistical metrics. If polynomial chaos expansions are chosen, `pc_method` further specifies whether point collocation (`"collocation"`) or spectral projection (`"spectral"`) methods are used to calculate the expansion coefficients. `single` specifies whether we perform the uncertainty quantification for a single parameter at the time, or consider all uncertain parameters at once. Performing the uncertainty quantification for one parameter at the time is a simple form of screening. The idea of such a screening is to use a computationally cheap method to reduce the number of uncertain parameters by setting the parameters that have the least effect on the model output to fixed values. We can then consider only the parameters with the greatest effect on the model output when performing the "full" uncertainty quantification and sensitivity analysis. This screening can be performed using both polynomial chaos expansions and the quasi-Monte Carlo method, but polynomial chaos expansions are almost always the faster choice. If nothing is specified, Uncertainpy by default uses polynomial chaos expansions based on point collocation with all uncertain parameters. The Rosenblatt transformation is automatically used if the input parameters are dependent.

The results from the uncertainty quantification are returned in `data`, as a `Data` object (see section 3.6). By default, the results are also automatically saved in a folder named `data`, and the figures are automatically plotted and saved in a folder named `figures`, both in the current directory. The returned `Data` object is therefore not necessarily needed.

As mentioned earlier, there is no guarantee that each set of sampled parameters produces a valid model or feature output. In such cases, Uncertainpy gives a warning which includes the number of runs that failed to return a valid output and performs the uncertainty quantification and sensitivity analysis using the reduced set of valid runs. However, if a large fraction of the simulations fail, the user could consider redefining the problem (e.g., by using narrower parameter distributions).

Polynomial chaos expansions are recommended as long as the number of uncertain parameters is small (typically < 20), as polynomial chaos expansions in these cases are much faster than the quasi-Monte Carlo method. Which of the polynomial chaos expansion methods to preferably use is problem dependent. In general, the pseudo-spectral method is faster than point collocation, but has a lower stability. We therefore recommend to use the point-collocation method.

The accuracy of the quasi-Monte Carlo method and polynomial chaos expansions is problem dependent and is determined by the chosen number of samples N, as well as the polynomial order p for polynomial chaos expansions. It is therefore a good practice to examine if the results from the uncertainty quantification and sensitivity analysis have converged (Eck et al., 2016). A simple method for doing this is to increase or decrease the number of samples or polynomial order, or both, and examine the difference between the current and previous results. If the differences are small enough, we can be reasonably certain that we have an accurate result.

3.2. Models

In order to perform the uncertainty quantification and sensitivity analysis of a model, Uncertainpy needs to set the parameters of the model, run the model using those parameters, and receive the model output. Uncertainpy has built-in support for NEURON and NEST models, found in the `NeuronModel` (section 3.2.4) and `NestModel` (section 3.2.5) classes respectively. It should be noted that while Uncertainpy is tailored toward neuroscience, it is not restricted to neuroscience models. Uncertainpy can be used on any model that meets the criteria in this section. Below, we first explain how to create custom models, before we explain how to use `NeuronModel` and `NestModel`.

3.2.1. The Model Class

Generally, models are created through the `Model` class. Among others, `Model` takes the argument `run` and the optional arguments `interpolate`, `labels`, `postprocess` and `ignore`.

```
model = un.Model(
     run=example_model,
     interpolate=True,
     labels=["xlabel", "ylabel"],
     postprocess=example_postprocess,
     ignore=False
)
```

The `run` argument must be a Python function that runs a simulation on a specific model for a given set of model parameters and returns the simulation output. In this paper we call such a function a model function. If we set `interpolate=True`, Uncertainpy automatically interpolates the model output to a regular form, meaning each model evaluation has the same number of measurement points (most commonly time points). An irregular model, on the other hand, has a varying number of measurement points between different evaluations (the output is on an irregular form), a typical example is a model that uses adaptive time steps. The uncertainty quantification requires the model output to be on a regular form, and we must set `interpolate=True` for irregular models. `labels` allows the user to specify a list of labels to be used on the axes when plotting the results. The `postprocess` argument is a Python function used to post-process the model output if required. We will go into details on the requirements of the `postprocess` and model functions below. Finally, if `ignore=True` we do not perform an uncertainty quantification of the model output. This is used if we want to examine features of the model, but are not interested in the model result itself.

3.2.2. Defining a Model Function

As explained above, the `run` argument is a Python function that runs a simulation of a specific model for a given set of model parameters, and returns the simulation output. An example outline of a model function is:

```
def example_model(parameter_1,
                  parameter_2):
    # An algorithm for the model,
    # or a script that runs an
    # external model, using the
    # given input parameters.

    # Returns the model output and
    # model time along with the
    # optional info object.
    return time, values, info
```

Such a model function has the following requirements:

1. **Input.** The model function takes a number of arguments which define the uncertain parameters of the model.
2. **Run the model.** The model must then be run using the parameters given as arguments.
3. **Output.** The model function must return at least two objects, the model time (or equivalent, if applicable) and model output. Additionally, any number of optional info objects can be returned. In Uncertainpy, we refer to the time object as `time`, the model output object as `values`, and the remaining objects as `info`.
   (a) **Time** (`time`). `time` can be interpreted as the x-axis of the model. It is used when interpolating (see below), and when certain features are calculated. We can return `None` if the model has no time associated with it.
   (b) **Model output** (`values`). The model output must either be regular (each model evaluation has the same number of measurement points), or it must be possible to interpolate or post-process the output (see section 3.2.3) to a regular form.
   (c) **Additional info** (`info`). Some of the methods provided by Uncertainpy, such as the later defined model post-processing, feature pre-processing, and feature calculations, require additional information from the model (e.g., the time when a neuron receives an external stimulus). This information can be passed on as any number of additional `info` objects returned after `time` and `values`. We recommend using a single dictionary as info object, with key-value pairs for the information, to make debugging easier. Uncertainpy always uses a single dictionary as the `info` object. Certain features require specific keys to be present in this dictionary.

The model itself does not need to be implemented in Python. Any simulator can be used, as long as we can set the model parameters and retrieve the simulation output via Python. As a shortcut, we can pass a model function to the `model` argument in `UncertaintyQuantification`, instead of first having to create a `Model` instance.

3.2.3. Defining a Post-process Function

The `postprocess` function is used to post-process the model output before it is used in the uncertainty quantification. Post-processing does not change the model output sent to the feature calculations. This is useful if we need to transform the model output to a regular form for the uncertainty quantification, but still need to preserve the original model output to reliably detect the model features. **Figure 2** illustrates how the objects returned by the model function are sent to both model `postprocess` and feature `preprocess` (see section 3.4).

An example outline of the `postprocess` function is:

```
def example_postprocess(time, values,
    info):
    # Post-process the result to a
    # regular form using time, values,
    # and info returned by the model
    # function.

    # Return the post-processed
    # model output and time.
    return time_postprocessed,
       values_postprocessed
```

The only time post-processing is required for Uncertainpy to work is when the model produces output that cannot be interpolated to a regular form by Uncertainpy. Post-processing is for example required for network models that give output in the form of spike trains, i.e., time values indicating when a given neuron fires. It should be noted that post-processing of spike trains is already implemented in Uncertainpy (see section 3.2.5). For most purposes, user-defined post-processing will not be necessary.

The requirements for the `postprocess` function are:

1. **Input.** The `postprocess` function must take the objects returned by the model function as input arguments.
2. **Post-processing.** The model time (`time`) and output (`values`) must be post-processed to a regular form, or to a form that can be interpolated to a regular form by Uncertainpy. If additional information is needed from the model, it can be passed along in the `info` object.
3. **Output.** The `postprocess` function must return two objects:

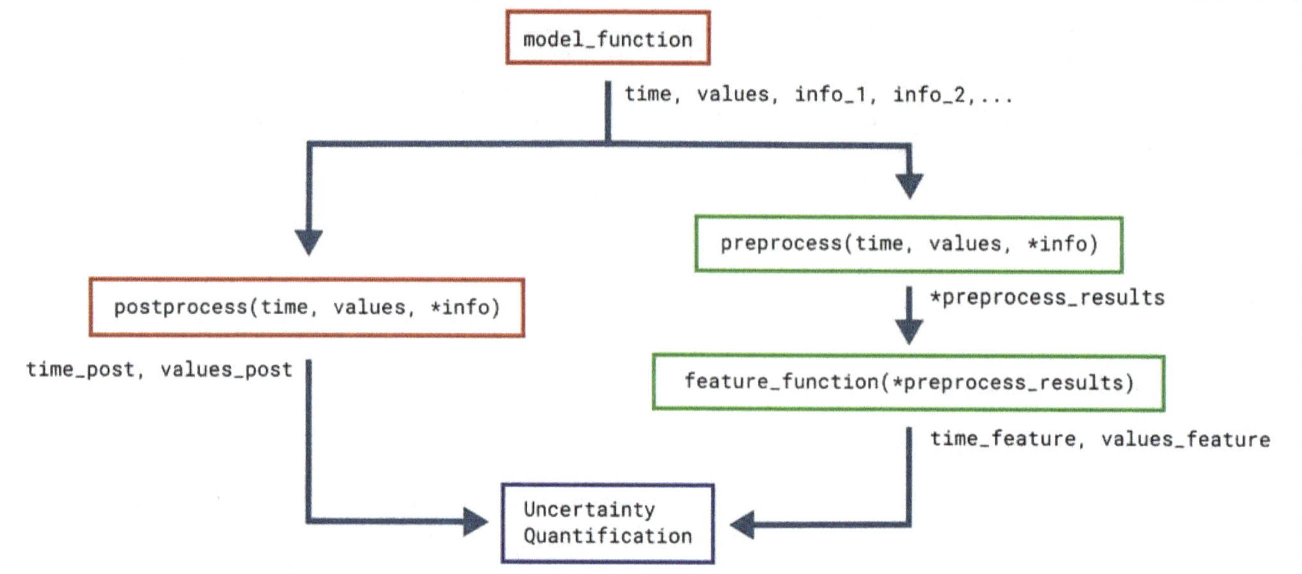

FIGURE 2 | Classes that affect the objects returned by the model. The Uncertainpy methods that use, change, and perform calculations on the objects returned by the model function (`time`, `values`, and the optional `info`). Functions associated with the model are in red while functions associated with features are in green.

(a) **Model time** (`time_postprocessed`). The first object is the post-processed time (or equivalent) of the model. We can return `None` if the model has no time. Note that the automatic interpolation can only be performed if a post-processed time is returned (if an interpolation is required).
(b) **Model output** (`values_postprocessed`). The second object is the post-processed model output.

3.2.4. NEURON Model Class

NEURON (Hines and Carnevale, 1997) is a widely used simulator for multi-compartmental neural models. Uncertainpy has support for NEURON models through the `NeuronModel` class, a subclass of `Model`. Among others, `NeuronModel` takes the arguments:

```
model = un.NeuronModel(
    file="mosinit.hoc",
    path="path/to/neuron_model",
    interpolate=True,
    stimulus_start=1000,              # ms
    stimulus_end=1900                 # ms
)
```

The `file` argument is the name of the hoc file that loads the NEURON model, which by default is `mosinit.hoc`. `path` is the path to the folder where the NEURON model is saved (the location of the `mosinit.hoc` file). `interpolate` indicates whether the NEURON model uses adaptive time steps and therefore should be interpolated. `stimulus_start` and `stimulus_end` denote the start and end time of any stimulus given to the neuron. `NeuronModel` loads the NEURON model from `file`, sets the parameters of the model, evaluates the model and returns the somatic membrane potential of the neuron (we record the voltage from the segment named `"soma"`). `NeuronModel` therefore does not require a model function to be defined. A case study of a NEURON model analyzed with Uncertainpy is found in section 4.3.

If changes are needed to the standard `NeuronModel`, such as measuring the voltage from other locations than the soma, the `Model` class with an appropriate model function could be used instead. Alternatively, `NeuronModel` can be subclassed and the existing methods customized as required. An example of the latter is shown in `uncertainpy/examples/bahl/`.

3.2.5. NEST Model Class

NEST (Peyser et al., 2017) is a simulator for large networks of spiking neurons. NEST models are supported through the `NestModel` class, another subclass of `Model`:

```
model = un.NestModel(
    run=nest_model_function,
    ignore=False
)
```

Unlike `NeuronModel`, `NestModel` requires the model function to be specified through the `run` argument. The NEST model function has the same requirements as a regular model function, except it is restricted to return only two objects: the final simulation time (denoted `simulation_end`), and a list of spike times for selected neurons in the network, which we refer to as spike trains (denoted `spiketrains`).

A spike train returned by a NEST model is a set of irregularly spaced time points where a neuron fired a spike. NEST models therefore require post-processing to make the model output regular. Such a post-processing is provided by the implemented `NestModel.postprocess` method, which converts a spike train to a list of zeros (no spike) and ones (a spike) for each time step in the simulation. For example: If a NEST simulation returns the spike train `[0, 2, 3.5]`, it means the neuron fired three spikes occurring at $t = 0, 2,$ and 3.5 ms, respectively. If the simulation has a time resolution of 0.5 ms and ends after 4 ms, `NestModel.postprocess` will return the post-processed spike train `[1, 0, 0, 0, 1, 0, 0, 1, 0]`, and the post-processed time array `[0, 0.5, 1, 1.5, 2, 2.5, 3, 3.5, 4]`. The final uncertainty quantification of a NEST network therefore predicts the probability for a spike to occur at any specific time point in the simulation. It should be noted that performing an uncertainty quantification of the post-processed NEST model output is computationally expensive. As such we recommend setting `ignore=True` as long as you are not interested in the uncertainty of the spike trains from the network. An Uncertainpy-based analysis of a NEST model is found in the case study in section 4.4.

3.3. Parameters of the Model

The parameters of a model are defined by two properties: They must have (i) a name and (ii) either a fixed value or a distribution. It is important that the name of a parameter is the same as the name given as the input argument in the model function. A parameter is considered uncertain if it is given a probability distribution, which are defined using Chaospy. 64 different univariate distributions are available in Chaospy, and Chaospy has support for easy creation of multivariate distributions. For a list of available distributions and detailed instructions on how to create probability distributions with Chaospy, see section 3.3 in Feinberg and Langtangen (2015).

The parameters are defined by the `Parameters` class. `Parameters` takes the argument `parameters`, which is a dictionary where the names of the parameters are the keys, and the fixed values or distributions of the parameters are the values. Here is an example of such a parameter dictionary with two parameters, where the first is named `name_1` and has a uniform probability distribution in the interval [8, 16], and the second is named `name_2` and has a fixed value of 42:

```
import chaospy as cp

parameters = {
    "name_1": cp.Uniform(8, 16),
    "name_2": 42
}
```

`Parameters` is now initialized as:

```
parameters = un.Parameters(parameters=
    parameters)
```

As a shortcut, we can pass the above parameter dictionary to the `parameters` argument in `UncertaintyQuantification`, instead of first having to create a `Parameters` instance.

If the parameters do not have separate univariate probability distributions, but a joint multivariate probability distribution, the multivariate distribution can be set by giving `Parameters` the optional argument `distribution`:

```
# Create the multivariate distribution
multivariate = cp.J(cp.Uniform(8, 16),
                    cp.Uniform(40, 44))

parameters = un.Parameters(
    parameters=parameters,
    distribution=multivariate
)
```

3.4. Features

As discussed in section 2.7, it is often more meaningful to examine the uncertainty in salient features of the model output, than to base the analysis directly on a point-to-point comparison of the raw output data (e.g., a voltage trace). Upon user request, Uncertainpy can identify and extract features of the model output. If we give the `features` argument to `UncertaintyQuantification`, Uncertainpy will perform uncertainty quantification and sensitivity analysis of the given features, in addition to the analysis of the raw output data (if desired).

Three sets of features come predefined with Uncertainpy, `SpikingFeatures`, `EfelFeatures`, and `NetworkFeatures`. Each feature class contains a set of features tailored toward one specific type of neuroscience models. We first explain how to create custom features, before explaining how to use the built-in features.

Features are defined through the `Features` class:

```
feature_functions = [example_feature]

features = un.Features(
    new_features=feature_functions,
    features_to_run=["example_feature"],
    preprocess=example_preprocess,
    interpolate=["example_feature"]
)
```

The `new_features` argument is a list of Python functions that each calculates a specific feature, whereas `features_to_run` specifies which of the features to perform uncertainty quantification of. If nothing is specified, the uncertainty quantification is by default performed on all features (`features_to_run="all"`). `preprocess` is a Python function that performs common calculations for all features. `interpolate` is a list of features that are irregular. As with models, Uncertainpy automatically interpolates the output of these features to a regular form. Below we first go into detail on the requirements of a feature function, and then the requirements of a `preprocess` function.

3.4.1. Feature Functions

A feature is given as a Python function. The outline of such a feature function is:

```
def example_feature(time, values, info):
    # Calculate the feature using
    # time, values, and info.
```

```
    # Return the feature time
    # and values.
    return time_feature, values_feature
```

Feature functions have the following requirements:

1. **Input.** The feature function takes the objects returned by the model function as input, except when a `preprocess` function is used (see below). In those cases, the feature function instead takes the objects returned by the `preprocess` function as input. `preprocess` is normally not used.
2. **Feature calculation.** The feature function calculates the value of a feature from the data given in `time`, `values` and optional `info` objects. As previously mentioned, in all built-in features in Uncertainpy, `info` is a dictionary containing required information as key-value pairs.
3. **Output.** The feature function must return two objects:
   (a) **Feature time** (`time_feature`). The time (or equivalent) of the feature. We can return `None` instead for features where this is not relevant.
   (b) **Feature values** (`values_feature`). The result of the feature calculation. As for the model output, the feature result must be regular, or able to be interpolated. If there are no feature result for a specific model evaluation (e.g., if the feature was spike width and there were no spikes), the feature function can return `None`. The specific feature evaluation is then discarded in the uncertainty calculations.

As with models, we can, as a shortcut, directly give a list of feature functions as the `feature` argument in `UncertaintyQuantification`, instead of first having to create a `Features` instance.

3.4.2. Feature Pre-processing

Some of the calculations needed to quantify features may overlap between different features. One example is finding the spike times from a voltage trace. The `preprocess` function is used to avoid having to perform the same calculations several times. An example outline of a `preprocess` function is:

```
def preprocess(time, values, info):
    # Perform all common feature
    # calculations using time, values,
    # and info returned by the model
    # function.

    # Return the pre-processed model
    # output and info.
    return time_preprocessed,
        values_preprocessed, info
```

The requirements for a `preprocess` function are:

1. **Input.** A `preprocess` function takes the objects returned by the model function as input.
2. **Pre-processing.** The model output (`time`, `values`, and additional `info` objects) are used to perform all pre-process calculations.
3. **Output.** The `preprocess` function can return any number of objects as output. The returned pre-process objects are used as input arguments to the feature functions, so the two must be compatible.

Figure 2 illustrates how the objects returned by the model function are passed to `preprocess`, and the returned pre-process objects are used as input arguments in all feature functions. This pre-processing makes feature functions have different required input arguments depending on the feature class they are added to. As mentioned earlier, Uncertainpy comes with three built-in feature classes. These classes all take the `new_features` argument, so custom features can be added to each set of features. These feature classes all perform a pre-processing and therefore have different requirements for the input arguments of new feature functions. Additionally, certain features require specific keys to be present in the `info` dictionary. Each class has a `reference_feature` method that states the requirements for feature functions of that class in its docstring.

3.4.3. Spiking Features

Here we introduce the `SpikingFeatures` class, which contains a set of features relevant for models of single neurons that receive an external stimulus and respond by producing a series of action potentials, also called spikes. Many of these features require the start time and end time of the stimulus, which must be returned as `info["stimulus_start"]` and `info["stimulus_end"]` in the model function. `info` is then used as an additional input argument in the calculation of each feature. A set of spiking features is created by:

```
features = SpikingFeatures()
```

`SpikingFeatures` implements a `preprocess` method, which locates spikes in the model output. This `preprocess` method can be customized; see the documentation on `SpikingFeatures`.

The features included in `SpikingFeatures` are briefly defined below. This set of features was taken from the previous work of Druckmann et al. (2007), with the addition of the number of action potentials during the stimulus period. We refer to the original publication for more detailed definitions.

1. `nr_spikes` – Number of action potentials (during stimulus period).
2. `spike_rate` – Action-potential firing rate (number of action potentials divided by stimulus duration).
3. `time_before_first_spike` – Time from stimulus onset to first elicited action potential.
4. `accommodation_index` – Accommodation index (normalized average difference in length of two consecutive interspike intervals).
5. `average_AP_overshoot` – Average action-potential peak voltage.

6. `average_AHP_depth` - Average afterhyperpolarization depth (average minimum voltage between action potentials).
7. `average_AP_width` - Average action-potential width taken at the midpoint between the onset and peak of the action potential.

The user may want to add custom features to the set of features in `SpikingFeatures`. The `SpikingFeatures.preprocess` method changes the input given to the feature functions, and as such each spiking feature function has the following input arguments:

1. The `time` array returned by the model simulation.
2. A `Spikes` object (`spikes`) which contain the spikes found in the model output.
3. An `info` dictionary with `info["stimulus_start"]` and `info["stimulus_end"]` set.

The `Spikes` object is the pre-processed version of the model output, used as a container for `Spike` objects. In turn, each `Spike` object contains information about a single spike. This information includes a brief voltage trace represented by a `time` and a voltage (`V`) array that only includes the selected spike. The information in `Spikes` is used to calculate each feature. As an example, let us create a feature that is the time at which the first spike in the voltage trace ends. Such a feature can be defined as follows:

```
def first_spike_ends(time, spikes, info)
    :
    # Get the first spike
    spike = spikes[0]

    # The last time point
    # in the spike
    values_feature = spike.t[-1]

    return None, values_feature
```

This feature may now be used as a feature function in the list given to the `new_features` argument.

From the set of both built-in and user-defined features, we may select subsets of features that we want to use in the analysis of a model. Let us say we are interested in how the model performs in terms of the three features: `nr_spikes`, `average_AHP_depth` and `first_spike_ends`. A spiking features object that calculates these features is created by:

```
features_to_run = [
    "nr_spikes",
    "average_AHP_depth",
    "first_spike_ends"
]

features = un.SpikingFeatures(
    new_features=[first_spike_ends],
    features_to_run=features_to_run
)
```

3.4.4. eFEL Features

A more extensive set of features for single neuron voltage traces is found in the Electrophys Feature Extraction Library (eFEL) (Blue Brain Project, 2015). A set of eFEL spiking features is created by:

```
features = EfelFeatures()
```

Uncertainpy has all features in the eFEL library in the `EfelFeatures` class. At the time of writing, eFEL contains 160 different features. Due to the high number of features, we do not list them here, but refer to the eFEL documentation[5] for detailed definitions, or the Uncertainpy documentation for a list of the features. `EfelFeatures` is used in the same way as `SpikingFeatures`.

3.4.5. Network Features

The last set of features implemented in Uncertainpy is found in the `NetworkFeatures` class:

```
features = NetworkFeatures()
```

This class contains a set of features relevant for the output of neural network models. These features are calculated using the *Elephant* Python package (NeuralEnsemble, 2017). The implemented features are:

1. `average_firing_rate` - Average firing rate (for a single recorded neuron).
2. `instantaneous_rate` - Instantaneous firing rate (averaged over all recorded neurons within a small time window).
3. `average_isi` - Average interspike interval (averaged over all recorded neurons).
4. `cv` - Coefficient of variation of the interspike interval (for a single recorded neuron).
5. `average_cv` - Average coefficient of variation of the interspike interval (averaged over all recorded neurons).
6. `local_variation` - Local variation (variability of interspike intervals for a single recorded neuron).
7. `average_local_variation` - Average local variation (variability of interspike intervals averaged over all recorded neurons).
8. `fanofactor` - Fanofactor (variability of spike trains).
9. `victor_purpura_dist` - Victor-Purpura distance (spike train dissimilarity between two recorded neurons).
10. `van_rossum_dist` - Van Rossum distance (spike train dissimilarity between two recorded neurons).
11. `binned_isi` - Histogram of the interspike intervals (for all recorded neurons).
12. `corrcoef` - Pairwise Pearson's correlation coefficients (between the binned spike trains of two recorded neurons).
13. `covariance` - Covariance (between the binned spike trains of two recorded neurons).

A few of these network features can be customized; see the documentation on `NetworkFeatures` for a further explanation.

[5]http://efel.readthedocs.io

The use of `NetworkFeatures` in Uncertainpy follows the same logic as the use of the other feature classes, and custom features can easily be included. As with `SpikingFeatures`, `NetworkFeatures` implements a `preprocess` method. This `preprocess` returns the following objects:

1. End time of the simulation (`end_time`).
2. A list of NEO (Garcia et al., 2014) spike trains (`spiketrains`).

Each feature function added to `NetworkFeatures` therefore requires these objects as input arguments. Note that the `info` object is not used.

3.5. Uncertainty Calculations in Uncertainpy

In this section, we describe how Uncertainpy performs the uncertainty calculations, as well as which options the user has to customize the calculations. Moreover, a detailed insight into this is not required to use Uncertainpy, as in most cases the default settings work fine. In addition to the customization options shown below, Uncertainpy has support for implementing entirely custom uncertainty-quantification and sensitivity-analysis methods. This is only recommended for expert users, as knowledge of both Uncertainpy and uncertainty quantification is needed. We do not go into detail here but refer to the Uncertainpy documentation for more information.

3.5.1. Quasi-Monte Carlo Method

To use the quasi-Monte Carlo method, we call `quantify` with `method="mc"`, and the optional argument `nr_mc_samples`:

```
data = UQ.quantify(
    method="mc",
    nr_mc_samples=10**4
)
```

The quasi-Monte Carlo method quasi-randomly draws $N_s = N(d+2)/2$ parameter samples, where $N =$ `nr_mc_samples` , and d is the number of uncertain parameters. This is the number of samples required by Saltelli's method to calculate the Sobol indices. By default `nr_mc_samples=10000`. These samples are drawn from a multivariate independent uniform distribution using Saltelli's sampling scheme, implemented in the SALib library (Saltelli et al., 2010; Herman and Usher, 2017). We use the Rosenblatt transformation to transform the samples from this uniform distribution to the parameter distribution given by the user. This transformation enables us to use Saltelli's sampling scheme for any parameter distribution.

The model is evaluated for each of these parameter samples, and features are calculated from each model evaluation (when applicable). To speed up the calculations, Uncertainpy uses the *multiprocess* Python package (McKerns et al., 2012) to perform this step in parallel. When model and feature calculations are done, Uncertainpy calculates the mean, variance, and 5th and 95th percentile (which gives the 90% prediction interval) for the model and each feature. This is done using a subset with N number of samples of the total set. We are unable to use the full set since not all samples are independent in Saltelli's sampling scheme. The Sobol indices are calculated using Saltelli's method and the complete set of samples. We use a modified version of the method in the SALib library, which is able to handle model evaluations with any number of dimensions.

Saltelli's method requires all model and feature evaluations to return a valid result. When this is not the case we use the workaround[6] suggested by Herman and Usher (2017), and replace invalid model and feature evaluations with the mean of that model or feature. This workaround introduces an error depending on the number of missing evaluations but enables us to still calculate the Sobol indices. If there are invalid model or feature evaluations, Uncertainpy gives a warning which includes the number of invalid evaluations.

3.5.2. Polynomial Chaos Expansions

To use polynomial chaos expansions we use `quantify` with the argument `method="pc"`, which takes a set of optional arguments (the specified values are the default):

```
data = UQ.quantify(
    method="pc",
    pc_method="collocation",
    rosenblatt="auto",
    polynomial_order=4,
    nr_collocation_nodes=None,
    quadrature_order=None,
    nr_pc_mc_samples=10**4
)
```

As previously mentioned, Uncertainpy allows the user to select between point collocation (`pc_method="collocation"`) and pseudo-spectral projections (`pc_method="spectral"`). The goal of both these methods is to create separate polynomial chaos expansions $\hat{U}_{\mathrm{model/feature}}$ for the model and each feature. The first step of both methods is the same: Uncertainpy starts by creating the orthogonal polynomial $\boldsymbol{\phi}_n$ using ρ_Q and the three-term recurrence relation if available, otherwise the discretized Stieltjes method (Stieltjes, 1884) is used. By default, Uncertainpy uses a fourth order polynomial expansion, as recommended by Eck et al. (2016). The polynomial order p can be changed with the `polynomial_order` argument. The polynomial $\boldsymbol{\phi}_n$ is the same for the model and all features, since they have the same uncertain input parameters, and therefore the same ρ_Q. Only the polynomial coefficients c_n differ between the model and each feature.

The two polynomial chaos methods differ in terms of how they calculate c_n. For point collocation Uncertainpy uses $N_s = 2(N_p + 1)$ collocation nodes, as recommended by Hosder et al. (2007), where N_p is the number of polynomial chaos expansion factors. The number of collocation nodes can be customized with `nr_collocation_nodes` (N_s), but the new number of nodes must be chosen carefully. The collocation nodes are sampled from ρ_Q using Hammersley sampling (Hammersley, 1960), also as recommended by Hosder et al. (2007). The model and features are calculated for each of the collocation nodes. As with the quasi-Monte Carlo method, this step is performed in parallel.

[6]https://github.com/SALib/SALib/issues/134

The polynomial coefficients c_n are calculated using the model and feature results, and Tikhonov regularization (Rifkin and Lippert, 2007).

For the pseudo-spectral projection, Uncertainpy chooses nodes and weights using a quadrature scheme, instead of choosing nodes from ρ_Q. The quadrature scheme used is Leja quadrature with a Smolyak sparse grid (Smolyak, 1963; Narayan and Jakeman, 2014). The Leja quadrature is by default of order two greater than the polynomial order, but this can be changed with `quadrature_order`. The model and features are calculated for each of the quadrature nodes. As before, this step is performed in parallel. The polynomial coefficients c_n are then calculated from the quadrature nodes, weights, and model and feature results.

When Uncertainpy has derived $\hat{U}$ for the model and features, it uses $\hat{U}$ to compute the mean, variance, first and total-order Sobol indices, as well as the average first and total-order Sobol indices. Finally, Uncertainpy uses $\hat{U}$ as a surrogate model and employs the quasi-Monte Carlo method with Hammersley sampling and `nr_pc_mc_samples=10**4` samples to find the 5th and 95th percentiles.

If the model parameters have a dependent joint multivariate distribution, the Rosenblatt transformation is by default automatically used. This can be changed by setting `rosenblatt=True` to always use the Rosenblatt transform, or `rosenblatt=False` to never use the Rosenblatt transformation. Note that the latter gives an error if you have dependent parameters. To perform this transformation Uncertainpy chooses a multivariate independent normal distribution ρ_R, which is used instead of ρ_Q to perform the polynomial chaos expansions. Both the point-collocation method and the pseudo-spectral method are performed as described above. The only difference is that we use ρ_R instead of ρ_Q, and use the Rosenblatt transformation to transform the selected nodes from $\boldsymbol{R}$ to $\mathbf{Q}$, before they are used in the model evaluation.

3.6. Data Format

All results from the uncertainty quantification and sensitivity analysis are returned as a `Data` object, as well as being stored in `UncertaintyQuantification.data`. The `Data` class works similarly to a Python dictionary. The names of the model and features are the keys, while the values are `DataFeature` objects that store each statistical metric in **Table 1** as attributes. Results can be saved and loaded through `Data.save` and `Data.load`, and are saved either as `HDF5` files (Collette, 2013) or `Exdir` structures (Dragly et al., 2018). `HDF5` files are used by default.

An example: If we have performed an uncertainty quantification of a spiking neuron model with the number of spikes as one of the features, we can load the results and get the variance of the number of spikes by:

```
data = un.Data()
data.load("filename")
variance = data["nr_spikes"].variance
```

TABLE 1 | Calculated values and statistical metrics, for the model and each feature stored in the `Data` class.

Calculated statistical metric	Symbol	Variable
Model and feature evaluations	U	`evaluations`
Model and feature times	t	`time`
Mean	$\mathbb{E}$	`mean`
Variance	$\mathbb{V}$	`variance`
5th percentile	P_5	`percentile_5`
95th percentile	P_{95}	`percentile_95`
First-order Sobol indices	S	`sobol_first`
Total-order Sobol indices	S_T	`sobol_total`
Average of the first-order Sobol indices	$\overline{S}$	`sobol_first_average`
Average of the total-order Sobol indices	$\overline{S}_T$	`sobol_total_average`

3.7. Visualization

Uncertainpy plots the results for all zero and one-dimensional statistical metrics, and some of the two-dimensional statistical metrics. An example of a zero-dimensional statistical metric is the mean of the average interspike interval of a neural network (**Figure 8**). An example of a one-dimensional statistical metric is the mean of the membrane potential over time for a multi-compartmental neuron (**Figure 4**). Lastly, an example of a two-dimensional statistical metric is the mean of the pairwise Pearson's correlation coefficient of a neural network (**Figure 9**). These visualizations are intended as a quick way to get an overview of the results, and not to create publication-ready plots. Custom plots of the data can easily be created by retrieving the results from the `Data` class.

3.8. Technical Aspects

Uncertainpy is open-source and found at https://github.com/simetenn/uncertainpy. Uncertainpy can easily be installed using `pip`:

```
pip install uncertainpy
```

or from source by cloning the Github repository:

```
$ git clone https://github.com/simetenn/
    uncertainpy
$ cd uncertainpy
$ sudo python setup.py install
```

Uncertainpy comes with an extensive test suite that can be run with the `test.py` script. For information on how to use `test.py`, run:

```
$ python test.py --help
```

4. EXAMPLE APPLICATIONS

In the current section, we demonstrate how to use Uncertainpy by applying it to four different case studies: (i) a simple model for the temperature of a cooling coffee cup implemented in Python, (ii) the original Hodgkin-Huxley model implemented in Python, (iii) a multi-compartmental model of a thalamic interneuron implemented in NEURON, and (iv) a sparsely connected recurrent network model implemented in NEST. The codes for all four case studies are available in `uncertainpy/examples/`, which generates all results shown in this paper. All the case studies can be run on a regular workstation computer. Uncertainpy does not create publication-ready figures, so custom plots have been created for the case studies. The code for creating all figures in this paper is found in a Jupyter Notebook in `uncertainpy/examples/paper_figures/`.

For simplicity, uniform distributions were assumed for all parameter uncertainties in the example studies. Further, the results for the case studies are calculated using point collocation. For the examples shown we used the default polynomial order of $p = 4$, but also confirmed that the results converged by increasing the polynomial order to $p = 5$, which gave similar results (results not shown).

The case studies were run in a Docker[7] container with Python 3, created from the Dockerfile `uncertainpy/.docker/Dockerfile_uncertainpy3`. A similar Dockerfile is available for Python 2. The used version of Uncertainpy is 1.0.1, commit `b7b3fa0`, and Zenodo[8] DOI `10.5281/zenodo.1300336`. We also used NEST 2.14.0, NEURON 7.5, and Chaospy commit `05fea24`. A requirements file that specifies the version of all used Python packages is located in `uncertainpy/examples/paper_figures/`.

4.1. Cooling Coffee Cup

To give a simple, first demonstration of Uncertainpy, we perform an uncertainty quantification and sensitivity analysis of a hot cup of coffee that follows Newton's law of cooling. We start with a model that has independent uncertain parameters, before we modify the model to have dependent parameters to show an example requiring the Rosenblatt transformation.

4.1.1. Cooling Coffee Cup With Independent Parameters

The temperature T of the cooling coffee cup is given by:

$$\frac{dT(t)}{dt} = -\kappa(T(t) - T_{env}), \tag{18}$$

where T_{env} is the temperature of the environment in units of °C. κ is a cooling constant in units of 1/min that is characteristic of the system and describes how fast the coffee cup radiates heat to the environment. We set the initial temperature to a fixed value, $T_0 = 95$°C, and assume that κ and T_{env} are uncertain parameters characterized by the uniform probability distributions:

$$\rho_\kappa = \text{Uniform}(0.025, 0.075), \tag{19}$$

$$\rho_{T_{env}} = \text{Uniform}(15, 25). \tag{20}$$

The following code is available in `uncertainpy/examples/coffee_cup/`. We start by importing the packages required to perform the uncertainty quantification:

```
import uncertainpy as un

# To create distributions
import chaospy as cp
# For the time array
import numpy as np
# To integrate our equation
from scipy.integrate import odeint
```

Next, we create the cooling coffee-cup model. To do this we define a Python function (`coffee_cup`) that takes the uncertain parameters `kappa` and `T_env` as input arguments, solves Equation (18) by integration using `scipy.integrate.odeint` over 200 min, and returns the resulting time and temperature arrays.

```
def coffee_cup(kappa, T_env):
    # Initial temperature and time array
    time = np.linspace(0, 200, 150)    #
        Minutes
    T_0 = 95                           #
        Celsius

    # The equation describing the model
    def f(T, time, kappa, T_env):
        return -kappa*(T - T_env)

    # Solving the equation by
        integration
    temperature = odeint(f, T_0, time,
        args=(kappa, T_env))[:, 0]

    # Return time and model output
    return time, temperature
```

We now use `coffee_cup` to create a `Model` object, and add labels:

```
model = un.Model(
    run=coffee_cup,
    labels=["Time (min)",
            "Temperature (C)"]
)
```

As previously mentioned, it is possible to use `coffee_cup` directly as the `model` argument in the `UncertaintyQuantification` class, however we would then be unable to specify the labels.

In the next step, we use Chaospy to assign distributions to the uncertain parameters κ and T_{env}, and use these distributions to create a parameter dictionary:

[7] https://www.docker.com/
[8] https://zenodo.org/

```
# Create the distributions
kappa_dist = cp.Uniform(0.025, 0.075)
T_env_dist = cp.Uniform(15, 25)

# Define the parameter dictionary
parameters = {"kappa": kappa_dist,
              "T_env": T_env_dist}
```

We can now set up the `UncertaintyQuantification`:

```
UQ = un.UncertaintyQuantification(
        model=model,
        parameters=parameters
)
```

With that, we are ready to calculate the uncertainty and sensitivity of the model. We use polynomial chaos expansions with point collocation, the default options of `quantify`, and set the seed for the random number generator to allow for precise reproduction of the results:

```
data = UQ.quantify(seed=10)
```

`quantify` calculates all statistical metrics discussed in sections 2.2 and 2.3, but here we only show the mean, standard deviation (square root of the variance), and 90% prediction interval (**Figure 3A**), and the first-order Sobol indices (**Figure 3B**). The reason we plot the standard deviation instead of the variance is to make it easier to compare it to the mean. As the mean (blue line) in **Figure 3A** shows, the cooling gives rise to an exponential decay in the temperature, toward the temperature of the environment T_{env}. From the sensitivity analysis (**Figure 3B**) we see that T is most sensitive to κ early in the simulation, and to T_{env} toward the end of the simulation. This is as expected since κ determines the rate of the cooling, while T_{env} determines the final temperature. After about 150 min, the cooling is essentially completed, and the uncertainty in T exclusively reflects the uncertainty of T_{env}.

4.1.2. Cooling Coffee Cup With Statistically Dependent Parameters

Uncertainpy can also perform uncertainty quantification and sensitivity analysis using polynomial chaos expansions on models with statistically dependent parameters. Here we use the cooling coffee-cup model to construct such an example. Let us parameterize the coffee cup differently:

$$\frac{dT(t)}{dt} = -\alpha\hat{\kappa}\left(T(t) - T_{env}\right). \qquad (21)$$

In order for the model to describe the same cooling process as before, the new variables α and $\hat{\kappa}$ should be dependent, so that $\alpha\hat{\kappa} = \kappa$. We can achieve this by demanding that $\rho_{\hat{\kappa}} = \rho_{\kappa}/\rho_{\alpha}$ (note that ρ_{α} should not include 0) and otherwise define the problem following the same procedure as in the original case study. Since this gives us a dependent distribution, Uncertainpy automatically uses the Rosenblatt transformation.

In this case, the distribution we assign to α does not affect the end result, as the distribution for $\hat{\kappa}$ will be scaled accordingly. Using the Rosenblatt transformation, an uncertainty quantification and sensitivity analysis of the dependent coffee-cup model therefore return the same results as seen in **Figure 3**, where the role of the original κ is taken over by $\hat{\kappa}$, while the sensitivity to the additional parameter α becomes strictly zero (we do not show the results here, but see the example in `uncertainpy/examples/coffee_cup_dependent/`).

4.2. Hodgkin-Huxley Model

From here on, we focus on case studies more relevant for neuroscience, starting with the original Hodgkin-Huxley model (Hodgkin and Huxley, 1952). An uncertainty analysis of this model has been performed previously (Torres Valderrama et al., 2015), and we here repeat a part of that study using Uncertainpy.

The original version of the Hodgkin-Huxley model has eleven parameters with the numerical values listed in **Table 2**.

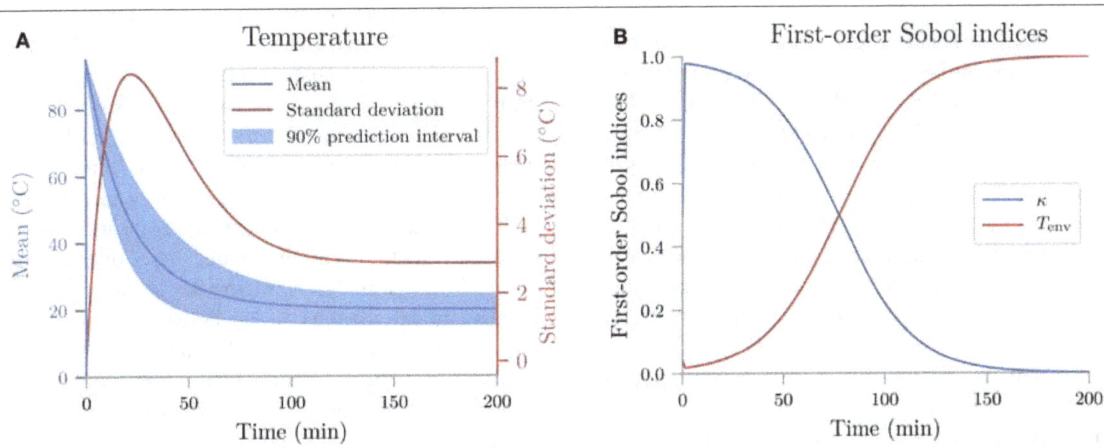

FIGURE 3 | The uncertainty quantification and sensitivity analysis of the cooling coffee-cup model. **(A)** The mean, standard deviation (square root of the variance) and 90% prediction interval of the temperature of the cooling coffee cup. **(B)** First-order Sobol indices of the cooling coffee-cup model.

TABLE 2 | Parameters in the original Hodgkin-Huxley model.

Parameter	Value	Unit	Meaning
V_0	−10	mV	Initial voltage
C_m	1	$\mu F/cm^2$	Membrane capacitance
$\bar{g}_{Na}$	120	mS/cm^2	Maximum sodium (Na) conductance
$\bar{g}_K$	36	mS/cm^2	Maximum potassium (K) conductance
$\bar{g}_L$	0.3	mS/cm^2	Maximum leak current conductance
E_{Na}	112	mV	Sodium equilibrium potential
E_K	−12	mV	Potassium equilibrium potential
E_L	10.613	mV	Leak current equilibrium potential
n_0	0.0011		Initial potassium activation gating variable
m_0	0.0003		Initial sodium activation gating variable
h_0	0.9998		Initial sodium inactivation gating variable

As in the previous study, we assume each of these parameters has a uniform distribution in the range ±10% around their original value. We use uncertainty quantification and sensitivity analysis to explore how these parameter uncertainties affect the model output, i.e., the action potential response of the neural membrane potential to an external current injection.

As in the cooling coffee-cup example, we implement the Hodgkin-Huxley model as a Python function and use polynomial chaos expansions with point collocation to calculate the uncertainty and sensitivity of the model (the code for this case study is found in `uncertainpy/examples/valderrama/`).

The uncertainty quantification of the Hodgkin-Huxley model is shown in **Figure 4A**, and the sensitivity analysis in **Figure 4B**. As we were not able to extract all implementation details in Torres Valderrama et al. (2015), our analysis is likely not an exact replica of the previous study, but the results obtained are quantitatively similar. Although the action potential is robust (within the selected parameter ranges), the onset and amplitude of the action potential vary between simulations. The variance (standard deviation) in the membrane potential is largest during the upstroke and peak of the action potential (**Figure 4A**), which occur in the time interval between $t = 8$ and 9 ms. This occurs mainly due to the difference in action potential timing.

The sensitivity analysis reveals that the variance in the membrane potential mainly is due to the uncertainty in two parameters: the maximum conductance of the K^+ channel, $\bar{g}_K$, and the Na^+ reversal potential, E_{Na} (**Figure 4B**). The low sensitivity to the remaining parameters means that most of the variability of the Hodgkin-Huxley model would be maintained if these remaining parameters were kept fixed. This result tells us that if we want to reduce the uncertainty in the model predictions, experiments should focus on measuring $\bar{g}_K$ and E_{Na} more precisely, while crude estimates of the remaining parameters will suffice. Of course, this conclusion only holds for the conditions considered in the current simulation, where the neuron is exposed to positive current injection starting at $t = 0$. If the neuron received no input, the membrane potential would show a much higher sensitivity to the leak current (E_L and $\bar{g}_L$) which are important for determining the resting potential of the neuron.

A sensitivity analysis such as that in **Figure 4B** may serve to give an insight into how different mechanisms are responsible for different aspects of the neuronal response. Some of the findings confirm what we would expect from a general knowledge of action potential firing (see figure 3.12 in Sterratt et al., 2011 for an overview). For example, it is not surprising that the action potential peak potential is most sensitive to the Na^+ reversal potential (E_{Na}), since this parameter is known to closely determine the peak value. Nor is it surprising that $\bar{g}_K$ is the most important parameter during the downstroke of the action potential, since the essential role of the K^+ channel is to repolarize the neuron.

Other parts of the analysis reveal some less intuitive relationships. For example, **Figure 4B** shows that the membrane potential during the upstroke of the action potential is most sensitive to $\bar{g}_K$. This may be surprising given that the Na^+ channel (parameterized by $\bar{g}_{Na}$ and E_{Na}) is responsible for depolarizing the neuron. This indicates that the all-or-nothing response of the Na^+ channel activation is rather robust, and that variance during the upstroke predominantly is due to the effects of the K^+ channel on the timing of the action-potential onset. Another unexpected observation is that E_{Na} has a high sensitivity within a time window after the peak of the action potential. This indicates that the Na^+ channel is not fully closed, and is involved in determining the potential at which the neuron lingers within this time window.

Another aspect of modeling where sensitivity analysis can be useful, is in exploring the dependence on initial conditions. When analyzing complex models, it is common to discard the initial part of the simulation from the analysis, i.e., one lets the model run for a time T before one starts to analyze its dynamics. The rationale behind this is that the model over time loses its dependence on (arbitrarily set) initial conditions of its dynamic variables, and reaches its inherent steady-state dynamics. In the example studied here, only the response for $T > 5$ ms is analyzed. **Figure 4B** shows that the Hodgkin-Huxley model then has a negligible sensitivity to the initial membrane potential (V_0) and initial activation states of the Na^+ channel (m_0) and K^+ channel (n_0), but maintains a sensitivity to the initial Na^+ inactivation state (h_0) through most of the simulation. Such a dependence on the initial condition of a state variable is typically unwanted and indicates that the model should have had more time to settle in before its response was analyzed.

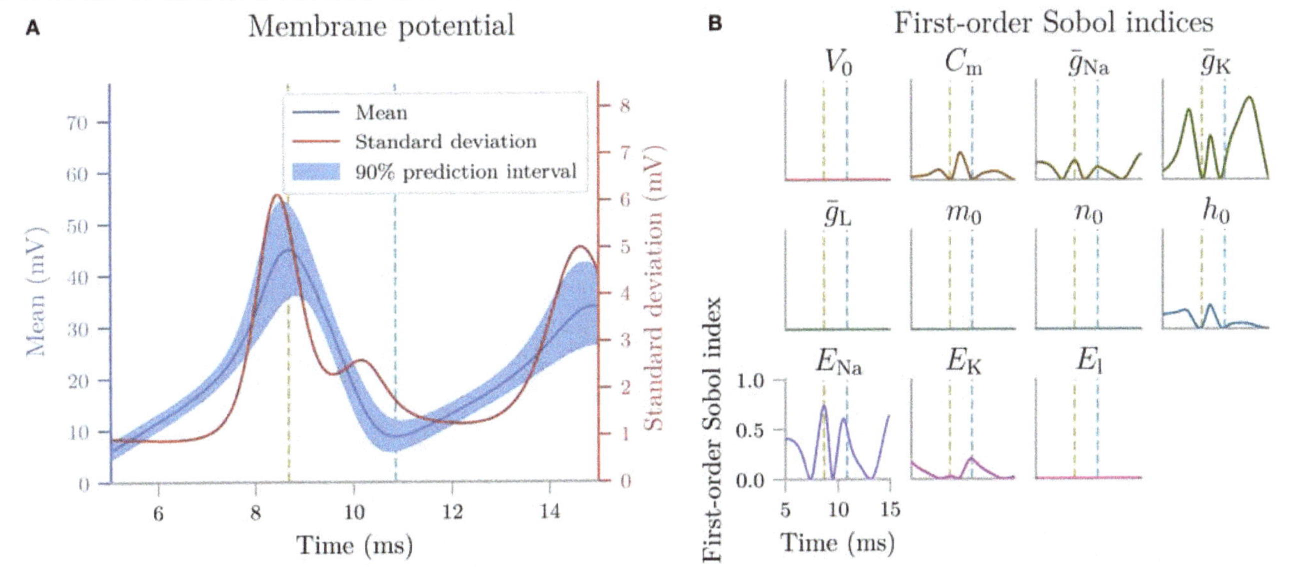

FIGURE 4 | The uncertainty quantification and sensitivity analysis of the Hodgkin-Huxley model, parameterized so it has a resting potential of 0 mV. The model was exposed to a continuous external stimulus of 140 μA/cm^2 starting at $t = 0$, and we examined the membrane potential in the time window between $t = 5$ and 15 ms. **(A)** Mean, standard deviation and 90% prediction interval for the membrane potential of the Hodgkin-Huxley model. **(B)** First-order Sobol indices of the uncertain parameters in the Hodgkin-Huxley model. The yellow line indicates the peak of the first action potential, while the cyan line indicates the minimum after the first action potential.

4.3. Multi-Compartmental Model of a Thalamic Interneuron

In the next case study, we illustrate how Uncertainpy can be used on models implemented in NEURON (Hines and Carnevale, 1997). For this study, we select a previously published model of an interneuron in the dorsal lateral geniculate nucleus (dLGN) of the thalamus (Halnes et al., 2011). Since the model is implemented in NEURON, the original model can be used directly with Uncertainpy by using the `NeuronModel` class. The code for this case study is found in `uncertainpy/examples/interneuron/`.

In the original modeling study, seven active ion channels were tuned (by trial and error) to capture the responses of thalamic interneurons to different current injections (Halnes et al., 2011). Here, we consider one of the stimulus conditions used in the original study, and examine how sensitive the interneuron response is to uncertain ion-channel conductances. The conductances in the original model are listed in **Table 3**, and we assume they have uniform distributions in the interval $\pm10\%$ around their original values.

The uncertainty quantification of the membrane potential in the soma of the interneuron is seen in **Figure 5A**. The variance (or standard deviation) indicates that the neuronal response varies strongly between the different parameterizations. To illustrate the variety of response characteristics hiding in the statistics in **Figure 5A**, four selected example simulations are shown in **Figure 5B**, all obtained by drawing the uncertain parameters from intervals $\pm10\%$ around their original values. In line with the discussion in section 2.7, the qualitative differences between the responses indicate that a feature-based analysis is more informative than a point-to-point comparison of the voltage traces.

TABLE 3 | Uncertain parameters in the thalamic interneuron model.

Parameter	Value	Unit	Variable	Meaning
g_{Na}	0.09	S/cm^2	gna	Max Na$^+$-conductance in soma
g_{Kdr}	0.37	S/cm^2	gkdr	Max direct-rectifying K$^+$-conductance in soma
g_{CaT}	1.17×10^{-5}	S/cm^2	gcat	Max T-type Ca^{2+}-conductance in soma
g_{CaL}	9×10^{-4}	S/cm^2	gcal	Max L-type Ca^{2+}-conductance in soma
g_h	1.1×10^{-4}	S/cm^2	ghbar	Max conductance of a non-specific hyperpolarization activated cation channel in soma
g_{AHP}	6.4×10^{-5}	S/cm^2	gahp	Max afterhyperpolarizing K$^+$-conductance in soma
g_{CAN}	2×10^{-8}	S/cm^2	gcanbar	Max conductance of a Ca^{2+}-activated non-specific cation channel in soma

For simplicity, we limited the analysis to only explore sensitivity to ion channel conductances, although the original model had some additional free parameters.

Since we examine a spiking neuron model, we want to use the features in the `SpikingFeatures` class for the feature-based analysis. `SpikingFeatures` needs to know the start

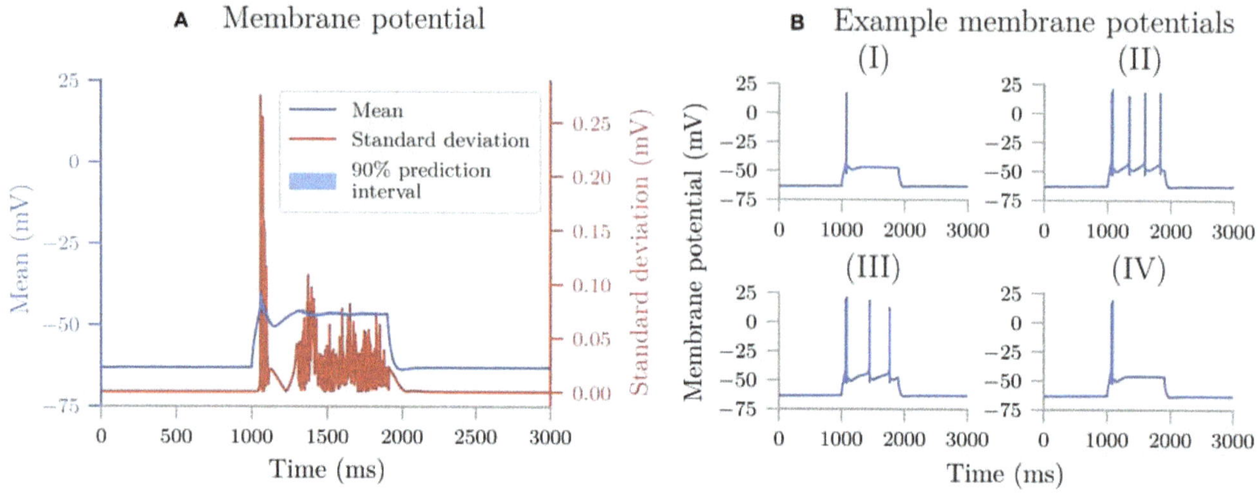

FIGURE 5 | Uncertainty quantification of the interneuron model. **(A)** The mean, standard deviation, and 90% prediction interval for the membrane potential of the interneuron model. **(B)** Four selected model outputs for different sets of parameters. The interneuron received a somatic current injection between 1,000 ms $< t <$ 1,900 ms, with a stimulus strength of 55 pA.

and end times of the stimulus to be able to calculate certain features. When we initialize `NeuronModel` we therefore specify the `stimulus_start` (set to 1,000 ms) and `stimulus_end` (set to 1,900 ms) arguments. Additionally, the interneuron model uses adaptive time steps, meaning we have to use `interpolate =True` (which is the default option of `NeuronModel`). We also specify the path to the folder where the neuron model is stored (for this example, it is `path="interneuron_modelDB/"`). As before, we use polynomial chaos expansions with point collocation to compute the statistical metrics for the model output and all features.

Figure 6 shows the sensitivity of the features in `SpikingFeatures` to the various ion-channel conductances (see section 3.4.3 for definitions of the features). For illustrative purposes, only the first-order Sobol indices are shown (although Uncertainpy by default calculates all statistical metrics from sections 2.2 and 2.3).

A feature-based sensitivity analysis such as in **Figure 6** gives valuable insight into the role of various biological mechanisms in determining the firing properties of a neuron. Some of the results confirm what we would expect from a general knowledge of neurodynamics. For example, it is not surprising that the spike rate (A), the number of action potentials elicited throughout the simulation (E), and the action-potential amplitude (F) are most sensitive to the Na^+ channel conductance g_{Na}, given the well-established role of the Na^+ channel in action-potential generation. Likewise, given the role of the K^+ channel in repolarizing the neuron after an action potential, it is not surprising that the action-potential width (D) is predominantly sensitive to g_{Kdr}.

The third most important parameter identified in this sensitivity analysis is the T-type Ca^{2+} conductance (g_{CaT}), known to be important for burst firing in thalamic interneurons (Zhu et al., 1999; Halnes et al., 2011; Allken et al., 2014). T-type Ca^{2+} channels are typically activated when the membrane potential makes a sudden step from low to high values, such as at the stimulus onset. Upon activation, T-type Ca^{2+} channels then evoke Ca^{2+} spikes which may act to boost the initial response of a neuron to an external stimulus. This explains why the timing of the first spike (C) has such a high sensitivity to g_{CaT}. Bursts are typically more pronounced under other stimulus conditions than the one used in the current simulations, but in some cases, the Ca^{2+} spike was large enough to evoke small, initial bursts of action potentials (see example simulations in **Figure 5B**, II–IV, where the initial responses are small bursts of two action potentials). The additional action potentials in neurons that elicit bursts serve to explain why the spike rate (A) and total number of action potentials (G) also are highly sensitive to g_{CaT}.

A perhaps less expected result is that the depth of the afterhyperpolarization (G) (voltage dip following an action potential) has such a low sensitivity to the two K^+ channels (g_{Kdr} and g_{AHP}) in the model, as these are the channels that have a direct effect on the hyperpolarization of the neuron. As for many of the features in **Figure 6**, there are complex interactions between several mechanisms and the limited analysis considered here can only hint at the possible underlying relationships. Part of the explanation may be that the afterhyperpolarization current (g_{AHP}) is Ca^{2+} activated, and is more limited by the availability of Ca^{2+} than by its own maximum conductance. This could serve to explain the high sensitivity to the Ca^{2+} channel g_{CaT}. Furthermore, the high sensitivity to g_{Na} implies that the Na^+ channel also is open during the down-stroke of the action potential, and counteracts the hyperpolarizing K^+ currents.

As **Figure 6** indicates, the variances of the `SpikingFeatures` are predominantly explained by the three model parameters g_{Na}, g_{Kdr} and g_{CaT}, with some contributions from g_{CaL}, g_{AHP} and negligible impact from the remaining

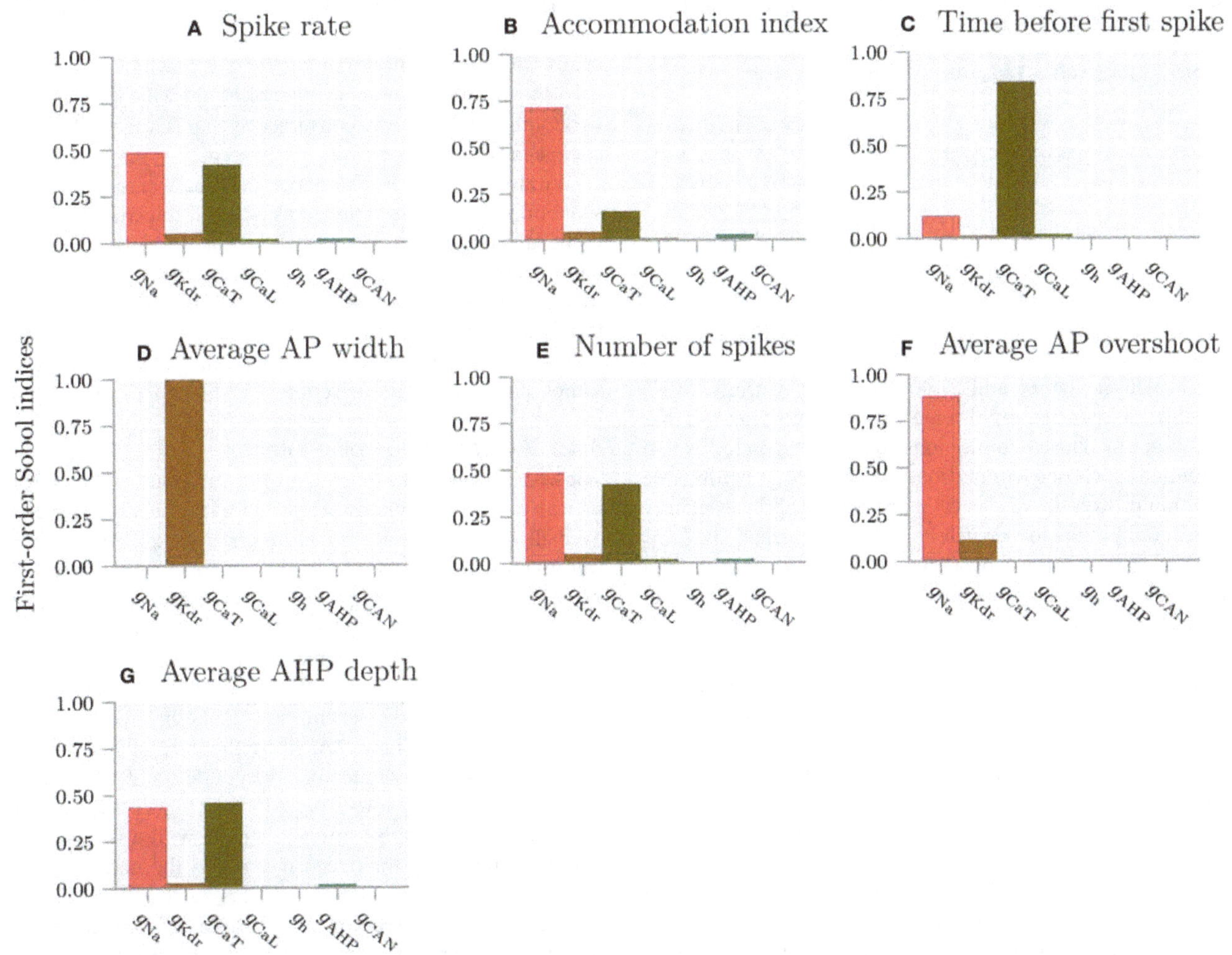

FIGURE 6 | The sensitivity for features of the interneuron model. First-order Sobol indices for features of the thalamic interneuron model. **(A)** Spike rate, that is, number of action potentials divided by stimulus duration. **(B)** Accommodation index, that is, the normalized average difference in length of two consecutive interspike intervals. **(C)** Time before first spike, that is, the time from stimulus onset to first elicited action potential. **(D)** Average AP width is the average action potential width taken at midpoint between the onset and peak of the action potential. **(E)** Number of spikes, that is, the number of action potentials during stimulus period. **(F)** Average AP overshoot is the average action-potential peak voltage. **(G)** Average AHP depth, that is, the average minimum voltage between action potentials.

parameters g_h and g_{CAN}. However, one should be cautious about generalizing insights found in an unexhaustive analysis such as the one presented here. Firstly, the presented analysis explores the sensitivity to variations within a ±10% range around the original parameter values, and thus spans a relatively local region of the parameter space. Additionally, this choice of distributions is a rather arbitrary choice and is unlikely to capture the actual uncertainty distributions. In reality, the uncertainty or biological variability, or both, in some of the parameters may have very different distributions, and an analysis that takes this into account could yield different results. Secondly, the above analysis was limited to a single stimulus protocol (a positive current step pulse of moderate magnitude to the soma), and a different stimulus protocol could activate a different set of neural mechanisms. For example, g_h denotes the conductance of a hyperpolarization-activated cation current, which would need a negative current injection to activate. It is therefore not surprising that our analysis shows zero sensitivity to this parameter.

Thirdly, the `SpikingFeatures` class contains a limited number of features, and other features (e.g., from the more comprehensive `EfelFeatures` class) can be sensitive to the parameters that were observed to be of less importance in the current example. We do not here consider additional features, stimulus protocols, or uncertainty distributions in the analysis, as the main purpose of this case study was to demonstrate the use of Uncertainpy on a detailed multi-compartmental model.

4.4. Recurrent Network of Integrate-and-Fire Neurons

In the last case study, we use Uncertainpy to perform a feature-based analysis of the sparsely connected recurrent network of integrate-and-fire neurons by Brunel (2000). We implement the Brunel network using NEST inside a Python function, and

TABLE 4 | Parameters in the Brunel network for the asynchronous irregular (AI) and synchronous regular (SR) state.

Parameter	Range SR	Range AI	Variable	Meaning
η	[1.5, 3.5]	[1.5, 3.5]	eta	External rate relative to threshold rate
g	[1, 3]	[5, 8]	g	Relative strength of inhibitory synapses
D	[1.5, 3]	[1.5, 3]	delay	Synaptic delay (ms)

Each parameter has a uniform distribution within the given range.

create 10,000 excitatory and 2,500 inhibitory neurons, with properties as specified by Brunel (2000). Each neuron has 1,000 randomly chosen connections to excitatory neurons and 250 randomly chosen connections to inhibitory neurons (a connection probability of $\epsilon = 0.1$). The weight of the excitatory synapses (amplitude of excitatory synaptic current) is $J = 0.1$ mV. We simulate the network for 1,000 ms, record the output from 20 of the excitatory neurons, and start the recording after 100 ms. The code for this case study is found in `uncertainpy/examples/brunel/`.

Three more parameters are needed to specify the Brunel model: (i) the external input rate (ν_{ext}) relative to the threshold rate (ν_{thr}) given as $\eta = \nu_{\text{ext}}/\nu_{\text{thr}}$, (ii) the relative strength of the inhibitory synapses compared to the excitatory synapses g, and (iii) the synaptic delay D. Depending on these parameters, the Brunel network may be in several different activity states. For the current case study we limit our analysis to two of these states, the synchronous regular (SR) state, where the neurons are almost completely synchronized, and the asynchronous irregular (AI) state, where the neurons fire mostly independently at low rates.

We create two sets of model parameters, one for the SR state and one for the AI state. For each set we assume that the uncertainties of the parameters η, g and D are characterized by uniform probability distributions within the ranges shown in **Table 4**. The parameter ranges are chosen so that all parameter combinations within the set give model behavior corresponding to one of the states. Two selected model results representative of the network in both states are shown in **Figure 7**, which illustrate the differences between the two states. **Figure 7** shows the recorded spike trains for the Brunel network in the SR state between 200 ms and 300 ms of the simulation. The results in this time window exemplifies network behavior during the entire simulation after spiking has started. Since the firing rate is very high in this state, only results for a limited time window are shown. **Figure 7B** shows the recorded spike trains for the Brunel network in the AI state for the entire simulation period.

We use the features in `NetworkFeatures` to examine features of the network dynamics. Of the 13 built-in network features in `NetworkFeatures`, we here only focus on two: the average interspike interval and the pairwise Pearson's correlation coefficient. These features are well suited to highlight the differences between the AI and SR network states, and to investigate how the details of the network dynamics depend on the model parameters within each of the states. We perform an uncertainty quantification and sensitivity analysis of the model and all features for each of the network states using polynomial chaos with point collocation. As for the previous examples we used the default polynomial order of $p = 4$ which was observed to be sufficient to achieve convergence, that is, the results did not change much when increasing p beyond 4.

We also explored the alternative situation where the excitatory synaptic weight J was included as a fourth uncertain parameter (with a similar relative spread as for the other uncertain parameters in **Table 4**). Here we observed that at least $p = 7$ (using the default number of collocation nodes) was needed to obtain accurate results. This illustrates that the required polynomial order, and by extension the required number of samples N_s, to get accurate results is problem dependent.

4.4.1. Average Interspike Interval

The average interspike interval is the average time it takes from a neuron produces a spike until it produces the next spike, averaged over all recorded neurons. The uncertainty quantification and sensitivity analysis of the average interspike interval of the Brunel network are shown in **Figure 8**. The average interspike interval is seen to differ strongly between the SR and AI states. In the high-firing SR state (**Figure 8A**), the mean of the average interspike interval is low, with a comparatively low standard deviation reflecting the synchronous firing in the network. We can observe this in **Figure 7A**, where the interspike intervals are short and do not vary much (i.e., very little standard deviation). In the comparatively low-firing AI state (**Figure 8B**), the mean of the average interspike interval is high, with a large standard deviation, reflecting the irregular firing in the network seen in **Figure 7B**.

The two states were also found to be different in terms of which parameters the average interspike interval is sensitive to. In the SR state the network is predominantly sensitive to the synaptic delay D. This reflects that in this state the neurons get very strong synaptic inputs so that the firing rate is mainly determined by the delay. In the AI state, the network is more balanced and "variance-driven", and the dynamics are to a large degree determined by the relative strength of the inhibitory synapses compared to the excitatory synapses g (Brunel, 2000). Thus the average interspike interval is observed in **Figure 7B** to, not surprisingly, be most sensitive to g. In the AI state the average interspike interval is quite long (~60 ms) so that an uncertainty in the synaptic delay of a couple of milliseconds (cf. **Table 4**) has little influence. Thus very little sensitivity to D is observed in this state.

4.4.2. Correlation Coefficient

The pairwise Pearson's correlation coefficient is a measure of how synchronous the spiking of a network is. This correlation coefficient measures the correlation between the spike trains of two neurons in the network. In **Figure 9** we examine how this correlation depends on parameter uncertainties by plotting the mean, standard deviation, and first-order Sobol indices for the pairwise Pearson's correlation coefficient in the SR and AI states.

As expected from examining **Figure 7**, the mean pairwise Pearson's correlation coefficient in the SR state (**Figure 9A**) is

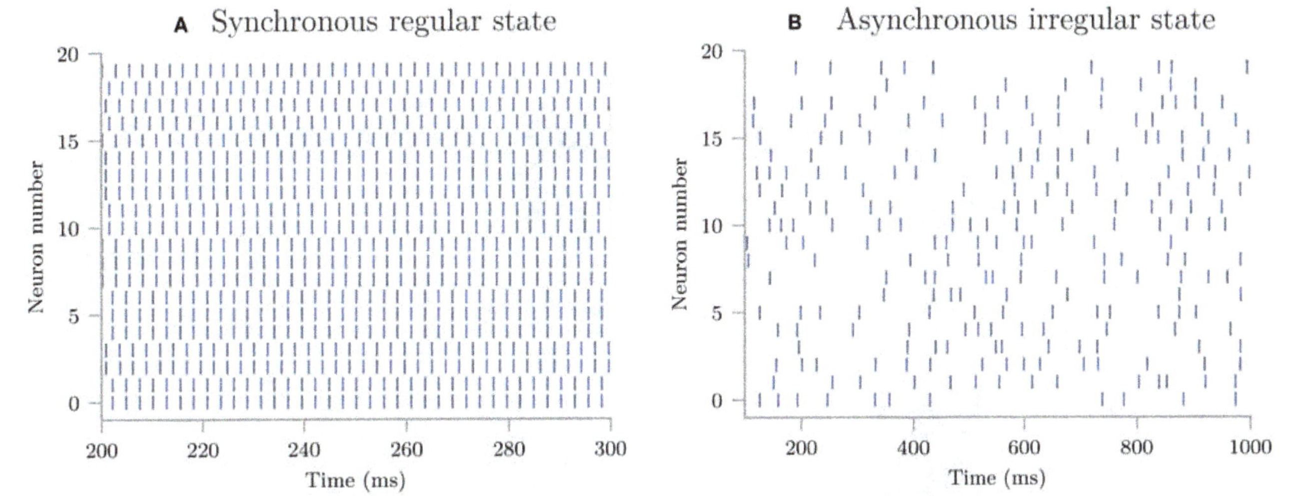

FIGURE 7 | Example model results for the Brunel network. **(A)** The recorded spike train for the Brunel network in the synchronous regular state between 200 and 300 ms of the simulation. **(B)** The recorded spike trains for the Brunel network in the asynchronous irregular state for the entire simulation period. The network has 10, 000 excitatory and 2, 500 inhibitory neurons, with properties as specified by Brunel (2000). Each neuron has 1, 000 randomly chosen connections to excitatory neurons and 250 randomly chosen connections to inhibitory neurons. We simulate the network for 1, 000 ms, record the output from 20 of the excitatory neurons, and start the recording after 100 ms.

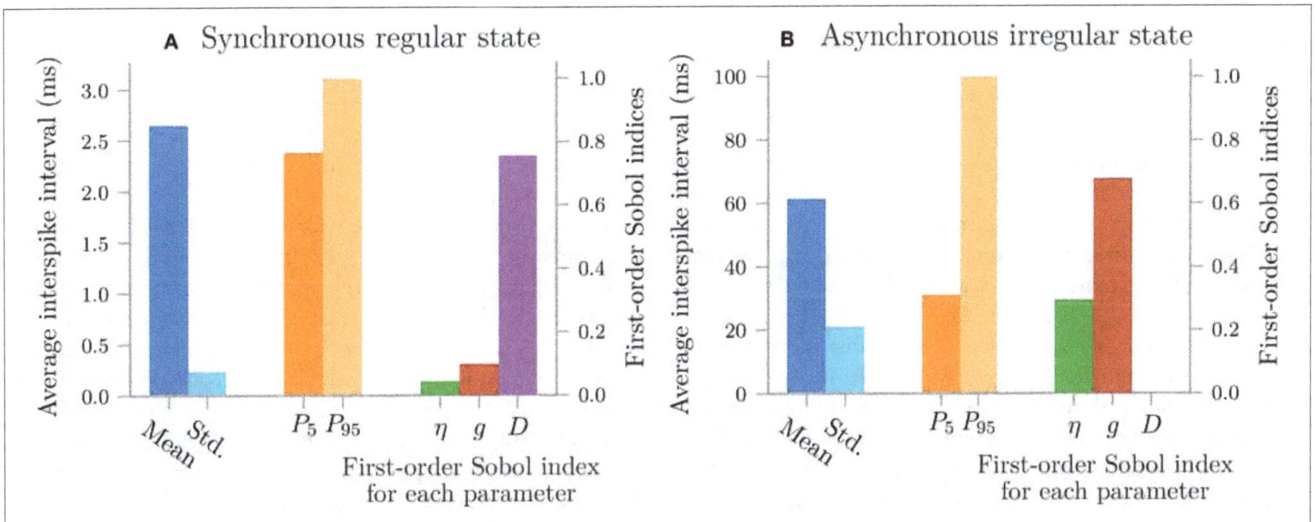

FIGURE 8 | The average interspike interval for the Brunel network in the two states. Mean, standard deviation, 90% prediction interval, and first-order Sobol indices of the average interspike interval of the Brunel network in the synchronous regular state **(A)**, and asynchronous irregular state **(B)**. The 90% prediction interval is indicated by the 5th and 95th percentiles, i.e., 90% of the average spike intervals are between P_5 and P_{95}.

much higher than in the AI state (**Figure 9D**). The first-order Sobol indices further show that the degree of synchronicity is by far most sensitive to the synaptic delay *D* when the network is in the SR state (**Figure 9C**), and most sensitive to the relative strength of inhibitory synapses *g* when the network is in the AI state (**Figure 9F**).

Thus, for both features investigated here (the average interspike interval and the mean pairwise Pearson's correlation coefficient), the conclusions regarding model sensitivity are the same. The SR state of the Brunel network is most sensitive to the synaptic delay *D*, while the AI state is most sensitive to the relative strength of inhibitory synapses *g*.

4.5. Comparing the Quasi-Monte Carlo Method to Polynomial Chaos Expansions

To compare the efficiency of the polynomial chaos expansions and the quasi-Monte Carlo method, we calculate the errors of the uncertainty quantification for the Hodgkin-Huxley model (section 4.2) using a varying number of model evaluations. The

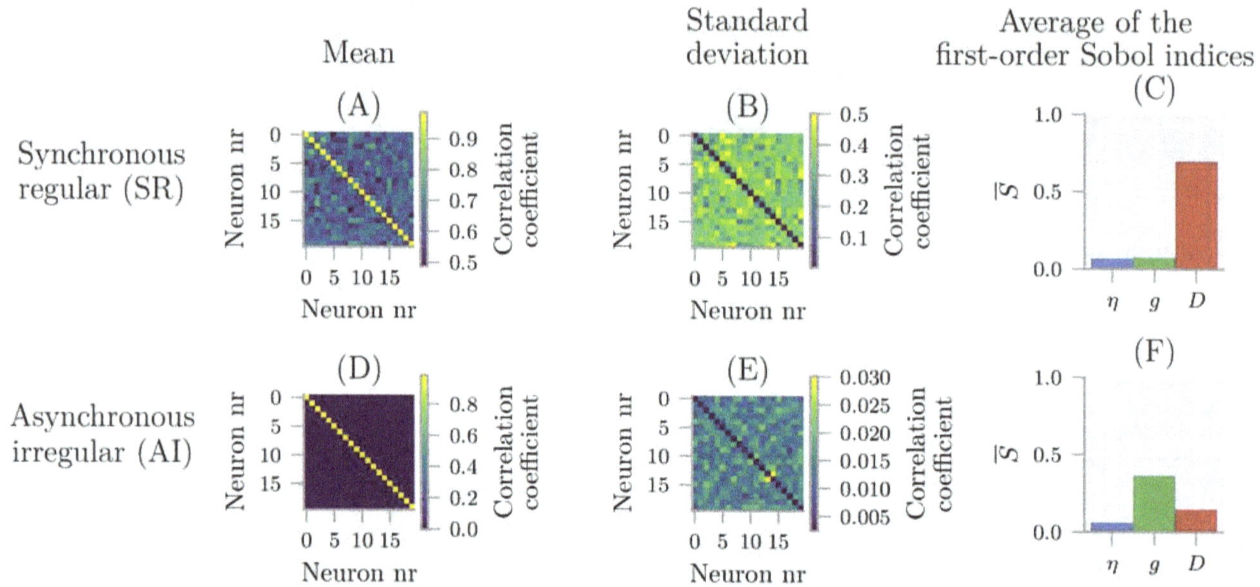

FIGURE 9 | The pairwise Pearson's correlation coefficient for the Brunel network in the two states. Mean **(A,D)**, standard deviation **(B,E)**, and first-order Sobol indices **(C,F)** for the pairwise Pearson's correlation coefficient of the Brunel network in the synchronous regular **(A–C)** and asynchronous irregular **(D–F)** states.

code for this comparison can be found in `uncertainpy/examples/mc_vs_pc`.

As efficiency measure we use the number of model evaluations N_s, since model evaluation generally is the computationally most costly step. We examine two versions of the Hodgkin-Huxley model to see how the efficiency of the two methods varies with the number of uncertain parameters. We use a reduced model with the three maximum conductances $\bar{g}_{\mathrm{Na}}$, $\bar{g}_{\mathrm{K}}$, and $\bar{g}_{\mathrm{L}}$ as uncertain parameters, and a complete model where all eleven parameters are uncertain. As in section 4.2, we assume each of these parameters to have a uniform distribution in the range ±10% around their original value. We use polynomial chaos expansions with the point-collocation method, where the number of evaluations equals the number of collocation nodes.

As error measure we use the average of the absolute relative error over time, which we simply will refer to as the error:

$$\varepsilon_X = \frac{1}{T}\int \frac{|X - X_{\mathrm{estimate}}|}{X} dt, \tag{22}$$

where "estimate" indicates the results from either the quasi-Monte Carlo method or the polynomial chaos expansions. T is the total simulation time in the model, disregarding the first 5 ms. X is either the mean $\mathbb{E}[Y]$, variance $\mathbb{V}[Y]$, or first-order Sobol indices S_i averaged over all parameters i.

Since an analytical solution for the Hodgkin-Huxley model is not available, we use the quasi-Monte Carlo method with 200,000 model evaluations to calculate the "exact" $\mathbb{E}[Y]$ and $\mathbb{V}[Y]$, and $100000(d+2)$ (where d is the number of uncertain parameters) model evaluations to calculate S_i. The quasi-Monte Carlo method is based on random sampling, so we calculate the average error of 50 re-runs for the quasi-Monte Carlo method, to get a more precise result.

The error of the mean, variance, and first-order Sobol indices of the two methods for the two variants of the model are shown in **Figure 10**. We clearly see that the polynomial chaos expansions are much faster than the quasi-Monte Carlo method for both test cases, that is, much fewer model evaluations N_s are needed to achieve a certain error.

Figure 10 shows the error for the Hodgkin-Huxley model with three uncertain parameters. In this case, the quasi-Monte Carlo method requires more than 200 times as many model evaluations as the polynomial chaos expansions to calculate the mean with an error of $\sim 10^{-5}$, and more than 2,500 times as many model evaluations to calculate the Sobol indices with an error of ~ 0.5.

Figure 10B shows the error for the Hodgkin-Huxley model with eleven uncertain parameters. By comparing with the results for three uncertain parameters, we observe that polynomial chaos expansions scale worse with the number of uncertain parameters than the quasi-Monte Carlo method. However, polynomial chaos expansions are still superior in regards to the required number of model evaluations. For the full Hodgkin-Huxley model, the quasi-Monte Carlo method needs more than ten times as many model evaluations as the polynomial chaos expansions to calculate the mean with an error of $\sim 2 \cdot 10^{-5}$. For the first-order Sobol indices the quasi-Monte Carlo method gives an error of more than 30 even after 65,000 evaluations. In contrast, the polynomial chaos expansions give an error of 0.26 after only 2,732 model evaluations.

4.6. Additional Examples

Additional examples for uncertainty quantification of the Izikevich neuron (Izhikevich, 2003), a reduced layer 5 pyramidal cell (Bahl et al., 2012), and a Hodgkin-Huxley model with shifted

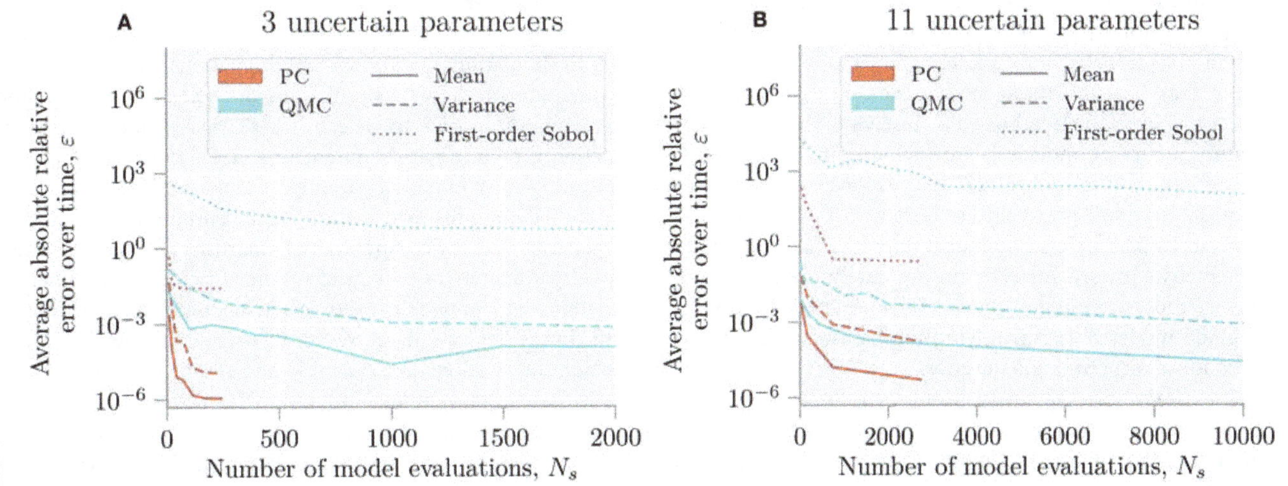

FIGURE 10 | The error of the mean, variance and (average) first-order Sobol indices for the quasi-Monte Carlo method (QMC) and polynomial chaos expansions (PC) used on the Hodgkin-Huxley model. The average of the absolute relative error over time of the mean (Equation 3), variance (Equation 4), and first-order Sobol indices (Equation 7) (averaged over all parameters i) of the Hodgkin-Huxley model with three **(A)** and eleven **(B)** uncertain parameters. The mean, variance and first-order Sobol indices are calculated using the quasi-Monte Carlo method with 50 re-runs, and polynomial chaos expansion with point collocation. The "exact" solutions are found using the quasi-Monte Carlo method with $N_S = 200000$ model evaluations to calculate the mean and variance, and $N_S = 100000(d + 2)$ model evaluations (where d is the number of uncertain parameters) to calculate the Sobol indices.

voltage (Sterratt et al., 2011) are found in `uncertainpy/examples/`.

5. DISCUSSION

A major challenge with models in neuroscience is that they tend to contain several uncertain parameters whose values are critical for the model behavior. In this paper we have presented Uncertainpy, a Python toolbox which quantifies how uncertainty in model parameters translates into uncertainty in the model output and how sensitive the model output is to changes in individual model parameters. Uncertainpy is tailored for neuroscience applications by its built-in capability for recognizing features in the model output.

The key aim of Uncertainpy is to make it quick and easy for the user to get started with uncertainty quantification and sensitivity analysis, without any need for detailed prior knowledge of uncertainty analysis. Uncertainpy is applicable to a wide range of different model types, as illustrated in the example applications. These included an uncertainty quantification and sensitivity analysis of four different models: a simple cooling coffee-cup model (section 4.1), the original Hodgkin-Huxley model for generation of action potentials (section 4.2), a multi-compartmental NEURON model of a thalamic interneuron (section 4.3), and a NEST model of a sparsely connected recurrent (Brunel) network of integrate-and-fire neurons (section 4.4). These analyses were mainly performed to illustrate the use of Uncertainpy, but also revealed both expected and unexpected features of the example models. However, we did not put any effort into estimating realistic distributions for the parameter uncertainties. The conclusions should therefore be treated with caution; see result sections for a detailed discussion.

To our knowledge, Uncertainpy is the first toolbox to use polynomial chaos expansions to perform uncertainty quantification and sensitivity analysis in neuroscience. Compared to the (quasi-)Monte Carlo method, polynomial chaos expansions dramatically reduce the number of model evaluations needed to get reliable statistics when the number of uncertain parameters is relatively low, typically smaller than about 20 (Xiu and Hesthaven, 2005; Crestaux et al., 2009; Eck et al., 2016). This was also observed in the present study where we in section 4.5 found that polynomial chaos expansions require one to three orders of magnitude fewer model evaluations than the quasi-Monte Carlo method when applied to the Hodgkin-Huxley model with three or eleven uncertain parameters. This gain in efficiency is especially important for models that require a long simulation time, where uncertainty quantification using the (quasi-)Monte Carlo method could require an unfeasible amount of computer time.

5.1. Application of Uncertainpy

Uncertainpy is a computationally efficient Python toolbox that enables uncertainty quantification and sensitivity analysis for computational models. It is tailored toward neuroscience applications by its built-in capability for calculating characteristic features of the model output. While Uncertainpy has a broad applicability, as demonstrated in this paper, certain limitations exist. The first, and perhaps most obvious, is that Uncertainpy does not deal with the problem of obtaining the distributions of the uncertain parameters.

It is also typically not obvious which model is best suited to describe a particular system. For example, when we construct a neural model we first have to decide which mechanisms (ion channels, ion pumps, synapses, network connectivity, etc.) to include in the model. Next, we select a set of mathematical equations that describe these mechanisms. Such choices are seldom trivial, and no methods for resolving this structural uncertainty aspect of modeling are included in Uncertainpy. Nevertheless, quantitative measures such as those obtained with Uncertainpy may still give valuable insight in the relationship between model parameters and model output, which can guide experimentalists toward focusing on accurately measuring the parameters most critical for the model output. Additionally, it can guide modelers by identifying mechanisms that can be sacrificed for model reduction purposes.

The accuracy of the quasi-Monte Carlo method and polynomial chaos expansions is problem dependent and is determined by the number of samples, as well as the polynomial order for polynomial chaos expansions. It is therefore a good practice to examine if the results from the uncertainty quantification and sensitivity analysis have converged (Eck et al., 2016). A simple method for checking the convergence is to change the number of samples or polynomial order, or both, and examine the differences between the results. We can be reasonably certain that the results are accurate once these differences are small enough.

5.2. Further Development of Uncertainpy

There are several ways that Uncertainpy can be further developed. If a model or features of a model are irregular, Uncertainpy performs an interpolation of the output to get the results on the regular form needed in the uncertainty quantification and sensitivity analysis. Currently, Uncertainpy only has support for interpolation of one-dimensional output (vectors), but this aspect can be improved.

The screening method available in Uncertainpy is unable to take interactions between parameters into account. More advanced screening methods able to do this exist (Morris, 1991; Campolongo et al., 2007) and could be implemented.

The built-in feature library in Uncertainpy can easily be expanded by adding additional features. The number of built-in simulators (at present NEST and NEURON) can also easily be extended. We encourage the users to add custom features and models through Github pull requests.

5.3. Outlook

In many fields of the physical sciences, the model parameters that go into simulations are known with high accuracy. For example, in quantum mechanical simulations of molecular systems, the masses of the nuclei and electrons, as well as the parameters describing their electrical interaction, are known so precisely that uncertainty in model parameters is not an issue (Marx and Hutter, 2009). This is not the case in computational biology in general, and in computational neuroscience in particular. Model parameters of biological systems often have an inherent variability and some may even be actively regulated and change with time. They can therefore not be precisely known. We thus consider uncertainty quantification and sensitivity analysis to be particularly important in computational biology.

Uncertainpy was developed with the aim of enabling such analysis, that is, to provide an easy-to-use tool for precise evaluation of the effect of uncertain model parameters on model predictions. Being an open-source Python toolbox, we hope that Uncertainpy can be further developed through a joint effort within the neuroscience community.

AUTHOR CONTRIBUTIONS

ST, GH, and GE conceived of and designed the project. ST designed, wrote, tested, and documented the software and performed analysis of the examples. ST, GH, and GE wrote and revised the paper.

FUNDING

This work was funded by the Research Council of Norway (DigiBrain, project no: 248828).

ACKNOWLEDGMENTS

We would like to acknowledge the vital contribution to the vision of this work by Hans-Petter Langtangen, who regretfully passed away before he could see the work completed. We would also like acknowledge the help from Jonathan Feinberg in teaching the basics of polynomial chaos expansions, as well as how to use Chaospy. Additionally, we would like to thank Svenn-Arne Dragly, Milad H. Mobarhan, and Andreas Våvang Solbrå for valuable discussions and feedback.

REFERENCES

Achard, P., and De Schutter, E. (2006). Complex parameter landscape for a complex neuron model. *PLoS Comput. Biol.* 2:e94. doi: 10.1371/journal.pcbi.0020094

Allken, V., Chepkoech, J.-L., Einevoll, G. T., and Halnes, G. (2014). The subcellular distribution of T-type Ca2+ channels in interneurons of the lateral geniculate nucleus. *PLoS ONE* 9:e107780. doi: 10.1371/journal.pone.0107780

Babtie, A. C., and Stumpf, M. P. H. (2017). How to deal with parameters for whole-cell modelling. *J. R. Soc Interface* 14. doi: 10.1098/rsif.2017.0237

Bahl, A., Stemmler, M., Herz, A., and Roth, A. (2012). Automated optimization of a reduced layer 5 pyramidal cell model based on experimental data. *J. Neurosci. Methods* 210, 22–34. doi: 10.1016/j.jneumeth.2012.04.006

Beck, M. B. (1987). Water quality modeling: a review of the analysis of uncertainty. *Water Resour. Res.* 23, 1393–1442.

Beer, R. D., Chiel, H. J., and Gallagher, J. C. (1999). Evolution and analysis of model CPGs for walking: II. General principles and individual variability. *J. Comput. Neurosci.* 7, 119–147.

Bhalla, U. S., and Bower, J. M. (1993). Exploring parameter space in detailed single neuron models: simulations of the mitral and granule cells of the olfactory bulb. *J. Neurophysiol.* 69, 1948–1965.

Blomquist, P., Devor, A., Indahl, U. G., Ulbert, I., Einevoll, G. T., and Dale, A. M. (2009). Estimation of thalamocortical and intracortical network models from joint thalamic single-electrode and cortical laminar-electrode recordings in the rat barrel system. *PLoS Comput. Biol.* 5:e1000328. doi: 10.1371/journal.pcbi.1000328

Blot, A., and Barbour, B. (2014). Ultra-rapid axon-axon ephaptic inhibition of cerebellar Purkinje cells by the pinceau. *Nat. Neurosci.* 17, 289–295. doi: 10.1038/nn.3624

Blue Brain Project (2015). *efel*. Available online at: https://github.com/BlueBrain/eFEL (Accessed June 16, 2018).

Borgonovo, E., and Plischke, E. (2016). Sensitivity analysis: a review of recent advances. *Eur. J. Oper. Res.* 248, 869–887. doi: 10.1016/j.ejor.2015.06.032

Brodland, G. W. (2015). How computational models can help unlock biological systems. *Semin. Cell Dev. Biol.* 47–48, 62–73. doi: 10.1016/j.semcdb.2015.07.001

Brunel, N. (2000). Dynamics of sparsely connected networks of excitatory and inhibitory spiking neurons. *J. Comput. Neurosci.* 8, 183–208. doi: 10.1023/A:1008925309027

Campolongo, F., Cariboni, J., and Saltelli, A. (2007). An effective screening design for sensitivity analysis of large models. *Environ. Model. Softw.* 22, 1509–1518. doi: 10.1016/j.envsoft.2006.10.004

Collette, A. (2013). *Python and HDF5*. Sebastopool, CA: O'Reilly.

Crestaux, T., Le Maître, O., and Martinez, J. M. (2009). Polynomial chaos expansion for sensitivity analysis. *Reliabil. Eng. Syst. Saf.* 94, 1161–1172. doi: 10.1016/j.ress.2008.10.008

Dayan, P., and Abbott, L. F. (2001). *Theoretical Neuroscience: Computational and Mathematical Modeling of Neural Systems*. Cambridge, MA: The MIT Press.

De Schutter, E., and Bower, J. M. (1994). An active membrane model of the cerebellar Purkinje cell II. Simulation of synaptic responses. *J. Neurophysiol.* 71, 401–419.

Degenring, D., Froemel, C., Dikta, G., and Takors, R. (2004). Sensitivity analysis for the reduction of complex metabolism models. *J. Process Control* 14, 729–745. doi: 10.1016/j.jprocont.2003.12.008

Dragly, S.-A., Hobbi Mobarhan, M., Lepperød, M. E., Tennøe, S., Fyhn, M., Hafting, T., et al. (2018). Experimental directory structure (exdir): an alternative to hdf5 without introducing a new file format. *Front. Neuroinformatics* 12:16. doi: 10.3389/fninf.2018.00016

Druckmann, S., Banitt, Y., Gidon, A. A., Schürmann, F., Markram, H., and Segev, I. (2007). A novel multiple objective optimization framework for constraining conductance-based neuron models by experimental data. *Front. Neurosci.* 1, 7–18. doi: 10.3389/neuro.01.1.1.001.2007

Eck, V. G., Donders, W. P., Sturdy, J., Feinberg, J., Delhaas, T., Hellevik, L. R., et al. (2016). A guide to uncertainty quantification and sensitivity analysis for cardiovascular applications. *Int. J. Numer. Methods Biomed. Eng.* 32:e02755. doi: 10.1002/cnm.2755

Edelman, G. M., and Gally, J. A. (2001). Degeneracy and complexity in biological systems. *Proc. Natl. Acad. Sci. U.S.A.* 98, 13763–13768. doi: 10.1073/pnas.231499798

Einevoll, G. T. (2009). Sharing with Python. *Front. Neurosci.* 3, 334–335. doi: 10.3389/neuro.01.037.2009

Feinberg, J., and Langtangen, H. P. (2015). Chaospy: an open source tool for designing methods of uncertainty quantification. *J. Comput. Sci.* 11, 46–57. doi: 10.1016/j.jocs.2015.08.008

Ferson, S., and Ginzburg, L. R. (1996). Different methods are needed to propagate ignorance and variability. *Reliabil. Eng. Syst. Saf.* 54, 133–144.

Ferson, S., Joslyn, C. A., Helton, J. C., Oberkampf, W. L., and Sentz, K. (2004). Summary from the epistemic uncertainty workshop: Consensus amid diversity. *Reliab. Eng. Syst. Saf.* 85, 355–369. doi: 10.1016/j.ress.2004.03.023

Garcia, S., Guarino, D., Jaillet, F., Jennings, T., Pröpper, R., Rautenberg, P. L., et al. (2014). Neo: an object model for handling electrophysiology data in multiple formats. *Front. Neuroinformatics* 8:10. doi: 10.3389/fninf.2014.00010

Glen, G., and Isaacs, K. (2012). Estimating Sobol sensitivity indices using correlations. *Environ. Model. Softw.* 37, 157–166. doi: 10.1016/j.envsoft.2012.03.014

Goldman, M. S., Golowasch, J., Marder, E., and Abbott, L. F. (2001). Global structure, robustness, and modulation of neuronal models. *J. Neurosci.* 21, 5229–5238. doi: 10.1523/JNEUROSCI.21-14-05229.2001

Golowasch, J., Goldman, M. S., Abbott, L. F., and Marder, E. (2002). Failure of averaging in the construction of a conductance-based neuron model. *J. Neurophysiol.* 87, 1129–1131. doi: 10.1152/jn.00412.2001

Gutenkunst, R. N., Waterfall, J. J., Casey, F. P., Brown, K. S., Myers, C. R., and Sethna, J. P. (2007). Universally sloppy parameter sensitivities in systems biology models. *PLoS Comput. Biol.* 3, 1871–1878. doi: 10.1371/journal.pcbi.0030189

Halnes, G., Augustinaite, S., Heggelund, P., Einevoll, G. T., and Migliore, M. (2011). A multi-compartment model for interneurons in the dorsal lateral geniculate nucleus. *PLoS Comput. Biol.* 7:e1002160. doi: 10.1371/journal.pcbi.1002160

Halnes, G., Liljenström, H., and Århem, P. (2007). Density dependent neurodynamics. *Biosystems* 89, 126–134. doi: 10.1016/j.biosystems.2006.06.010

Halnes, G., Ulfhielm, E., Eklöf Ljunggren, E., Kotaleski, J. H., and Rospars, J. P. (2009). Modelling and sensitivity analysis of the reactions involving receptor, G-protein and effector in vertebrate olfactory receptor neurons. *J. Comput. Neurosci.* 27, 471–491. doi: 10.1007/s10827-009-0162-6

Hamby, D. M. (1994). A review of techniques for parameter sensitivity analysis of environmental models. *Environ. Monit. Assess.* 32, 135–154.

Hammersley, J. M. (1960). Monte carlo methods for solving multivariable problems. *Ann. N. Y. Acad. Sci.* 86, 844–874.

Hay, E., Schürmann, F., Markram, H., and Segev, I. (2013). Preserving axosomatic spiking features despite diverse dendritic morphology. *J. Neurophysiol.* 109, 2972–2981. doi: 10.1152/jn.00048.2013

Herman, J., and Usher, W. (2017). SALib: an open-source python library for sensitivity analysis. *J. Open Source Softw.* 2:97. doi: 10.21105/joss.00097

Hines, M. L., and Carnevale, N. T. (1997). The NEURON Simulation Environment. *Neural Comput.* 9, 1179–1209.

Hodgkin, A. L., and Huxley, A. F. (1952). A quantitative description of membrane current and its application to conduction and excitation in nerve. *J. Physiol.* 117, 500–544.

Homma, T., and Saltelli, A. (1996). Importance measures in global sensitivity analysis of nonlinear models. *Reliabil. Eng. Syst. Saf.* 52, 1–17.

Hora, S. C. (1996). Aleatory and epistemic uncertainty in probability elicitation with an example from hazardous waste management. *Reliabil. Eng. Syst. Saf.* 54, 217–223.

Hosder, S., Walters, R., and Balch, M. (2007). Efficient sampling for non-intrusive polynomial chaos applications with multiple uncertain input variables. in *48th AIAA/ASME/ASCE/AHS/ASC Structures, Structural Dynamics, and Materials Conference* (Honolulu, HI).

Izhikevich, E. M. (2003). Simple model of spiking neurons. *IEEE Trans. Neural Netw* 14, 1569–1572. doi: 10.1109/TNN.2003.820440

Izhikevich, E. M., and Edelman, G. M. (2008). Large-scale model of mammalian thalamocortical systems. *Proc. Natl. Acad. Sci. U.S.A.* 105, 3593–3598. doi: 10.1073/pnas.0712231105

Kiureghian, A. D., and Ditlevsen, O. (2009). Aleatory or epistemic? Does it matter? *Struct. Saf.* 31, 105–112. doi: 10.1016/j.strusafe.2008.06.020

Koch, C., and Segev, I. (eds.) (1998). *Methods in Neuronal Modeling: From Ions to Networks, 2nd Edn*. Cambridge, MA: MIT Press.

Kuchibhotla, K. V., Gill, J. V., Lindsay, G. W., Papadoyannis, E. S., Field, R. E., Sten, T. A., et al. (2017). Parallel processing by cortical inhibition enables context-dependent behavior. *Nat. Neurosci.* 20, 62–71. doi: 10.1038/nn.4436

Leamer, E. (1985). Sensitivity analyses would help. *Am. Econ. Rev.* 75, 308–313.

Lemieux, C. (2009). *Monte Carlo and Quasi-Monte Carlo Sampling. Springer Series in Statistics*. Dordrecht: Springer.

Marder, E., and Goaillard, J. M. (2006). Variability, compensation and homeostasis in neuron and network function. *Nat. Rev. Neurosci.* 7, 563–574. doi: 10.1038/nrn1949

Marder, E., and Taylor, A. L. (2011). Multiple models to capture the variability in biological neurons and networks. *Nat. Neurosci.* 14, 133–138. doi: 10.1038/nn.2735

Marino, S., Hogue, I. B., Ray, C. J., and Kirschner, D. E. (2008). A methodology for performing global uncertainty and sensitivity analysis in systems biology. *J. Theor. Biol.* 254, 178–196. doi: 10.1016/j.jtbi.2008.04.011

Markram, H., Muller, E., Ramaswamy, S., Reimann, M. W., Abdellah, M., Sanchez, C. A.,et al. (2015). Reconstruction and simulation of neocortical microcircuitry. *Cell* 163, 456–492. doi: 10.1016/j.cell.2015.09.029

Marx, D., and Hutter, J. (2009). *Ab initio Molecular Dynamics: Basic Theory and Advanced Method*. Cambridge, UK: Cambridge University Press.

McKerns, M. M., Strand, L., Sullivan, T., Fang, A., and Aivazis, M. A. G. (2012). Building a framework for predictive science. *CoRR*, (Scipy):1–12.

Merolla, P. A., Arthur, J. V., Alvarez-Icaza, R., Cassidy, A. S., Sawada, J., Akopyan, F., et al. (2014). A million spiking-neuron integrated circuit with a scalable communication network and interface. *Science* 345, 668–673. doi: 10.1126/science.1254642

Morris, M. D. (1991). Factorial sampling plans for preliminary computational experiments. *Technometrics* 33, 161–174.

Muller, E., Bednar, J. A., Diesmann, M., Gewaltig, M.-O., Hines, M., and Davison, A. P. (2015). Python in neuroscience. *Front. Neuroinformatics* 9:11. doi: 10.3389/fninf.2015.00011

Mullins, J., Ling, Y., Mahadevan, S., Sun, L., and Strachan, A. (2016). Separation of aleatory and epistemic uncertainty in probabilistic model validation. *Reliabil. Eng. Syst. Saf.* 147, 49–59. doi: 10.1016/j.ress.2015.10.003

Najm, H. N. (2009). Uncertainty quantification and polynomial chaos techniques in computational fluid dynamics. *Annu. Rev. Fluid Mech.* 41, 35–52. doi: 10.1146/annurev.fluid.010908.165248

Narayan, A., and Jakeman, J. (2014). Adaptive Leja sparse grid constructions for stochastic collocation and high-dimensional approximation. *SIAM J. Sci. Comput.* 36, A2952–A2983. doi: 10.1137/140966368

NeuralEnsemble (2017). *Elephant - electrophysiology analysis toolkit*. Available online at: https://github.com/NeuralEnsemble/elephant (Accessed June 16, 2018).

Oberkampf, W. L., DeLand, S. M., Rutherford, B. M., Diegert, K. V., and Alvin, K. F. (2002). Error and uncertainty in modeling and simulation. *Reliabil. Eng. Syst. Saf.* 75, 333–357. doi: 10.1016/S0951-8320(01)00120-X

O'Donnell, C., Gonçalves, J. T., Portera-Cailliau, C., and Sejnowski, T. J. (2017). Beyond excitation/inhibition imbalance in multidimensional models of neural circuit changes in brain disorders. *eLife* 6:e26724. doi: 10.7554/eLife.26724

Oliphant, T. E. (2007). Python for scientific computing. *Comput. Sci. Eng.* 9, 10–20. doi: 10.1109/MCSE.2007.58

Peyser, A., Sinha, A., Vennemo, S. B., Ippen, T., Jordan, J., Graber, S., et al. (2017). *Nest 2.14.0*.

Prinz, A. A., Bucher, D., and Marder, E. (2004). Similar network activity from disparate circuit parameters. *Nat. Neurosci.* 7, 1345–1352. doi: 10.1038/nn1352

Rifkin, R. M., and Lippert, R. A. (2007). *Notes on Regularized Least Squares*. Cambridge, MA: Massachusetts Institute of Technology.

Rosenblatt, M. (1952). Remarks on a Multivariate Transformation. *Ann. Math. Stat.* 23, 470–472.

Rossa, A., Liechti, K., Zappa, M., Bruen, M., Germann, U., Haase, G., et al. (2011). The COST 731 Action: a review on uncertainty propagation in advanced hydro-meteorological forecast systems. *Atmos. Res.* 100, 150–167. doi: 10.1016/j.atmosres.2010.11.016

Saltelli, A. (2002a). Making best use of model valuations to compute sensitivity indices. *Comput. Phys. Commun.* 145, 280–297. doi: 10.1016/S0010-4655(02)00280-1

Saltelli, A. (2002b). Sensitivity analysis for importance assessment. *Risk Anal.* 22, 579–590. doi: 10.1111/0272-4332.00040

Saltelli, A., Annoni, P., Azzini, I., Campolongo, F., Ratto, M., and Tarantola, S. (2010). Variance based sensitivity analysis of model output. Design and estimator for the total sensitivity index. *Comput. Phys. Commun.* 181, 259–270. doi: 10.1016/j.cpc.2009.09.018

Saltelli, A., Ratto, M., Andres, T., Campolongo, F., Cariboni, J., Gatelli, D., et al. (2007). *Global Sensitivity Analysis. The Primer*. Chichester, UK: Wiley.

Schulz, D. J., Goaillard, J.-M., and Marder, E. (2007). Quantitative expression profiling of identified neurons reveals cell-specific constraints on highly variable levels of gene expression. *Proc. Natl. Acad. Sci. U.S.A.* 104, 13187–13191. doi: 10.1073/pnas.0705827104

Sharp, D., and Wood-Schultz, M. (2003). Qmu and nuclear weapons certification: What's under the hood? *Los Alamos Sci.* 28, 47–53.

Smolyak, S. (1963). Quadrature and interpolation formulas for tensor products of certain classes of functions. *Dokl. Akad. Nauk SSSR* 148, 1042–1045.

Snowden, T. J., van der Graaf, P. H., and Tindall, M. J. (2017). Methods of model reduction for large-scale biological systems: a survey of current methods and trends. *Bull. Math. Biol.* 79, 1449–1486. doi: 10.1007/s11538-017-0277-2

Sobol, I. M. (1967). On the distribution of points in a cube and the approximate evaluation of integrals. *USSR Comput. Math. Math. Phys.* 7, 86–112.

Sobol, I. M. (1990). Sensitivity analysis for nonlinear mathematical models. *Matematicheskoe Modelirovanie* 2, 112–118.

Sterratt, D., Graham, B., Gillies, A., and Willshaw, D. (2011). *Principles of Computational Modelling in Neuroscience*. Cambridge, UK: Cambridge University Press.

Stieltjes, T. J. (1884). Quelques recherches sur la théorie des quadratures dites mécaniques. *Ann. Sci. 'École Normale Supérieure* 1, 409–426.

Sudret, B. (2008). Global sensitivity analysis using polynomial chaos expansions. *Reliab. Eng. Syst. Saf.* 93, 964–979. doi: 10.1016/j.ress.2007.04.002

Taylor, A. L., Goaillard, J.-M., and Marder, E. (2009). How multiple conductances determine electrophysiological properties in a multicompartment model. *J. Neurosci.* 29, 5573–5586. doi: 10.1523/JNEUROSCI.4438-08.2009

Tobin, A.-E. (2006). Endogenous and half-center bursting in morphologically inspired models of leech heart interneurons. *J. Neurophysiol.* 96, 2089–2106. doi: 10.1152/jn.00025.2006

Torres Valderrama, A., Witteveen, J., Navarro, M., and Blom, J. (2015). Uncertainty propagation in nerve impulses through the action potential mechanism. *J. Math. Neurosci.* 5:3. doi: 10.1186/2190-8567-5-3

Turanyi, T., and Turányi, T. (1990). Sensitivity analysis of comprex kinetic systems. Tools and applications. *J. Math. Chem.* 5, 203–248.

Van Geit, W., De Schutter, E., and Achard, P. (2008). Automated neuron model optimization techniques: A review. *Biol. Cybern.* 99, 241–251. doi: 10.1007/s00422-008-0257-6

Wang, H., and Sheen, D. A. (2015). Combustion kinetic model uncertainty quantification, propagation and minimization. *Prog. Energy Combust. Sci.* 47, 1–31. doi: 10.1016/j.pecs.2014.10.002

Xiu, D. (2010). *Numerical Methods for Stochastic Computations: A Spectral Method Approach*. Princeton, NJ: Princeton University Press.

Xiu, D., and Hesthaven, J. S. (2005). High-order collocation methods for differential equations with random inputs. *SIAM J. Sci. Comput.* 27, 1118–1139. doi: 10.1137/040615201

Yildirim, B., and Karniadakis, G. E. (2015). Stochastic simulations of ocean waves: an uncertainty quantification study. *Ocean Model.* 86, 15–35. doi: 10.1016/j.ocemod.2014.12.001

Zhu, J. J., Uhlrich, D. J., and Lytton, W. W. (1999). Burst firing in identified rat geniculate interneurons. *Neuroscience* 91, 1445–1460.

Zi, Z. (2011). Sensitivity analysis approaches applied to systems biology models. *IET Syst. Biol.* 5, 336–346. doi: 10.1049/iet-syb.2011.0015

Permissions

All chapters in this book were first published by Frontiers; hereby published with permission under the Creative Commons Attribution License or equivalent. Every chapter published in this book has been scrutinized by our experts. Their significance has been extensively debated. The topics covered herein carry significant findings which will fuel the growth of the discipline. They may even be implemented as practical applications or may be referred to as a beginning point for another development.

The contributors of this book come from diverse backgrounds, making this book a truly international effort. This book will bring forth new frontiers with its revolutionizing research information and detailed analysis of the nascent developments around the world.

We would like to thank all the contributing authors for lending their expertise to make the book truly unique. They have played a crucial role in the development of this book. Without their invaluable contributions this book wouldn't have been possible. They have made vital efforts to compile up to date information on the varied aspects of this subject to make this book a valuable addition to the collection of many professionals and students.

This book was conceptualized with the vision of imparting up-to-date information and advanced data in this field. To ensure the same, a matchless editorial board was set up. Every individual on the board went through rigorous rounds of assessment to prove their worth. After which they invested a large part of their time researching and compiling the most relevant data for our readers.

The editorial board has been involved in producing this book since its inception. They have spent rigorous hours researching and exploring the diverse topics which have resulted in the successful publishing of this book. They have passed on their knowledge of decades through this book. To expedite this challenging task, the publisher supported the team at every step. A small team of assistant editors was also appointed to further simplify the editing procedure and attain best results for the readers.

Apart from the editorial board, the designing team has also invested a significant amount of their time in understanding the subject and creating the most relevant covers. They scrutinized every image to scout for the most suitable representation of the subject and create an appropriate cover for the book.

The publishing team has been an ardent support to the editorial, designing and production team. Their endless efforts to recruit the best for this project, has resulted in the accomplishment of this book. They are a veteran in the field of academics and their pool of knowledge is as vast as their experience in printing. Their expertise and guidance has proved useful at every step. Their uncompromising quality standards have made this book an exceptional effort. Their encouragement from time to time has been an inspiration for everyone.

The publisher and the editorial board hope that this book will prove to be a valuable piece of knowledge for researchers, students, practitioners and scholars across the globe.

List of Contributors

Hans E. Plesser
Faculty of Science and Technology, Norwegian University of Life Sciences, Ås, Norway
Institute for Neuroscience and Medicine (INM-6), Jülich Research Centre, Jülich, Germany

Tiina Manninen, Jugoslava Aćimović, Riikka Havela, Heidi Teppola and Marja-Leena Linne
Computational Neuroscience Group, BioMediTech Institute and Faculty of Biomedical Sciences and Engineering, Tampere University of Technology, Tampere, Finland
Laboratory of Signal Processing, Tampere University of Technology, Tampere, Finland

Gubbi Vani HarshaRani and Upinder S. Bhalla
National Centre for Biological Sciences, Tata Institute of Fundamental Research, Bangalore, India

Nisha A. Viswan
National Centre for Biological Sciences, Tata Institute of Fundamental Research, Bangalore, India
The University of Trans-Disciplinary Health Sciences and Technology, Bangalore, India

Melanie I. Stefan
Centre for Discovery Brain Sciences, University of Edinburgh, Edinburgh, United Kingdom
ZJU-UoE Institute, Zhejiang University, Hangzhou, China

Zbigniew Ję drzejewski-Szmek and Joanna Ję drzejewska-Szmek
Krasnow Institute of Advanced Study, George Mason University, Fairfax, VA, United States

Karina P. Abrahao and David M. Lovinger
Laboratory for Integrative Neuroscience, Section on Synaptic Pharmacology, National Institute on Alcohol Abuse and Alcoholism, National Institutes of Health, Rockville, MD, United States

Kim T. Blackwell
Krasnow Institute of Advanced Study, George Mason University, Fairfax, VA, United States
Department of Bioengineering, Volgenau School of Engineering, George Mason University, Fairfax, VA, United States

Andrew Drach
The Institute for Computational Engineering and Sciences, The University of Texas at Austin, Austin, TX, United States

Lealem Mulugeta
InSilico Labs LLC, Houston, TX, United States

Ahmet Erdemir
Department of Biomedical Engineering and Computational Biomodeling (CoBi) Core, Lerner Research Institute, Cleveland Clinic, Cleveland, OH, United States

C. A. Hunt
Department of Bioengineering and Therapeutic Sciences, University of California, San Francisco, San Francisco, CA, United States

Marc Horner
ANSYS, Inc., Evanston, IL, United States

Joy P. Ku
Department of Bioengineering, Stanford University, Stanford, CA, United States

Jerry G. Myers Jr.
NASA Glenn Research Center, Cleveland, OH, United States

Rajanikanth Vadigepalli
Department of Pathology, Anatomy and Cell Biology, Daniel Baugh Institute for Functional Genomics and Computational Biology, Thomas Jefferson University, Philadelphia, PA, United States

William W. Lytton
Department of Neurology, SUNY Downstate Medical Center, The State University of New York, New York, NY, United States
Department of Physiology and Pharmacology, SUNY Downstate Medical Center, The State University of New York, New York, NY, United States
Department of Neurology, Kings County Hospital Center, New York, NY, United States

Na Zhao, Xi-Ze Jia, Xu-Feng Zhou, Xin-Ping Deng, Jue Wang and Yu-Feng Zang
Center for Cognition and Brain Disorders, Institutes of Psychological Sciences, Hangzhou Normal University, Hangzhou,China
Zhejiang Key Laboratory for Research in Assessment of Cognitive Impairments, Hangzhou, China

Christian Nowke, Benjamin Weyers, Bernd Hentschel and Torsten W. Kuhlen
Visual Computing Institute, RWTH Aachen University, JARA-HPC, Aachen, Germany

Hong-Jian He, Jianhui Zhong and Li-Xia Yuan
Center for Brain Imaging Science and Technology, Key Laboratory for Biomedical Engineering of Ministry of Education, College of Biomedical Engineering and Instrumental Science, Zhejiang University, Hangzhou, China

Susanne Kunkel
Faculty of Science and Technology, Norwegian University of Life Sciences, Ås, Norway
Department of Computational Science and Technology, School of Computer Science and Communication, KTH Royal Institute of Technology, Stockholm, Sweden

Abigail Morrison
SimLab Neuroscience, Jülich Supercomputing Centre (JSC), Institute for Advanced Simulation, JARA, Forschungszentrum Jülich GmbH, Jülich, Germany
Institute of Neuroscience and Medicine, Institute for Advanced Simulation, JARA Institute Brain Structure-Function Relationships, Forschungszentrum Jülich GmbH, Jülich, Germany
Institute of Cognitive Neuroscience, Faculty of Psychology, Ruhr-University Bochum, Bochum, Germany
Institute of Neuroscience and Medicine (INM-6) and Institute for Advanced Simulation (IAS-6) and JARA BRAIN Institute I, Jülich Research Centre, Jülich, Germany

Guido Trensch
Simulation Lab Neuroscience, Jülich Supercomputing Centre, Institute for Advanced Simulation, JARA, Jülich Research Centre, Jülich, Germany

Robin Gutzen, Inga Blundell and Michael Denker
Institute of Neuroscience and Medicine (INM-6) and Institute for Advanced Simulation (IAS-6) and JARA Institute Brain Structure-Function Relationships (INM-10), Jülich Research Centre, Jülich, Germany

Abigail Morrison
Simulation Lab Neuroscience, Jülich Supercomputing Centre, Institute for Advanced Simulation, JARA, Jülich Research Centre, Jülich, Germany
Institute of Neuroscience and Medicine (INM-6) and Institute for Advanced Simulation (IAS-6) and JARA Institute Brain Structure-Function Relationships (INM-10), Jülich Research Centre, Jülich, Germany
Faculty of Psychology, Institute of Cognitive Neuroscience, Ruhr-University Bochum, Bochum, Germany

Fabien C. Y. Benureau and Nicolas P. Rougier
INRIA Bordeaux Sud-Ouest, Talence, France
Institut des Maladies Neurodégénératives, Université de Bordeaux, Centre National de la Recherche Scientifique UMR 5293, Bordeaux, France
LaBRI, Université de Bordeaux, Bordeaux INP, Centre National de la Recherche Scientifique UMR 5800, Talence, France

Hananel Hazan, Daniel J. Saunders, Hassaan Khan, Devdhar Patel, Darpan T. Sanghavi, Hava T. Siegelmann and Robert Kozma
Biologically Inspired Neural and Dynamical Systems Laboratory, College of Computer and Information Sciences, University of Massachusetts Amherst, Amherst, MA, United States

Robin Pauli and Philipp Weidel
Institute of Neuroscience and Medicine (INM-6) and Institute for Advanced Simulation (IAS-6) and JARA BRAIN Institute I, Jülich Research Centre, Jülich, Germany

Sandra Diaz-Pier and Alexander Peyser
SimLab Neuroscience, Jülich Supercomputing Centre (JSC), Institute for Advanced Simulation, JARA, Forschungszentrum Jülich GmbH, Jülich, Germany

Michael L. Hines
Department of Neuroscience, Yale University, New Haven, CT, United States

J. H. Newton
Department of Neuroscience, Yale University, New Haven, CT, United States
SUNY Downstate Medical Center, The State University of New York, New York, NY, United States

Robert A. McDougal
Department of Neuroscience, Yale University, New Haven, CT, United States
Center for Medical Informatics, Yale University, New Haven, CT, United States

William W. Lytton
SUNY Downstate Medical Center, The State University of New York, New York, NY, United States
Neurology, Kings County Hospital Center, Brooklyn, NY, United States

Simen Tennøe
Centre for Integrative Neuroplasticity, University of Oslo, Oslo, Norway
Department of Informatics, University of Oslo, Oslo, Norway

Romain Brette and Marcel Stimberg
Sorbonne Université, INSERM, CNRS, Institut de la Vision, Paris, France

Pramod Kumbhar
Blue Brain Project, EPFL, Campus Biotech, Geneva, Switzerland

Geir Halnes
Centre for Integrative Neuroplasticity, University of Oslo, Oslo, Norway
Faculty of Science and Technology, Norwegian University of Life Sciences, Ås, Norway

Gaute T. Einevoll
Centre for Integrative Neuroplasticity, University of Oslo, Oslo, Norway
Faculty of Science and Technology, Norwegian University of Life Sciences, Ås, Norway
Department of Physics, University of Oslo, Oslo, Norway

Index

www.ingramcontent.com/pod-product-compliance
Lightning Source LLC
LaVergne TN
LVHW082224200926
848484LV00008B/2300